SPIRAL STABILIZATION OF THE SPINE

MUSCLE CHAINS

Manual
Movement therapy

for a herniated intervertebral disc without surgery
for post spinal surgery complications
for scoliosis without a brace or surgery

www.spiralstabilization.com

Method
Spiral stabilization of the spine

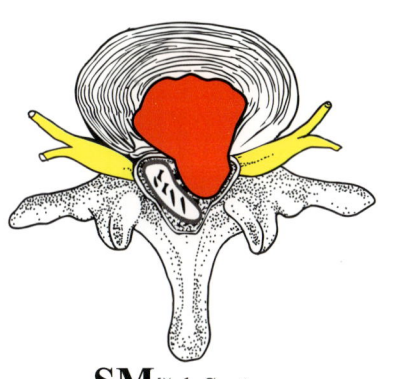

SMíšek System
Richard Smíšek, M.D.
Kateřina Smíšková, M.D.
Zuzana Smíšková, M.D.

Spiral stabilization of the spine is our original method for treating disorders of the spine and, above all, for preventing them through sufficient regeneration.

The name "Spiral stabilization of the spine" and the logo are protected by trademark with our written permission.
All rights are reserved, in particular for reproduction and distribution and for the right to translate materials into other languages.
No part of the work may be reproduced in any form without the written permission of the author.

© Dr. Richard Smíšek

ISBN: 978-80-87568-68-2
Published by Dr. Richard Smíšek
January 2016

SPIRAL MUSCLE CHAINS
STABILIZATION OF MOVEMENT

SA - serratus anterior
PM - pectoralis major

TR - trapezius
LD - latisimus dorsi

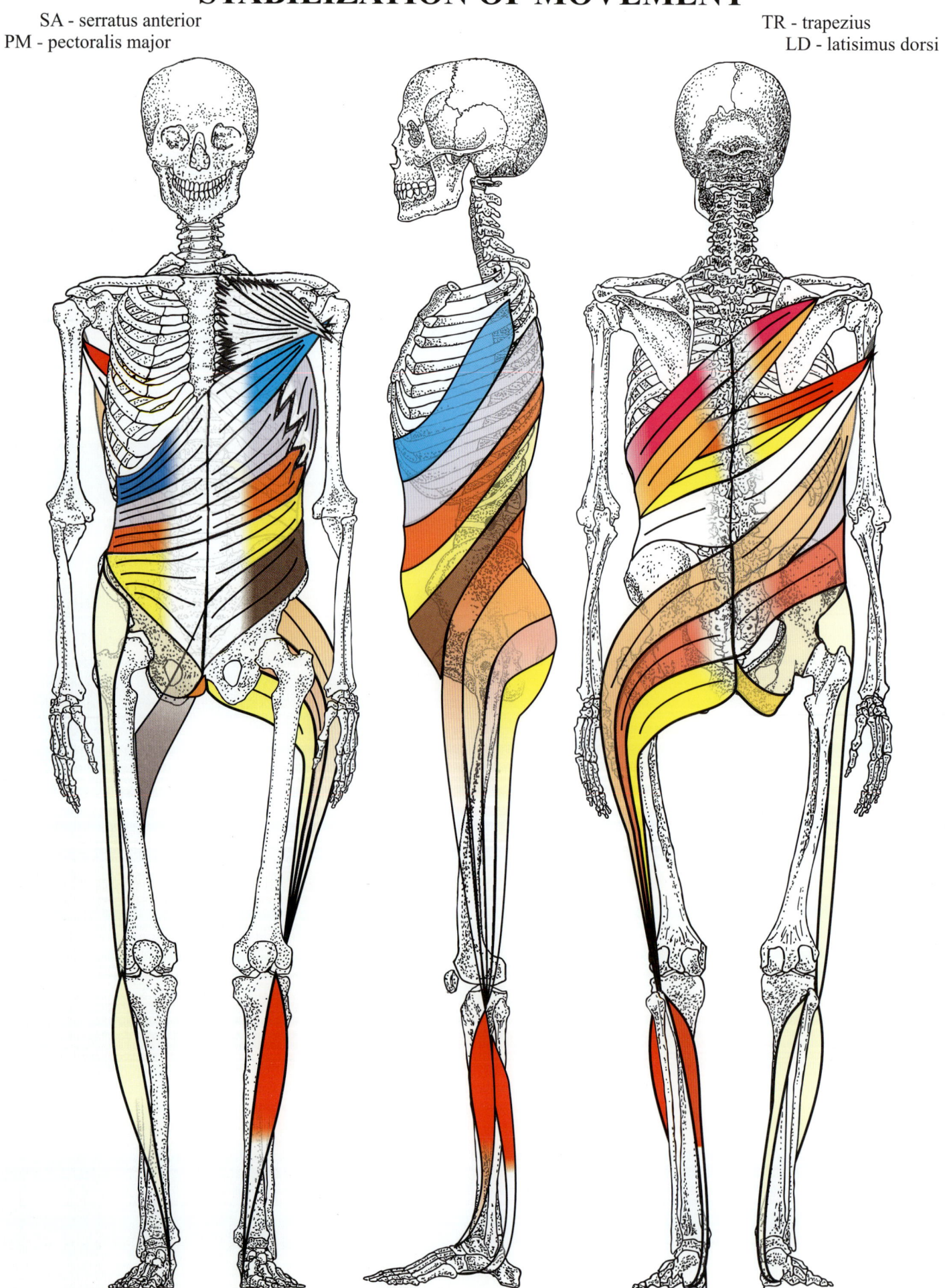

VERTICAL MUSCLE CHAINS
STABILIZATION OF REST

RA - rectus abdominis
IP - iliopsoas

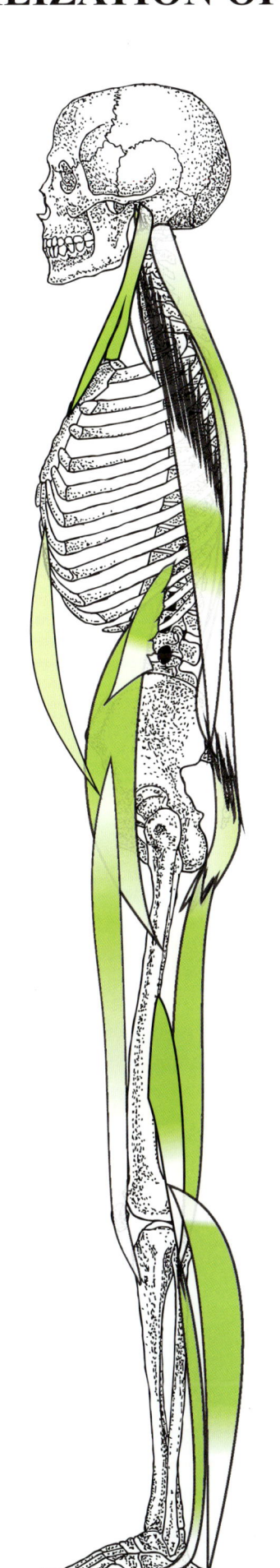

ES - erector spinae
QL - quadratus lumborum

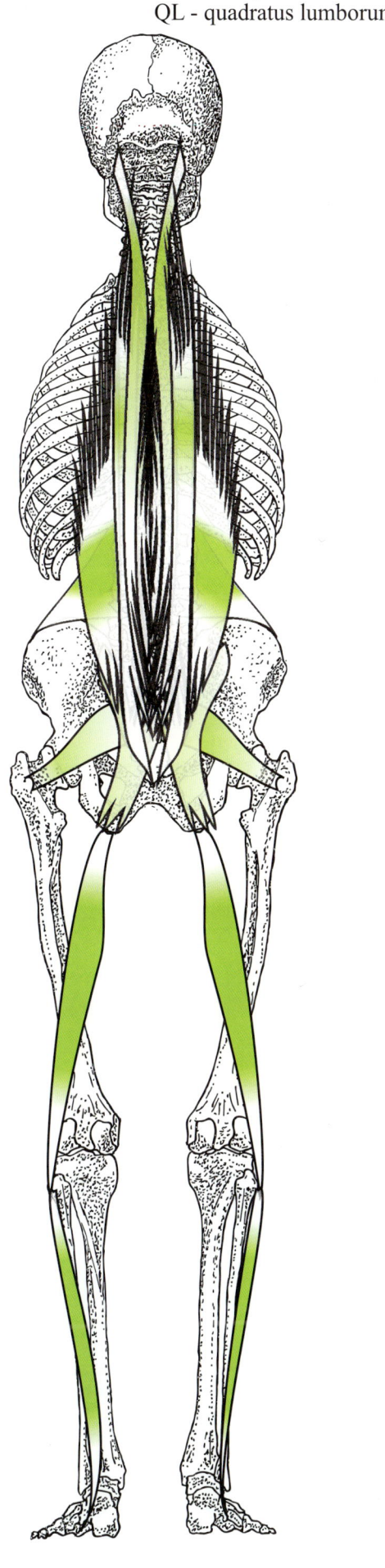

CAUSE OF BACK PAIN

Tension in the verticals   **Weakening of the spirals**

TREATMENT OF BACK PAIN

Relaxation of the verticals   **Strengthening of the spirals**

The path to health

In general:
- To restore the function of the agonists and integrate them into the spiral muscles chains.
- To inhibit the antagonists.
- To increase the extent of movement to the physiological extent necessary for walking.
- To walk.
- To integrate movement patterns into everyday life - lifestyle.

Specifically:
- To engage the oblique abdominal muscles and the transverse muscle through the spiral muscle chains.
- To activate the TR - trapezius and LD - latissimus dorsi chains to the full extent.
- To stretch the muscles of the anterior and upper muscles groups of the shoulder girdle while relaxed and in reciprocal inhibition.
- To relax the paravertebral muscles in reciprocal inhibition and to relax them.
- To engage the m. gluteus maximus through the spiral muscle chains.
- To stretch the muscles of the anterior muscle group of the pelvic girdle while relaxed and in reciprocal inhibition.
- To train the coordination and stabilization of the gait, stabilization by the TR - trapezius, LD - latissimus dorsi, SA - serratus anterior and PM - pectoralis major muscle chains.
- To walk with correct coordination and stabilization.
- To integrate optimal movement patterns into everyday life - lifestyle.

Examples of disc disruption

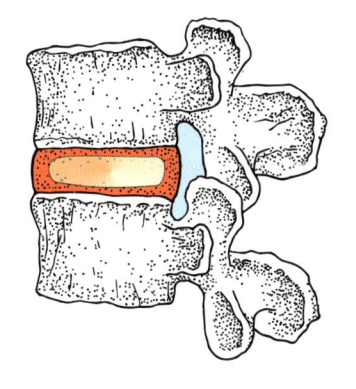

Healthy intervertebral disc

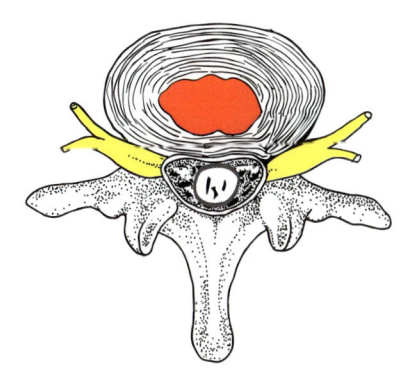

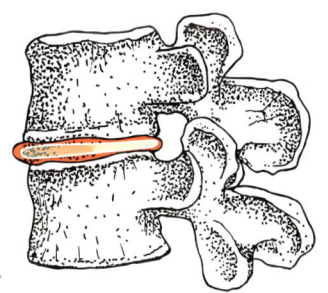

Circular protrusion of a degenerated disc

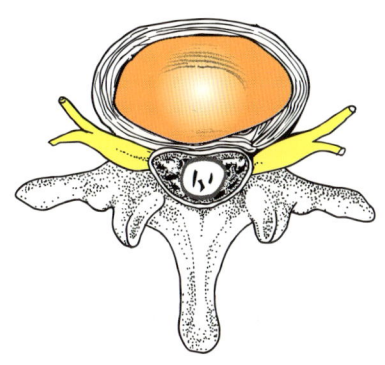

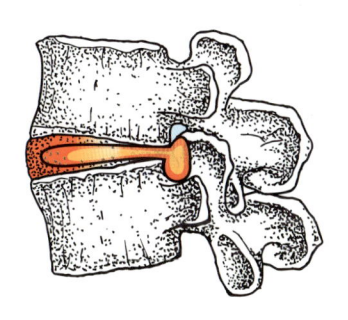

Foraminal herniation of a disc

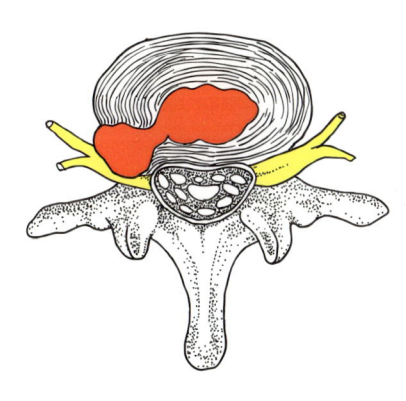

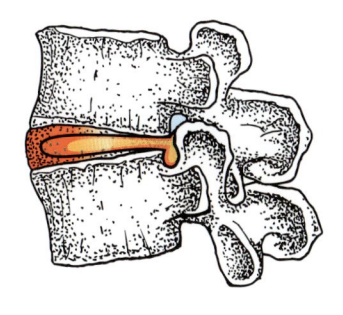

Dorsolateral herniation of a disc

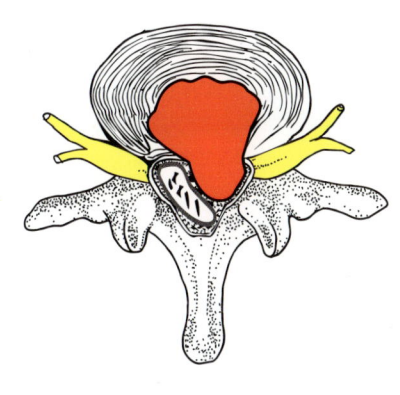

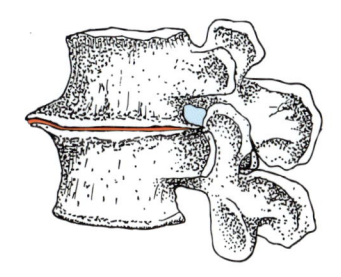

Spinal stenosis
Spondylosis
Spondylarthrosis

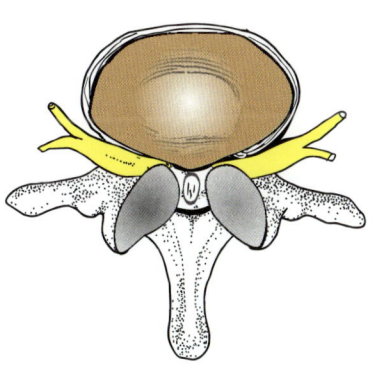

Contents:

1) Herniation of an intervertebral disc in the lumbar region:
- acute phase..5
- subacute phase..11
- reconvalescent phase..13
- resorption...17

2) Examples of the successful treatment of a herniated disc..23

3) Examination of the muscles at rest and in motion...35

4) Muscles with a tendency to tension and shortening in the vertical muscle chains:
- muscles of the trunk - posterior muscle group:
   - paravertebral posterior lower muscle group..41
   - paravertebral posterior upper muscle group..73
- muscles of the shoulder girdle anterior muscle group...91
- muscles of the pelvic girdle anterior muscle group - hip flexors...............................107

5) Muscles with a tendency to weakening, spiral muscle chains:
- muscles of the shoulder girdle - posterior lower muscle group..................................131
- muscles of the shoulder girdle - lateral muscle group...149
- muscles of the shoulder girdle - anterior muscle group...161
- muscles of the trunk - anterior muscle group - abdominal muscles...........................169
- muscles of the pelvic girdle - posterior muscle group...181

6) Principles of muscle relaxation...189

7) Complications following an operation on an intervertebral disc...................................199

8) Eliminating a disorder of spiral stabilization..211

9) Parameters for measuring the extent and coordination of movement............................217

Testimonial for the Spiral Stabilisation technique:

Having been in the profession for nearly 30 years I was looking for some CPD points
when I visited the Back Pain Show in 2013. I met and instantly liked Dr Smisek, his enthusiasm,
knowledge and passion for his system was infectious. The system has helped me in the clinical field
and in a very short time has given patients a great set of tools for self-help which I have been advocating.
Like all things that work the application is relatively simple but the theory and depth of knowledge is vast.
This is a system that should be given the utmost respect and applied universally to help those suffering
from pain. My only regret is that I did not do this 10 years ago.

Anthony Padgett
MMACP MCSP SRP GradDipPhys
Chartered Manipulative Physiotherapist- UK

MANUAL TECHNIQUES AND EXERCISE ACCORDING TO MUSCLE ANALYSIS

Herniation of an intervertebral disc in the lumbar region

Acute phase

Manual techniques

Main principles of therapy:
- relaxation of the muscles which compress the spine
- simple traction of the spine

Contraindicated - prohibited techniques:
- flexion techniques
- extension techniques
- rotation techniques
- lateroflexion techniques
- impact techniques
- mobilization techniques

Manual techniques - lying - one limb in a hoist
M. iliocostalis lumborum - massage, relaxation, passive stretching

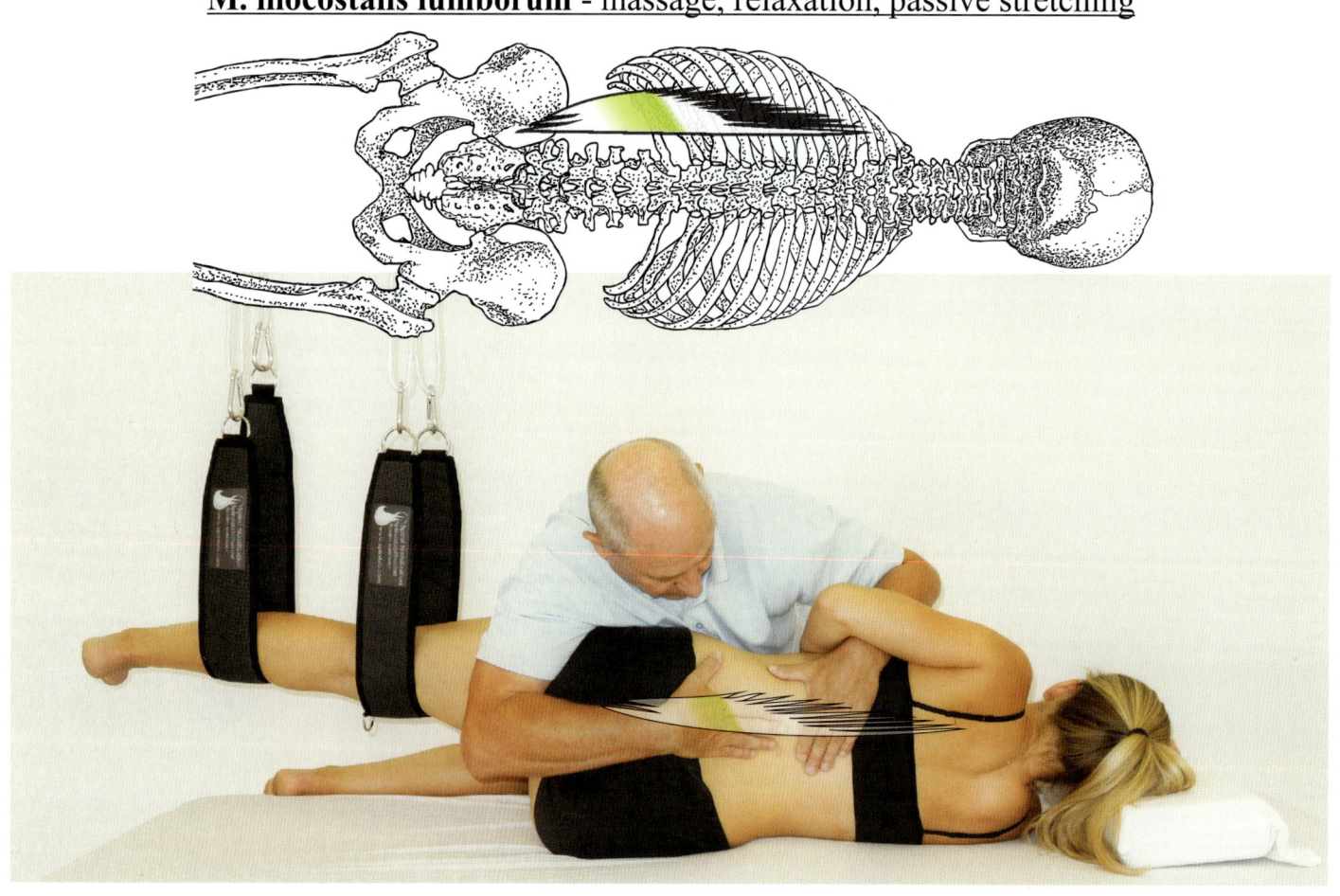

M. longissimus thoracis - massage, relaxation, passive stretching

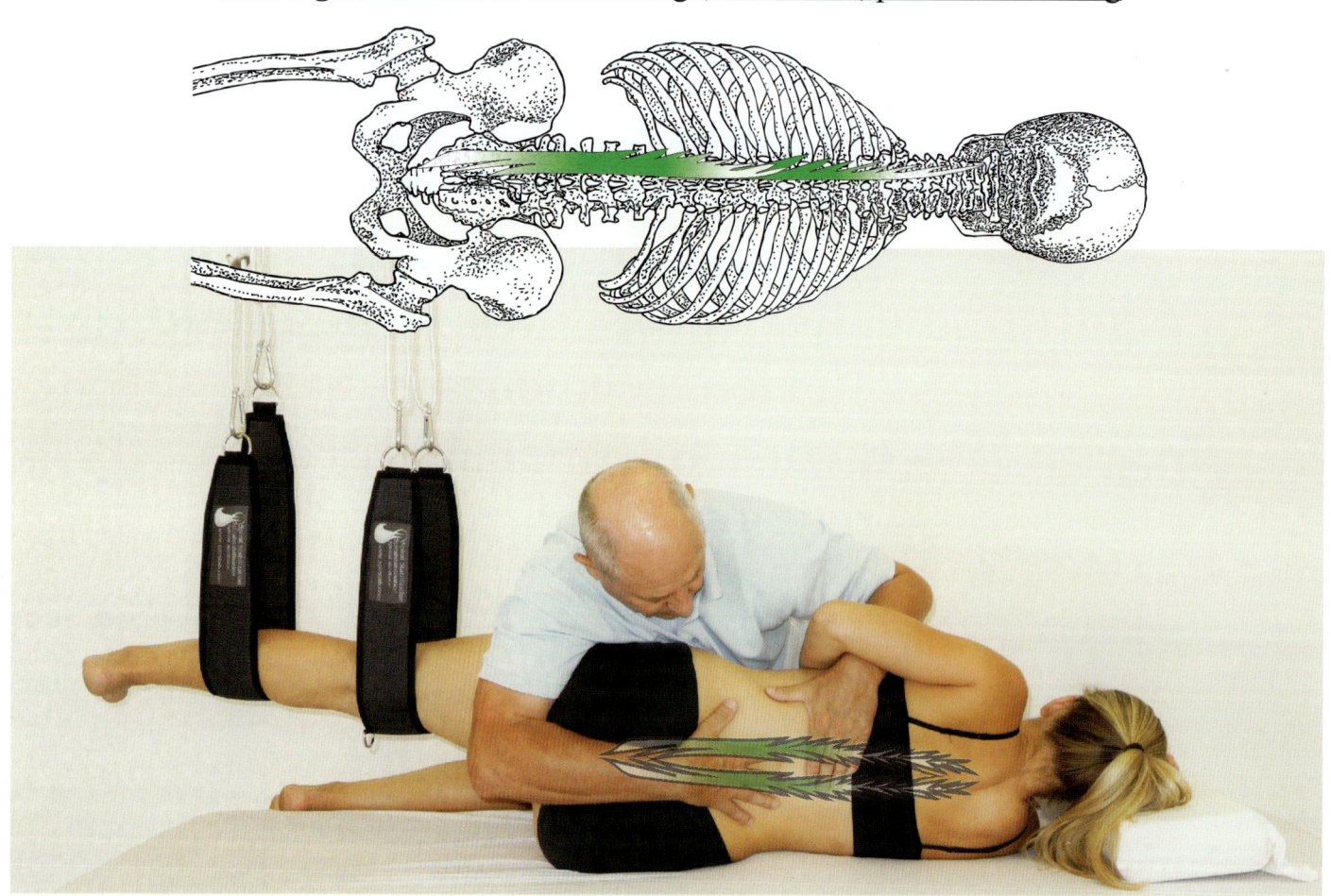

Manual techniques - lying - one limb in a hoist
M. quadratus lumborum - massage, relaxation, passive stretching

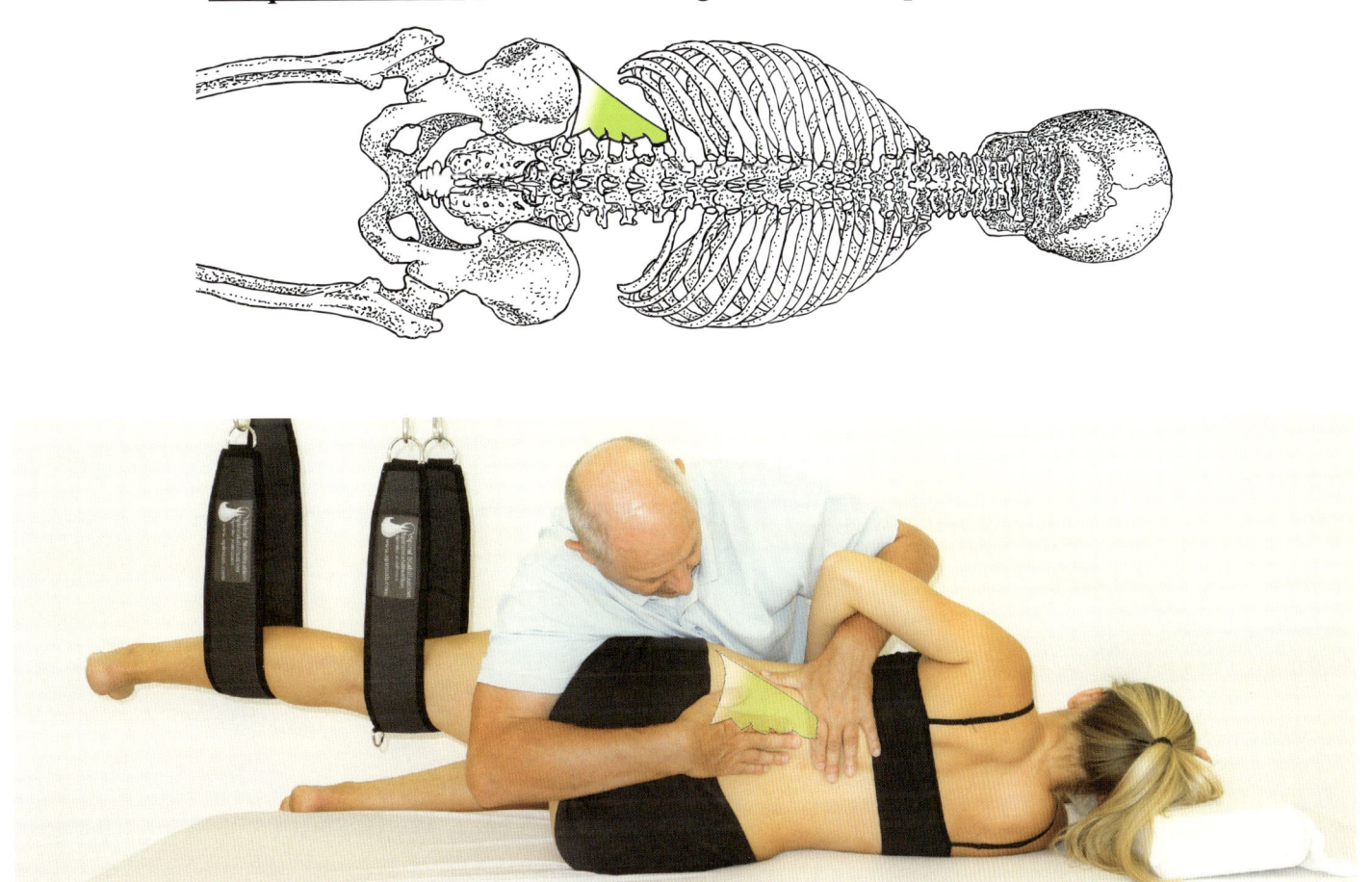

M. multifidus - massage, relaxation, passive stretching

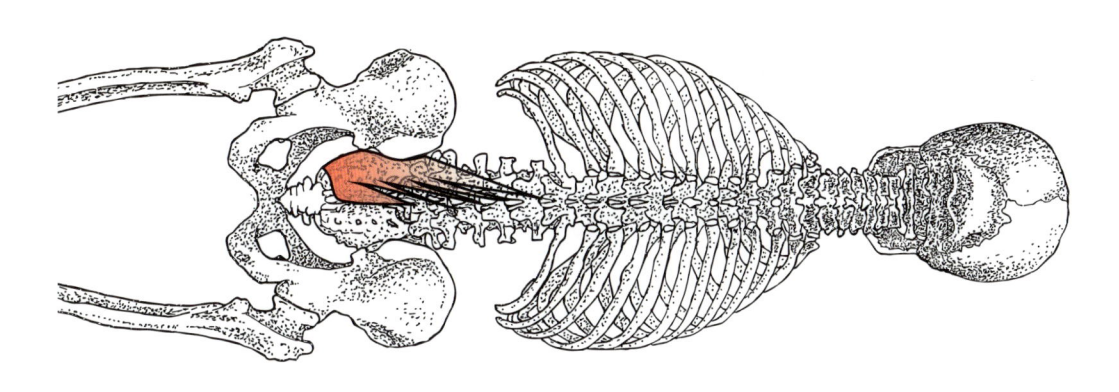

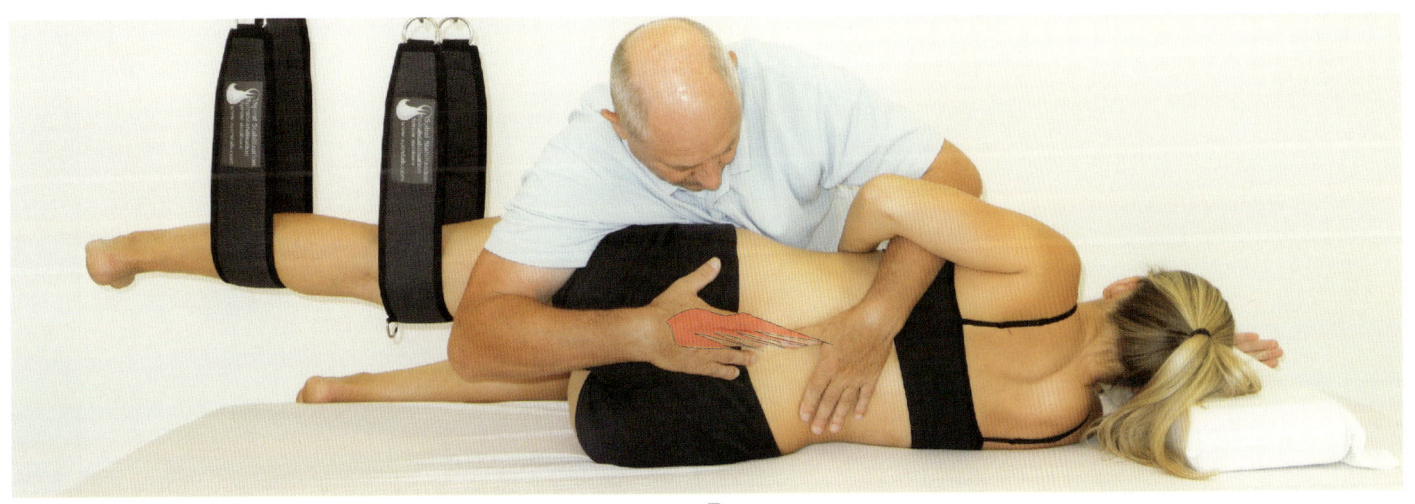

제3차 SSM 척추측만증 국제워크샵

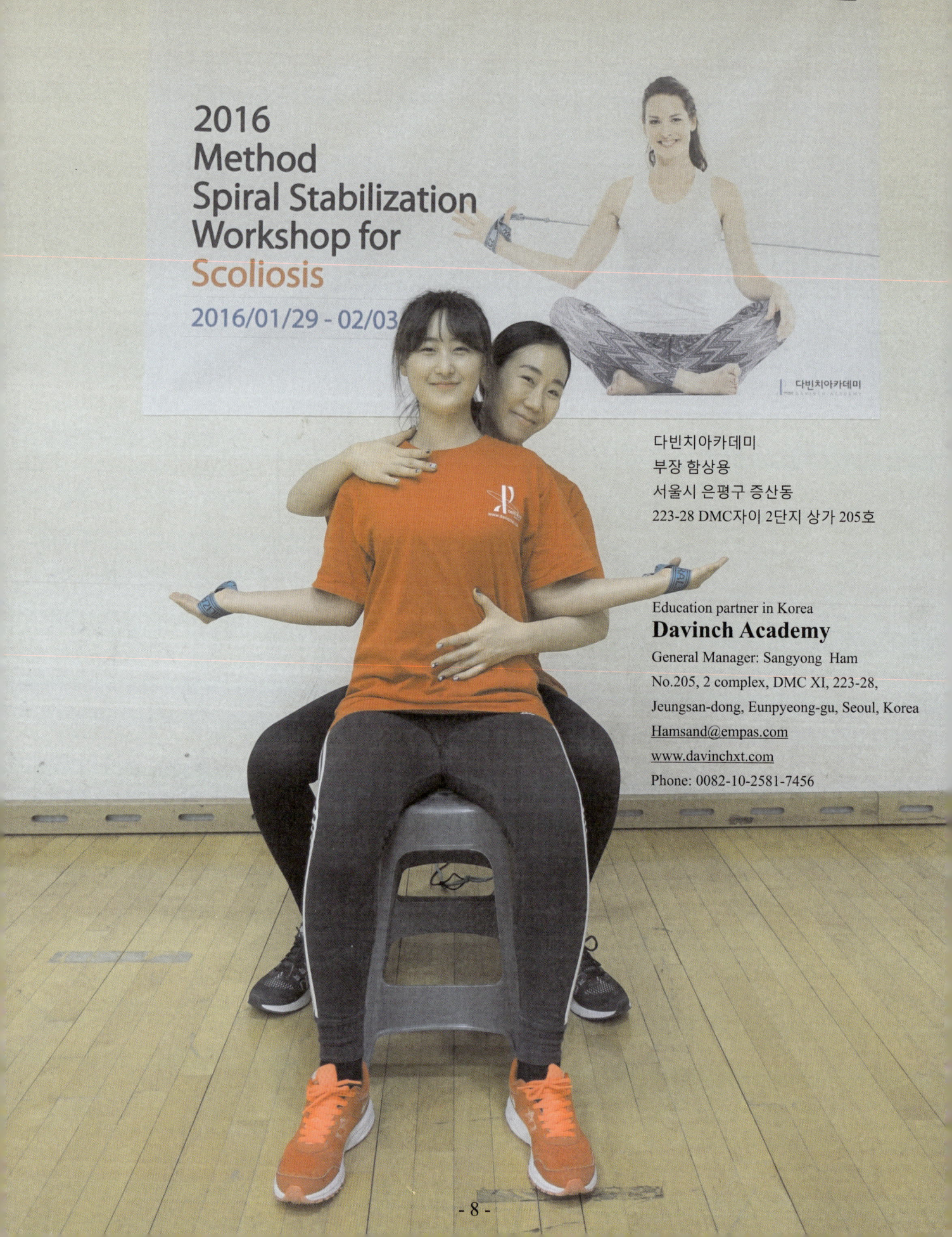

2016
Method
Spiral Stabilization
Workshop for
Scoliosis
2016/01/29 - 02/03

다빈치아카데미
부장 함상용
서울시 은평구 증산동
223-28 DMC자이 2단지 상가 205호

Education partner in Korea
Davinch Academy
General Manager: Sangyong Ham
No.205, 2 complex, DMC XI, 223-28,
Jeungsan-dong, Eunpyeong-gu, Seoul, Korea
Hamsand@empas.com
www.davinchxt.com
Phone: 0082-10-2581-7456

MANUAL TECHNIQUES AND EXERCISE ACCORDING TO MUSCLE ANALYSIS

Herniation of an intervertebral disc in the lumbar region

Acute phase

Exercises

Main principles:
- activation of the muscles which stretch the spine
- simple traction of the spine

Contraindicated - prohibited exercises:
- exercises which compress the spine
- flexion exercises
- extension exercises
- rotation exercises
- lateroflexion exercises
- mobilization exercises

Exercise 1 basic performance
Standing on both legs, backward pull with both arms

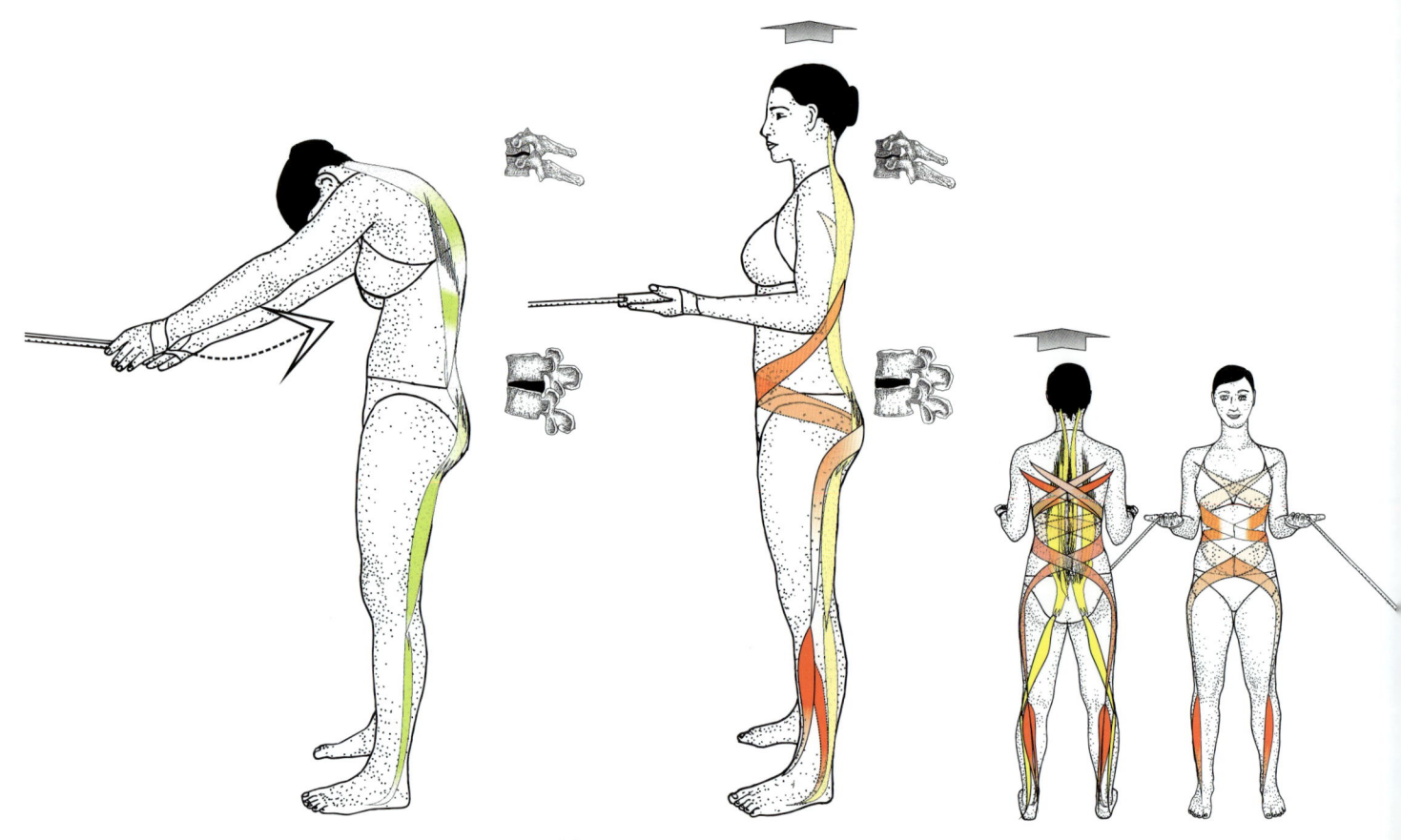

Stabilization through TR, LD

Exercise 2 basic performance
Standing on both legs, sideways pull with one arm

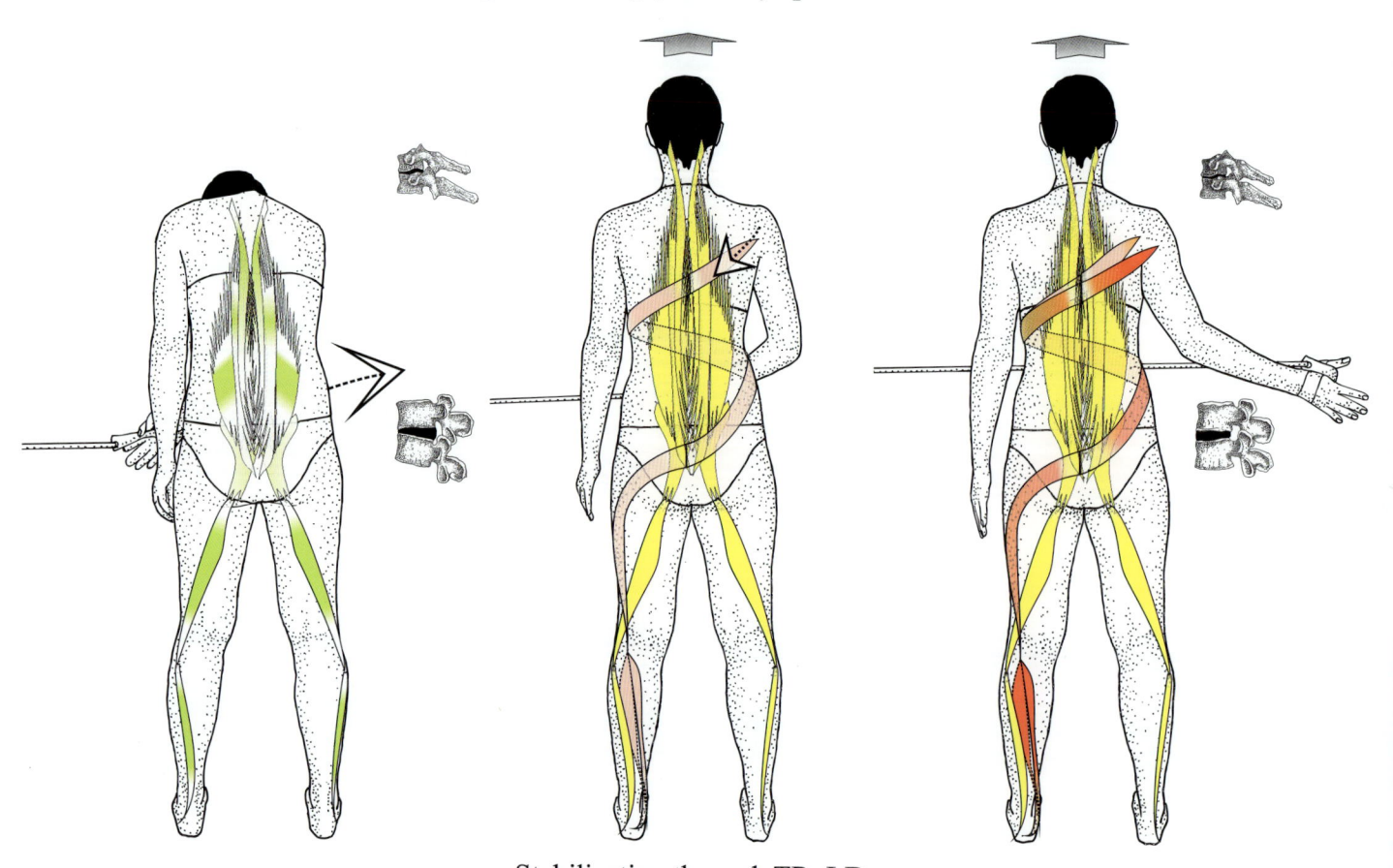

Stabilization through TR, LD

MANUAL TECHNIQUES AND EXERCISE ACCORDING TO MUSCLE ANALYSIS

Herniation of an intervertebral disc in the lumbar region

Subacute phase

Exercises

Main principles:
- traction of the spine
- slight stretching of the paravertebral muscles in reciprocal inhibition

Contraindicated - prohibited exercises:
- exercises which compress the spine
- extension exercises
- rotation exercises

Exercise 3 basic performance
**Standing on both legs, opening the arms backwards
and pulling the shoulder blades towards each other**

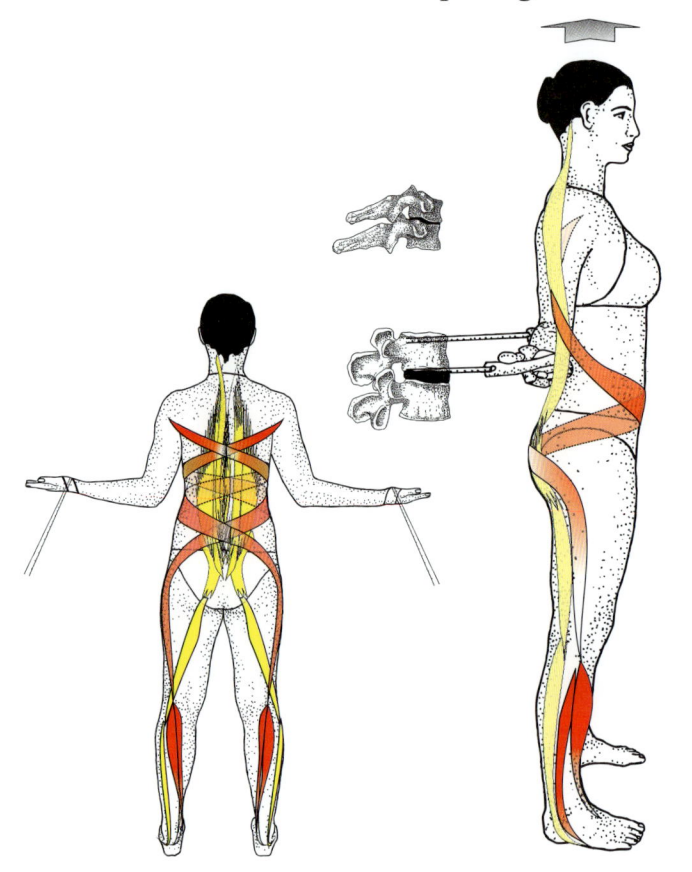

Stabilization through TR, LD

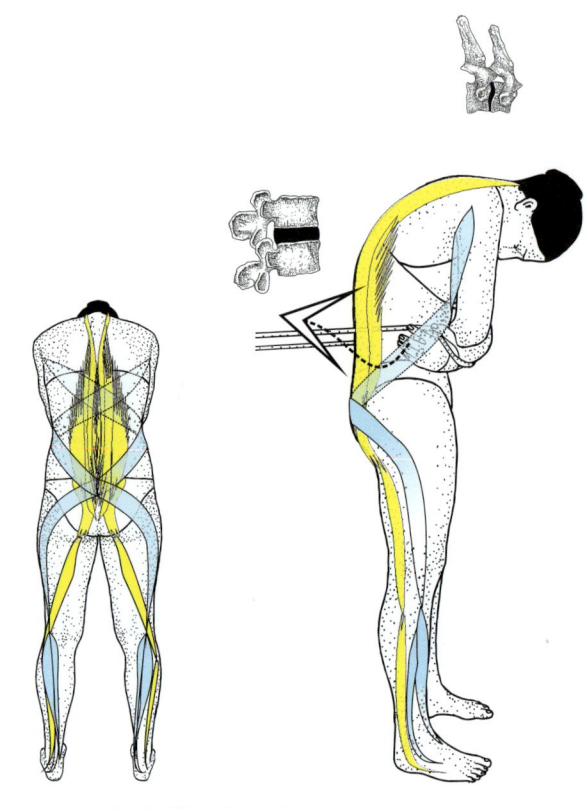

Stabilization through PM

Exercise 4 basic performance
**Kneeling on both knees, opening the arms backwards,
pulling the shoulder blades together, pushing the pelvis forward**

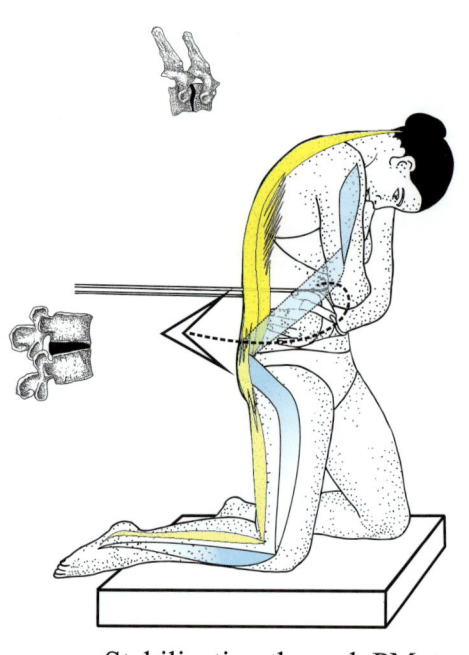

Stabilization through PM

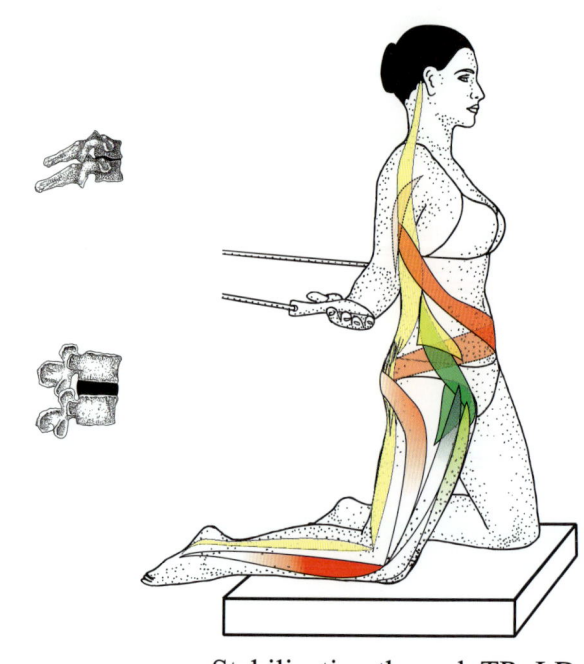

Stabilization through TR, LD

MANUAL TECHNIQUES AND EXERCISE ACCORDING TO MUSCLE ANALYSIS

Herniation of an intervertebral disc in the lumbar region

Recovery phase

Exercises

Main prinicples:
- traction of the spine
- vigorous stretching of the paravertebral muscles in reciprocal inhibition

Contraindicated - prohibited exercises:
- exercises which compress the spine
- extension exercises
- rotation exercises
- lateroflexion exercises

Exercise 1 advanced performance
Standing with one leg placed forward on the mat, backward pull with both arms

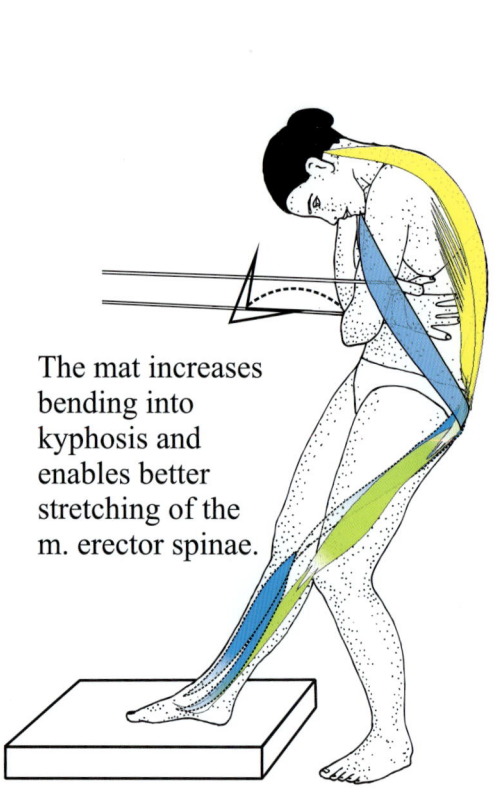

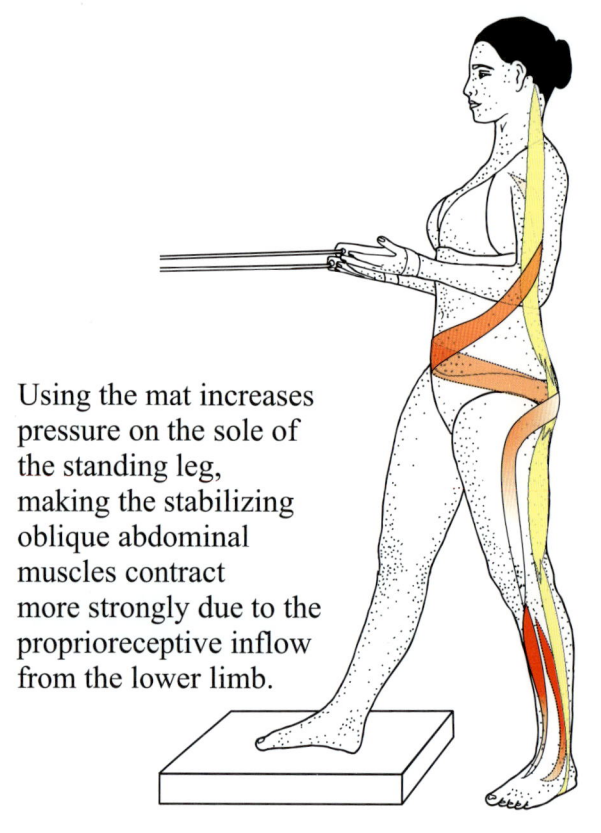

The mat increases bending into kyphosis and enables better stretching of the m. erector spinae.

Using the mat increases pressure on the sole of the standing leg, making the stabilizing oblique abdominal muscles contract more strongly due to the proprioceptive inflow from the lower limb.

Stabilization through PM

Stabilization through TR, LD

Exercise 2 advanced performance
Standing with one leg placed forward on the mat, sideways pull with one arm

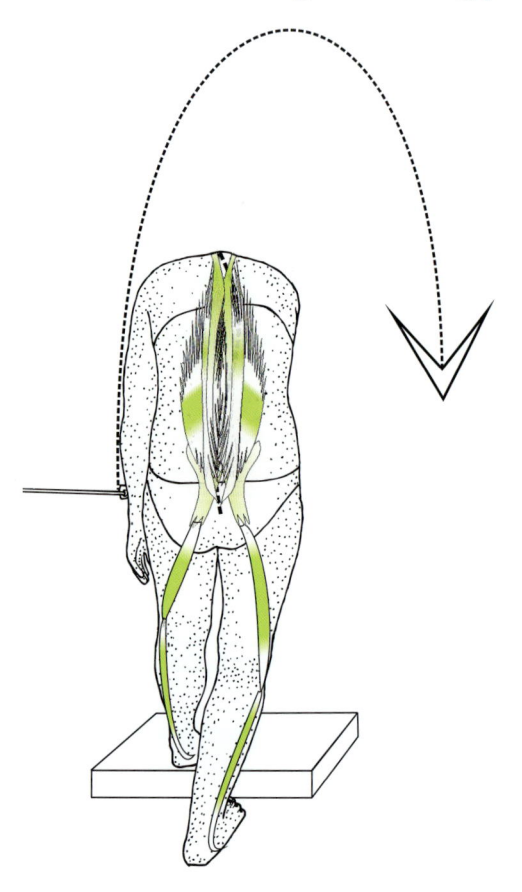

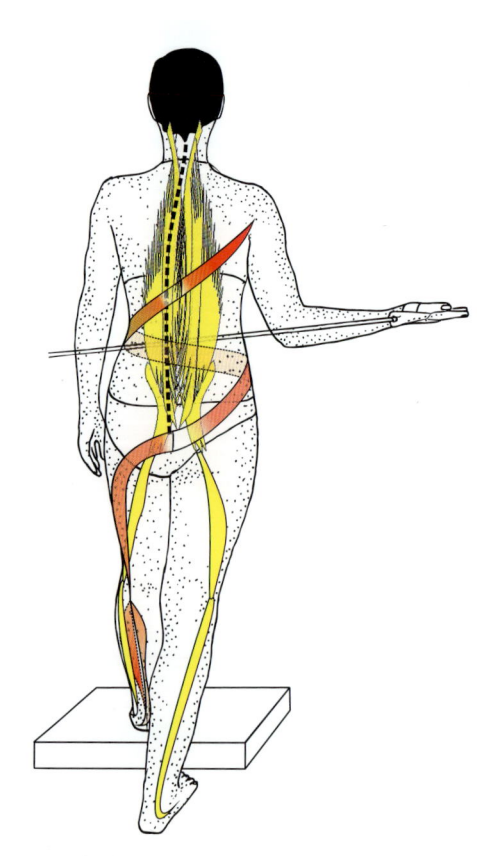

Stabilization through TR, LD

Exercise 3 advanced performance
Standing with on leg placed forward on the mat, arms opened backwards and shoulder blades pulled towards each other

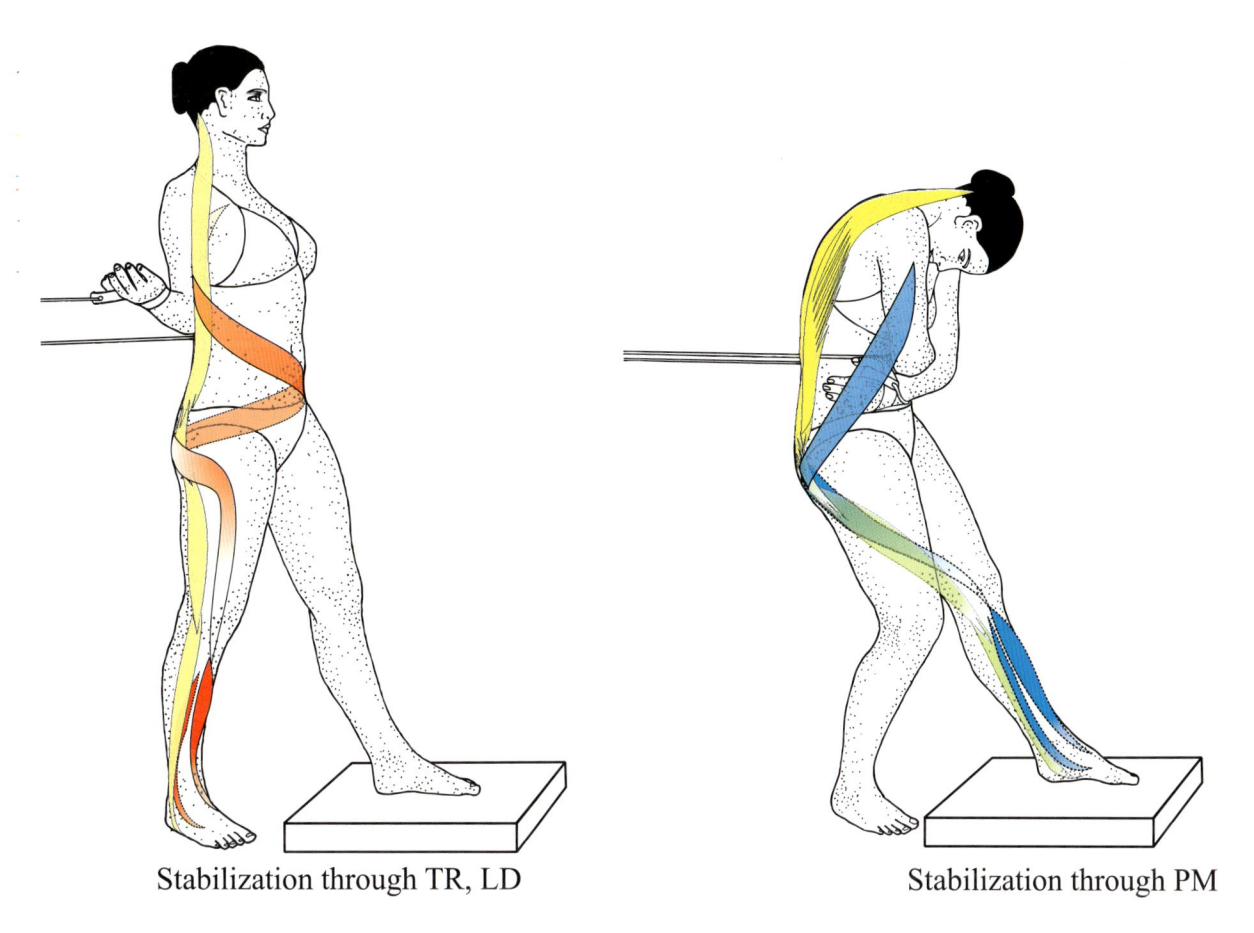

Stabilization through TR, LD

Stabilization through PM

Exercise 4 advanced performance
Kneeling position with one leg in front, arms opened backwards, shoulder blades pulled towards each other, pelvis pushed forward

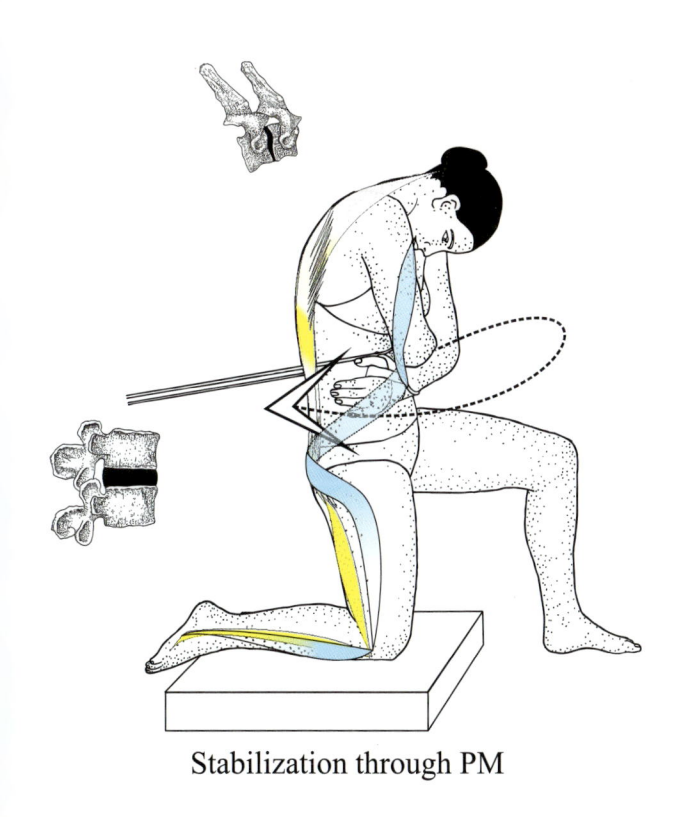

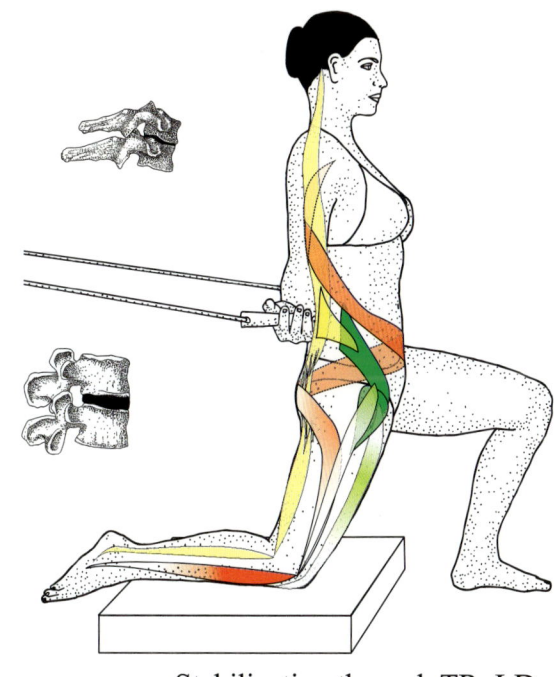

Stabilization through PM

Stabilization through TR, LD

Exercise 11 advanced performance

**Standing on one leg, firm support from the barre,
double extension - stretching the arms at the shoulder and the legs at the hip**

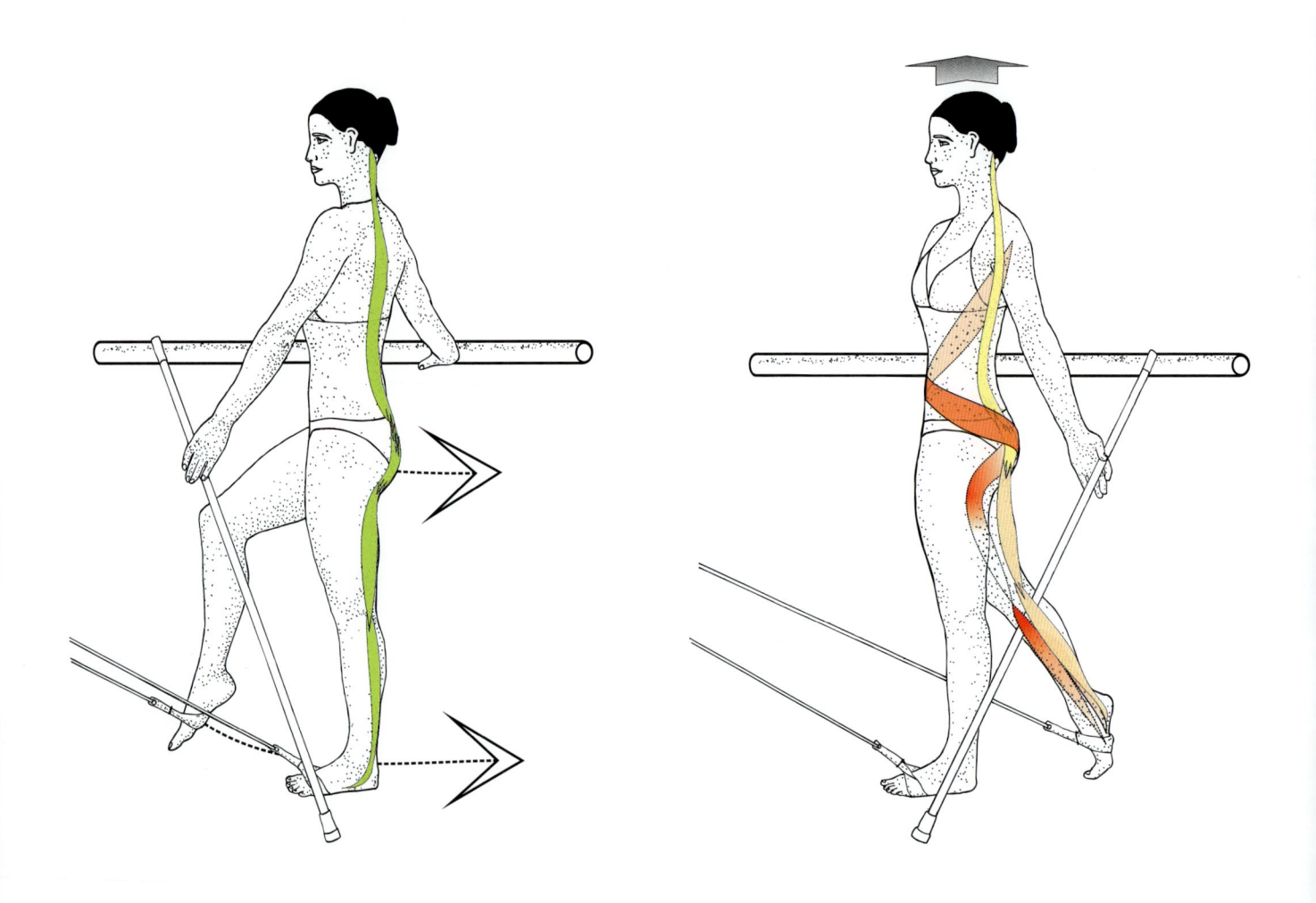

MANUAL TECHNIQUES AND EXERCISE ACCORDING TO MUSCLE ANALYSIS

Herniation of an intervertebral disc in the lumbar region

Resorption phase

Exercise

main principles:
- traction of the spine
- vigorous stretching of the paravertebral muscles in reciprocal inhibition
- rotation of the spine in upward stretching

Contraindicated - prohibited exercises:
- exercises which compress the spine
- extension exercises

Spirally stabilized gait

Exercise 1 advanced performance with rotation

Standing with one leg placed forward on the mat, backward pull with one arm, rotation of the trunk

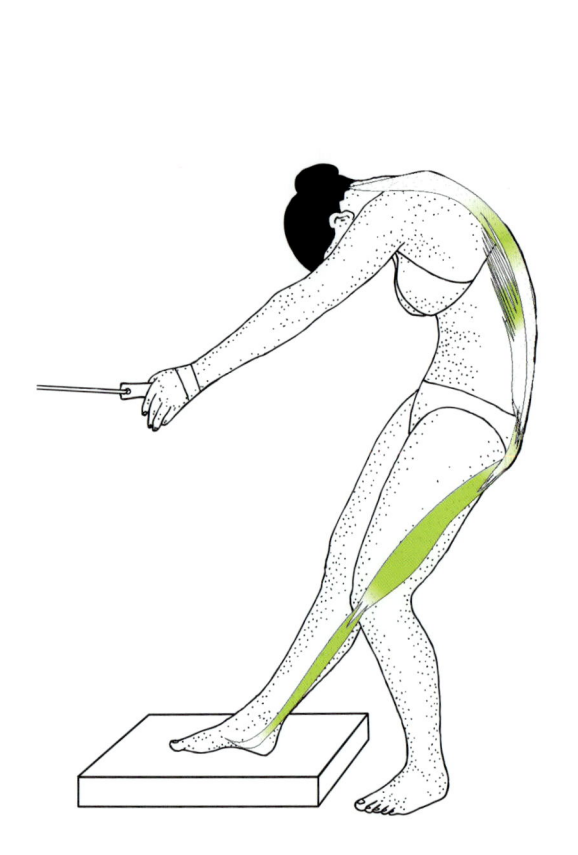

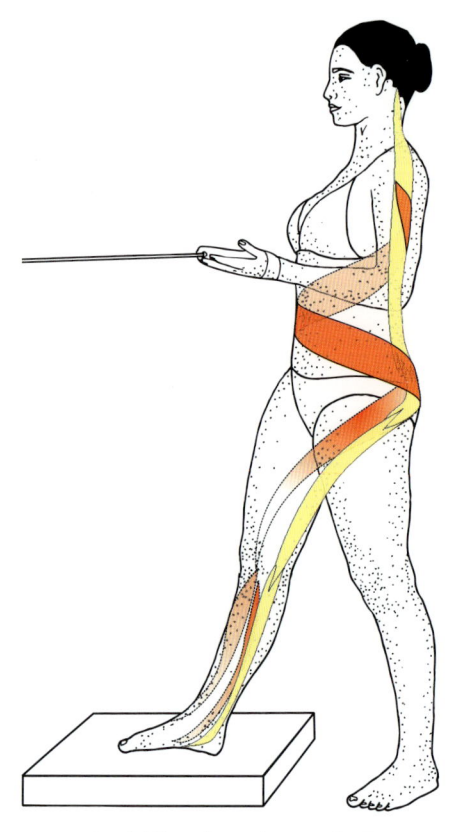

Stabilization through TR, LD

Exercise 2 advanced performance with rotation

Standing with one leg placed forward on the mat, sideways pull with one arm and oblique backward downward pull with one arm, rotation of the trunk

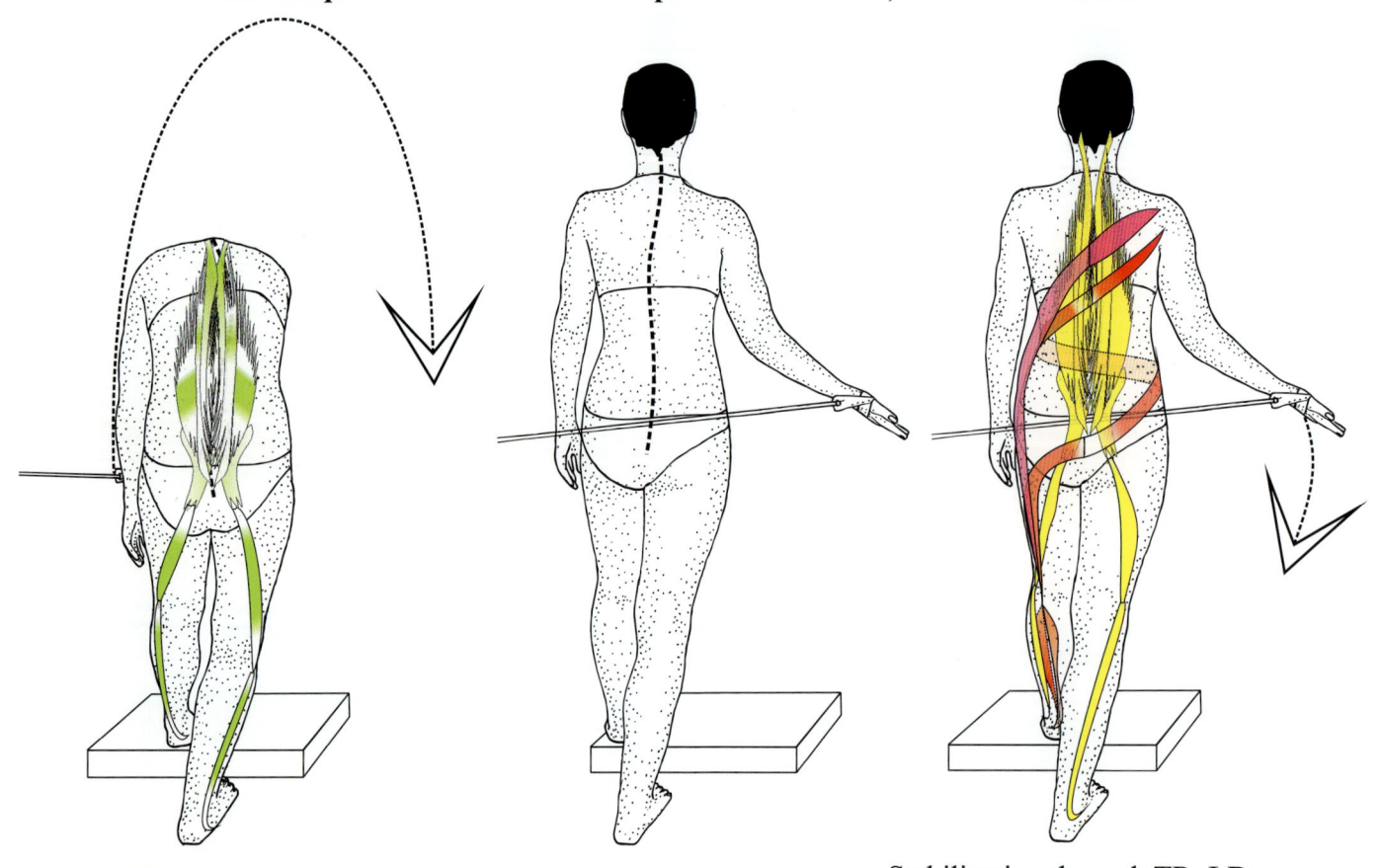

Stabilization through TR, LD

Exercise 6 - advanced performance with rotation

**Standing with one leg placed forward on the mat,
forward circles with one arm, rotation of the trunk**

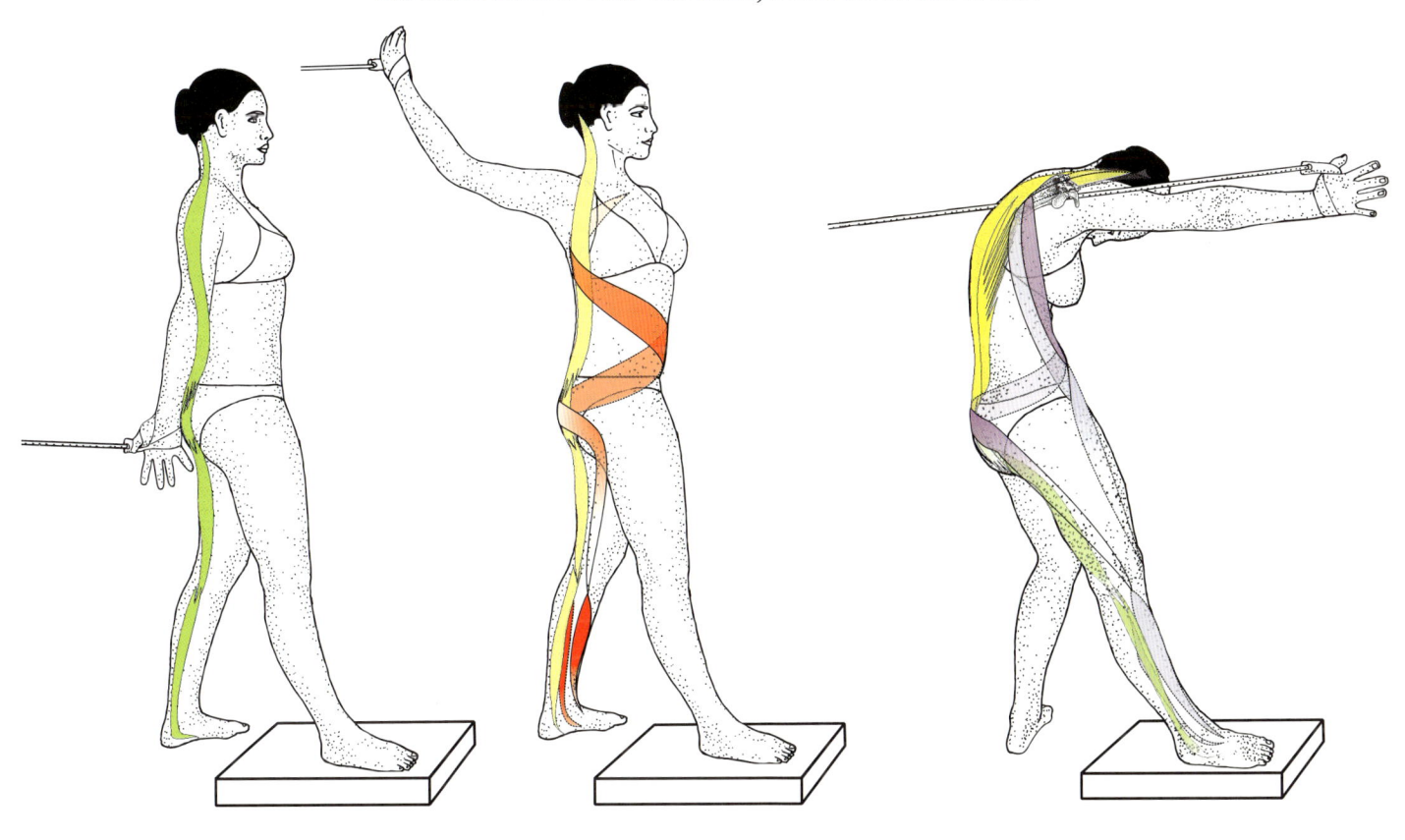

Stabilization through TR, LD   Stabilization through SA

Exercise 10 - advanced performance with rotation

**Standing with one leg place forward on the mat,
one arm is pulled forward in front of the centre of the abdomen, rotation of the trunk**

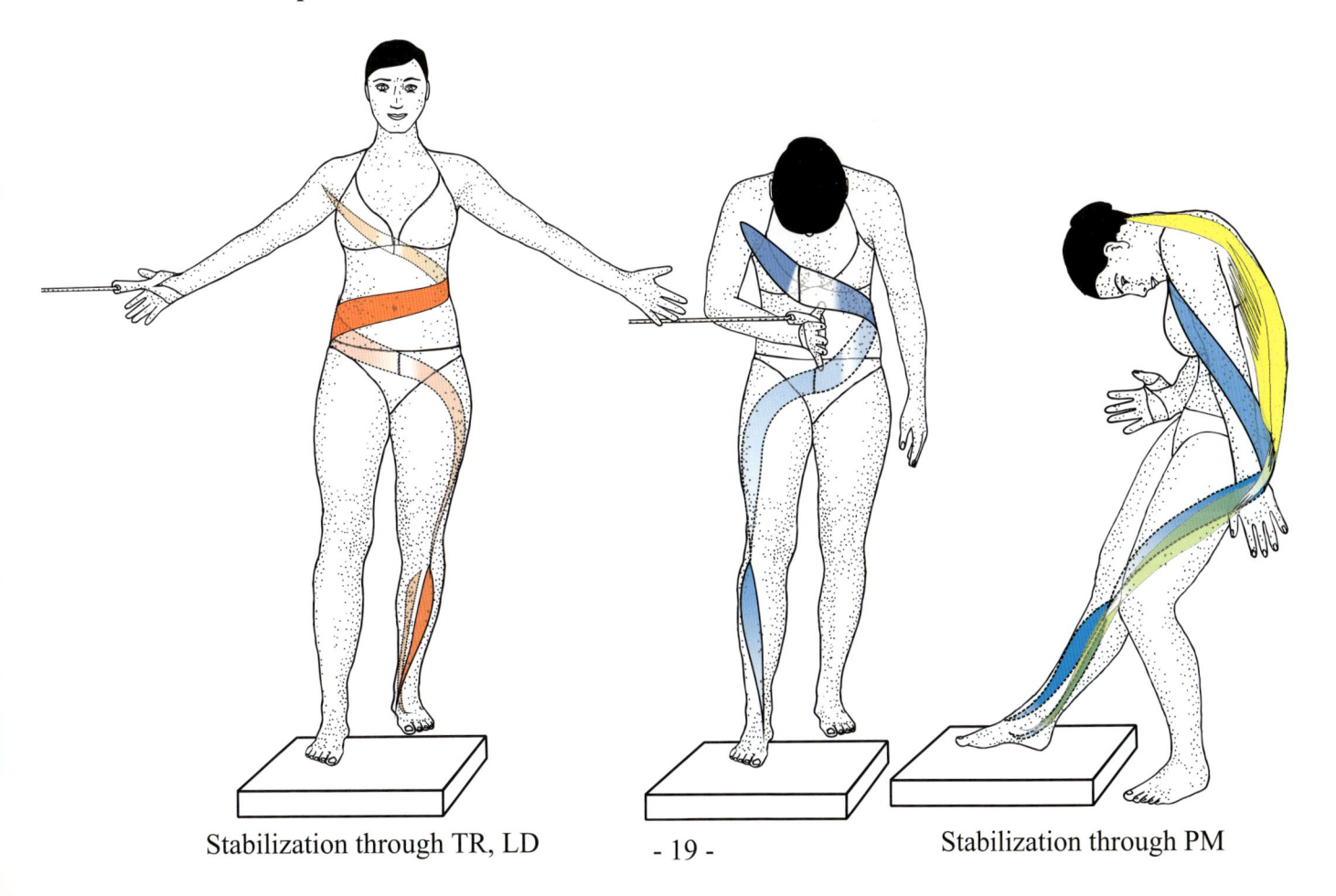

Stabilization through TR, LD   Stabilization through PM

Exercise 11 - advanced performance with rotation

Standing, alternating extension of the arms with alternation of the standing leg - marking time, rotation of the trunk

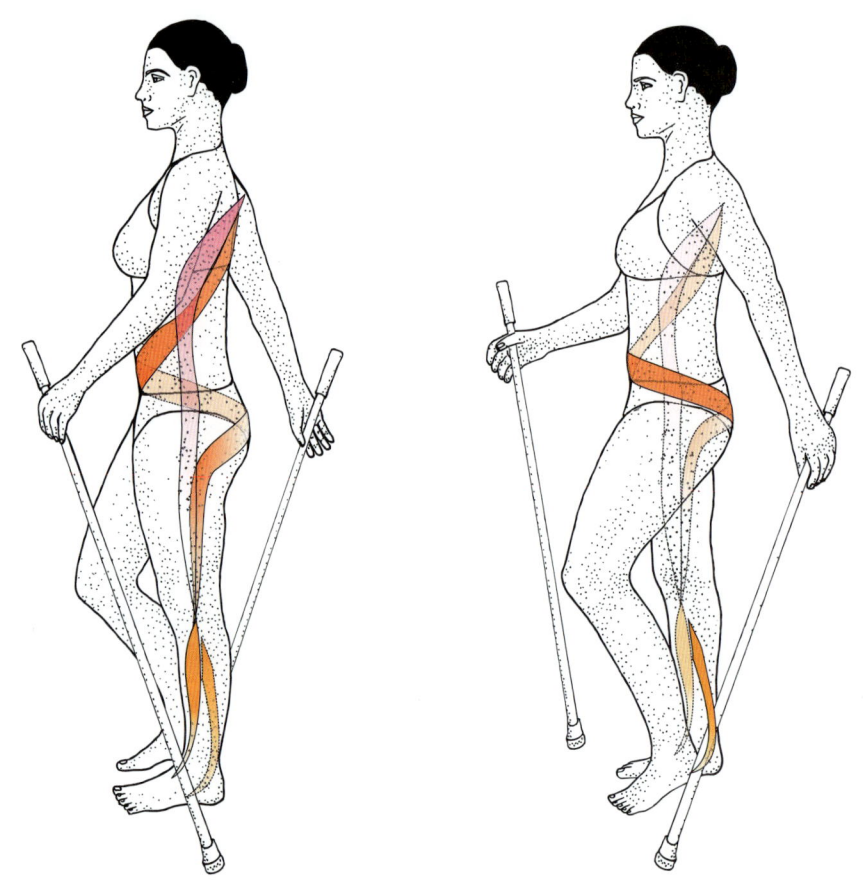

Exercise 11 advanced performance with rotation

Standing on one leg, mobile support from the pole, double extension - stretching the arms at the shoulder and the legs at the hip with counter-rotation of the pelvis and trunk

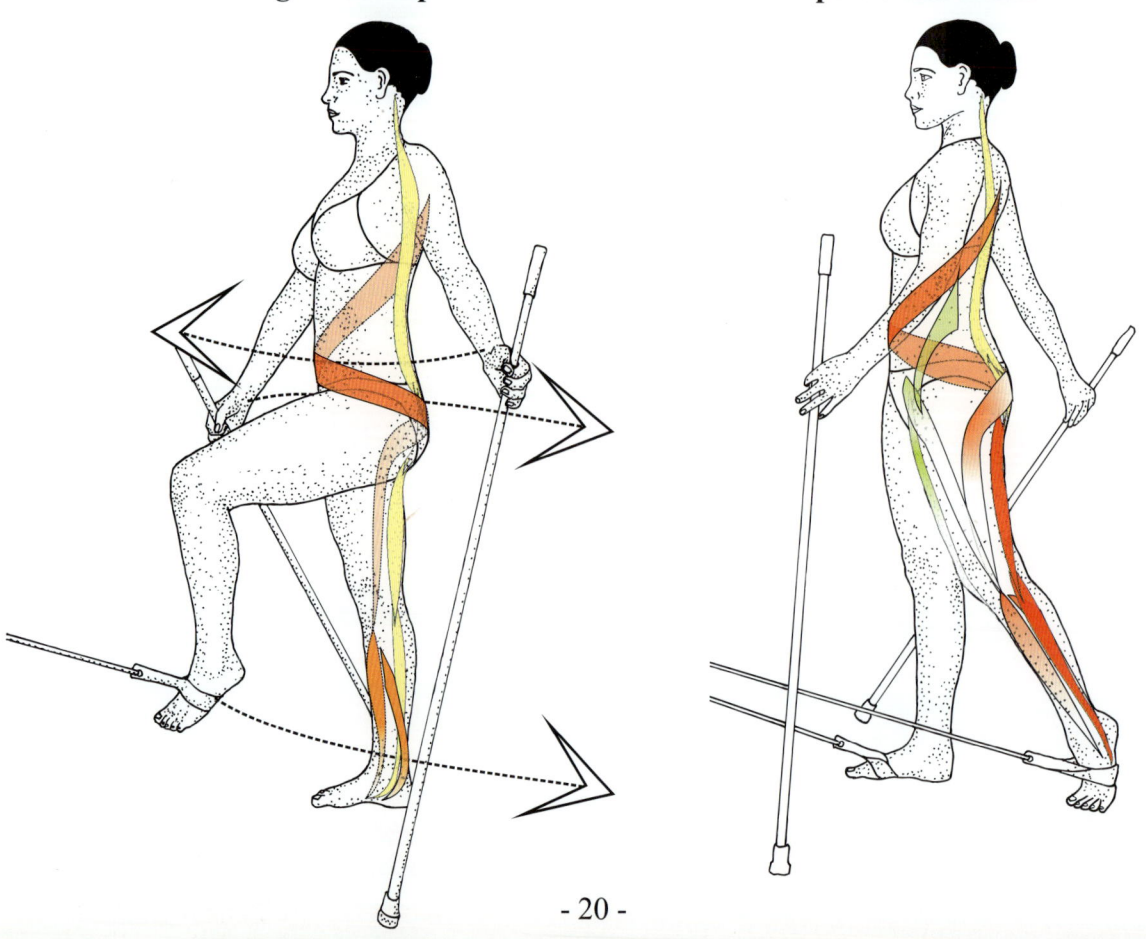

Spirally stabilized gait with counter-rotation of the pelvis and trunk

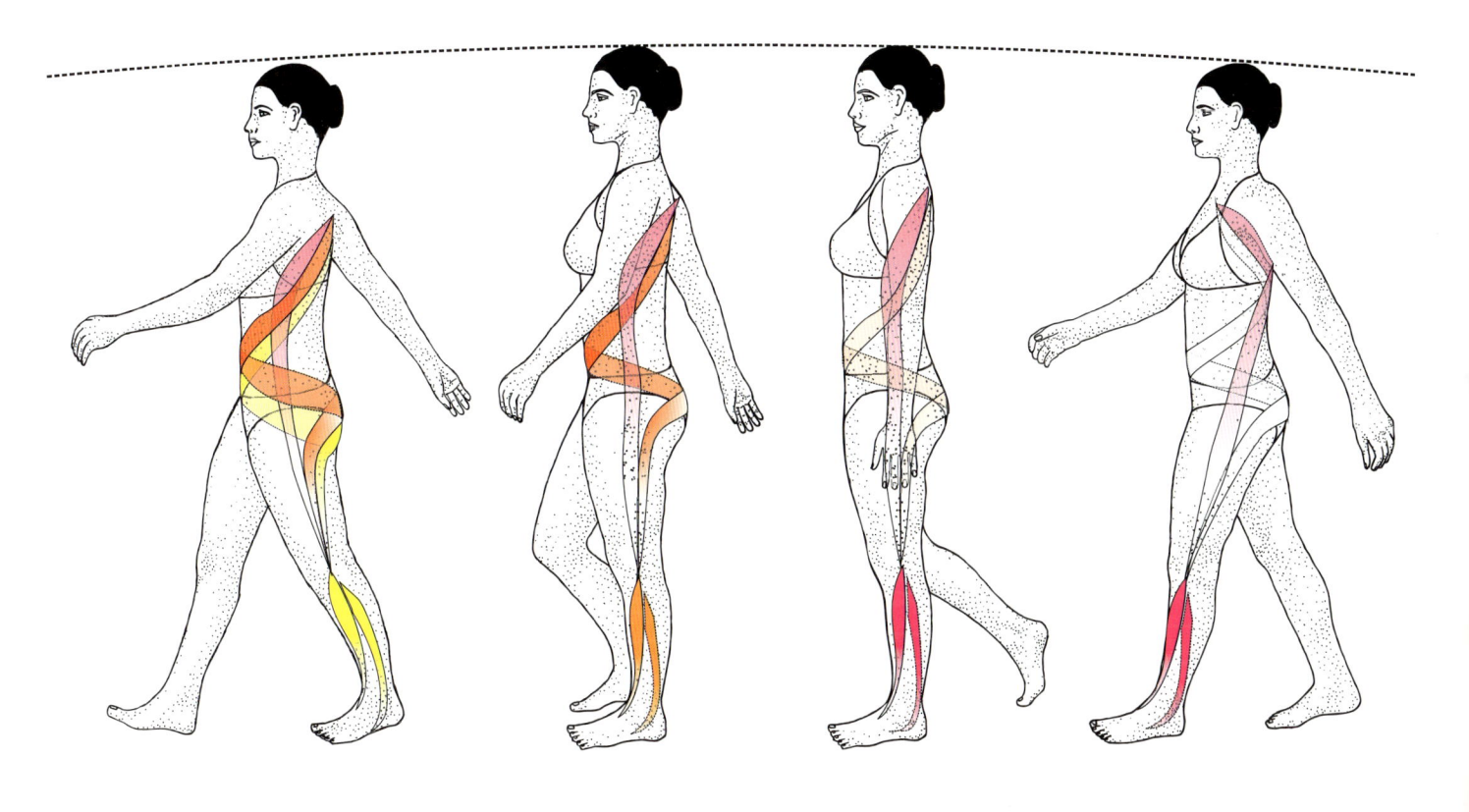

Stabilization through
TR-C, D, LD-B, C

Stabilization through
TR-C, LD-B

Stabilization through
TR-B, LD-A

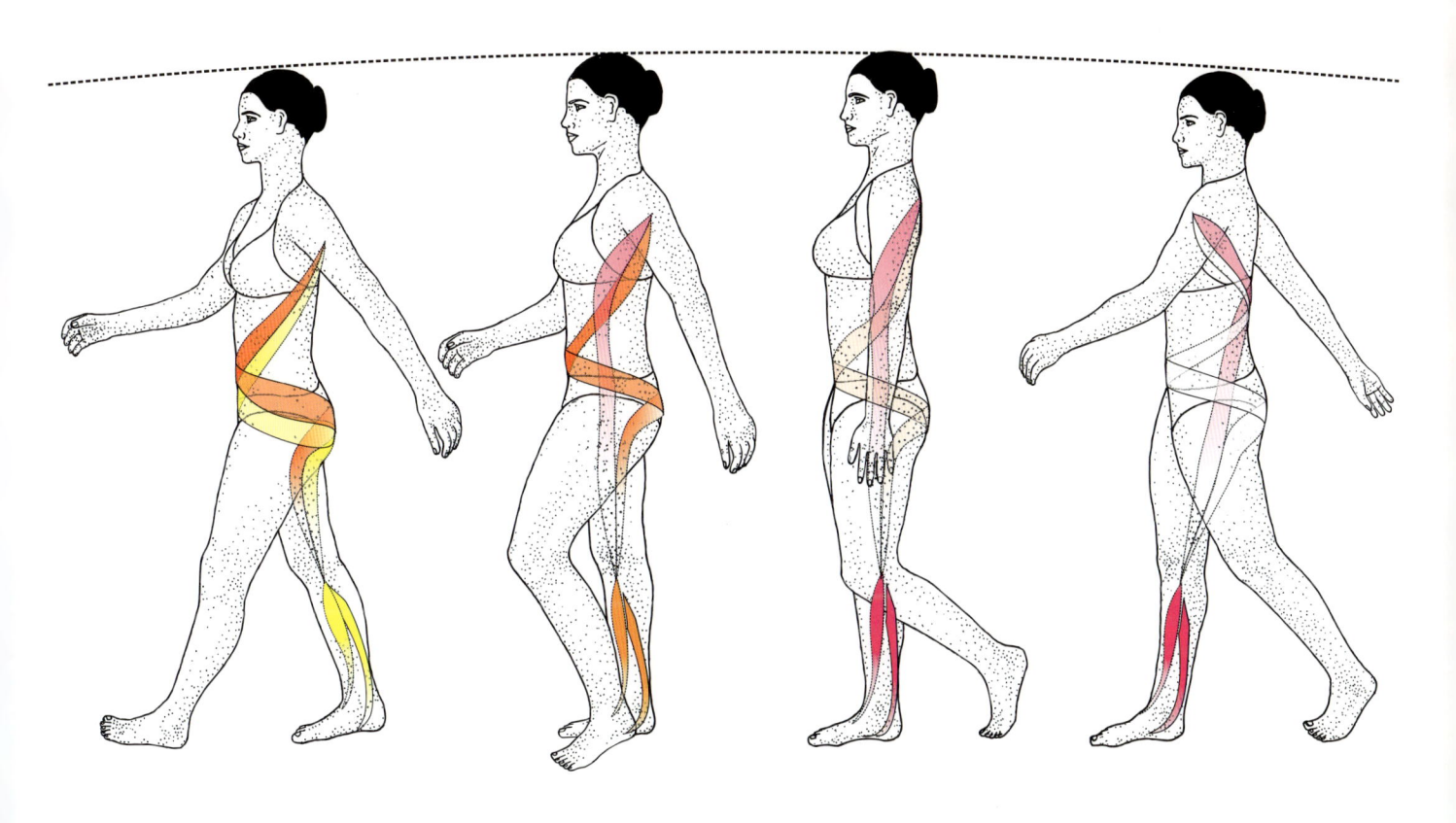

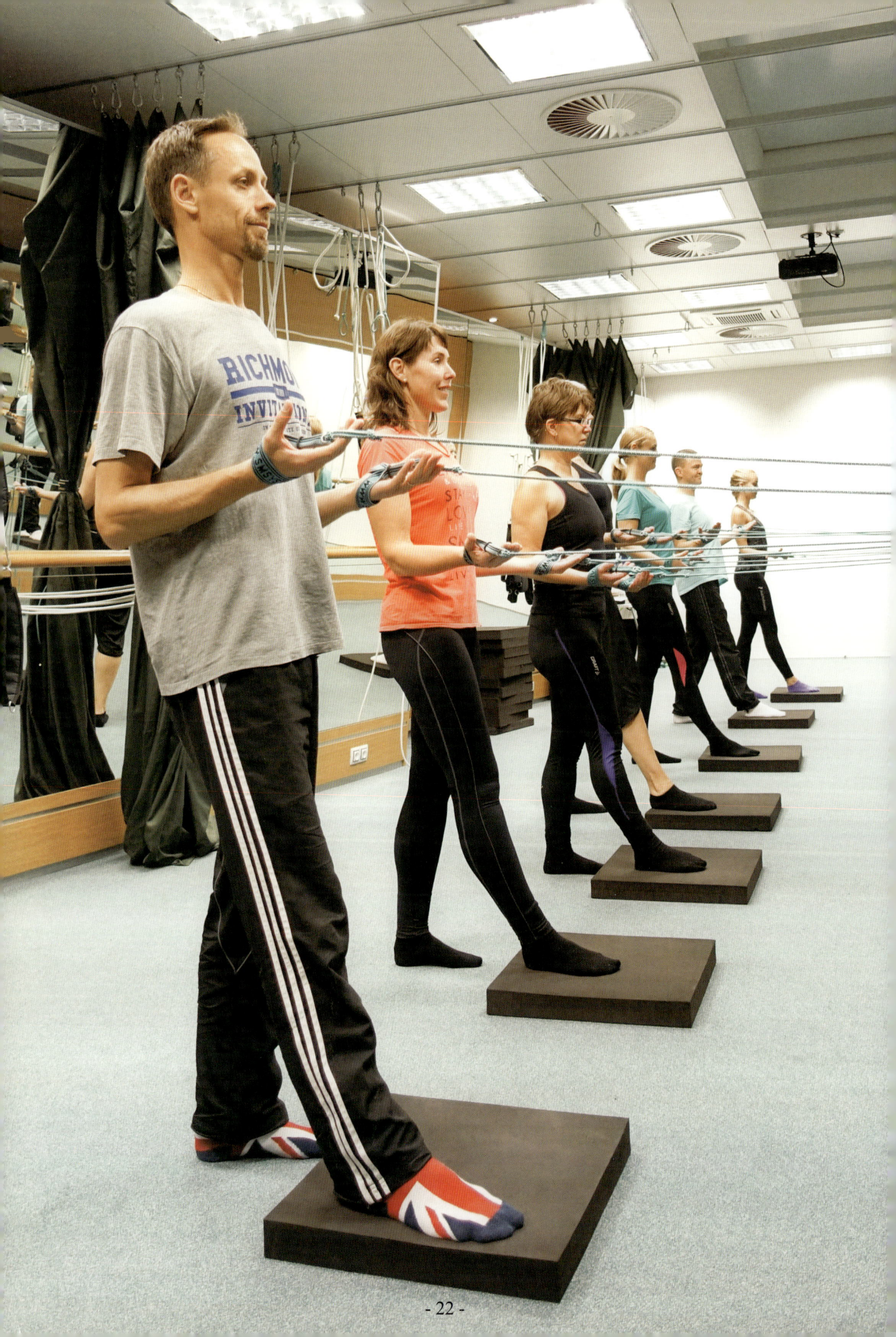

Examples of the successful treatment of a herniated disc

Example of the successful treatment of herniated disc L3/4

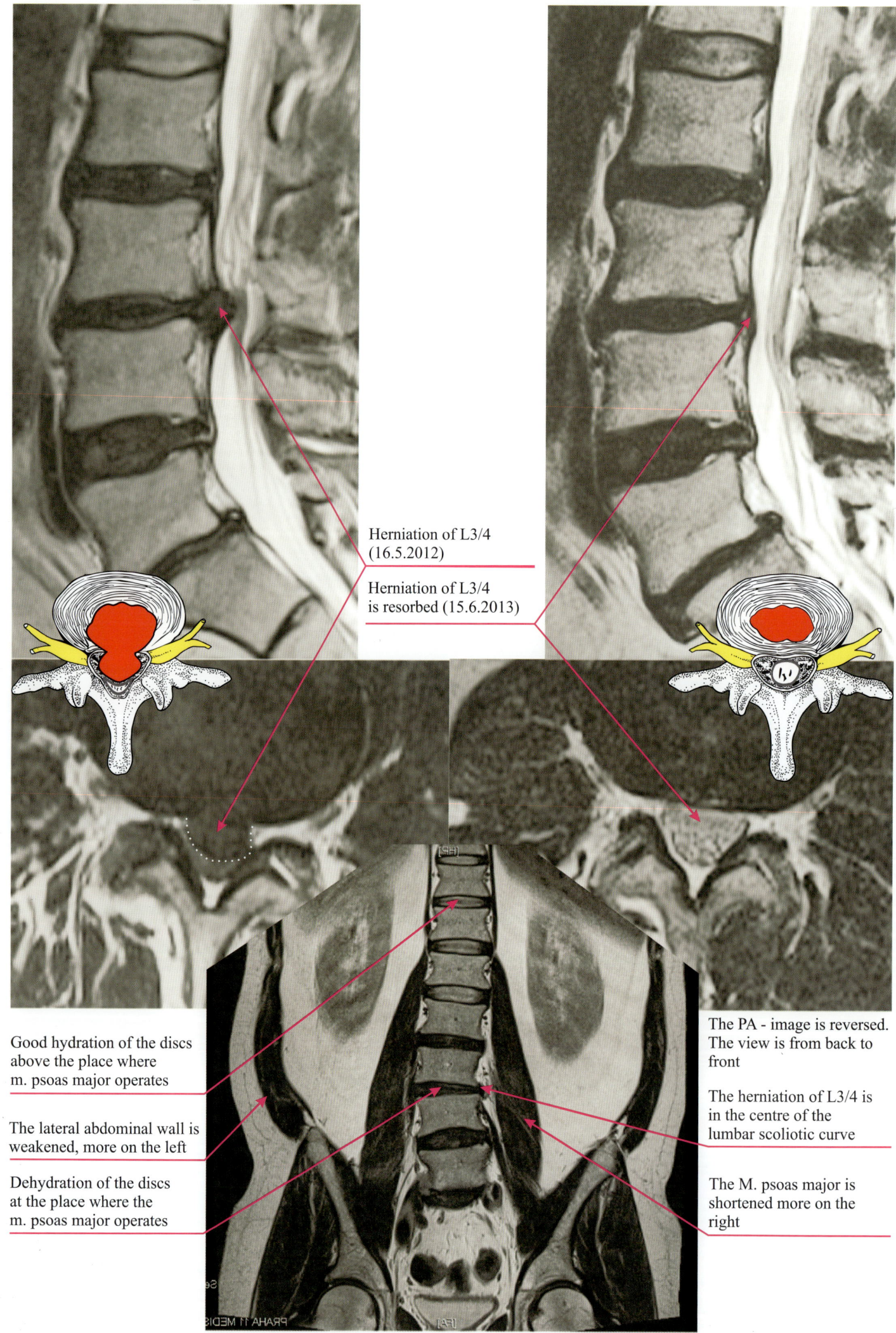

Herniation of L3/4 (16.5.2012)

Herniation of L3/4 is resorbed (15.6.2013)

Good hydration of the discs above the place where m. psoas major operates

The lateral abdominal wall is weakened, more on the left

Dehydration of the discs at the place where the m. psoas major operates

The PA - image is reversed. The view is from back to front

The herniation of L3/4 is in the centre of the lumbar scoliotic curve

The M. psoas major is shortened more on the right

Example of the successful treatment of herniated disc L3/4

Stabilization of lateral abdominal wall

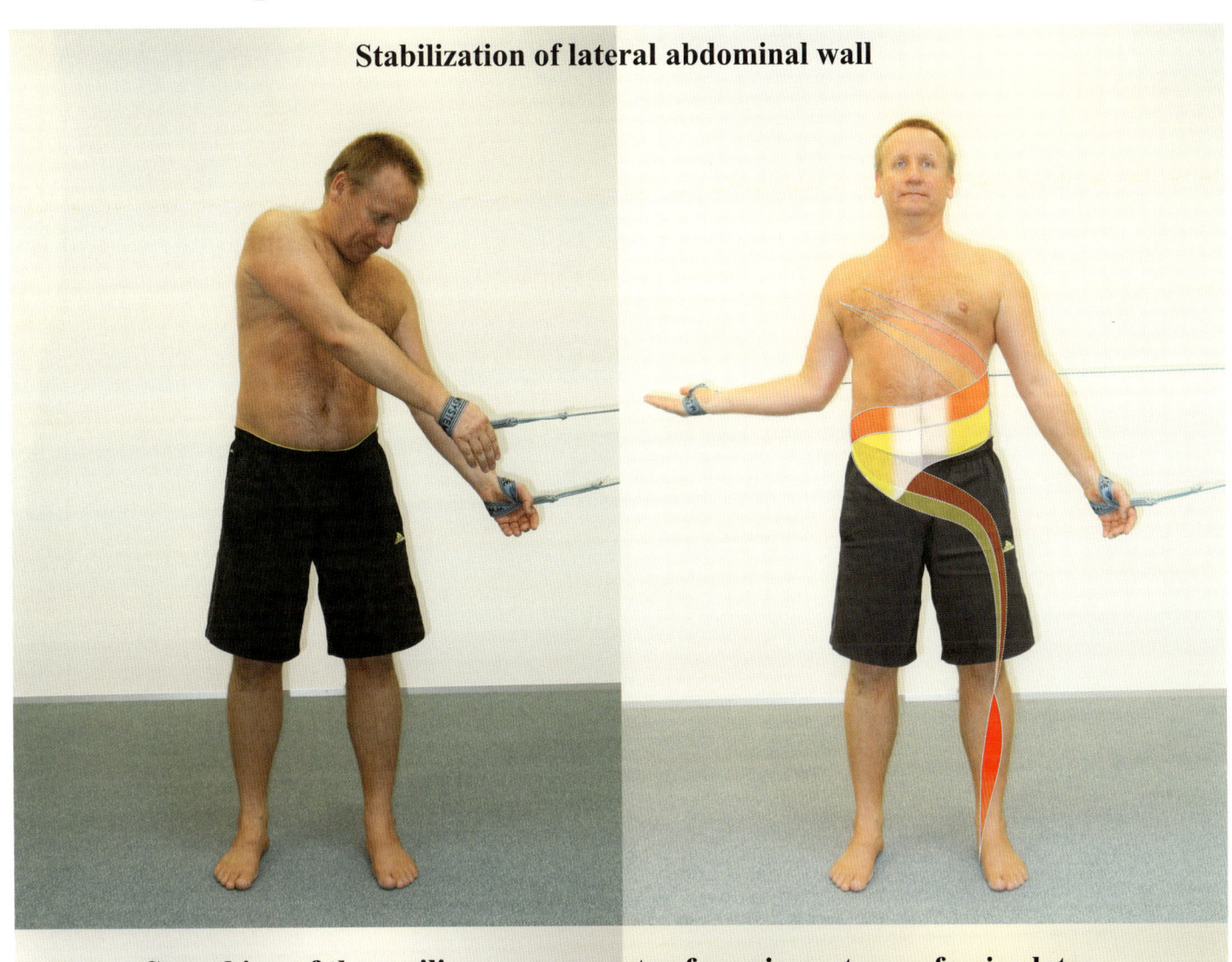

Stretching of the m. iliopsoas, m. rectus femoris, m. tensor fasciae latae
in a body spirally stabilized by the TR and LD chains

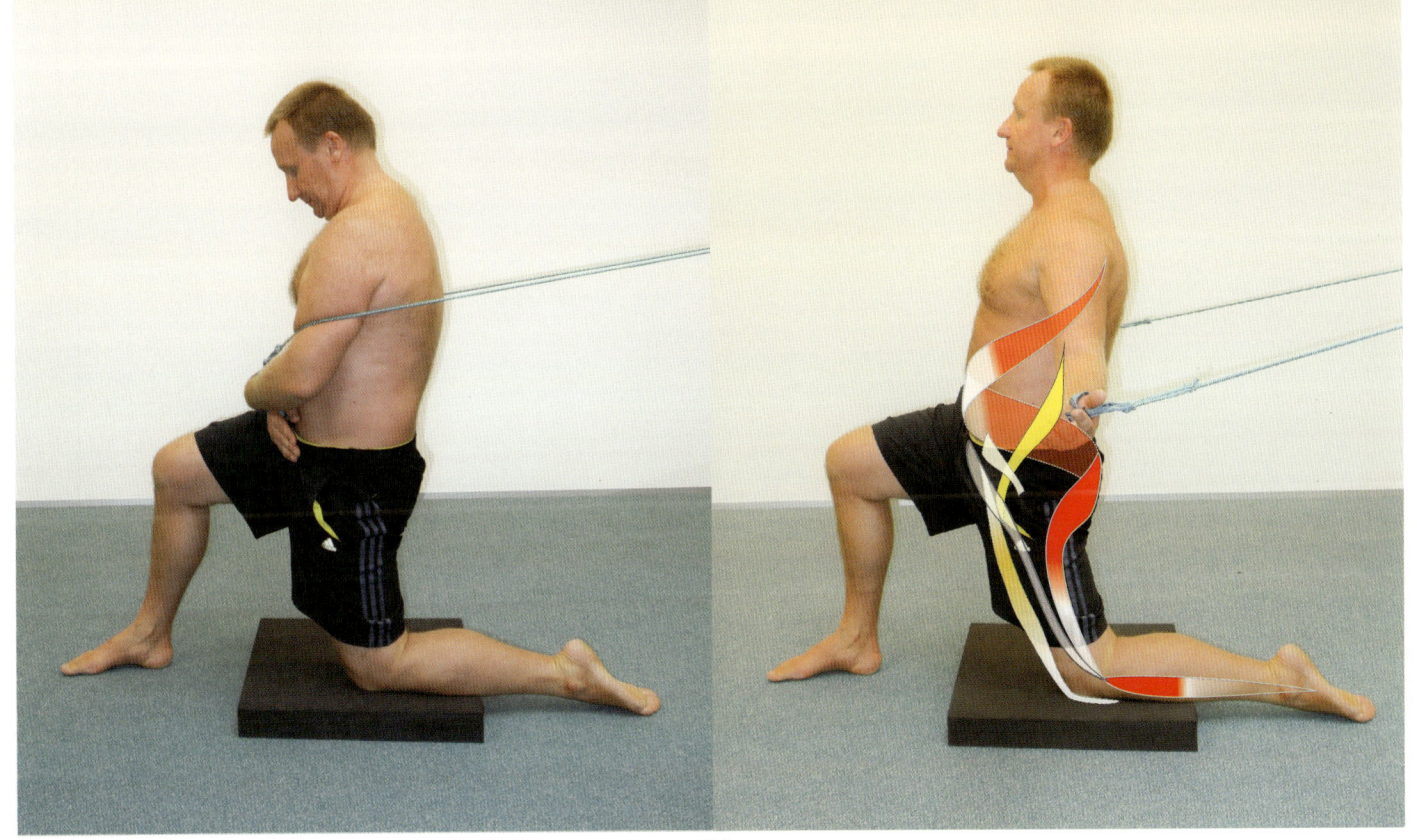

Example of the successful treatment of herniated disc L4/5

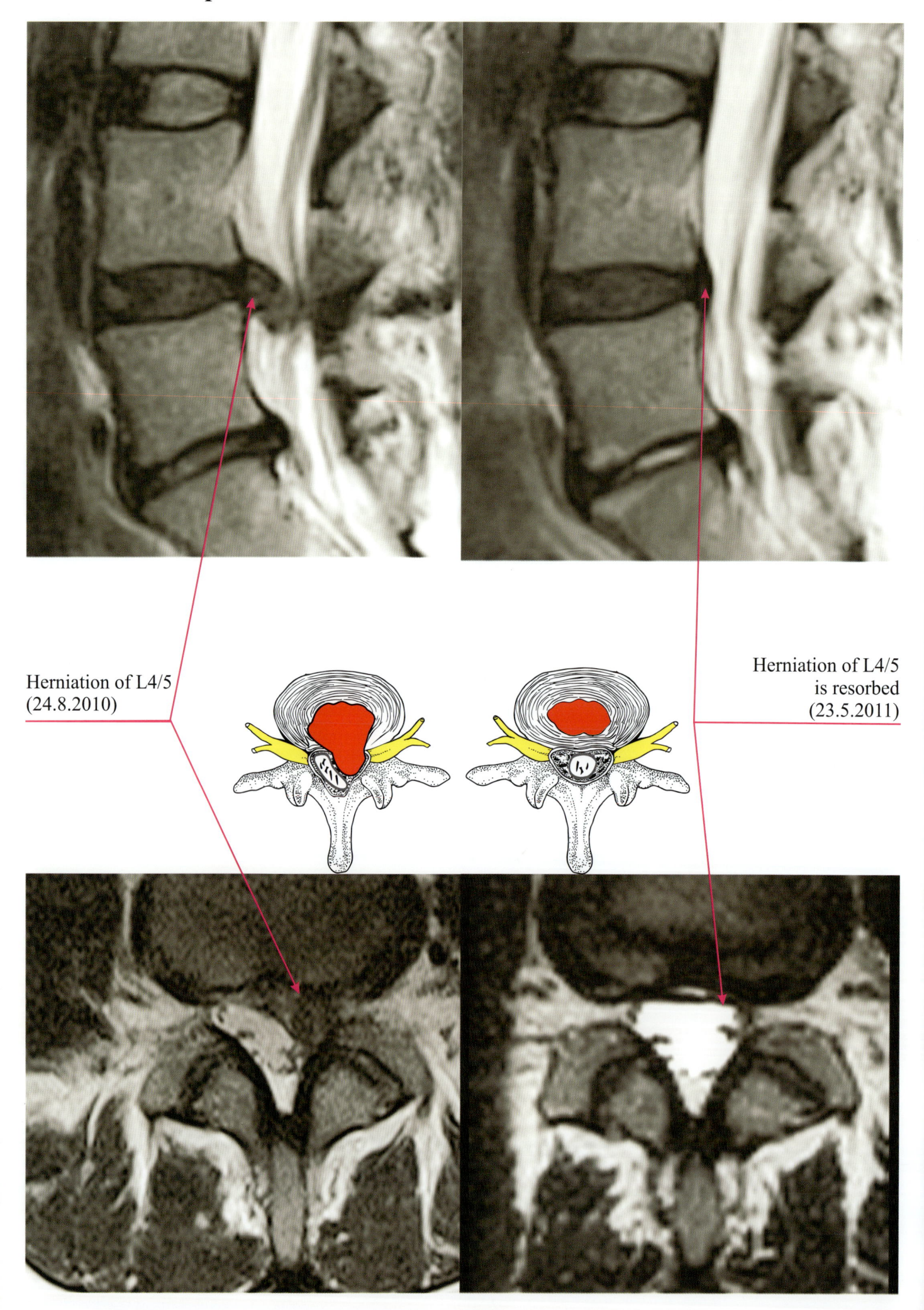

Herniation of L4/5
(24.8.2010)

Herniation of L4/5
is resorbed
(23.5.2011)

- 26 -

Example of the successful treatment of herniated disc L4/5

Stabilization of the abdominal wall by the TR and LD spirals

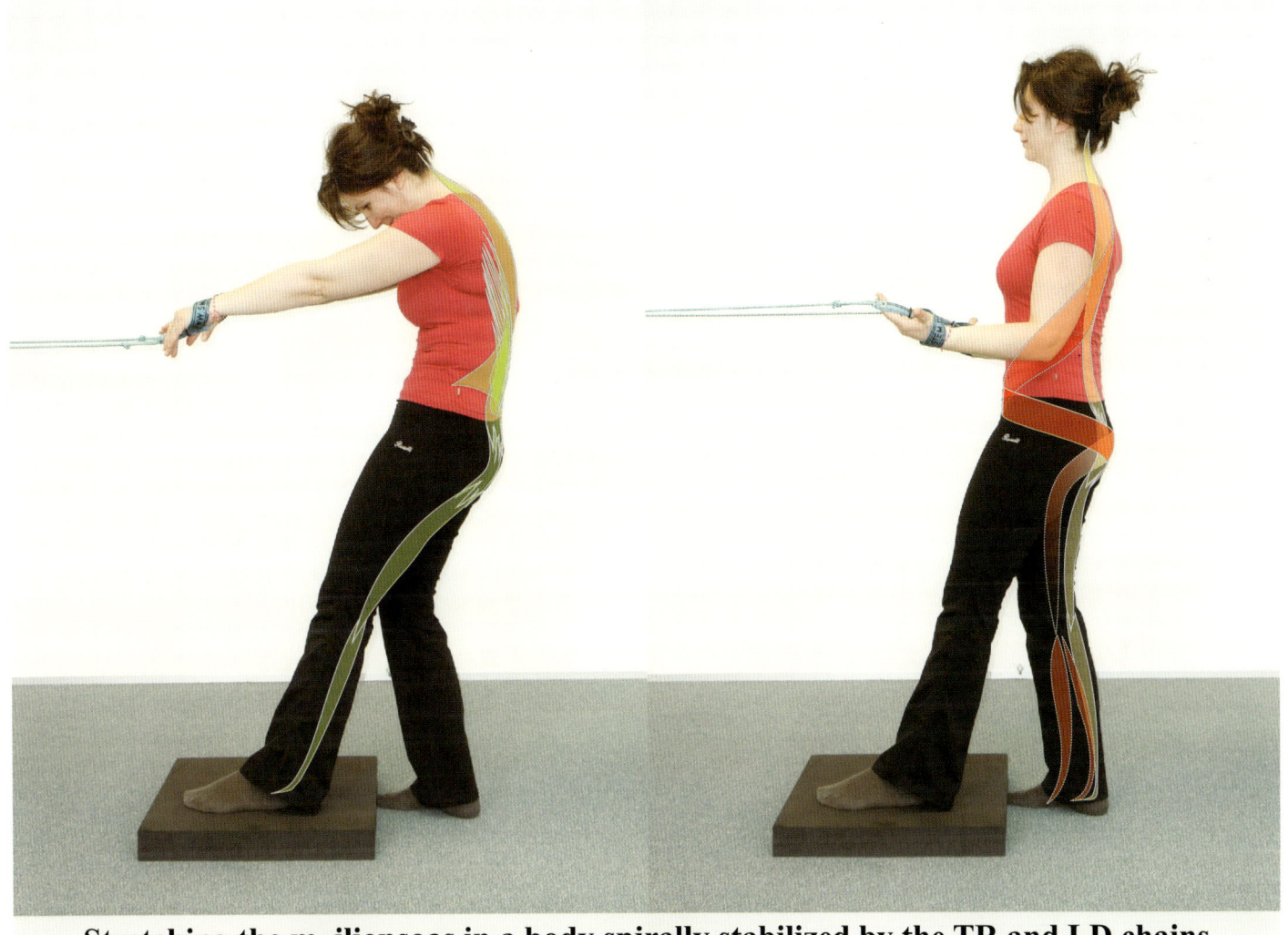

Stretching the m. iliopsoas in a body spirally stabilized by the TR and LD chains

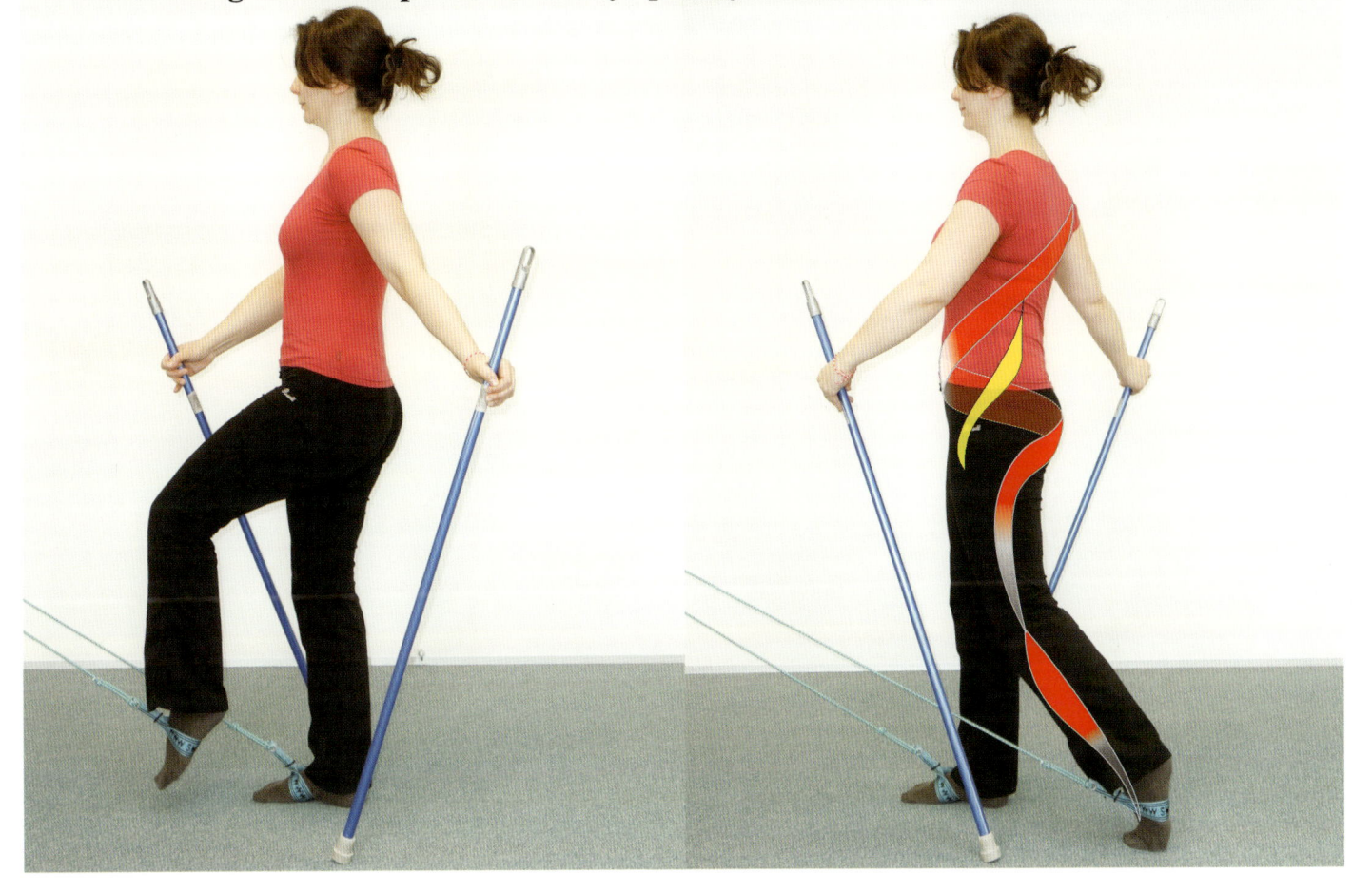

Example of the successful treatment of herniated disc L5/S1

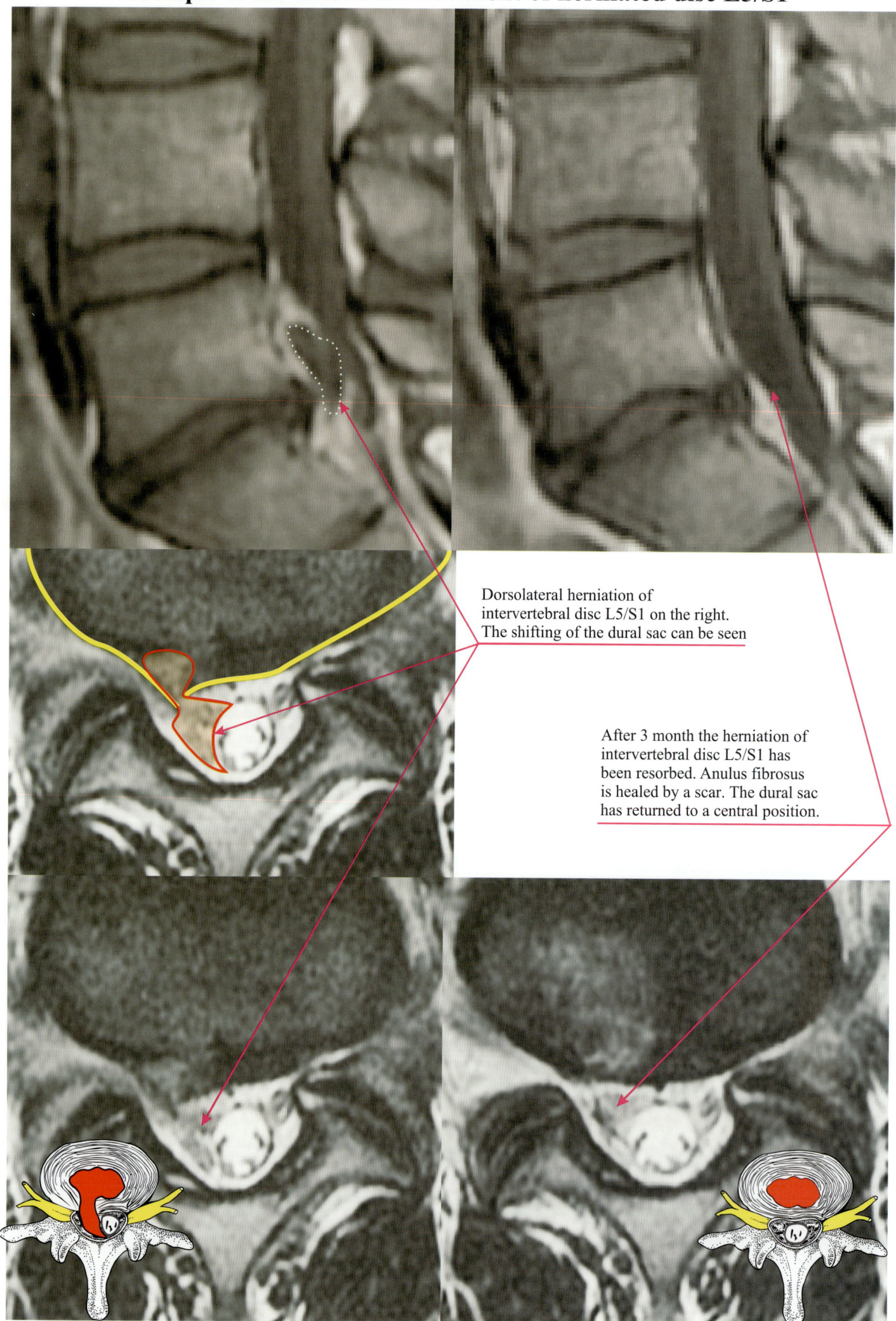

Dorsolateral herniation of intervertebral disc L5/S1 on the right. The shifting of the dural sac can be seen

After 3 month the herniation of intervertebral disc L5/S1 has been resorbed. Anulus fibrosus is healed by a scar. The dural sac has returned to a central position.

Example of the successful treatment of herniated disc L5/S1

M. quadratus lumborum
M. iliocostalis lumborum

M. multifidus

Stretching paravertebral muscles and spine

Stabilization of abdominal wall
The phenomenon of narrowing the waist

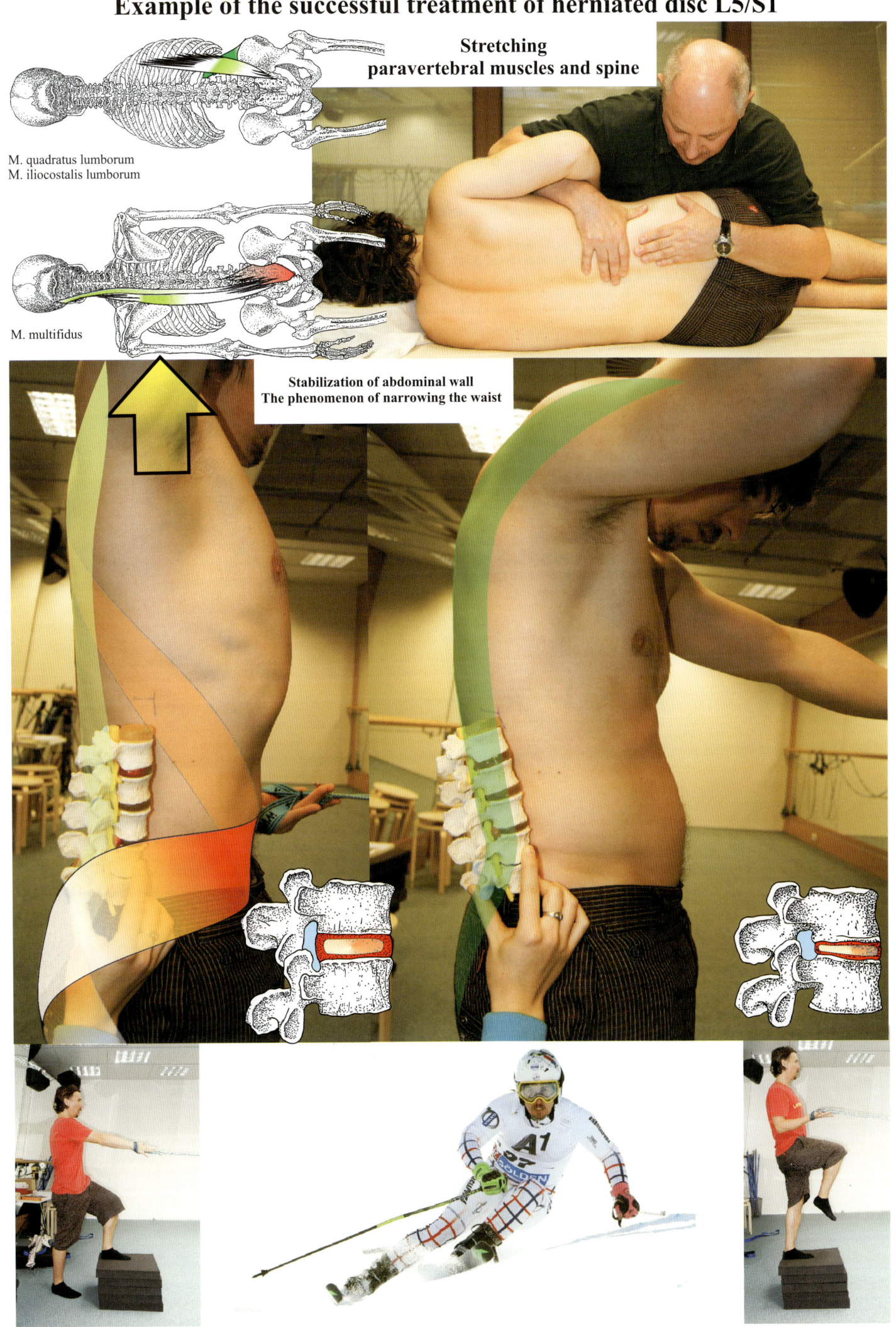

- 29 -

Example of the successful treatment of herniated disc L5/S1

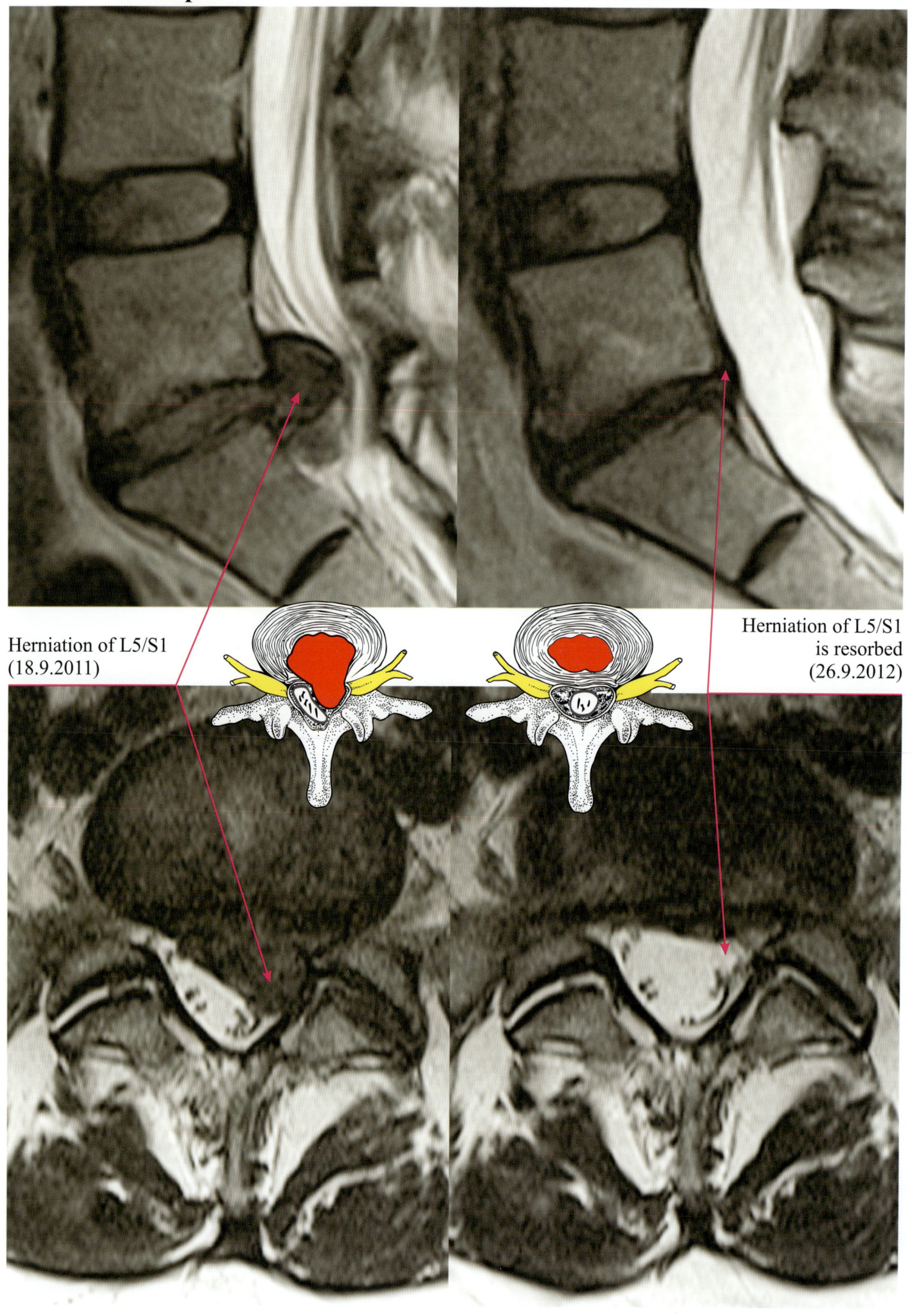

Herniation of L5/S1
(18.9.2011)

Herniation of L5/S1
is resorbed
(26.9.2012)

Example of the successful treatment of herniated disc L5/S1

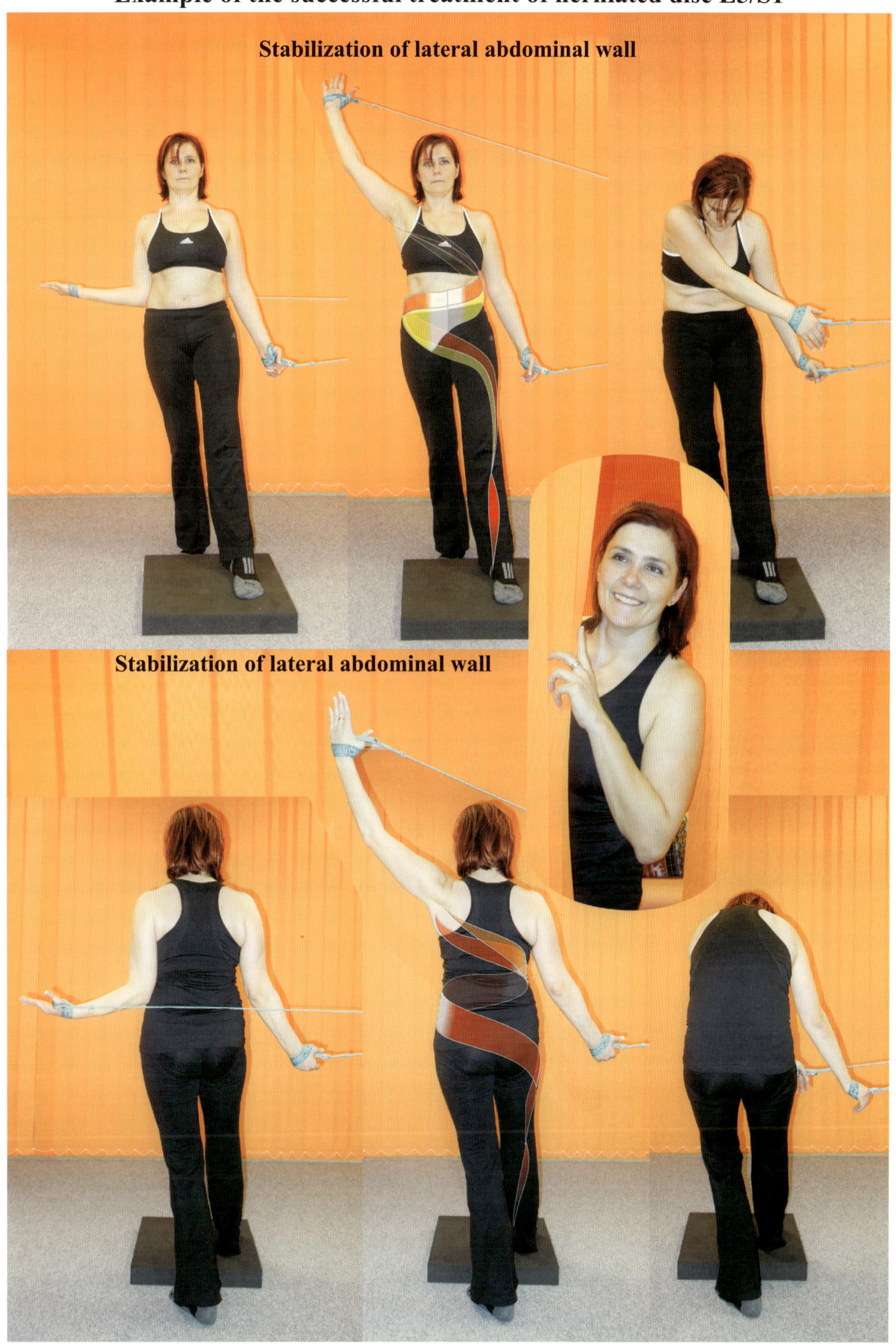

Stabilization of lateral abdominal wall

Stabilization of lateral abdominal wall

Loss of muscle tissue in the paravertebral muscles due to the herniation of disc L5/S1

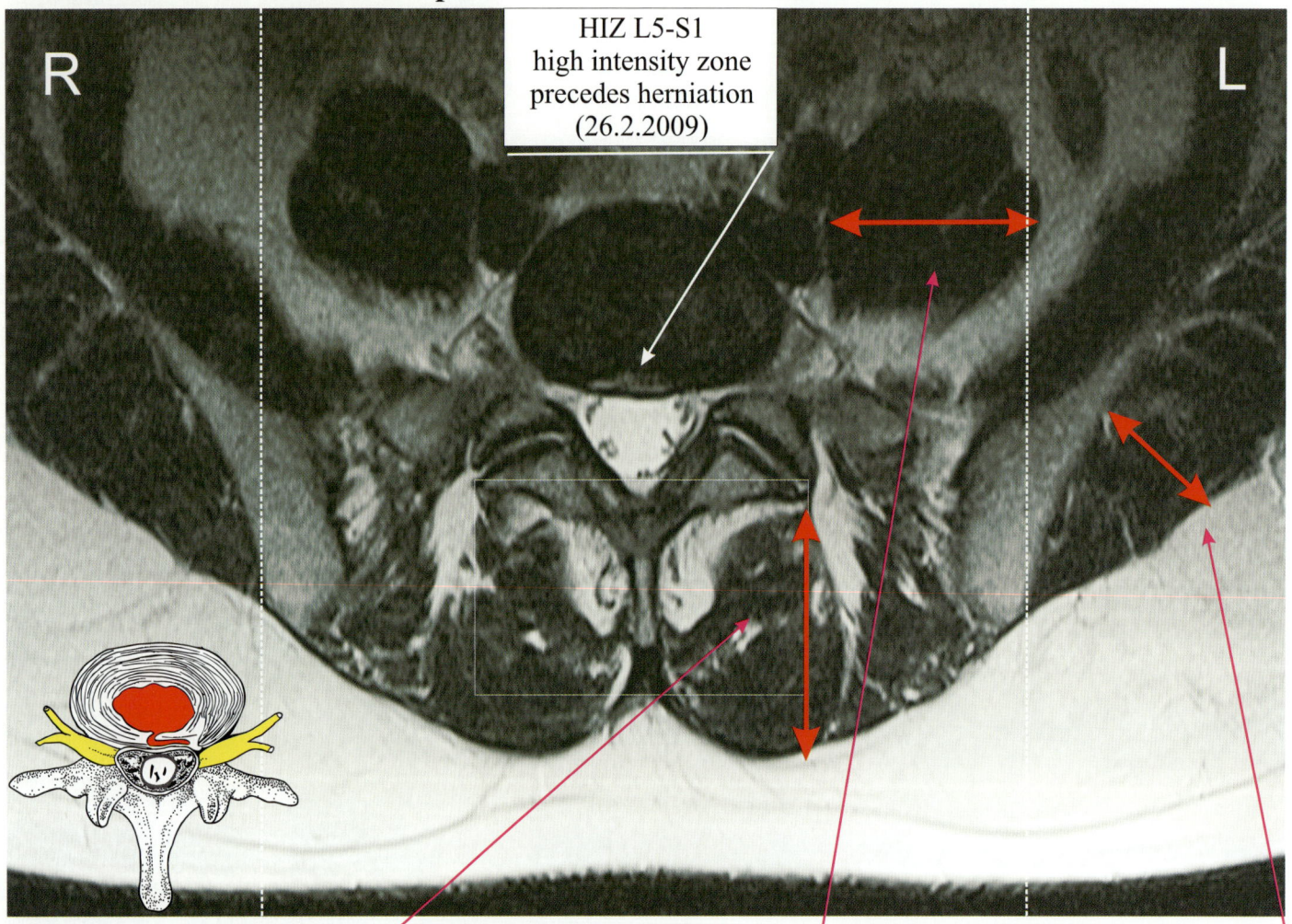

HIZ L5-S1 high intensity zone precedes herniation (26.2.2009)

R   L

Atrophy of m. multifidus on both sides (18.9.2011)

Atrophy of m. psoas major on both sides (18.9.2011)

Atrophy of m. gluteus maximus on the left (18.9.2011)

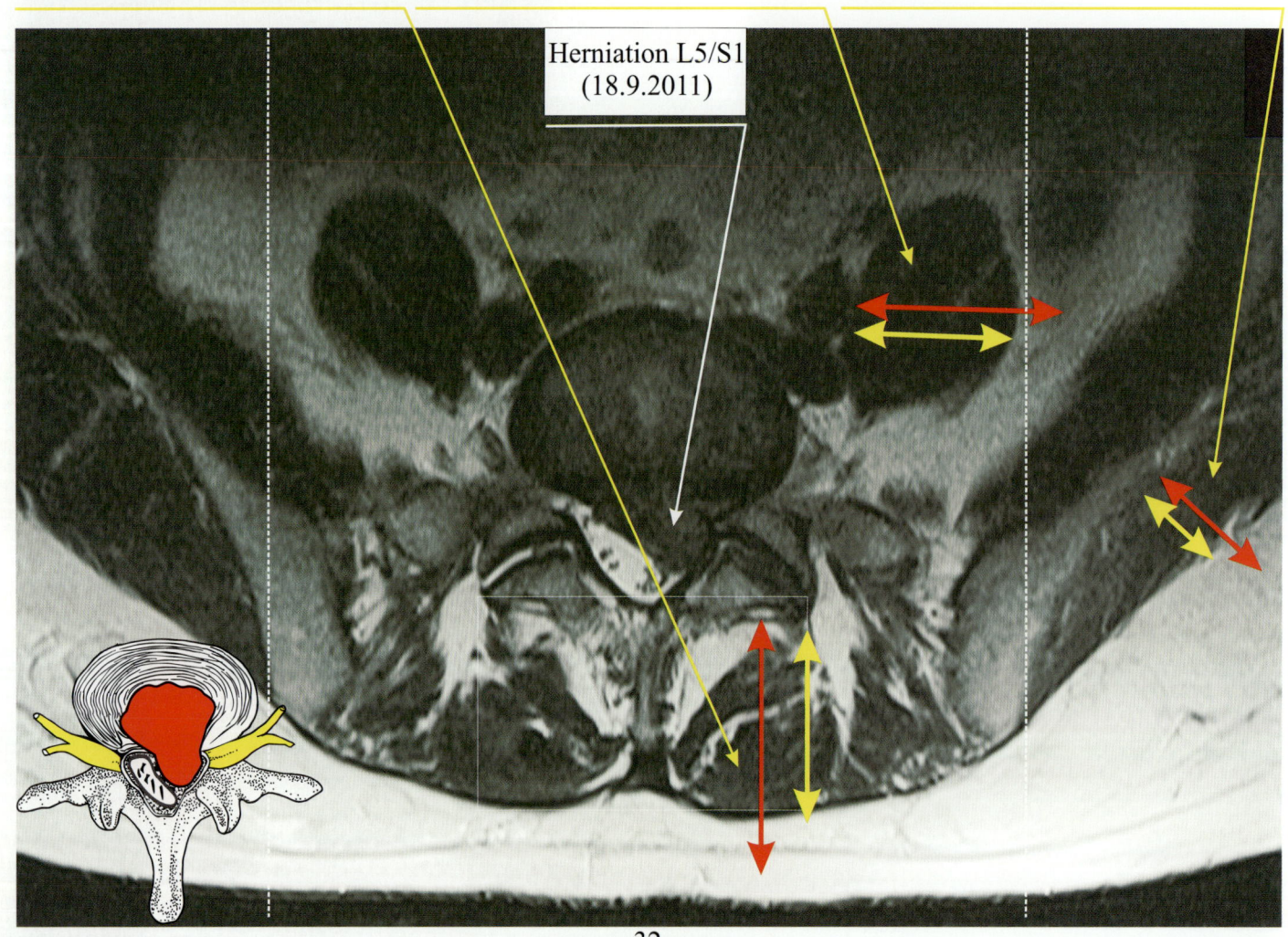

Herniation L5/S1 (18.9.2011)

Example of the successful treatment of herniated disc L5/S1

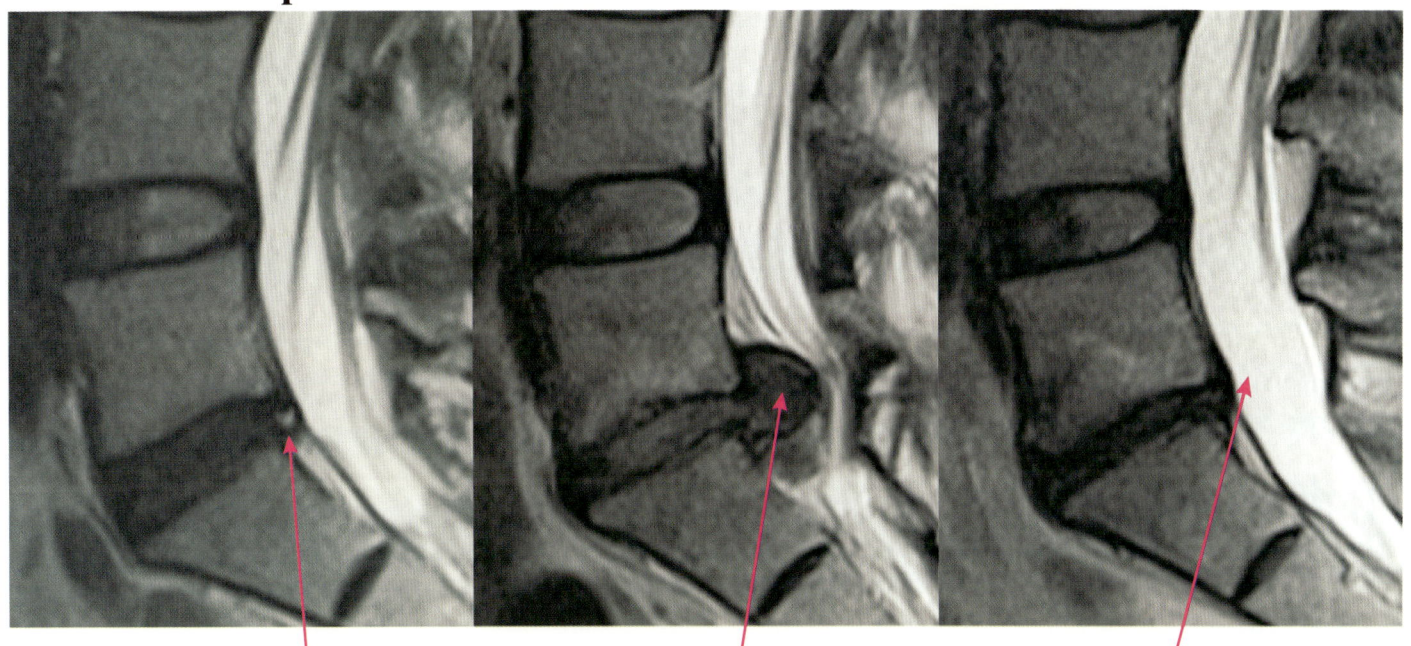

HIZ L5-S1
high intensity zone
precedes herniation
(26.2.2009)

Herniation L5/S1
(18.9.2011)

Herniation of L5/S1 is
resorbed (26.9.2012)

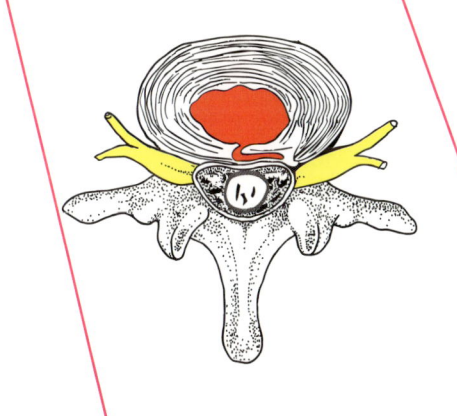

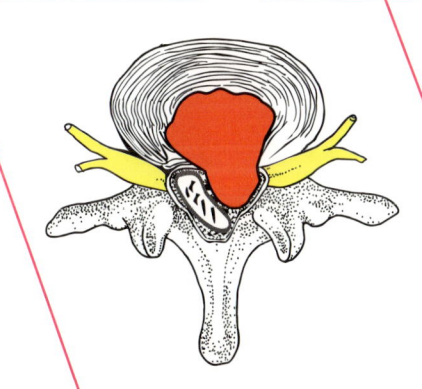

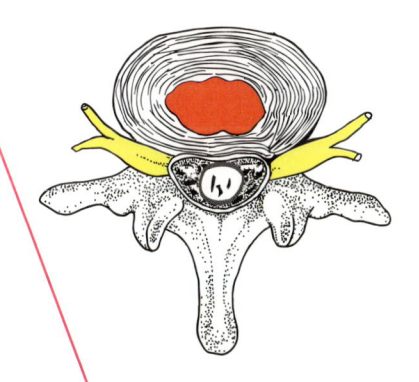

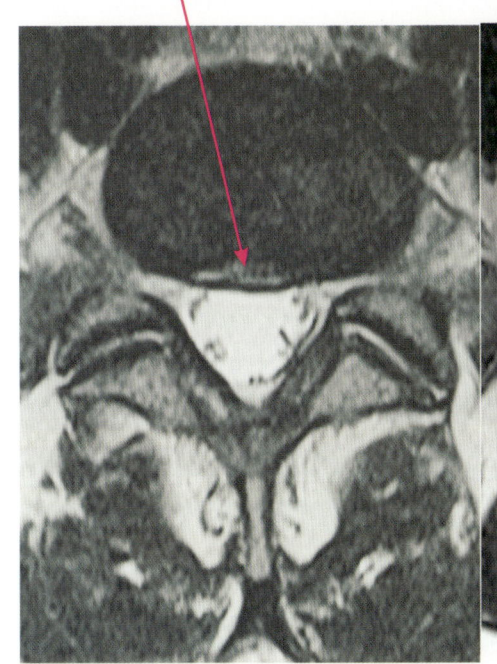

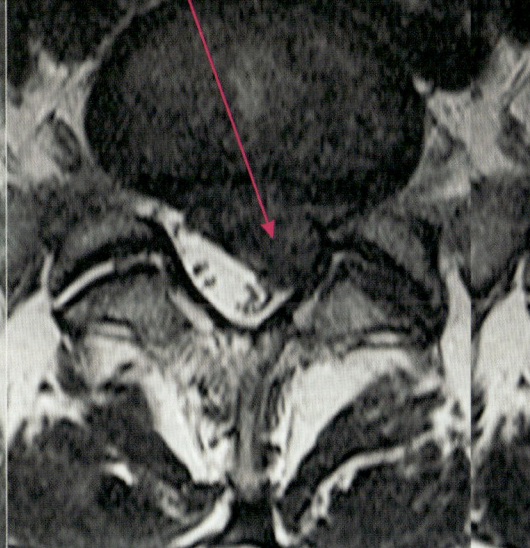

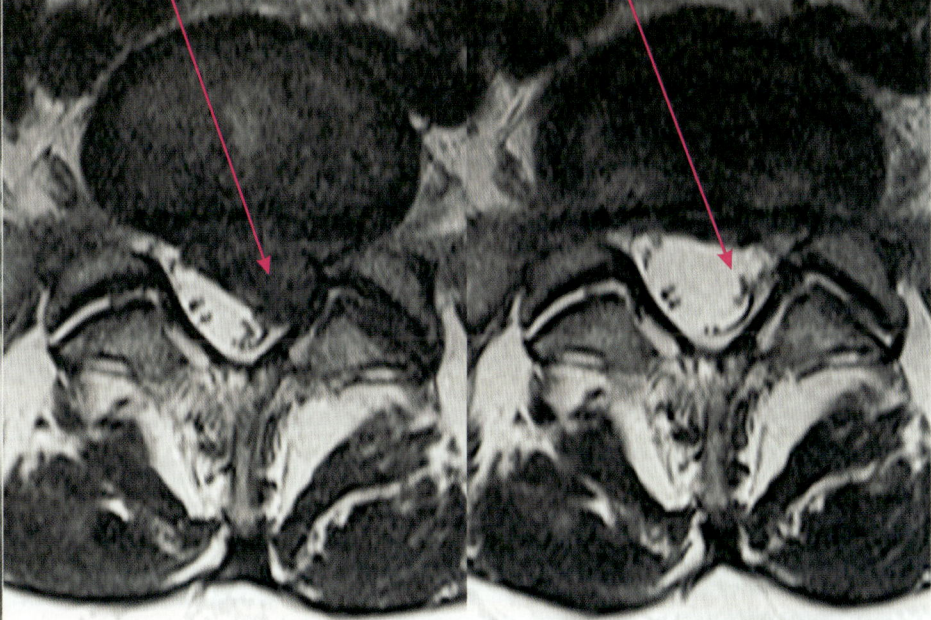

HIZ precedes the herniation of disc L5/S1
HIZ must immediately be treated intensively to avoid disc herniation!!!
HIZ is most often hidden under the diagnosis of nonspecific lumbago!!!

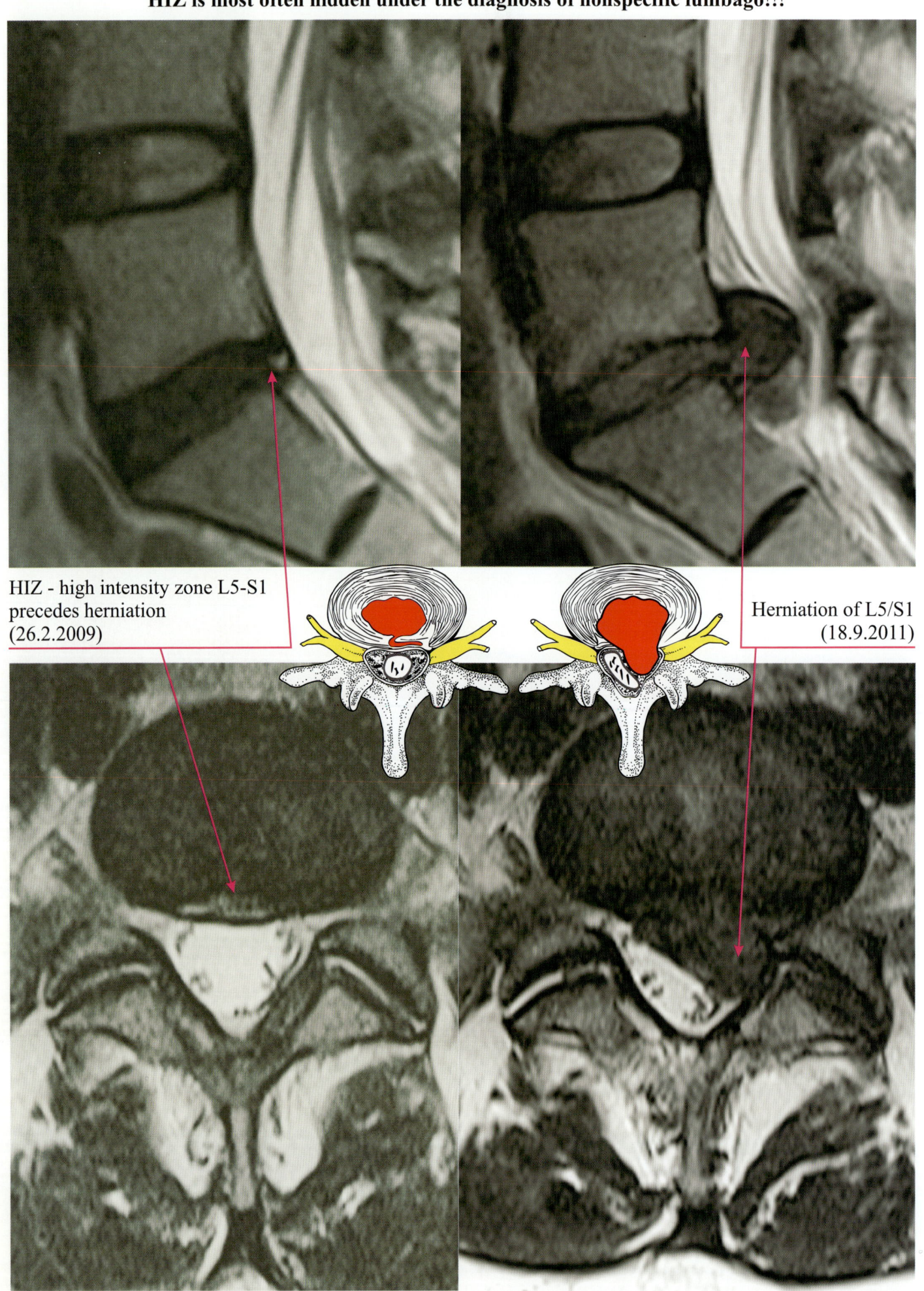

HIZ - high intensity zone L5-S1 precedes herniation (26.2.2009)

Herniation of L5/S1 (18.9.2011)

Examination of the muscles at rest and in motion

EXAMINATION OF TENSE AND WEAKENED MUSCLES

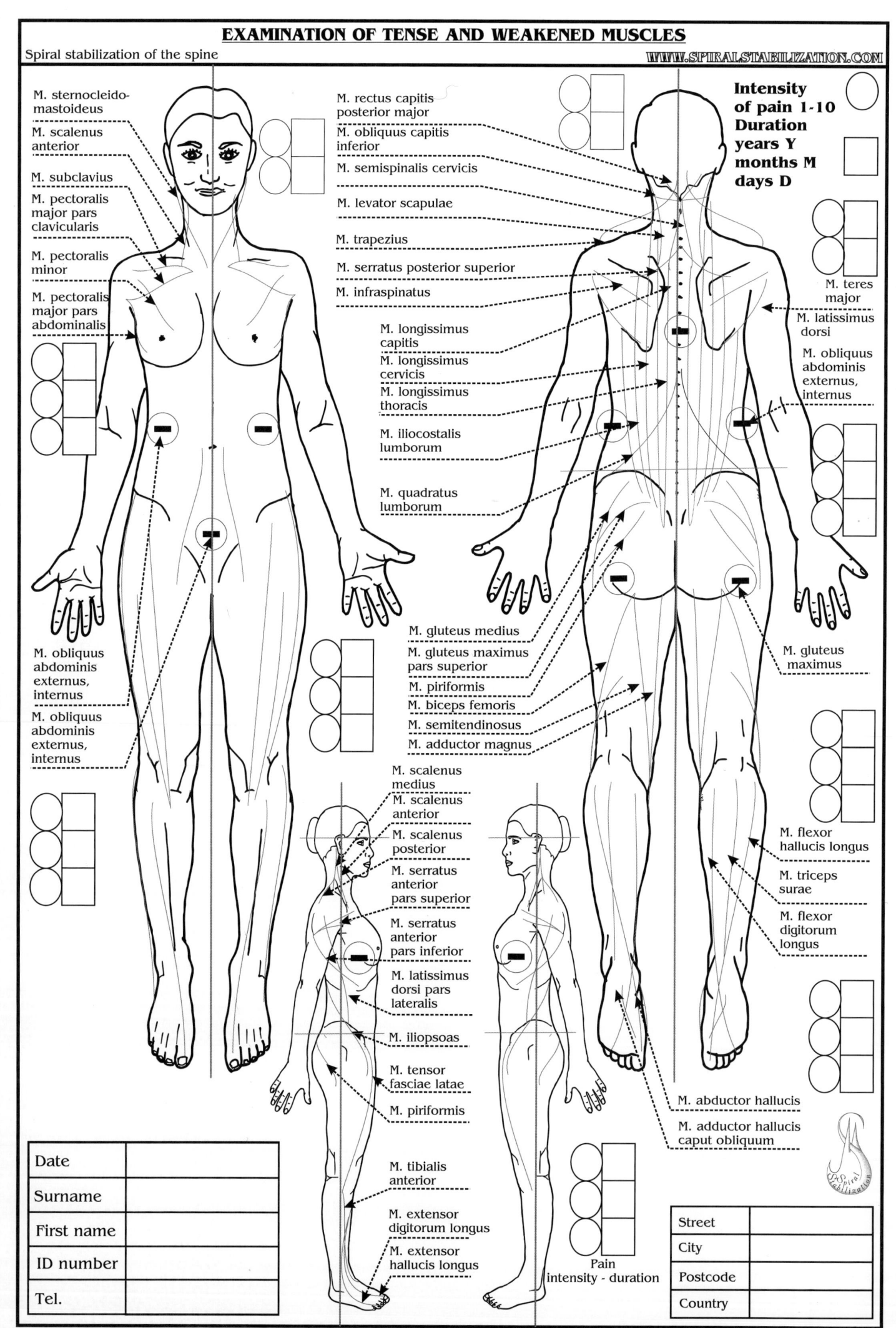

Spiral stabilization of the spine
WWW.SPIRALSTABILIZATION.COM

Intensity of pain 1-10
Duration years Y months M days D

- M. sternocleido-mastoideus
- M. scalenus anterior
- M. subclavius
- M. pectoralis major pars clavicularis
- M. pectoralis minor
- M. pectoralis major pars abdominalis
- M. obliquus abdominis externus, internus
- M. obliquus abdominis externus, internus

- M. rectus capitis posterior major
- M. obliquus capitis inferior
- M. semispinalis cervicis
- M. levator scapulae
- M. trapezius
- M. serratus posterior superior
- M. infraspinatus
- M. longissimus capitis
- M. longissimus cervicis
- M. longissimus thoracis
- M. iliocostalis lumborum
- M. quadratus lumborum

- M. teres major
- M. latissimus dorsi
- M. obliquus abdominis externus, internus

- M. gluteus medius
- M. gluteus maximus pars superior
- M. piriformis
- M. biceps femoris
- M. semitendinosus
- M. adductor magnus

- M. gluteus maximus
- M. flexor hallucis longus
- M. triceps surae
- M. flexor digitorum longus

- M. scalenus medius
- M. scalenus anterior
- M. scalenus posterior
- M. serratus anterior pars superior
- M. serratus anterior pars inferior
- M. latissimus dorsi pars lateralis
- M. iliopsoas
- M. tensor fasciae latae
- M. piriformis
- M. tibialis anterior
- M. extensor digitorum longus
- M. extensor hallucis longus

- M. abductor hallucis
- M. adductor hallucis caput obliquum

Pain intensity - duration

Date	
Surname	
First name	
ID number	
Tel.	

Street	
City	
Postcode	
Country	

- 36 -

PAIN, MUSCLE TENSION, MUSCLE WEAKENING, LOSS OF SENSATION, LOSS OF MOBILITY, CHANGE OF SHAPE

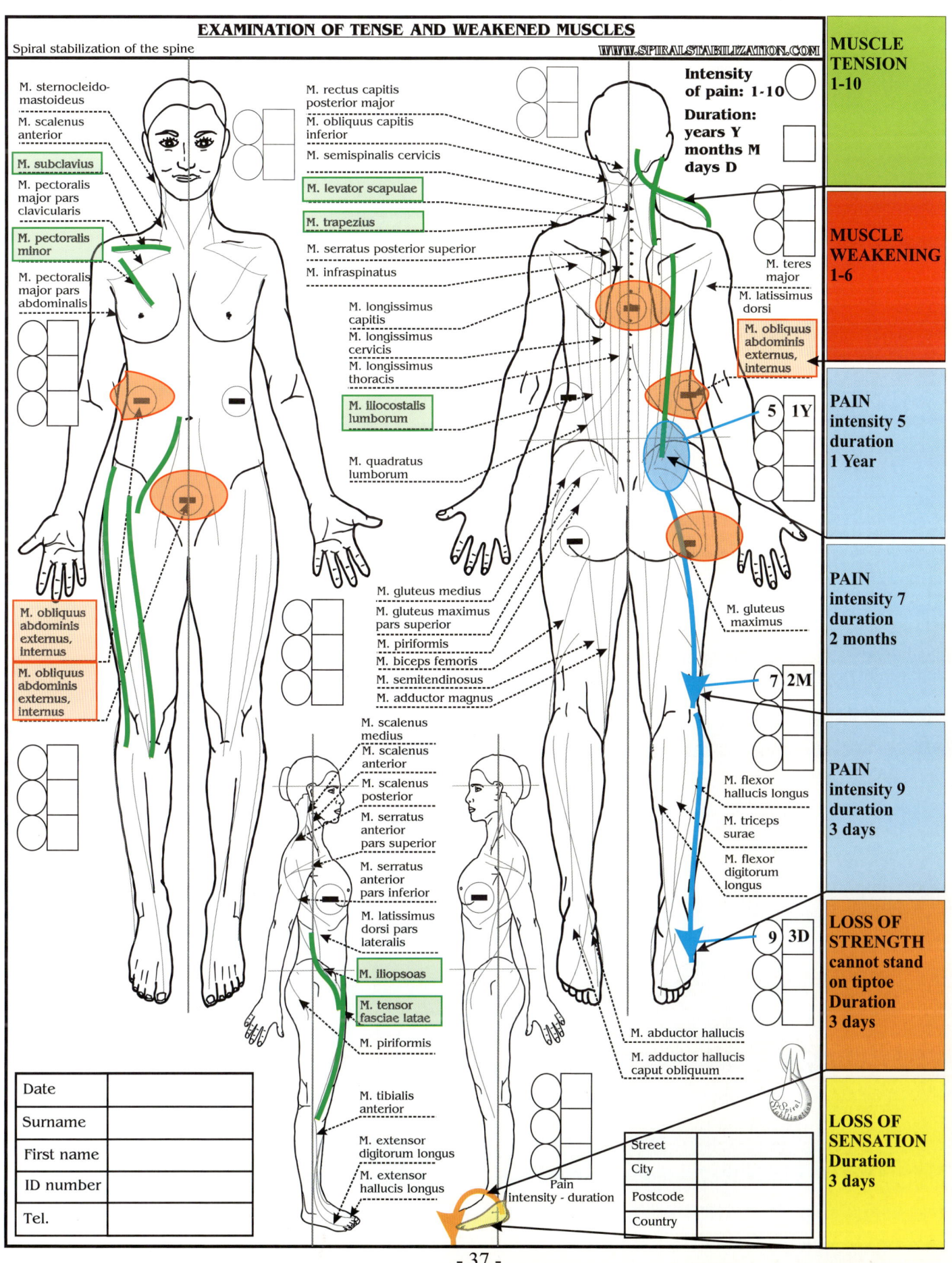

EXAMINATION OF TENSE AND WEAKENED MUSCLES

Spiral stabilization of the spine
www.spiralstabilization.com

Intensity of pain: 1-10
Duration: years Y months M days D

Anterior labels (left figure):
- M. sternocleido-mastoideus
- M. scalenus anterior
- M. subclavius
- M. pectoralis major pars clavicularis
- M. pectoralis minor
- M. pectoralis major pars abdominalis
- M. rectus capitis posterior major
- M. obliquus capitis inferior
- M. semispinalis cervicis
- M. levator scapulae
- M. trapezius
- M. serratus posterior superior
- M. infraspinatus
- M. longissimus capitis
- M. longissimus cervicis
- M. longissimus thoracis
- M. iliocostalis lumborum
- M. quadratus lumborum
- M. obliquus abdominis externus, internus
- M. obliquus abdominis externus, internus

Posterior labels (right figure):
- M. teres major
- M. latissimus dorsi
- M. obliquus abdominis externus, internus
- M. gluteus medius
- M. gluteus maximus pars superior
- M. piriformis
- M. biceps femoris
- M. semitendinosus
- M. adductor magnus
- M. gluteus maximus
- M. flexor hallucis longus
- M. triceps surae
- M. flexor digitorum longus
- M. abductor hallucis
- M. adductor hallucis caput obliquum

Side view labels:
- M. scalenus medius
- M. scalenus anterior
- M. scalenus posterior
- M. serratus anterior pars superior
- M. serratus anterior pars inferior
- M. latissimus dorsi pars lateralis
- M. iliopsoas
- M. tensor fasciae latae
- M. piriformis
- M. tibialis anterior
- M. extensor digitorum longus
- M. extensor hallucis longus

Pain intensity - duration

Date	
Surname	
First name	
ID number	
Tel.	

Street	
City	
Postcode	
Country	

Legend

MUSCLE TENSION 1-10

MUSCLE WEAKENING 1-6

PAIN intensity 5 duration 1 Year — 5 | 1Y

PAIN intensity 7 duration 2 months — 7 | 2M

PAIN intensity 9 duration 3 days — 9 | 3D

LOSS OF STRENGTH cannot stand on tiptoe Duration 3 days

LOSS OF SENSATION Duration 3 days

- 37 -

EXAMINING EXTENSION

EXTENSION (backward movement of the arm) IN THE SHOULDER GIRDLE

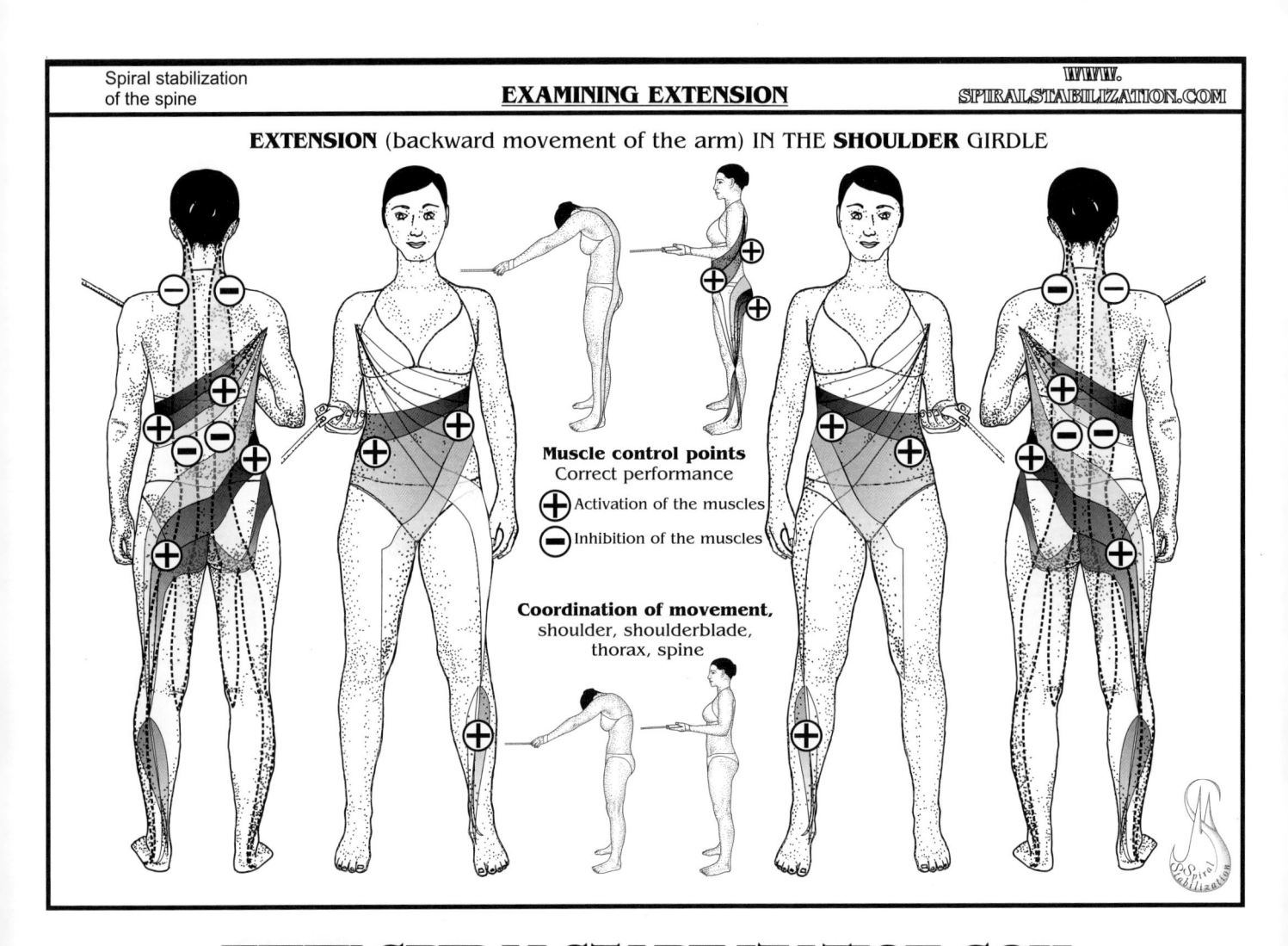

Muscle control points
Correct performance
⊕ Activation of the muscles
⊖ Inhibition of the muscles

Coordination of movement,
shoulder, shoulderblade, thorax, spine

EXAMINING EXTENSION

EXTENSION (backward movement of the arm and leg) IN THE SHOULDER AND PELVIC GIRDLES

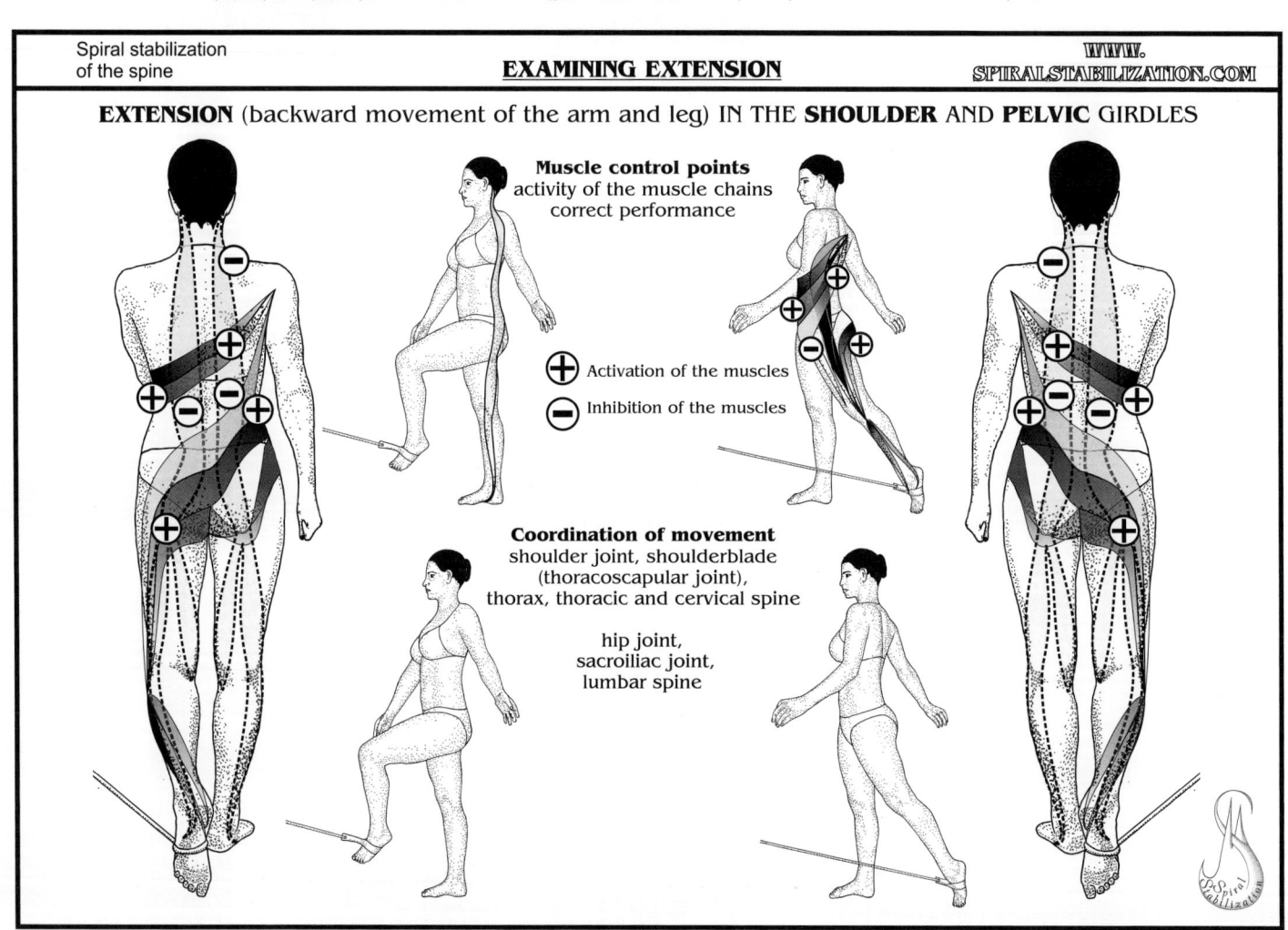

Muscle control points
activity of the muscle chains
correct performance

⊕ Activation of the muscles
⊖ Inhibition of the muscles

Coordination of movement
shoulder joint, shoulderblade
(thoracoscapular joint),
thorax, thoracic and cervical spine

hip joint,
sacroiliac joint,
lumbar spine

EXAMINING EXTENSION

EXTENSION (backward movement of the arm) IN THE SHOULDER GIRDLE

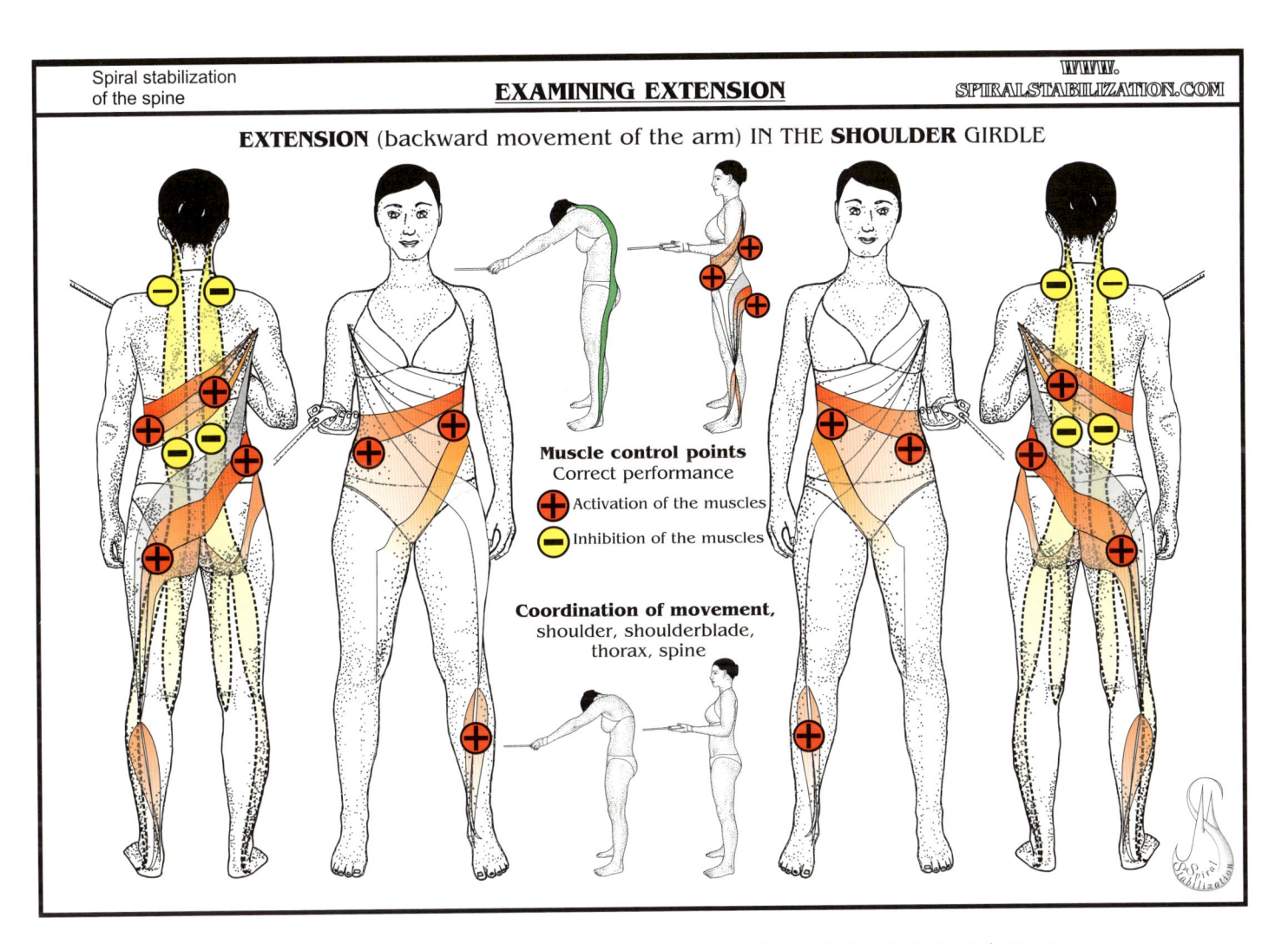

Muscle control points
Correct performance

⊕ Activation of the muscles
⊖ Inhibition of the muscles

Coordination of movement,
shoulder, shoulderblade, thorax, spine

EXAMINING EXTENSION

EXTENSION (backward movement of the arm and leg) IN THE SHOULDER AND PELVIC GIRDLES

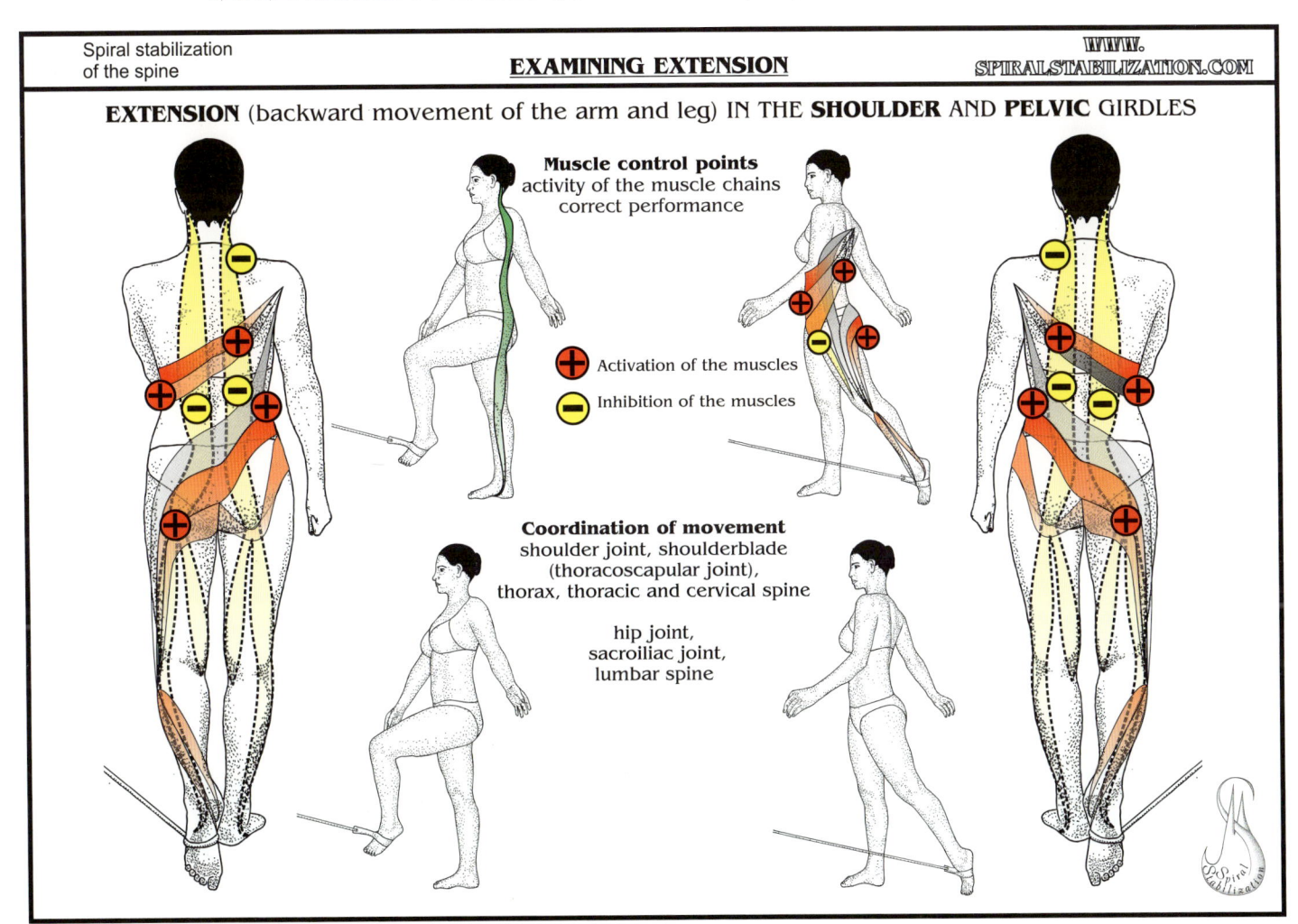

Muscle control points
activity of the muscle chains
correct performance

⊕ Activation of the muscles
⊖ Inhibition of the muscles

Coordination of movement
shoulder joint, shoulderblade
(thoracoscapular joint),
thorax, thoracic and cervical spine

hip joint,
sacroiliac joint,
lumbar spine

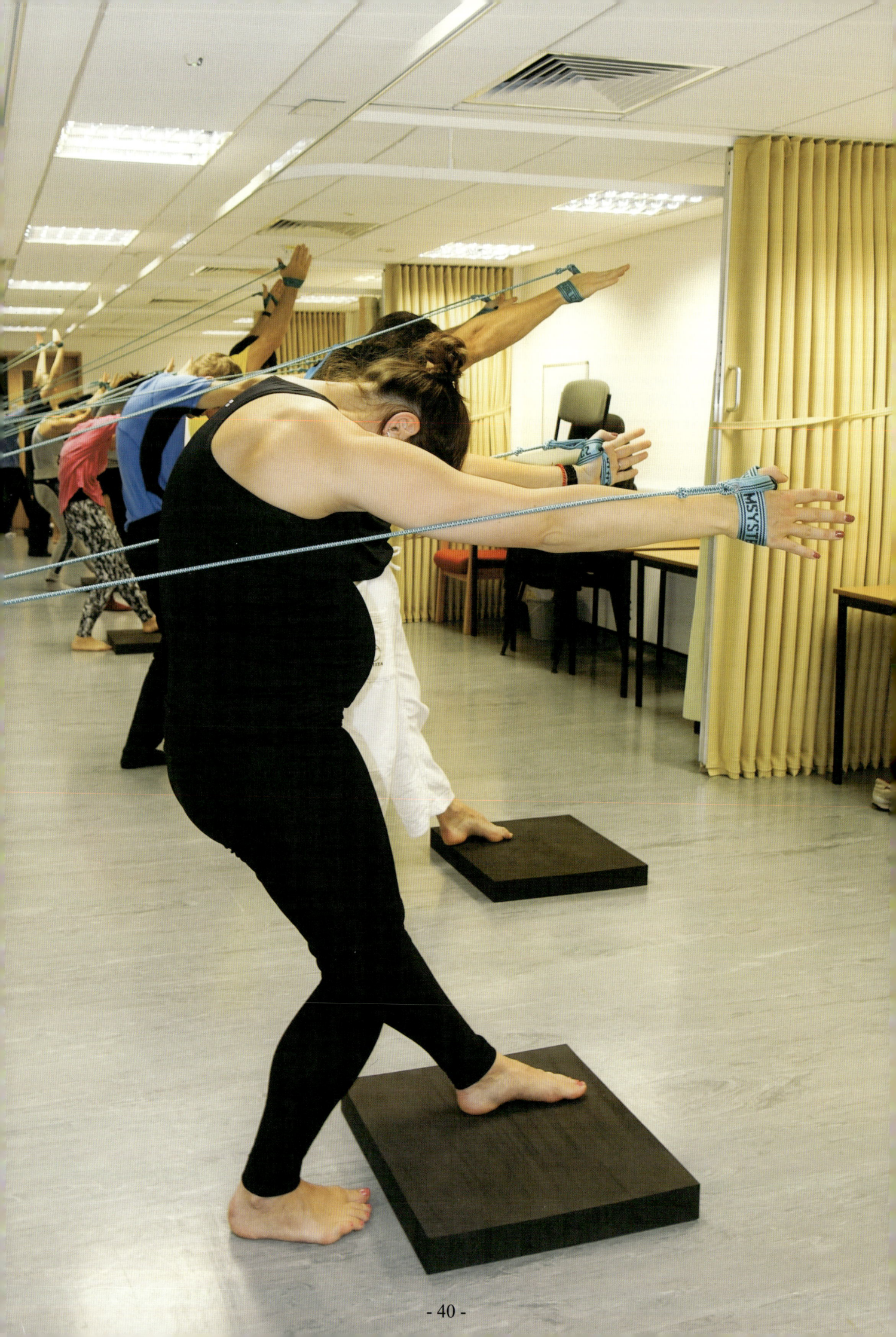

MANUAL TECHNIQUES AND EXERCISE ACCORDING TO MUSCLE ANALYSIS

Trunk and pelvis
Paravertebral muscles
The posterior lower muscle group

Muscles with a tendency towards tension and shortening:

M. erector spinae
M. iliocostalis
M. longissimus thoracis
M. longissimus cervicis
M. longissimus capitis
M. quadratus lumborum
M. multifidus

Anatomy
M. erector spinae

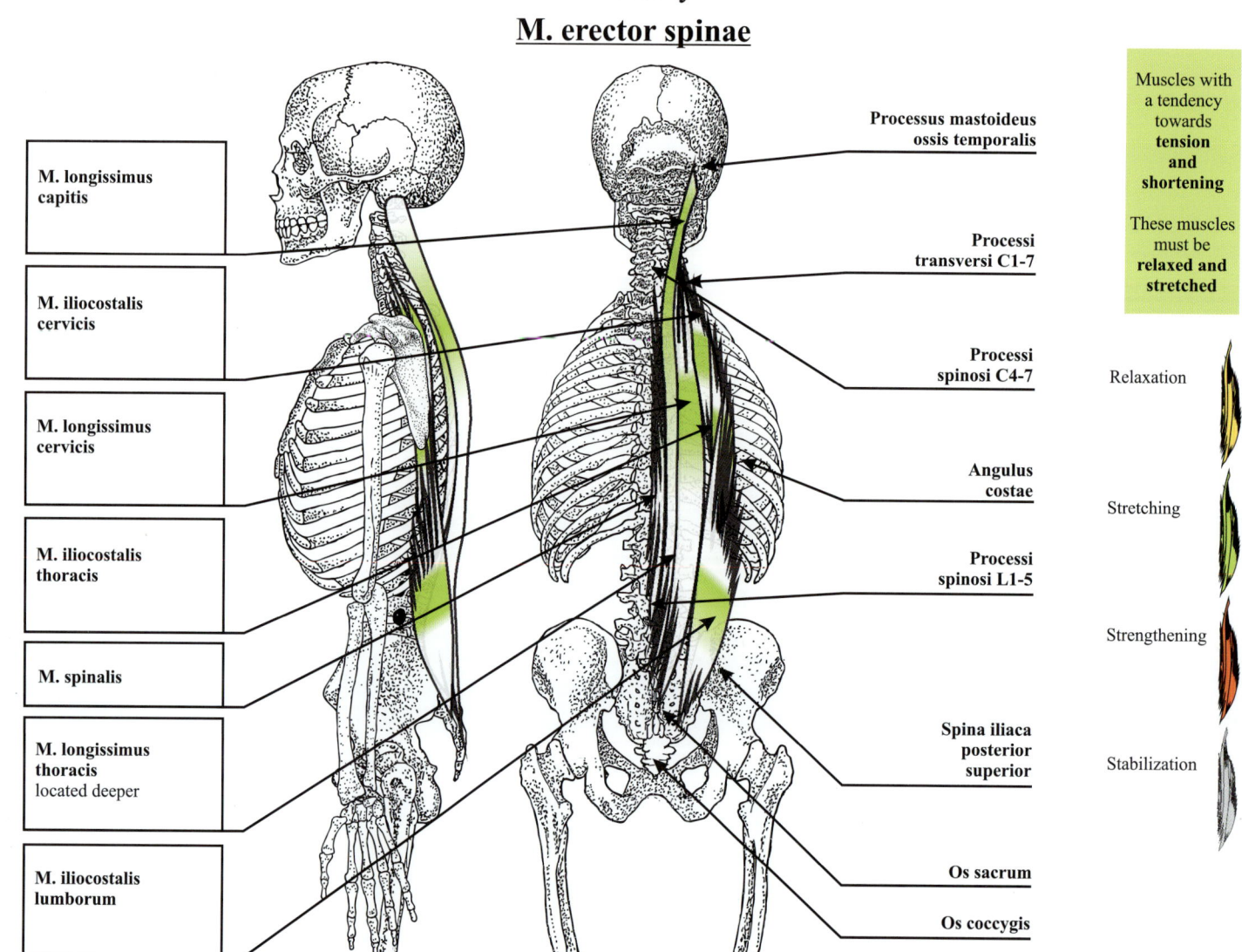

Labels (left side):
- M. longissimus capitis
- M. iliocostalis cervicis
- M. longissimus cervicis
- M. iliocostalis thoracis
- M. spinalis
- M. longissimus thoracis (located deeper)
- M. iliocostalis lumborum

Labels (right side):
- Processus mastoideus ossis temporalis
- Processi transversi C1-7
- Processi spinosi C4-7
- Angulus costae
- Processi spinosi L1-5
- Spina iliaca posterior superior
- Os sacrum
- Os coccygis

Muscles with a tendency towards tension and shortening

These muscles must be relaxed and stretched

- Relaxation
- Stretching
- Strengthening
- Stabilization

M. erector spinae

- **M. iliocostalis**
  - M. iliocostalis lumborum
  - M. iliocostalis thoracis
  - M. iliocostalis cervicis

- **M. longissimus**
  - M. longissimus thoracis
  - M. longissimus cervicis
  - M. longissimus capitis

- **M. spinalis**

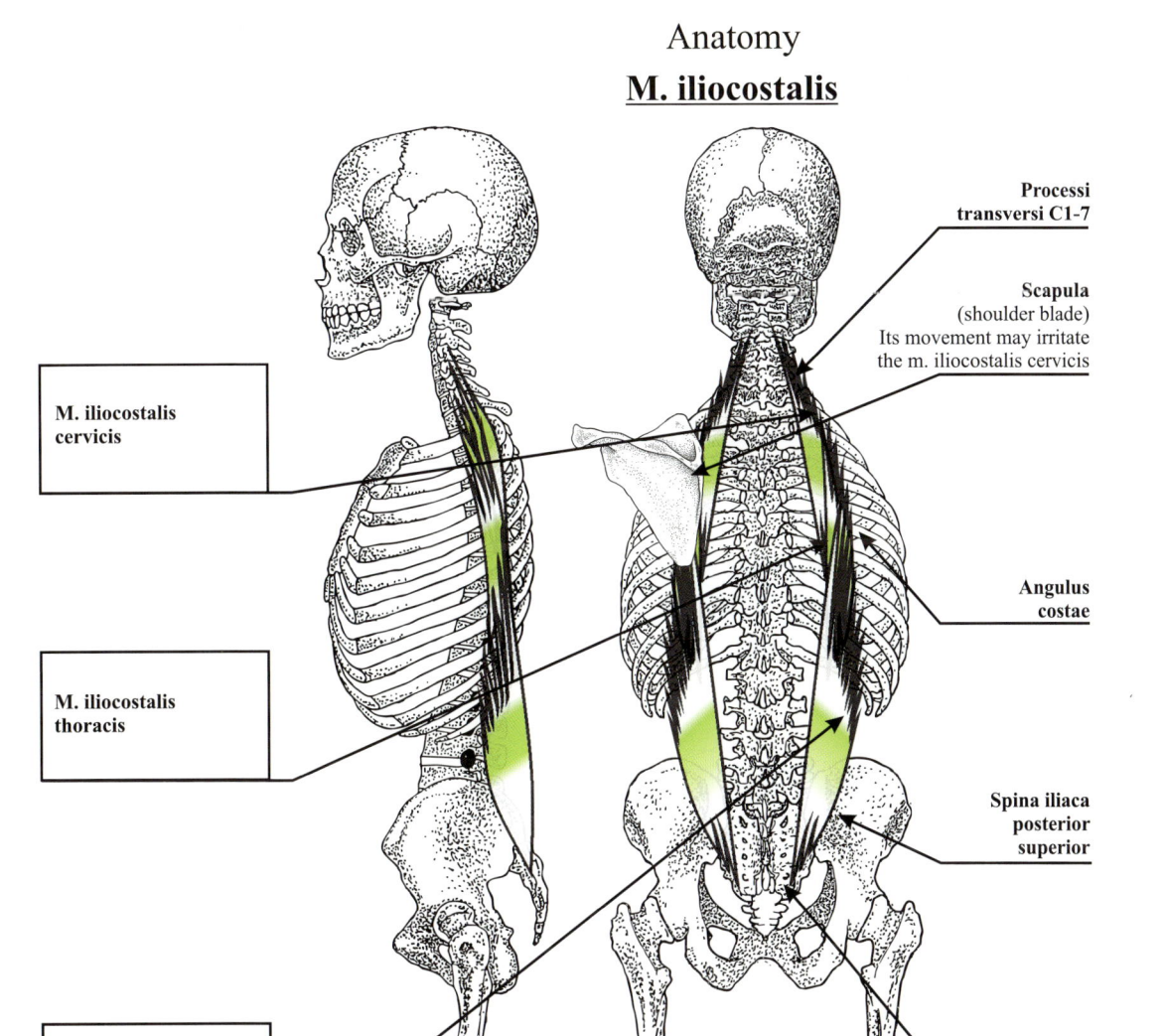

Anatomy
M. iliocostalis

Labels on diagram:
- M. iliocostalis cervicis
- M. iliocostalis thoracis
- M. iliocostalis lumborum
- Processi transversi C1-7
- Scapula (shoulder blade) Its movement may irritate the m. iliocostalis cervicis
- Angulus costae
- Spina iliaca posterior superior
- Os sacrum

Muscles with a tendency towards **tension and shortening**

These muscles must be **relaxed and stretched**

- Relaxation
- Stretching
- Strengthening
- Stabilization

M. iliocostalis
Function of the whole muscle:
- extension of the trunk from a forward bend (bilateral contraction)
- lateral flexion (sideways bend), (unilateral contraction)

Innervation:
- lateral branches of the rr. dorsales of the spinal nerves C8-L1

M. iliocostalis lumborum
Origin:
- crista iliaca
- spina iliaca posterior superior
- os sacrum

Insertion:
- 6.-12. angulus costae

M. iliocostalis thoracis
Origin:
- 7.-12. angulus costae

Insertion:
- 1.-6. angulus costae

M. iliocostalis cervicis
Origin:
- 3.-7. angulus costae

Insertion:
- processi transversi C4-C6

Muscle chains
Vertical muscle chain **ES - erector spinae**
The ES chain is activated at rest.

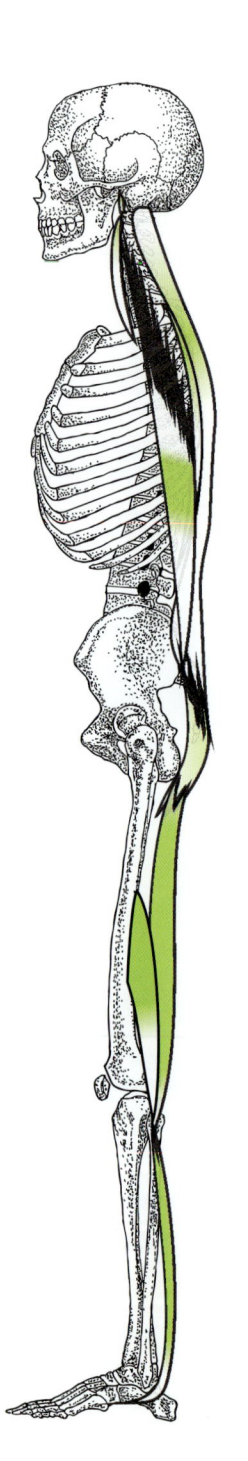

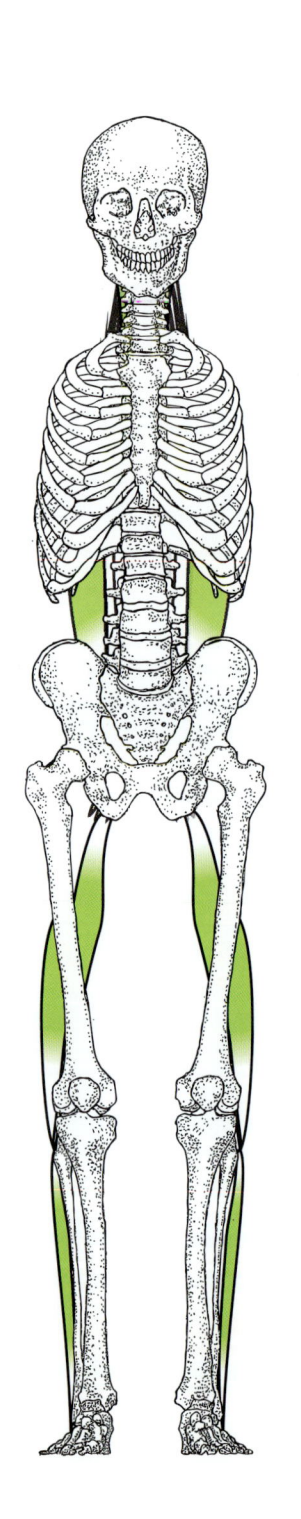

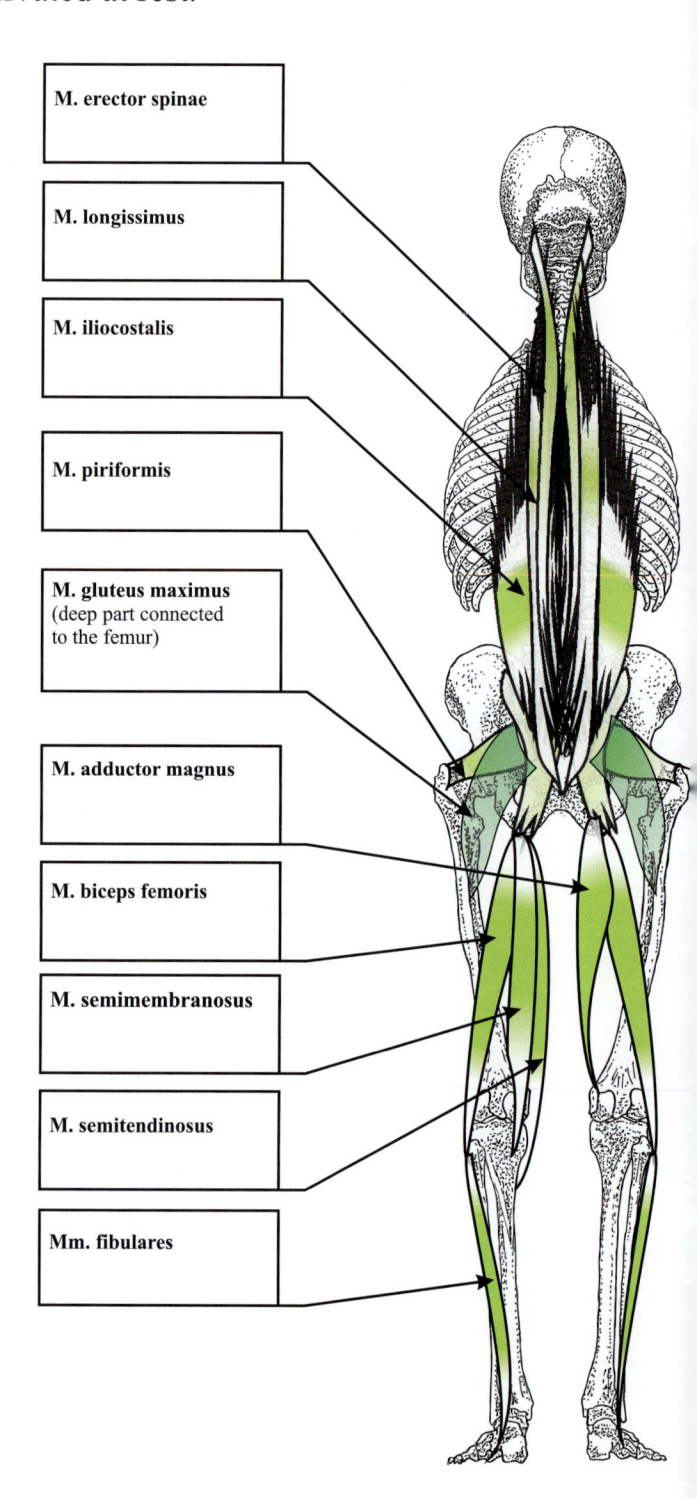

- M. erector spinae
- M. longissimus
- M. iliocostalis
- M. piriformis
- M. gluteus maximus (deep part connected to the femur)
- M. adductor magnus
- M. biceps femoris
- M. semimembranosus
- M. semitendinosus
- Mm. fibulares

Manual techniques lying on one side
M. iliocostalis lumborum - massage, relaxation, passive stretching

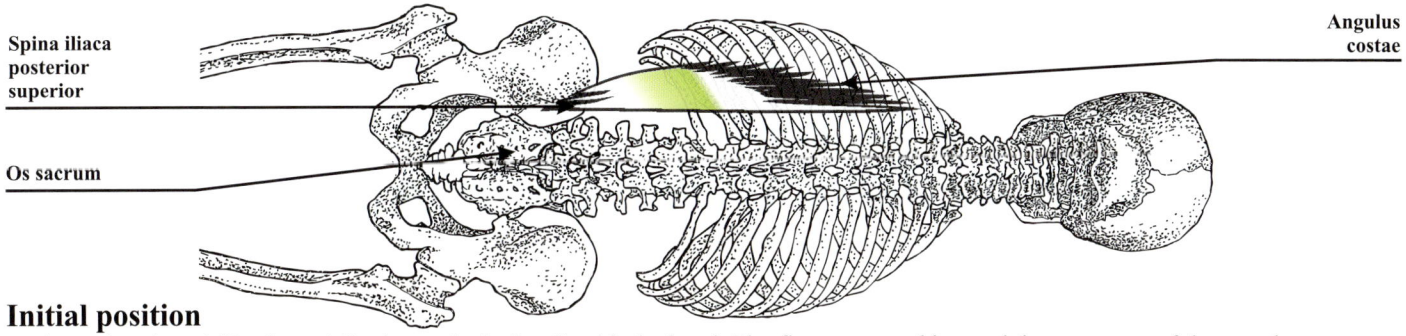

Spina iliaca posterior superior

Os sacrum

Angulus costae

Initial position

The patient is stabilized cranially (towards the head) with the hand. The fingers extend beyond the processes of the vertebrae. The forearm follows the surface of the body. The arm balances the position of the chest.

The pelvis is stabilized from in front by the chest resting against the patient's thigh, the therapist's axila (armpit) follows the surface of the pelvis from above, the forearm is placed against the sacral bone, and the fingers are gently placed on the surface of the m. iliocostalis lumborum.

When the therapist's little finger is lying on the processes of the vertebrae, the middle finger finds the tension TP - trigger point in the muscle fibres which are oriented towards the shoulder blade. The fingers must not bend. The patient breathes in.

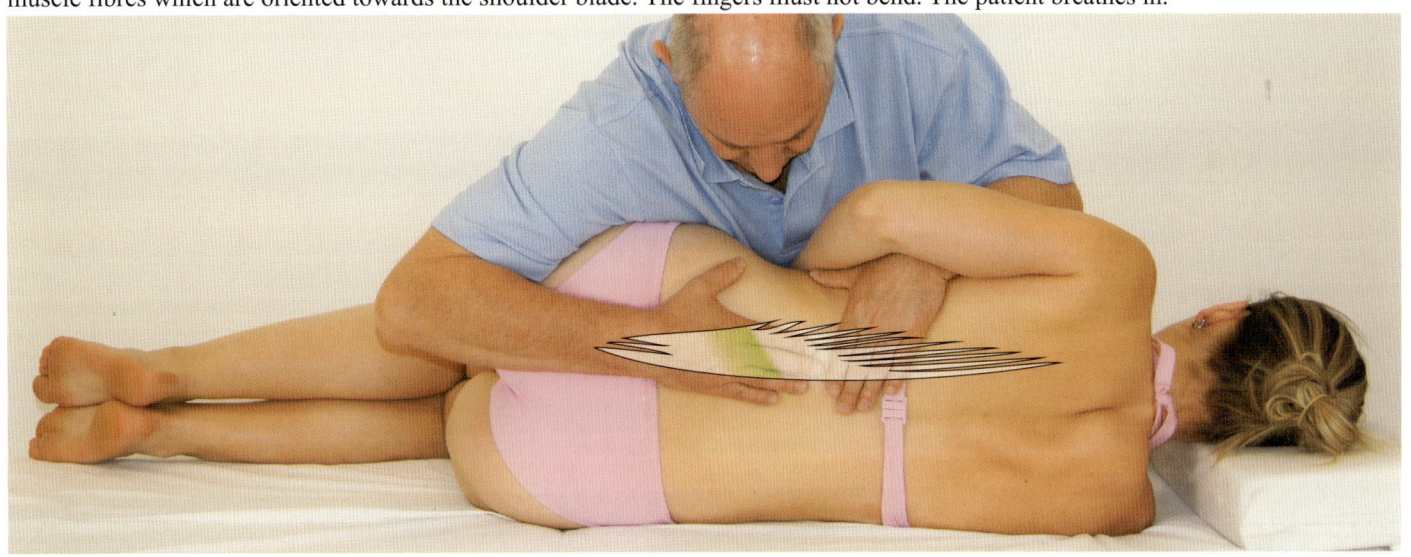

Performance

The cranial arm (nearer the head) stabilizes and stays in place (punctum fixum - fixed point). The therapist transfers the weight to the patient's pelvis and evenly shifts the pelvis caudally (towards the feet) - (punctum mobile - mobile point). He strengthens the shift by stretching his left leg. The pelvis must not tilt forwards or backwards or rotate. Massage of the m. ilocostalis lumborum is initiated by shifting the pelvis caudally (towards the feet). The patient breathes out slowly. The pulling movement is slackened and the stretching is repeated six times. At the end of the technique the therapist pauses for about 3 seconds.

PIR (post isometric relaxation). The extension is held and the patient breathes in. This causes a counter-pressure. The patient relaxes while breathing out, thus achieving further stretching. The process is repeated three times. This technique stretches the lumbar discs, and the intervertebral joints and opens the foramina.

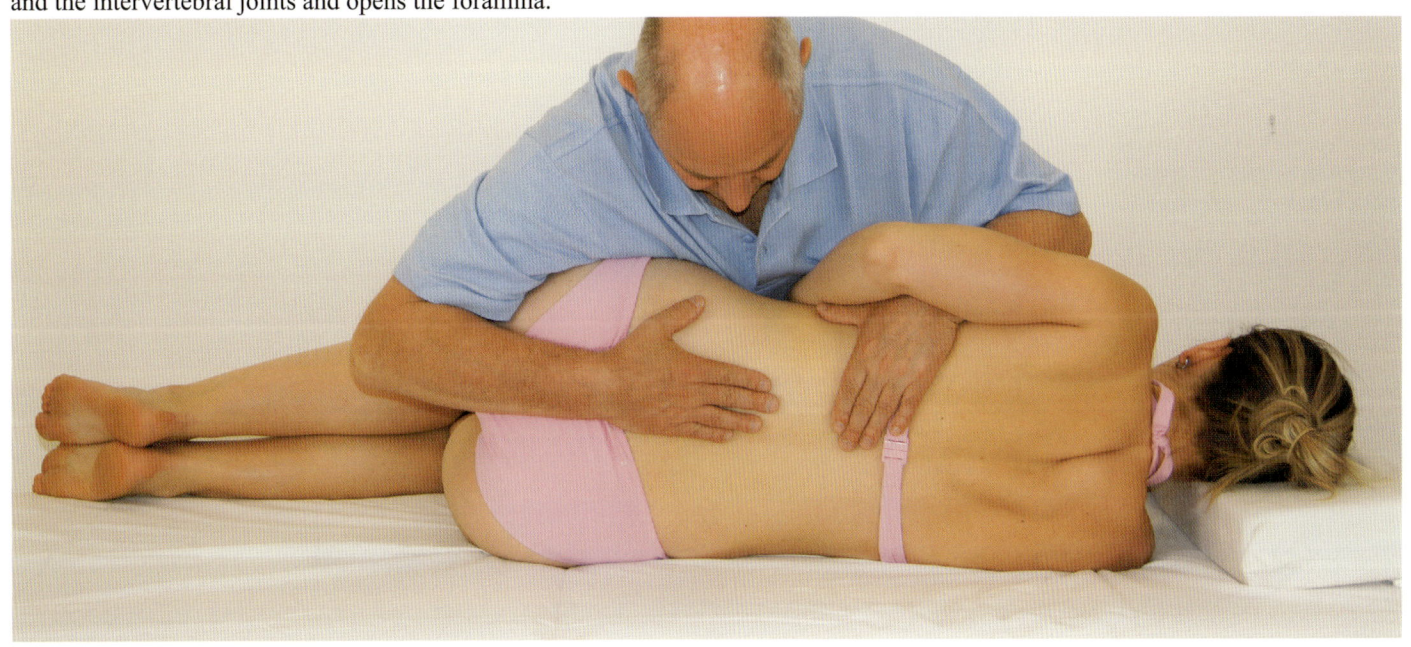

Manual techniques - lying - one limb in a hoist
M. iliocostalis lumborum - massage, relaxation, passive stretching

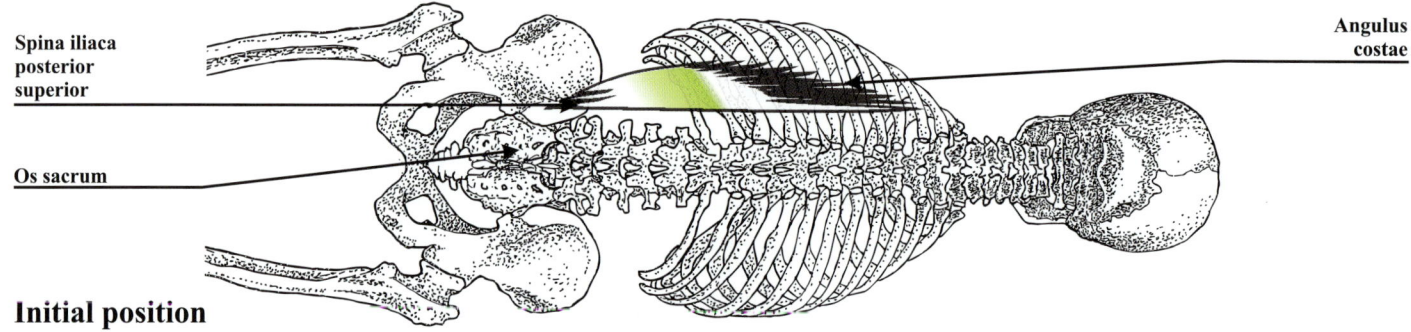

Spina iliaca posterior superior

Os sacrum

Angulus costae

Initial position

The patient's trunk is stabilized cranially (towards the head), by the arm. The fingers extend beyond the processes of the vertebrae. The forearm follows the surface of the body. The arm balances the position of the chest.

The pelvis is stabilized from in front by the chest resting against the patient's thigh. The therapist's axila (armpit) follows the surface of the pelvis from above, the forearm is placed against the sacral bone and the fingers are placed gently on the surface of the m. iliocostalis lumborum.

When the therapist's little finger is resting on the processes of the vertebrae, the middle finger finds the tension - TP - in the muscle fibres which are oriented towards the shoulder blade. The fingers must not bend. The patient breathes in.

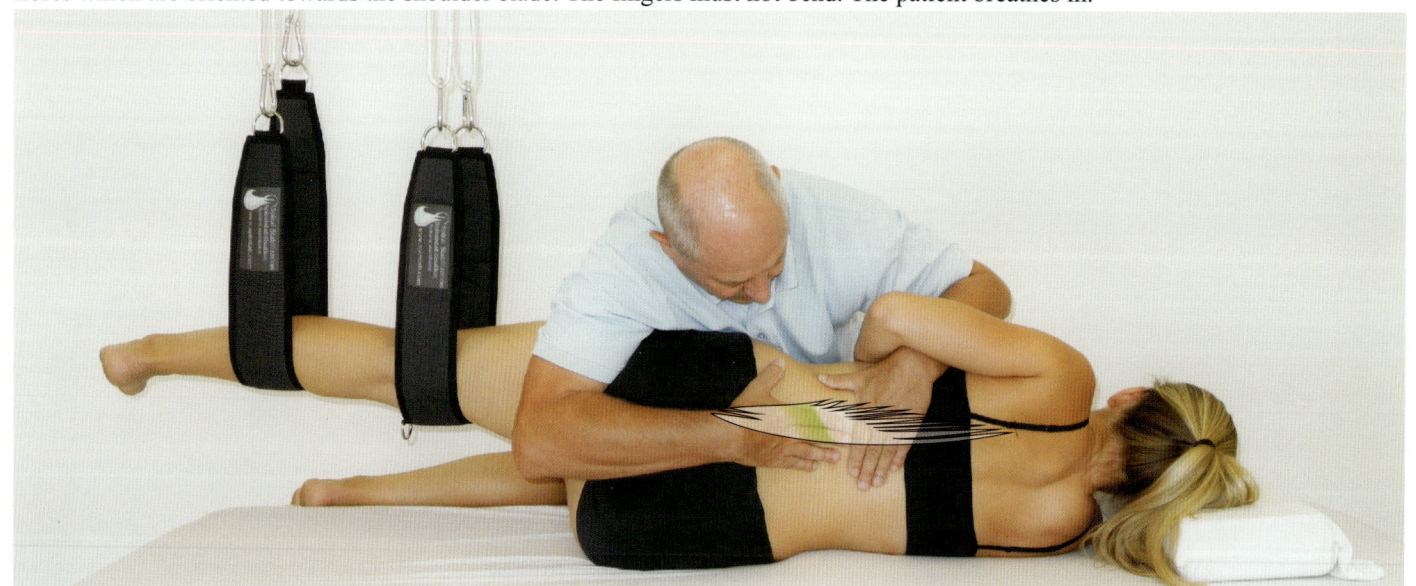

Performance

The cranial arm (nearer the head) stabilizes and remains in place (punctum fixum - fixed point).
The therapist shifts the weight to the patient's pelvis and evenly shifts the pelvis caudally (towards the feet) (punctum mobile - mobile point). The shift is strengthened by stretching his left leg. The pelvis must not bend forwards or backwards or rotate. The massage is initiated by shifting the pelvis caudally (towards the feet). The patient breathes out slowly. The pulling is slackened and the stretching is repeated six times. At the end of the technique the therapist pauses for about 3 seconds.

PIR. The extension is held and the patient breathes in. This causes a counter-pressure.
The patient relaxes while breathing out, thus achieving further stretching. The processes is repeated three times.
This technique stretches the lumbar discs and the intervertebral joints and opens the foramina.

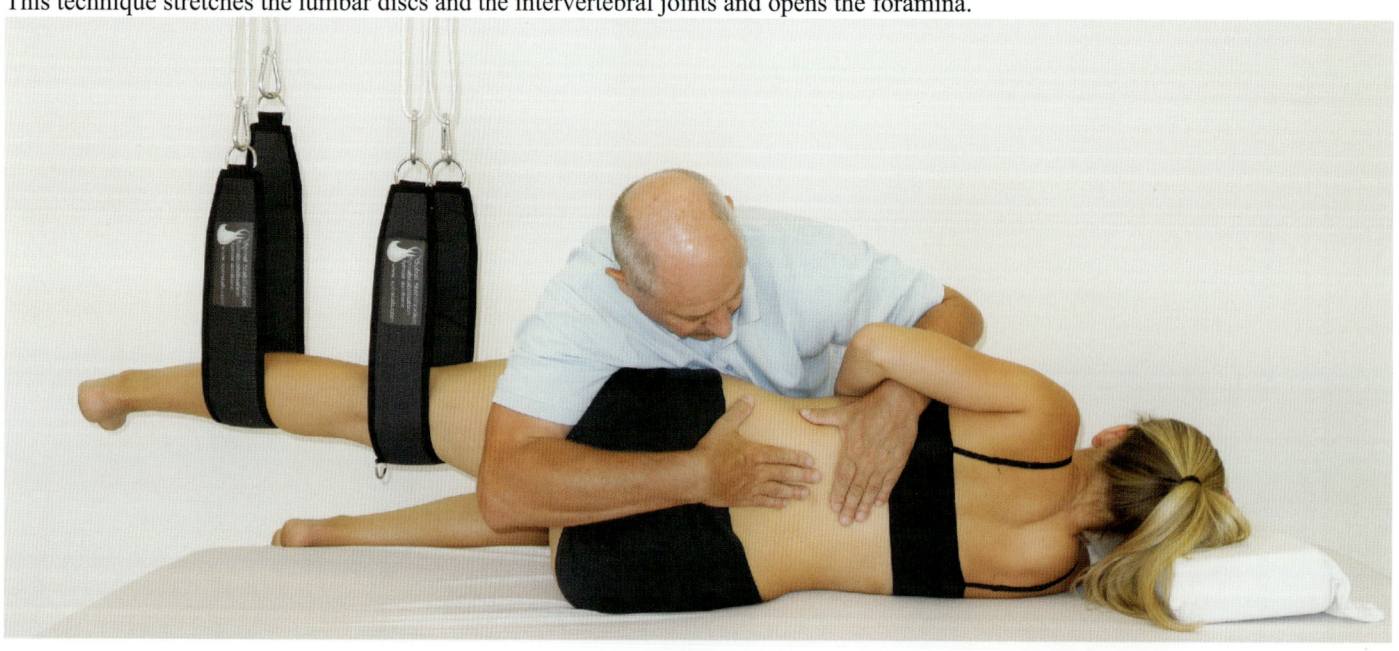

Manual techniques - lying - one limb in a hoist
M. iliocostalis lumborum - massage, relaxation, passive stretching

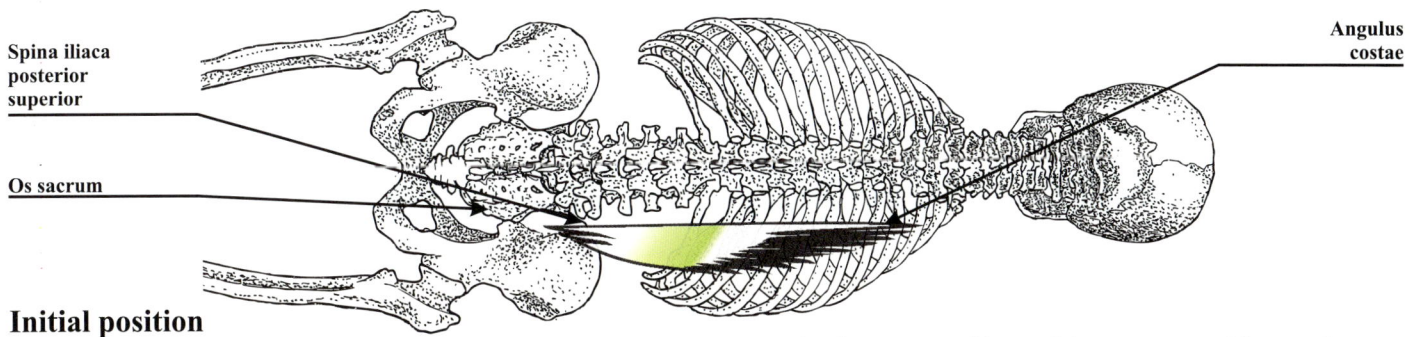

Spina iliaca posterior superior

Os sacrum

Angulus costae

Initial position

The patient's trunk is stabilized cranially (towards the head) by the arm. The fingers extend beyond the processes of the vertebrae. The forearm follows the surface of the body. The arm balances the position of the chest.

The pelvis is stabilized from in front by the chest resting against the patient's thigh. The therapists's axila (armpit) follows the surface of the pelvis from above. The forearm is placed against the sacral bone and the fingers are placed gently on the surface of the m. iliocostalis lumborum.

When the therapists's little finger is resting on the processes of the vertebrae, the middle finger finds the tension - TP - in the muscle fibres oriented towards the shoulder blade. The fingers must not bend. The patient breathes in.

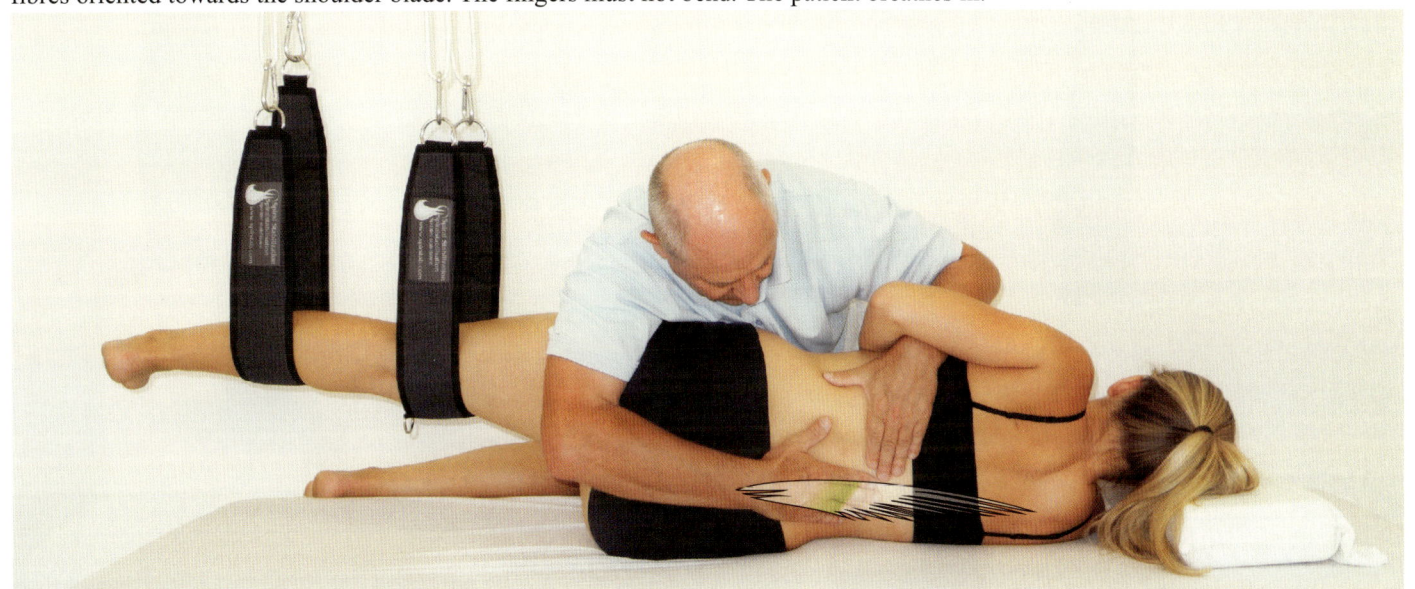

Performance

The cranial arm (nearer the head) stabilizes and stays in place (punctum fixum). The therapist shifts the weight to the patient's pelvis and evenly shifts the pelvis caudally (towards the feet) - (punctum mobile). The shift is strengthened by stretching the left leg. The pelvis must not bend forwards or backwards or rotate. The massage of the m. ilocostalis lumborum is initiated by shifting the pelvis caudally (towards the feet). The patient breathes out slowly. The pulling is slackened and the stretching is repeated 6 times. At the end of the technique the therapist pauses for about 3 seconds.

PIR. The extension is held and the patient breathes in. This causes a counter-pressure. The patient relaxes while breathing out. The process is repeated 3 times. The technique stretches the lumbar discs and the intervertebral joints and opens the foramina.

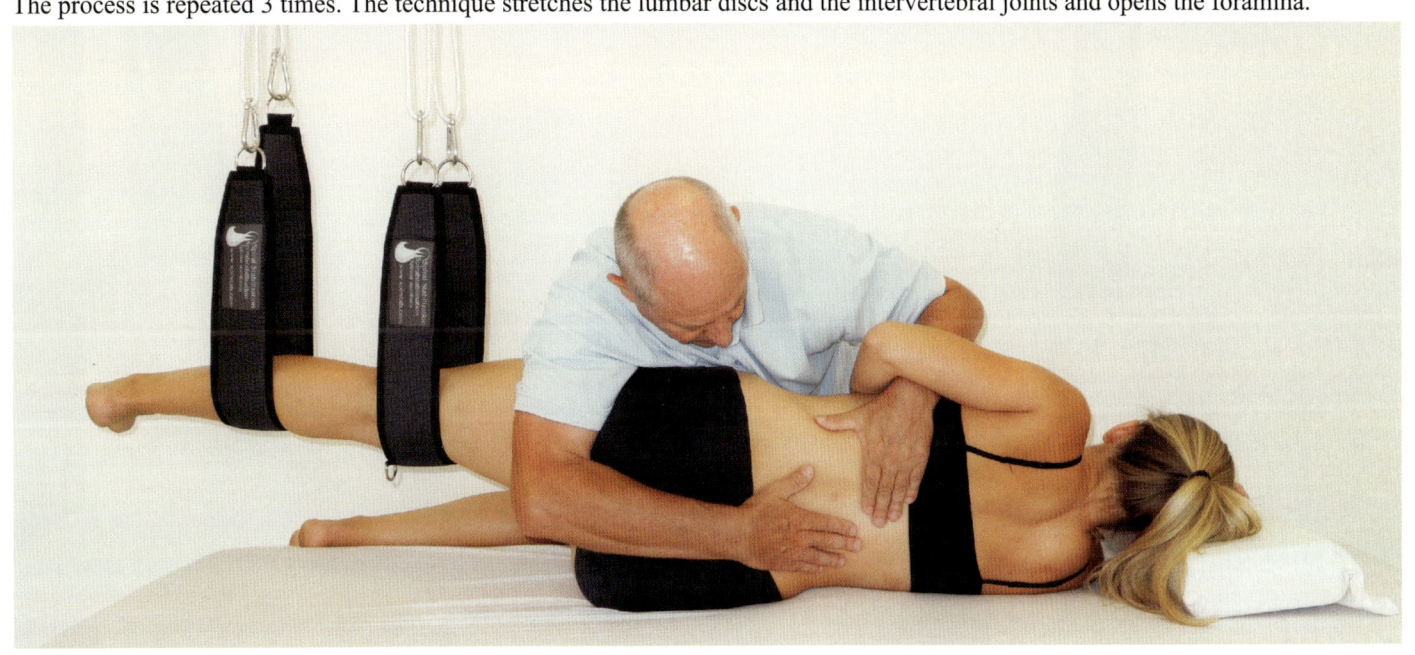

Manual techniques - lying - limbs in a hoist
M. iliocostalis lumborum - massage, relaxation, passive stretching

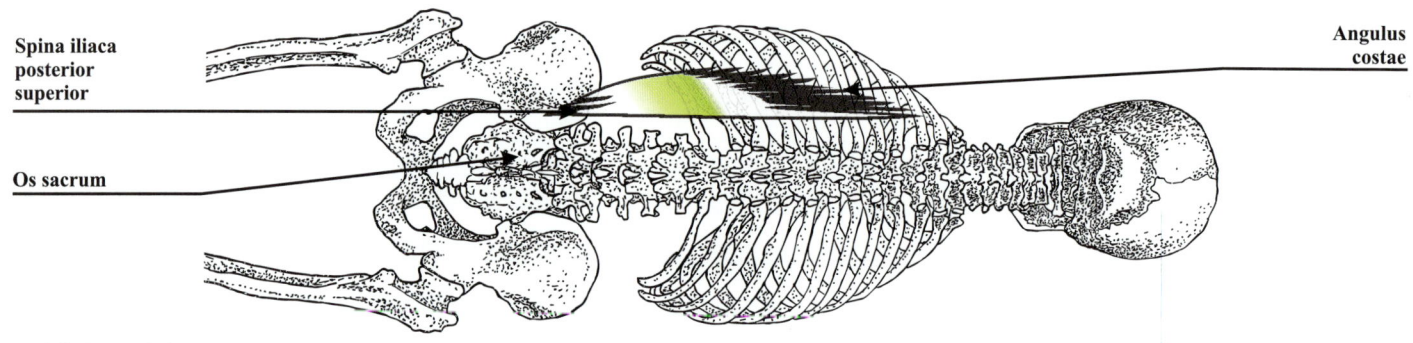

Spina iliaca posterior superior

Os sacrum

Angulus costae

Initial position

The therapist kneels behind the patient facing the head. He stabilizes the patient's pelvis from behind with his thigh and own pelvis. The patient is in kyphosis (a long, extended arch facing forward).

The palm of the therapist's left hand stabilizes while the fingers support the sternum.

The left thumb is placed along the 10th rib. The right hand moves along the 10th rib dorsally towards the spine. The process of the 10th vertebra is in the centre of the palm. The thumb supports the rib. The patient breathes in.

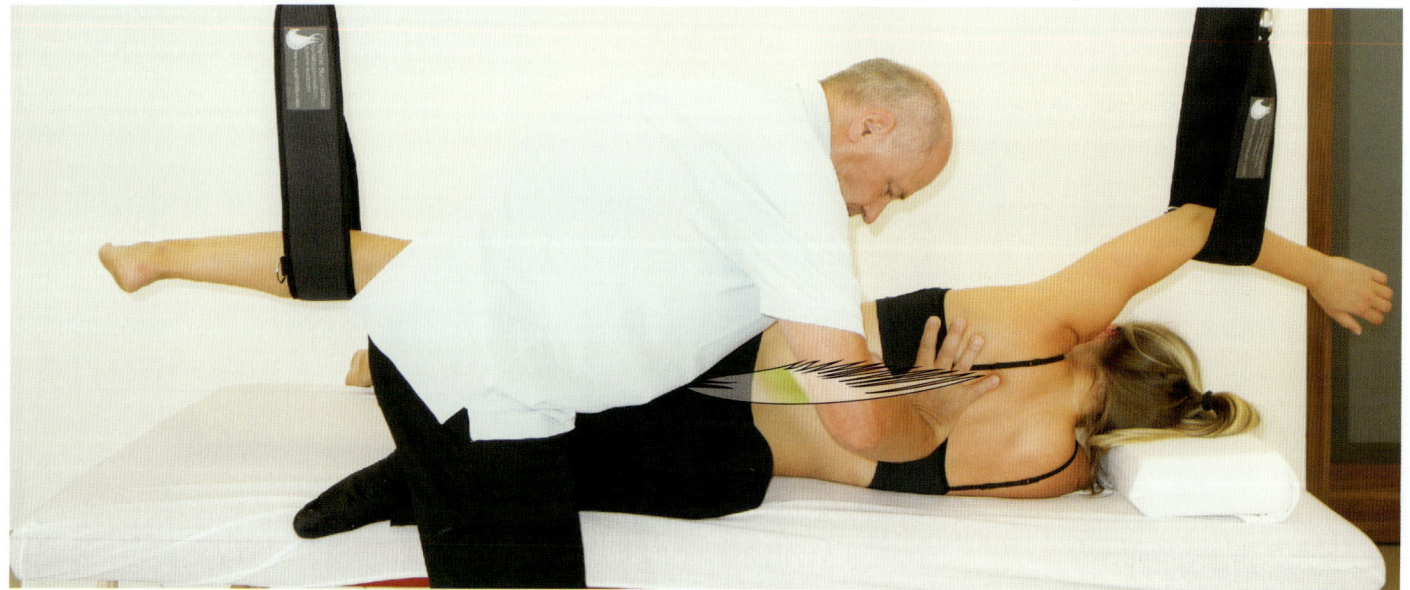

Performance

The therapist's arms and trunk direct the 10th rib first dorsally then cranially. The patient breathes out slowly. The pulling is slackened and the stretching is repeated 6 times. At the end of the technique the therapist pauses for about 3 seconds.

PIR. The extension is held and the patient breathes in. This causes a counter-pressure. The patient relaxes while breathing out, thus achieving further stretching. The process is repeated 3 times. This techniques stretches the m. iliocostalis and mobilizes the ribs. The technique is repeated for all the ribs.

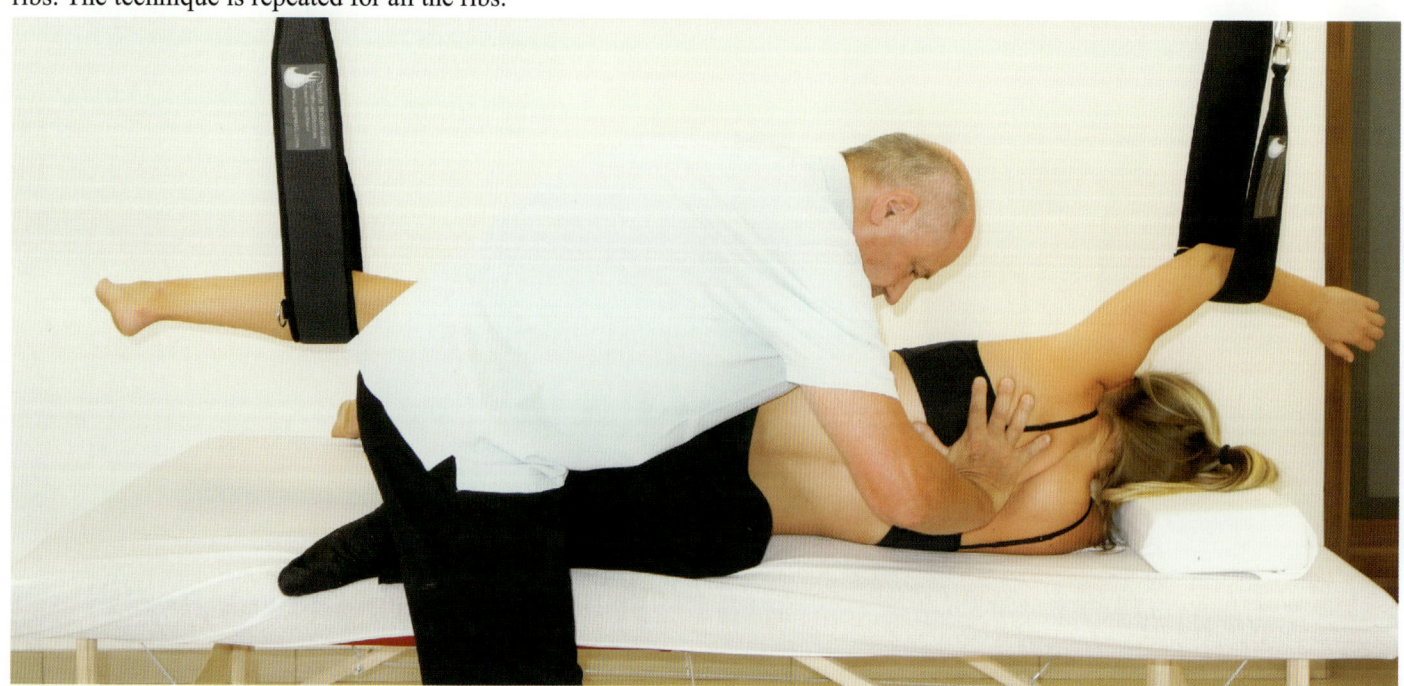

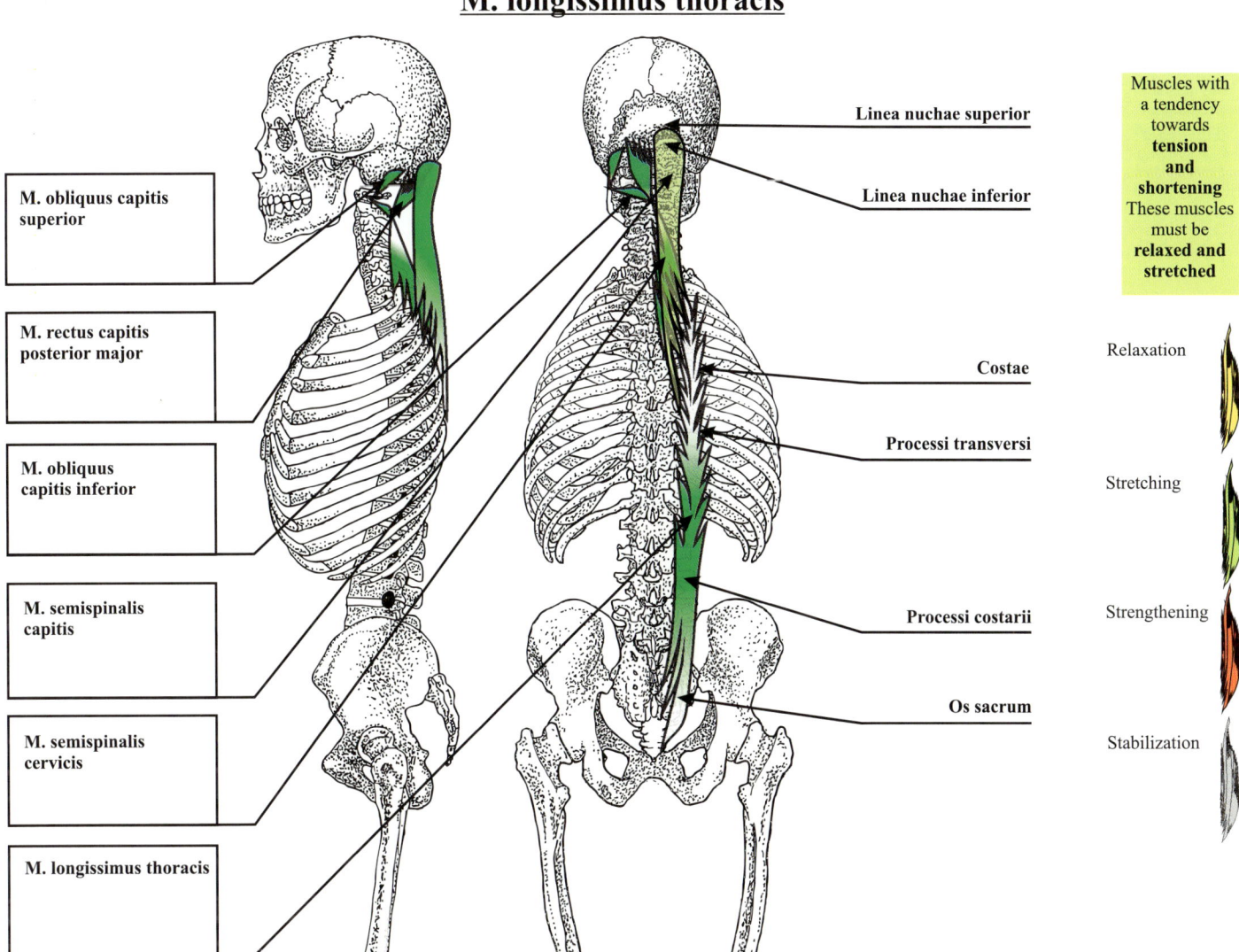

Anatomy
M. longissimus thoracis

- M. obliquus capitis superior
- M. rectus capitis posterior major
- M. obliquus capitis inferior
- M. semispinalis capitis
- M. semispinalis cervicis
- M. longissimus thoracis

- Linea nuchae superior
- Linea nuchae inferior
- Costae
- Processi transversi
- Processi costarii
- Os sacrum

Muscles with a tendency towards **tension and shortening**
These muscles must be **relaxed and stretched**

- Relaxation
- Stretching
- Strengthening
- Stabilization

M. longissimus
M. longissimus thoracis
Origin:
- os sacrum
- processi spinosi L1-5
- processi transversi Th6-12

Insertion:
- lateral projections - 2nd-12th ribs near the spine
- medial projections - processi transversi Th2-12

Function:
- extension of the trunk (straightening) from a forward bend (bilateral contraction)
- lateral flexion (sideways bend), (unilateral contraction)

Manual techniques - lying - one limb in a hoist
M. longissimus thoracis - massage, relaxation, passive stretching

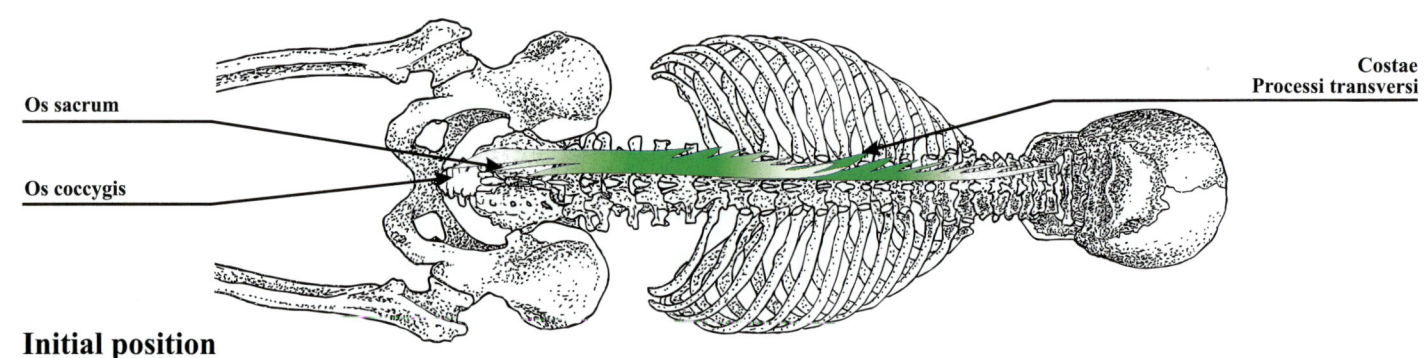

Os sacrum

Os coccygis

Costae
Processi transversi

Initial position
The patient's trunk is stabilized cranially by the arm. The fingers extend beyond the processes of the vertebrae. The forearm follows the surface of the body. The arm balances the position of the chest. The pelvis is stabilized from in front by the chest resting against the patient's thigh. The therapist's axila (armpit) follows the surface of the pelvis from above, the forearm is placed against the sacral bone and the fingers are placed gently on the surface of the m. longissimus thoracis on both sides of the processi spinosi. The fingers must not bend and must not press on the processi spinosi. The patient breathes in.

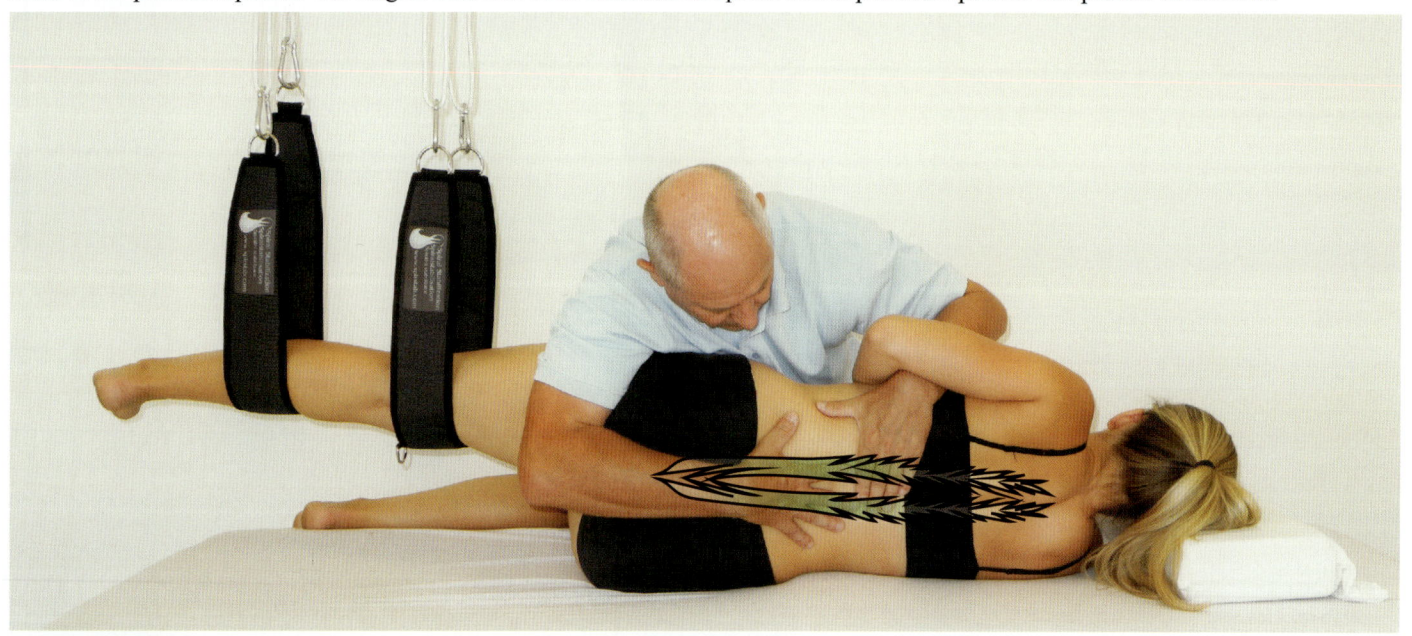

Performance
The cranial arm stabilizes and stays in place (punctum fixum). The therapist shifts the weight to the patient's thigh and evenly shifts the pelvis caudally (punctum mobile). The shift is strengthened by stretching the left leg. The pelvis must not bend forwards or backwards or rotate. Massage of the m. longissimus thoracis is initiated by shifting the pelvis caudally.
The patient breathes out slowly. The pulling is slackened and the stretching is repeated 6 times. At the end of the technique the therapist pauses for about 3 seconds.
PIR. The extension is held and the patient breathes in. This causes a counter-pressure. While breathing out, the patient achieves further stretching. The process is repeated 3 times. This technique stretches the lumbar discs and intervertebral joints and opens the foramina.

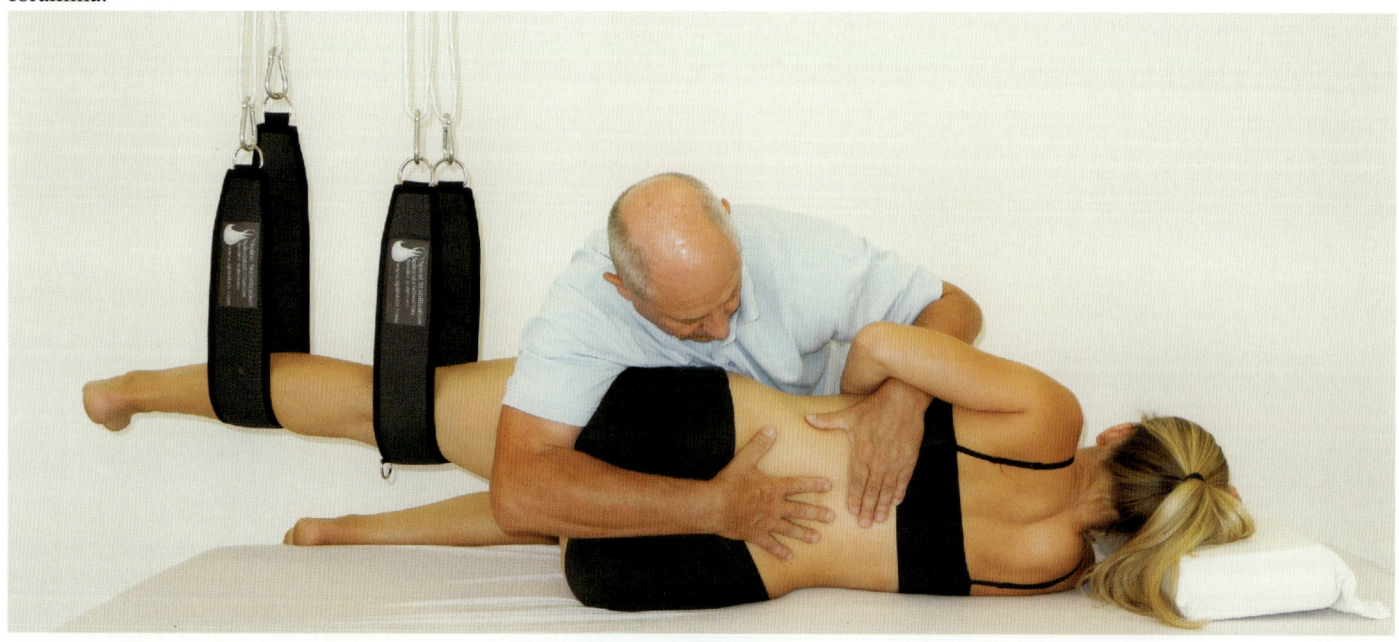

Anatomy
M. quadratus lumborum, m. iliacus

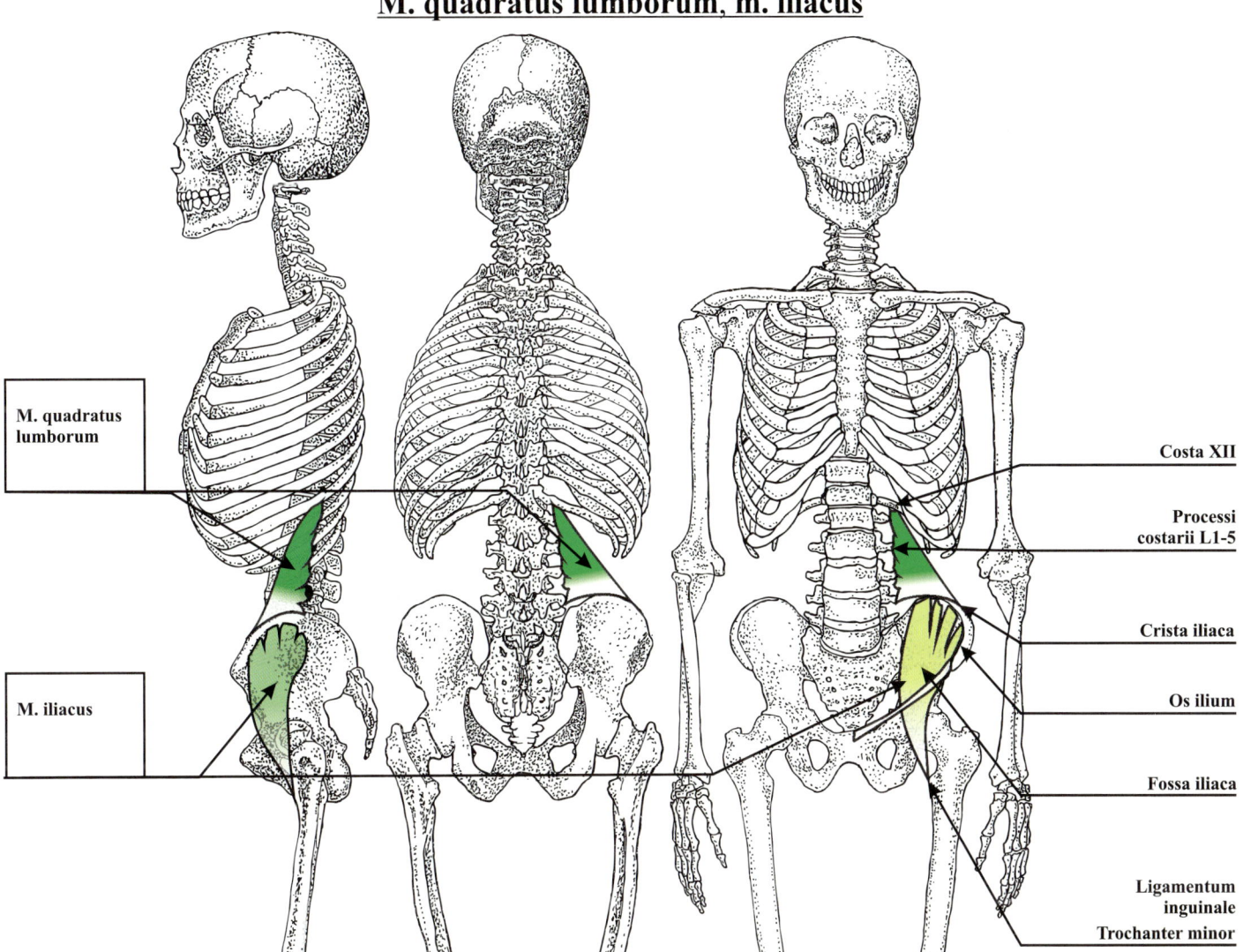

Costa XII
Processi costarii L1-5
Crista iliaca
Os ilium
Fossa iliaca
Ligamentum inguinale
Trochanter minor

M. quadratus lumborum
Origin:
- crista iliaca, labium int.
- lig. iliolumbale
Insertion:
- costa XII. (12th rib)
- processi costarii L1-5
Function: - lumbar spine
  - bilateral activity:
- extension (stretching)
- fixes the 12th rib during inhalation
- creates lordosis
  - unilateral activity
- lateral flexion (sideways bend)
Innervation:
- n. subcostalis - n. intercostalis XII
- plexus lumbalis

M. iliacus
Origin:
- fossa iliaca
Insertion:
- trochanter minor
Function: - hip:
- flexion (bending) of the hip joint
- outward rotation of the thigh
- it arches the spine in flexion,
- an effort to straighten creates hyperlordosis
- straightening the trunk from a position lying on the back
Innervation:
- n. femoralis (L2-4)
- direct branches from the plexus lumbalis

Muscles with a tendency towards **tension and shortening**

These muscles must be **relaxed and stretched**

Relaxation

Stretching

Strengthening

Stabilization

Muscle chains
Vertical muscle chain QL - quadratus lumborum
The QL chain is activated at rest

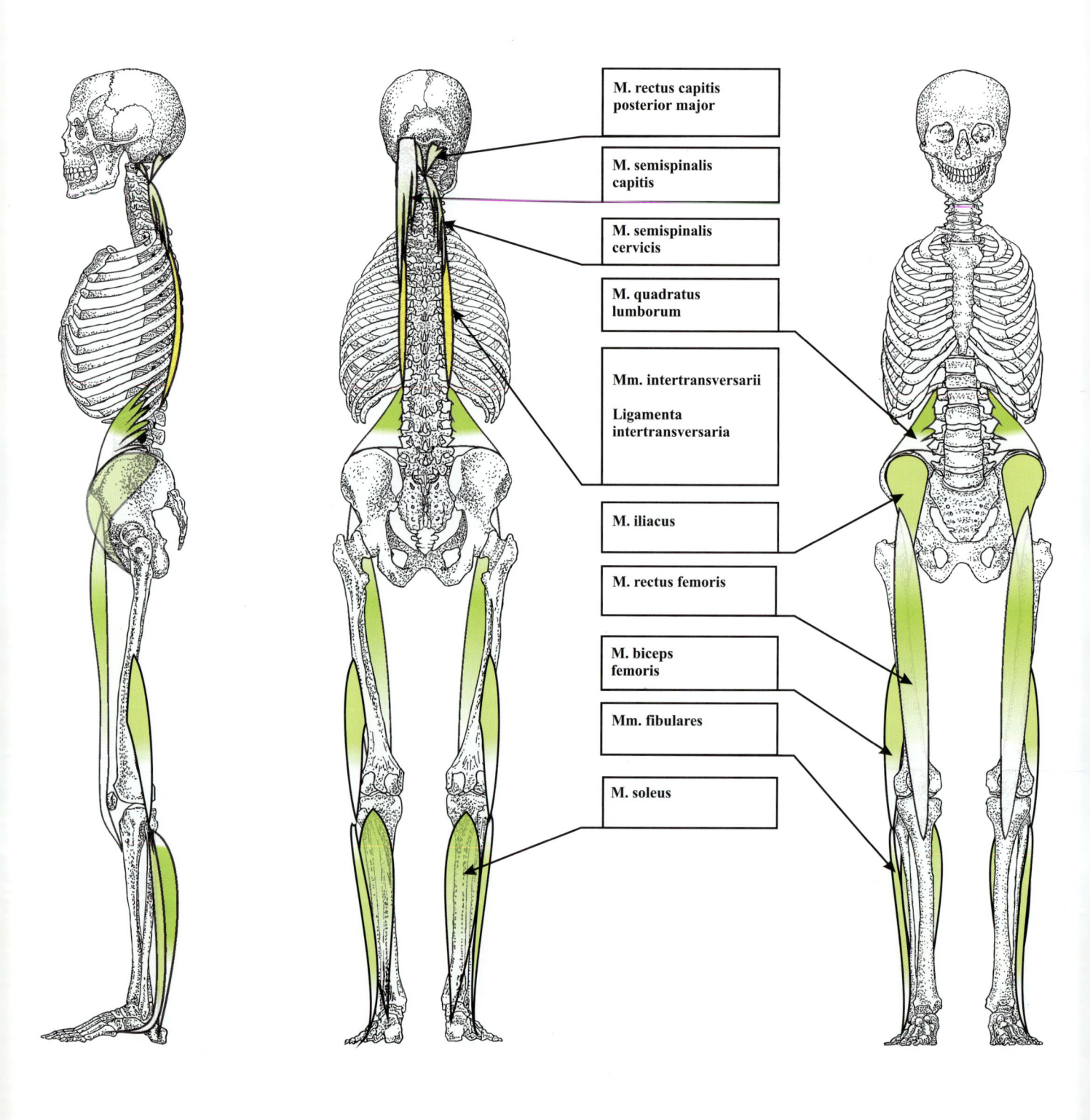

- M. rectus capitis posterior major
- M. semispinalis capitis
- M. semispinalis cervicis
- M. quadratus lumborum
- Mm. intertransversarii
- Ligamenta intertransversaria
- M. iliacus
- M. rectus femoris
- M. biceps femoris
- Mm. fibulares
- M. soleus

Manual techniques lying on one side
M. quadratus lumborum - massage, relaxation, passive stretching

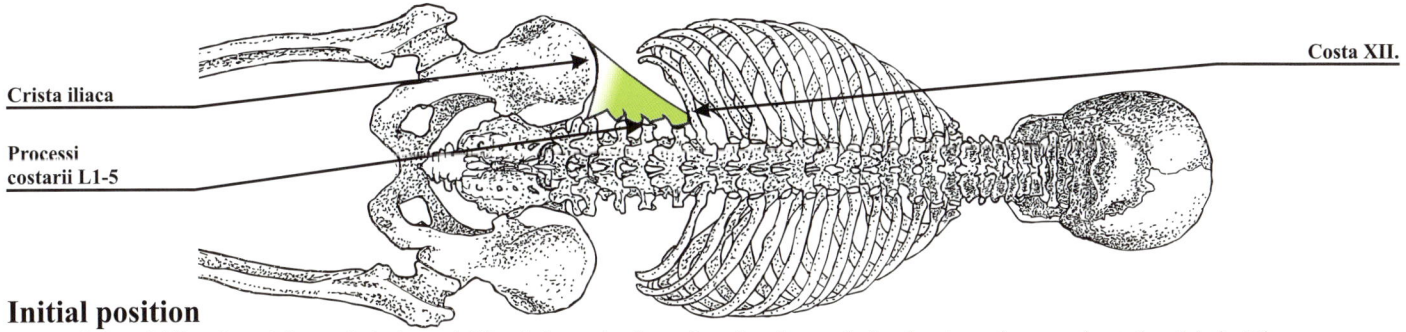

Crista iliaca

Processi costarii L1-5

Costa XII.

Initial position
Caudal stabilization. The pelvis is stabilized from in front by the therapist's chest resting against the thigh. The therapist's axila (armpit) follows the surface of the pelvis from above. The right forearm is placed against the sacral bone and the fingers are gently placed on the surface of the m. iliocostalis. The fingers must not bend. The patient breathes in.
The left hand moves from in front under the crista iliaca with the thumb extended, and whole thenar engages with the surface of the body. It moves slowly cranially and medially until the palm reaches the ribs.

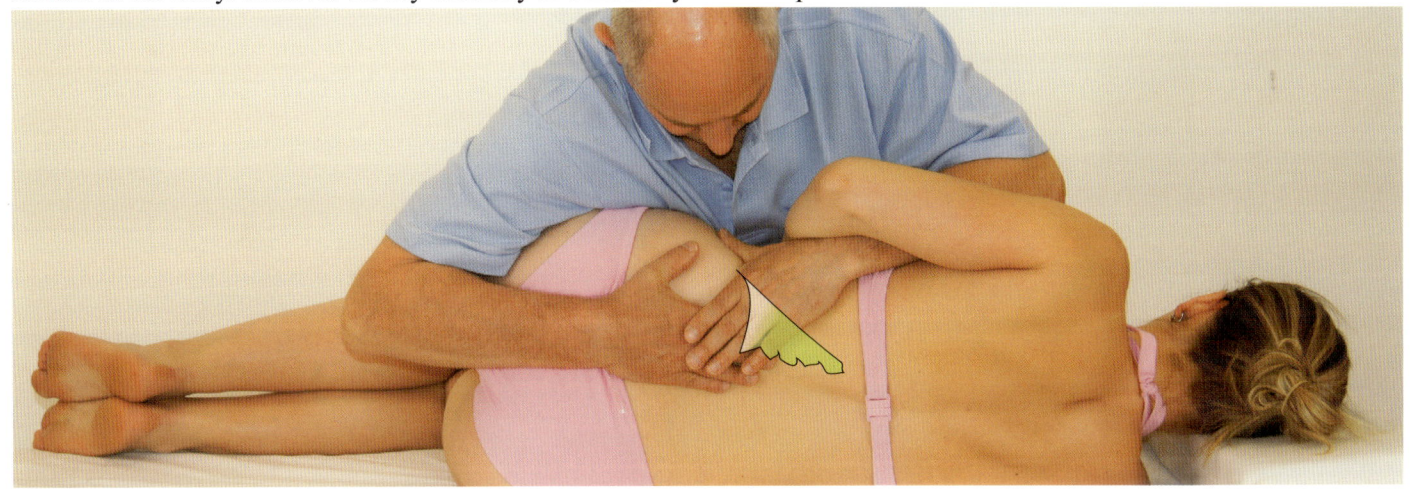

Performance
The cranial arm stabilizes and stays in place resting against the ribs (punctum fixum). The therapist shifts the weight to the patient's pelvis and evenly shifts the pelvis caudally (punctum mobile). The shift is strengthened by stretching the lower leg. The pelvis must not bend forwards or backwards or rotate. The left thumb is placed against the m. quadratus lumborum. Massage is initiated by a caudal movement of the pelvis. The thumb must not bend. The patient breathes out slowly. The pulling is slackened and the stretching is repeated 6 times. At the end of the technique the therapist pauses for about 3 second.
PIR. The extension is held and the patient breathes in. This causes a counter-pressure. While breathing out, the patient achieves further stretching. The process is repeated 3 times. This technique stretches the lumbar discs and intervertebral joints and opens the foramina.

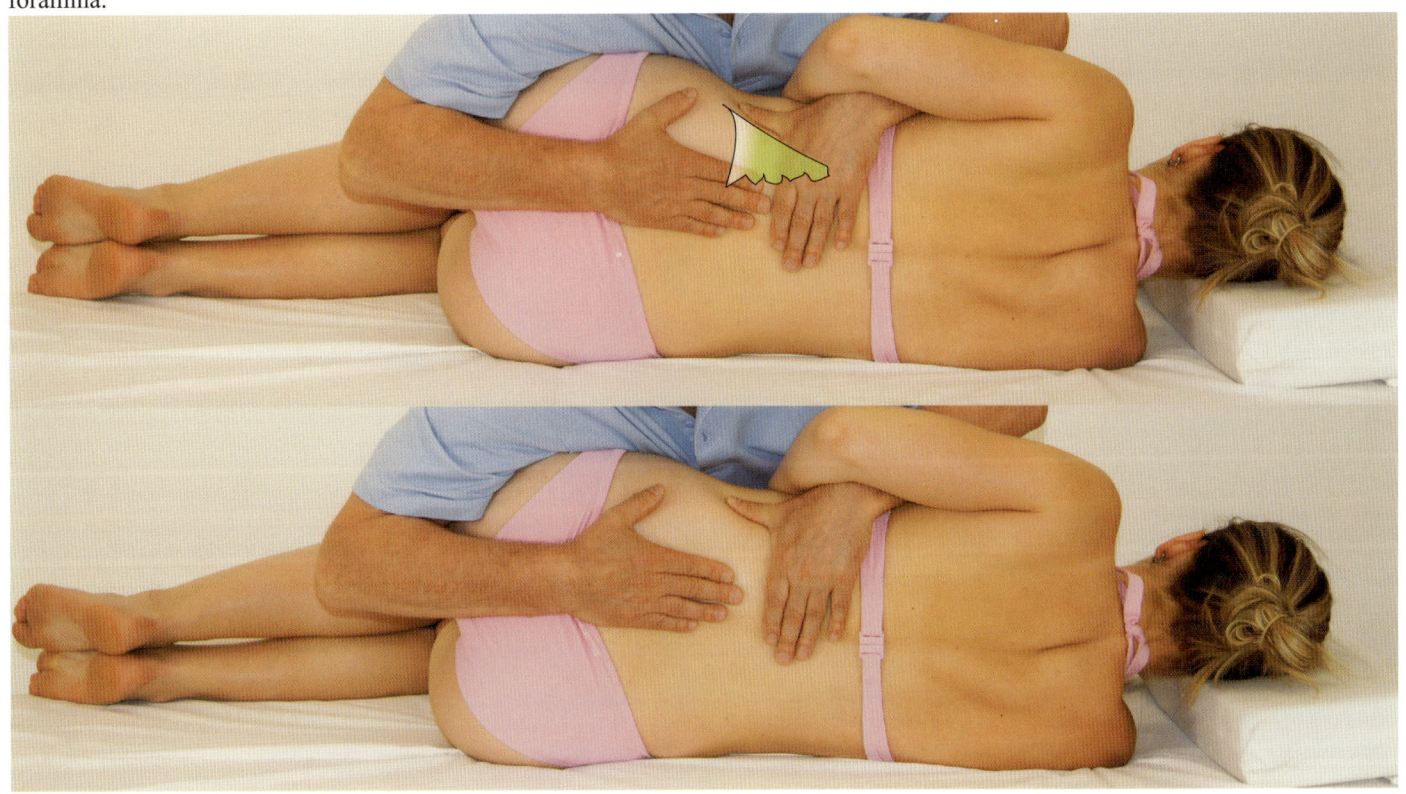

Manual techniques - lying - one limb in a hoist
M. quadratus lumborum - massage, relaxation, passive stretching

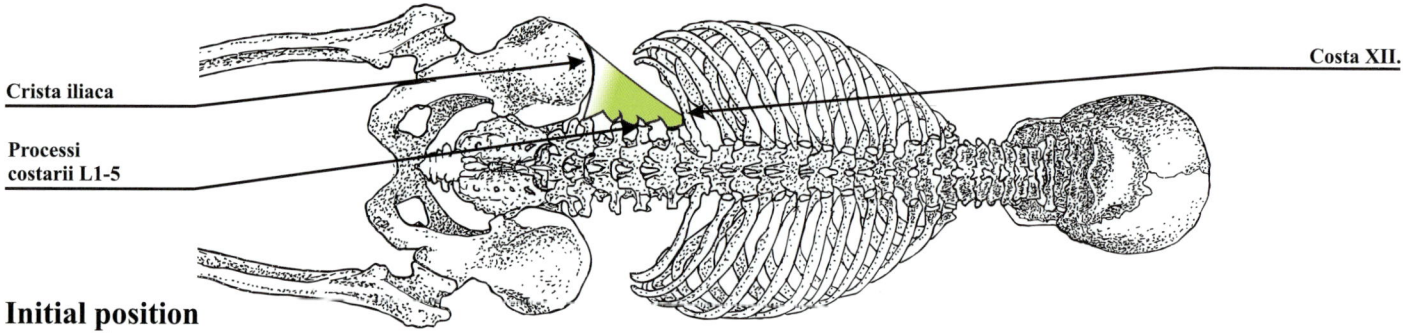

Crista iliaca

Processi costarii L1-5

Costa XII.

Initial position
Caudal stabilization. The pelvis is stabilized from in front by the therapist's chest resting on the thigh. The therapist's axila follows the surface of the pelvis from above, the right forearm is placed against the sacral bone and the fingers are placed gently on the surface of the m. iliocostalis. The fingers must not bend. The patient breathes in.

The left hand moves from in front under the crista iliaca with the thumb extended. The whole thenar engages the surface of the body. It moves slowly cranially and medially until the palm reaches the ribs.

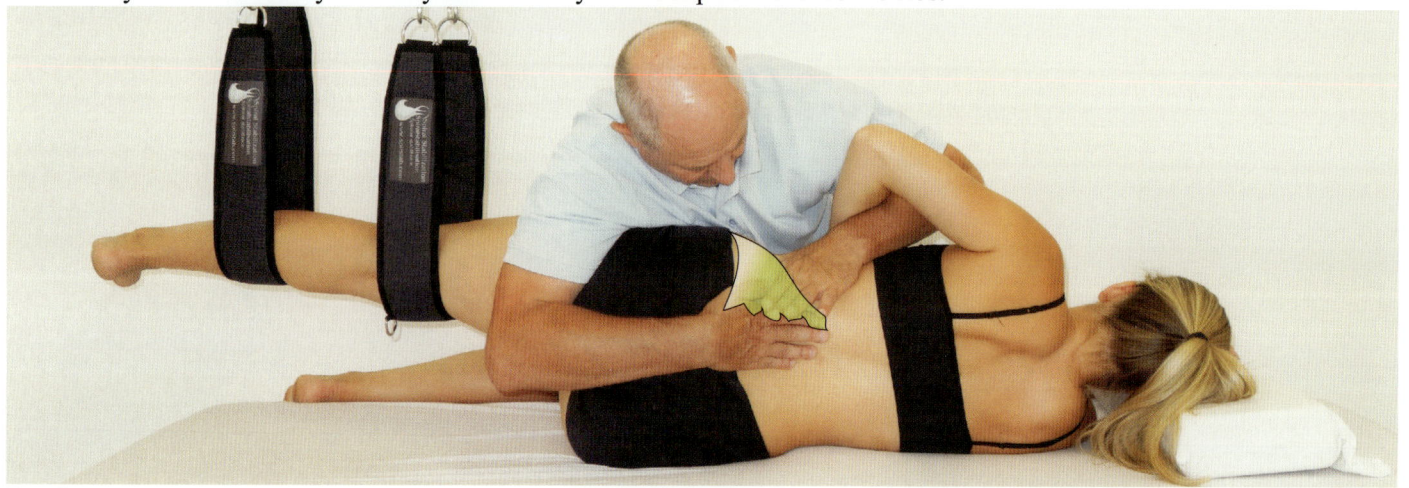

Performance
The cranial left arm stabilizes and remains in place resting against the ribs (punctum fixum). The therapist shifts the weight to the patient's pelvis and evenly shifts the pelvis caudally (punctum mobile). The shift is strengthened by stretching the lower leg. The pelvis must not bend forwards or backwards or rotate. The left thumb is placed against the m. quadratus lumborum. Massage is initiated by the caudal movement of the pelvis. The thumb must not bend. The patient breathes out slowly. The pulling is slackened and the stretching is repeated 6 times. At the end of the technique the therapist pauses for about 3 seconds.

PIR. The extension is held and the patient breathes in. This causes a counter-pressure. When breathing out, the patient achieves further stretching. The process is repeated 3 times. This technique stretches the lumbar discs and intervertebral joints and opens the foramina.

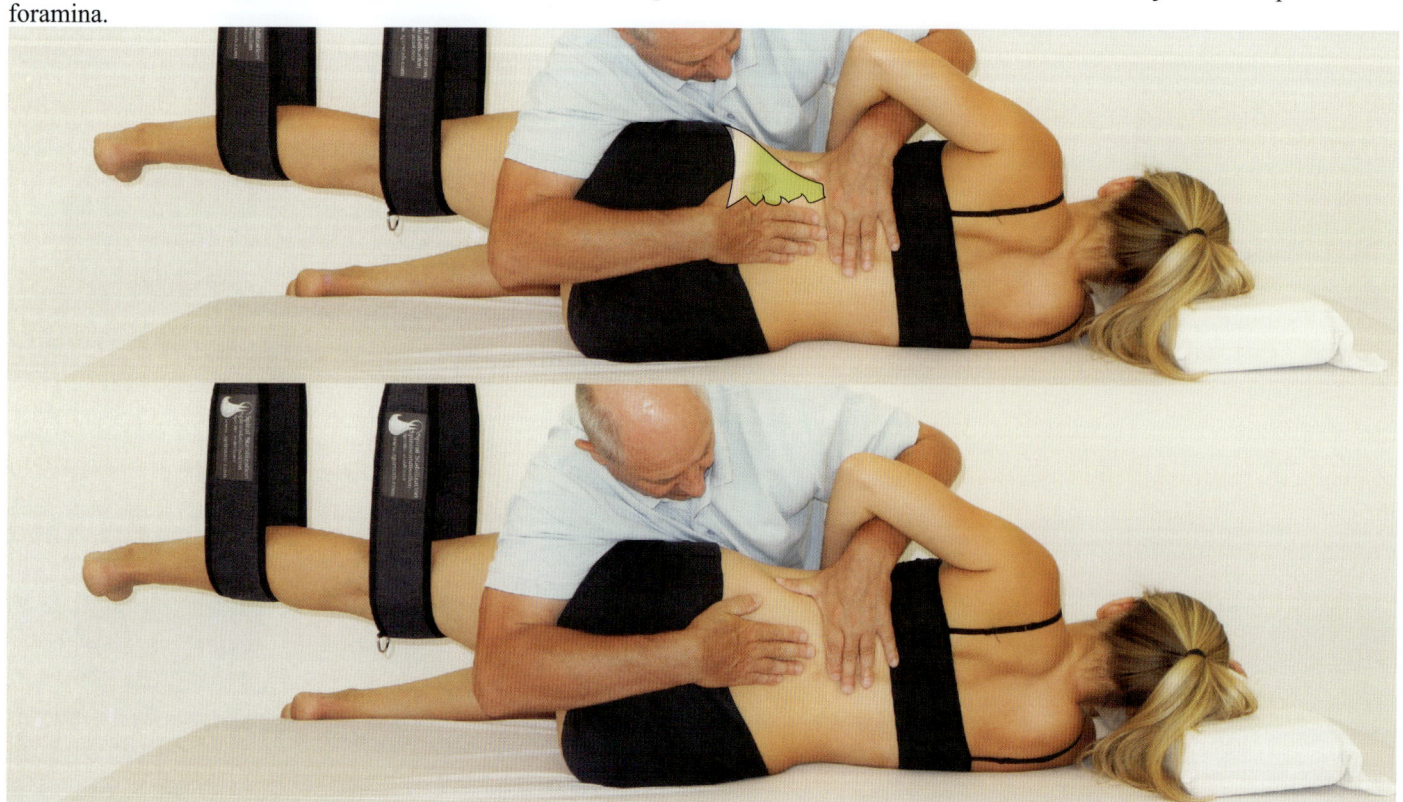

Anatomy
M. longissimus capitis, cervicis, m. multifidus

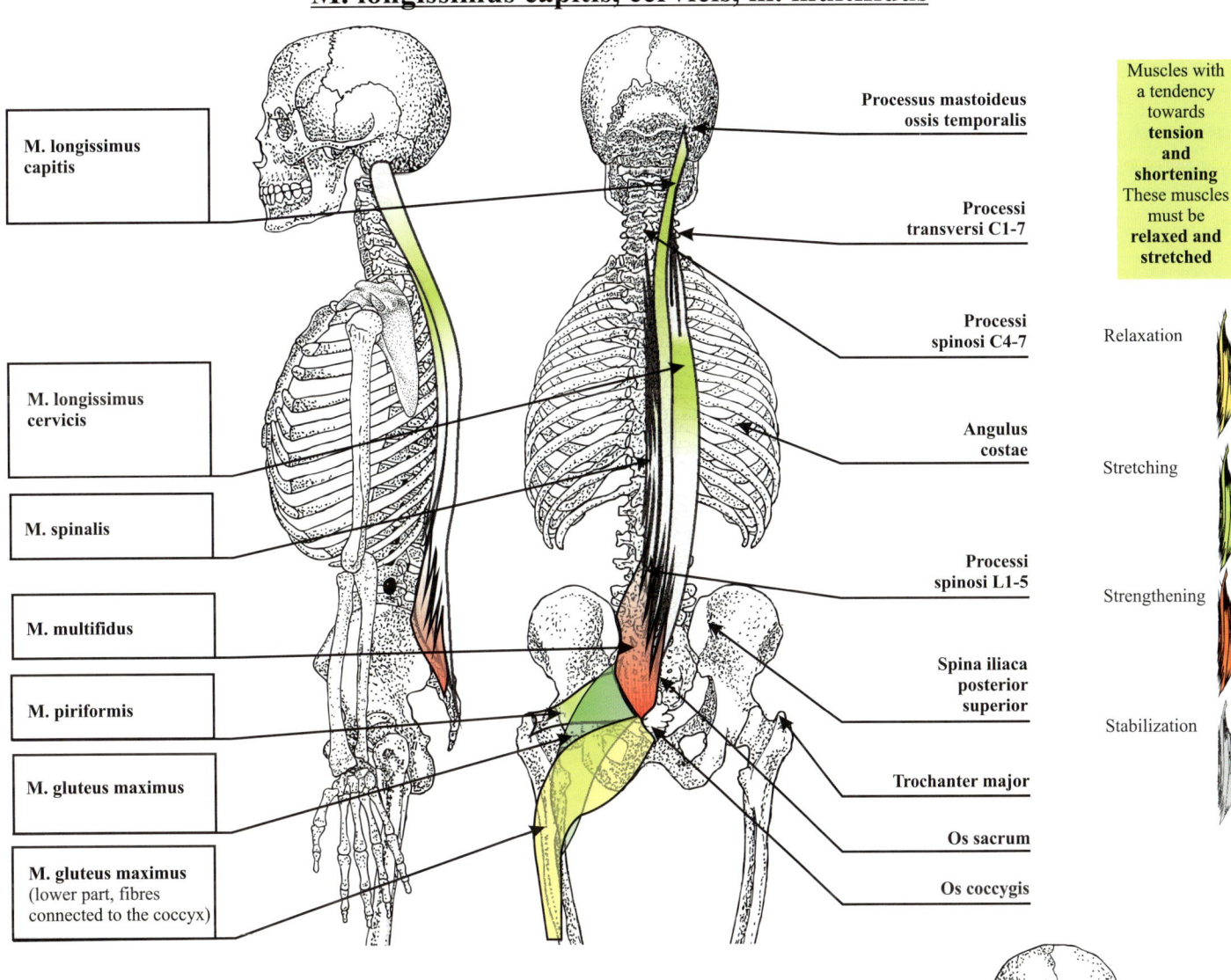

M. longissimus capitis

M. longissimus cervicis

M. spinalis

M. multifidus

M. piriformis

M. gluteus maximus

M. gluteus maximus (lower part, fibres connected to the coccyx)

Processus mastoideus ossis temporalis
Processi transversi C1-7
Processi spinosi C4-7
Angulus costae
Processi spinosi L1-5
Spina iliaca posterior superior
Trochanter major
Os sacrum
Os coccygis

Muscles with a tendency towards **tension and shortening** These muscles must be **relaxed and stretched**

Relaxation
Stretching
Strengthening
Stabilization

M. longissimus
M. longissimus cervicis
Origin:
- os sacrum
- processi spinosi L4, 5
Insertion:
- processi transversi C2-5

M. longissimus capitis
Origin:
- processi spinosi L1-3
Insertion:
- processus mastoideus
Function:
- extension of the head (lifting and tilting), (bilateral contraction)
- rotation (unilateral contraction)
- tilt to the corresponding side (unilateral contraction)
Innervation:
- lateral branches rr. dorsales of spinal nerves C1-L5

Mm. multifidi
Origin:
- processi transversi L, Th, C2
- os sacrum
Insertion:
- processi spinosi Th2-5, C4-7
Function: - bilateral contraction
- extension of the trunk
 - unilateral contraction
- lateral flexion to the corresponding side
- rotation to the contralateral side
Innervation:
- rr. dorsales of spinal nerves (C-L)

M. trapezius pars ascendens

M. multifidus

M. gluteus maximus

M. spinalis
Origin:
- processi spinosi L1-5
Insertion:
- processi spinosi Th2-5, C4-7
Function:
- extension of the trunk (bilateral contraction)
- lateral flexion (unilateral contraction)
Innervation:
- lateral branches rr. dorsales of spinal nerves C8-L1

Manual techniques lying on one side
M. multifidus - massage, relaxation, passive stretching,

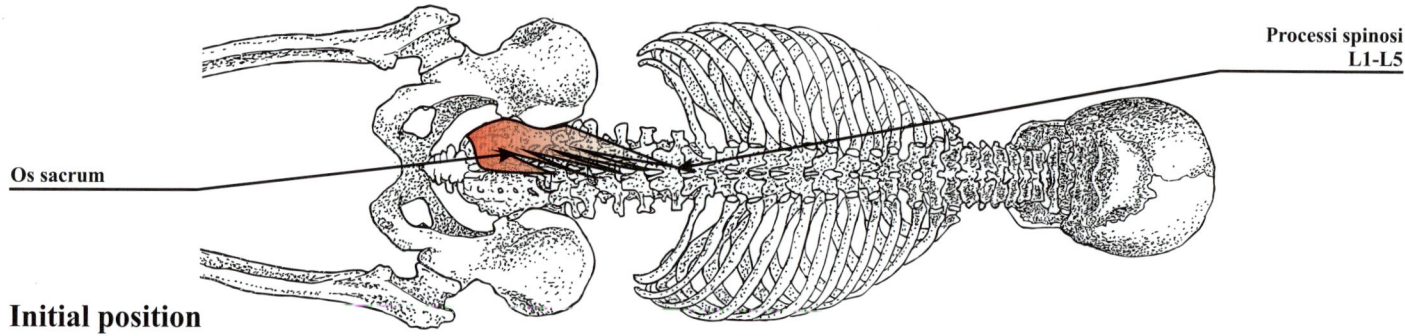

Os sacrum

Processi spinosi L1-L5

Initial position
Cranial stabilization. The thumb and whole thenar of the left hand rest on the spinous process from the side.

Caudal stabilization. The pelvis is stabilized from in front by the therapist's chest resting on the thigh, the therapist's axila (armpit) follows the surface of the pelvis from above, the right forearm is placed against the sacral bone and the fingers are placed gently against the surface of the m. multifidus. The middle finger is pressed from the side against the caudal procesus spinosus. The fingers must not bend. The patient breathes in.

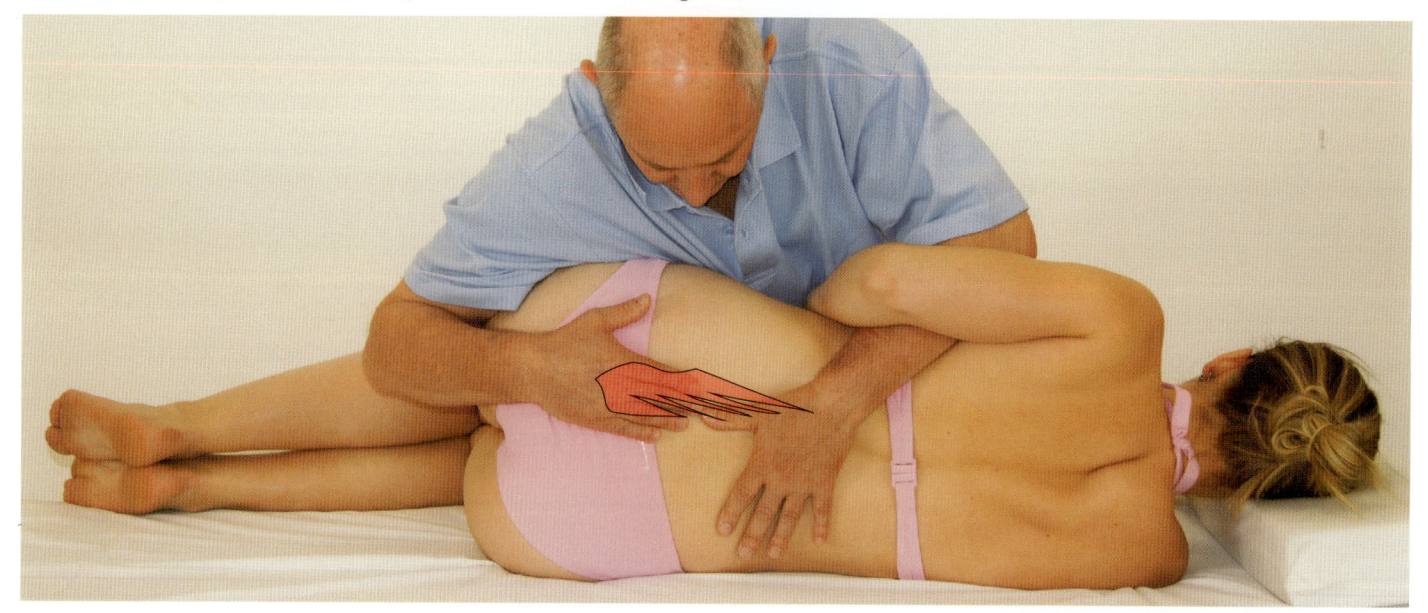

Performance
The cranial left arm stabilizes and stays in place (punctum fixum). The therapist shifts the weight to the patient's pelvis and evenly shifts the pelvis caudally (punctum mobile). The shift is strengthened by stretching the lower legs. The pelvis must not bend forwards or backwards or rotate. Massage of the m.multifidus is initiated by shifting the pelvis caudally. In segment L5/S1 the segment is first stretched, then the lordosis is slightly straightened by gentle flexion. The patient breathes out slowly. The pulling is slackened and the stretching is repeated 6 times. At the end of the technique the therapist pauses for about 3 seconds.

PIR. The extension is held and the patient breathes in. This causes a counter-pressure. When breathing out, the patient achieves further stretching. The process is repeated 3 times. This technique stretches a specific disc as well as stretching the intervertebral joints and opening the foramen.

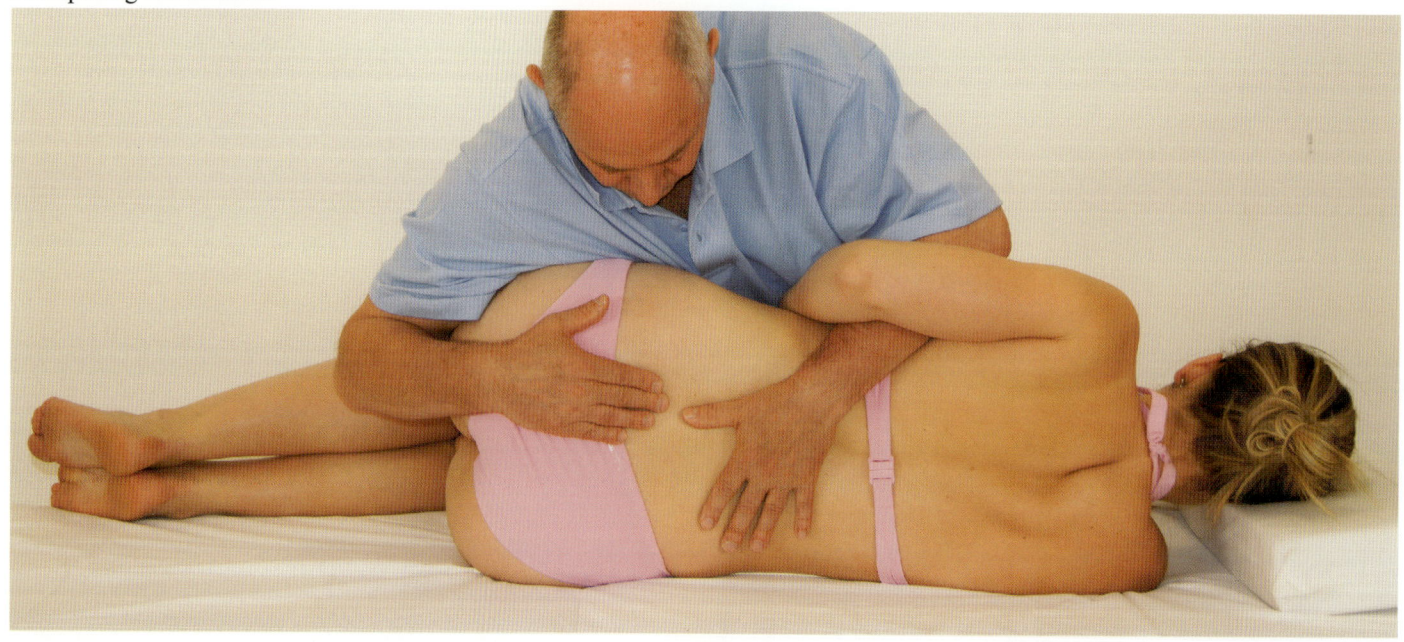

Manual techniques - lying - one limb in a hoist
M. multifidus - massage, relaxation, passive stretching

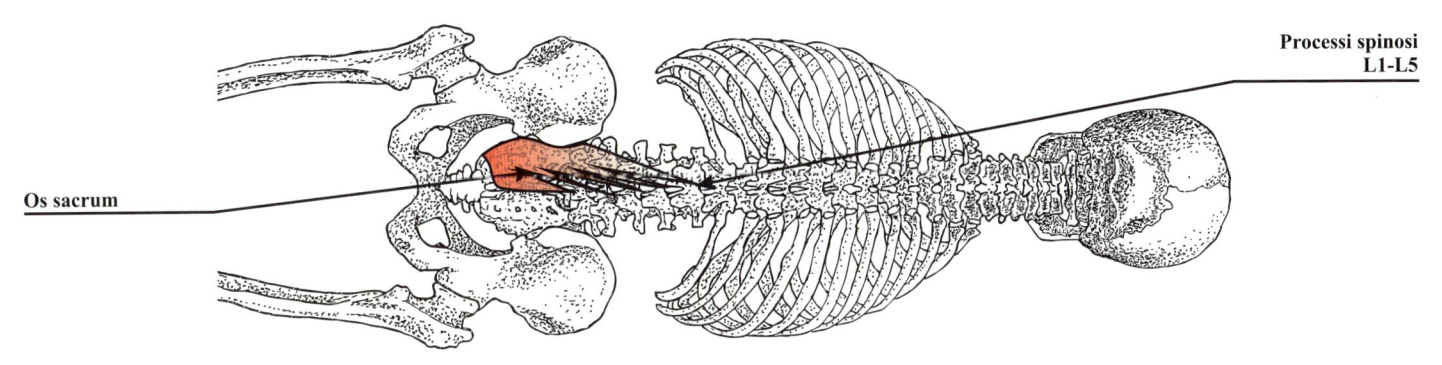

Processi spinosi L1-L5

Os sacrum

Initial position
Cranial stabilization. The thumb and whole thenar of the left hand rest on the processi spinosi from the side.
Caudal stabilization. The pelvis is stabilized from in front by the therapist's chest resting on the thigh. The therapist's axila (armpit) follows the surface of the pelvis from above, the right forearm is placed against the sacral bone and the fingers are placed gently against the caudal procesus spinosus. The fingers must not bend. The patient breathes in.

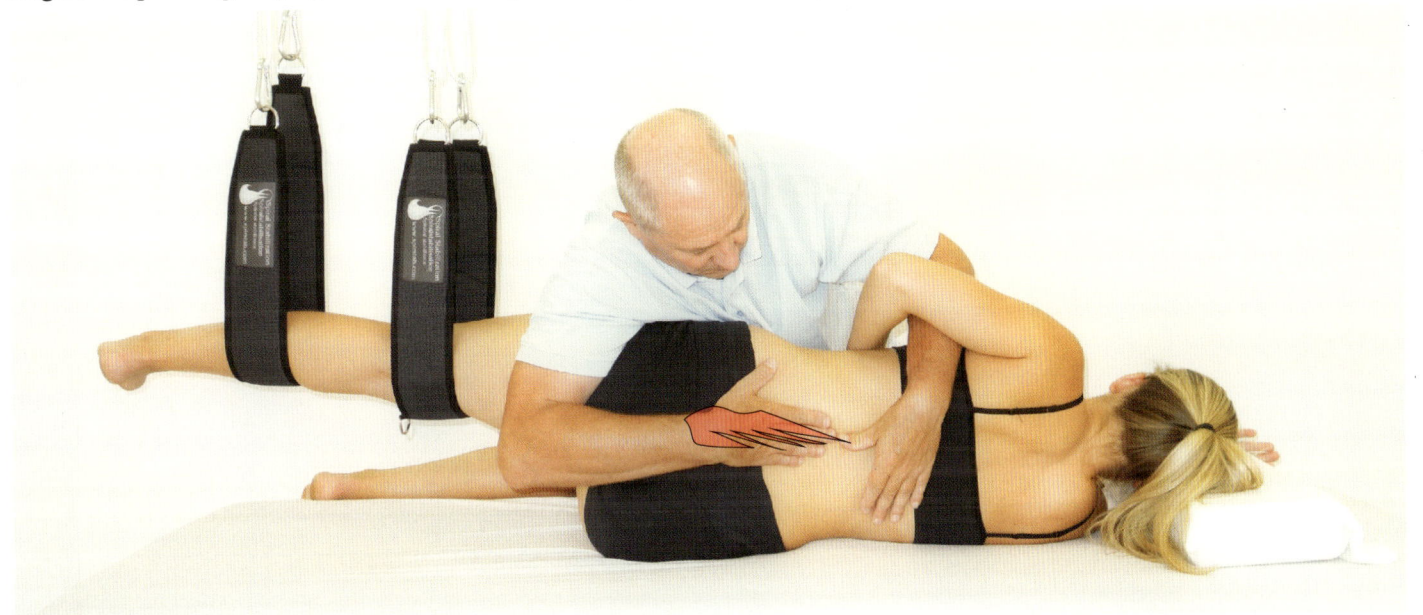

Performance
The cranial left arm stabilizes and stays in place (punctum fixum). The therapist shifts the weight to the patient's pelvis and evenly shifts the pelvis caudally (punctum mobile). The shift is strengthening by stretching the legs. The pelvis must not bend forwards or backwards or rotate. Massage of the m. multifidus is initiated by shifting the pelvis caudally. The patient breathes out slowly.
The pulling is slackened and the stretching is repeated 6 times. At the end of the technique the therapist pauses for about 3 seconds.
PIR. The extension is held and the patient breathes in. This causes a counter-pressure. When breathing out, the patient achieves further stretching. The process is repeated 3 times. The technique stretches a specific disc as well as stretching the intervertebral joints and opening the foramen.

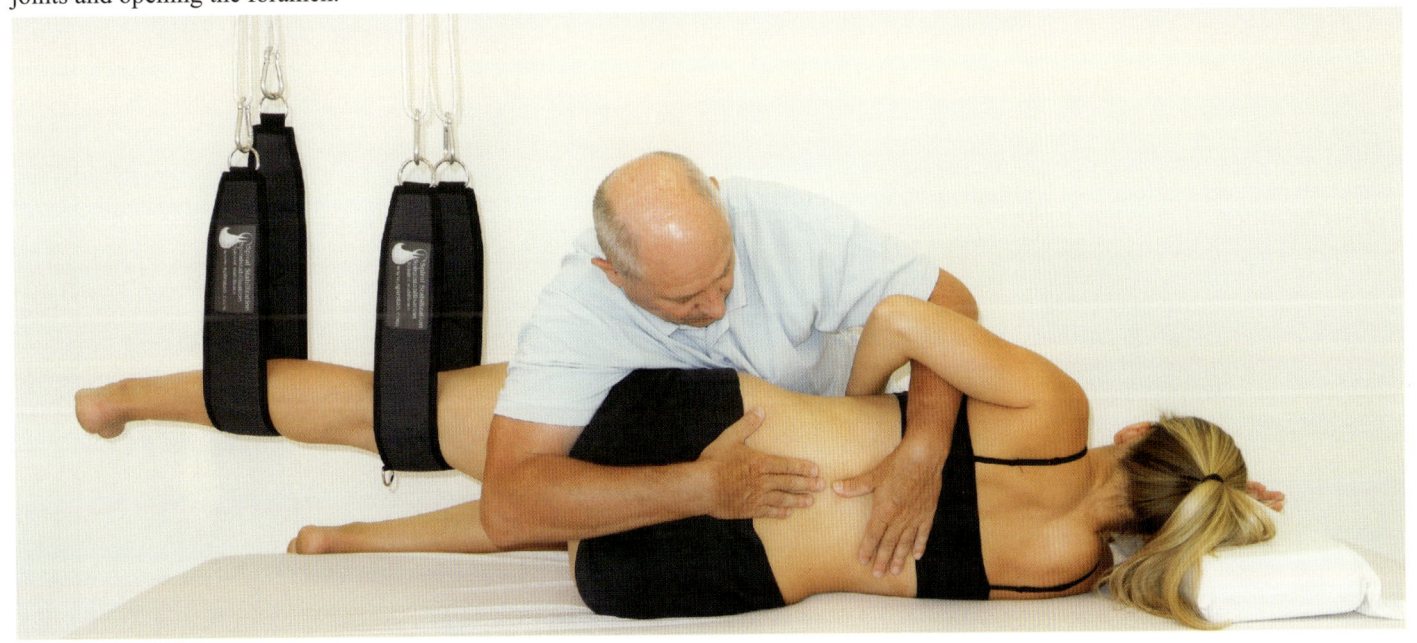

Manual techniques - lying - one limb in a hoist
M. multifidus - massage, relaxation, passive stretching

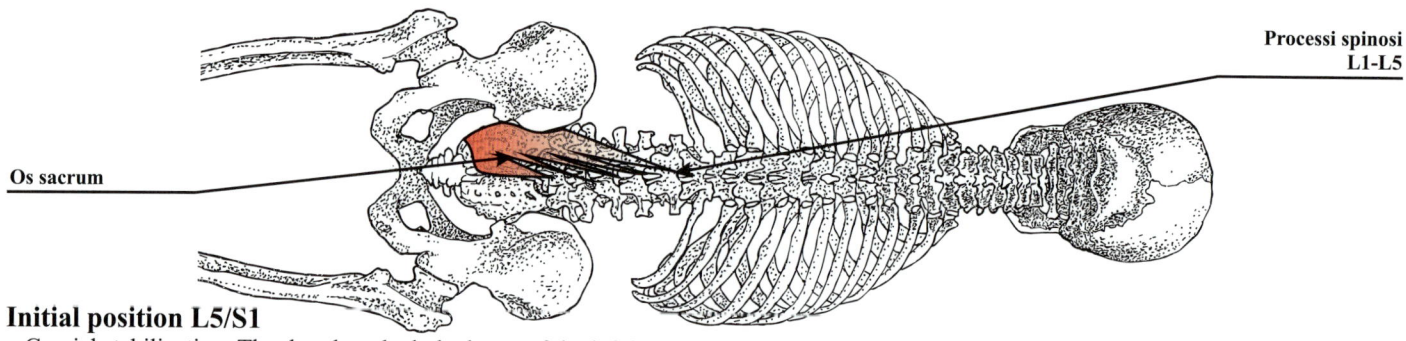

Os sacrum

Processi spinosi L1-L5

Initial position L5/S1
Cranial stabilization. The thumb and whole thenar of the left hand rest on the procesus spinosus of L5 from the side and the higher processes. Caudal stabilization. The pelvis is stabilized from in front by the therapists's chest resting on the thigh. The therapist's axila (armpit) follows the surface of the pelvis from above, the right forearm is placed against the sacral bone and the fingers are placed gently against the surface of the m. multifidus. The middle finger is pressed from the side against the os sacrum. The fingers must not bend. The patient breathes in.

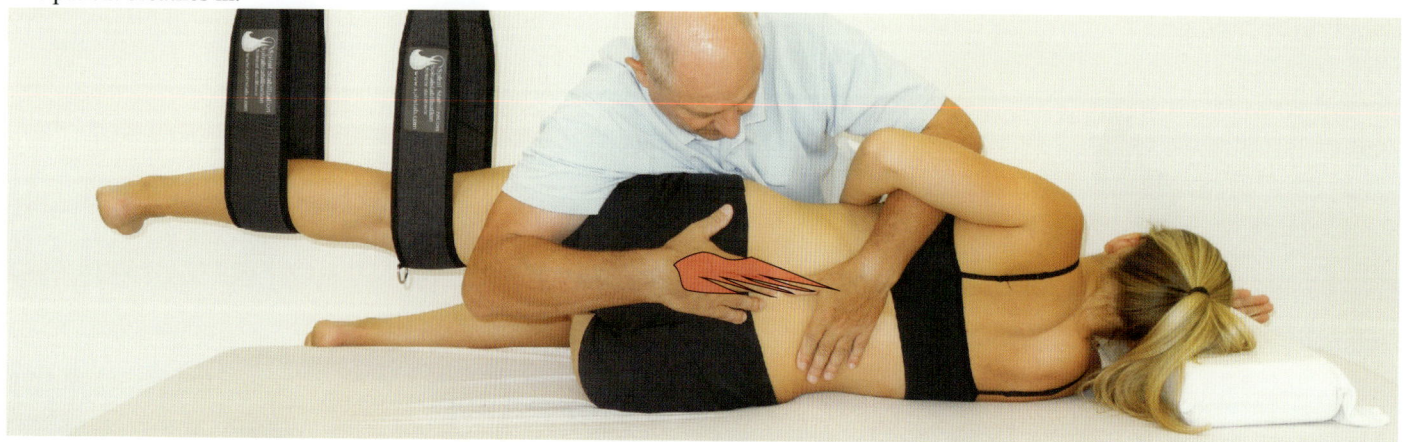

Performance
The cranial left arm stabilized and stays in place (punctum fixum). The therapist shifts the weight to the patient's pelvis and evenly shifts the pelvis caudally (punctum mobile). The shift is strengthened by stretching the legs. The pelvis must not bend forwards or backwards or rotate. Massage of the m. multifidus is initiated by shifting the pelvis caudally. The patient breathes out slowly. The pulling is slackened and the stretching is repeated 6 times. At the end of the technique the therapist pauses for about 3 seconds.
PIR. The extension is held and the patient breathes in. This causes a counter-pressure. When breathing out, the patient achieves further stretching. The process is repreated 3 times. This technique stretches a specific disc as well as stretching the intervertebral joints and opening the foramen.

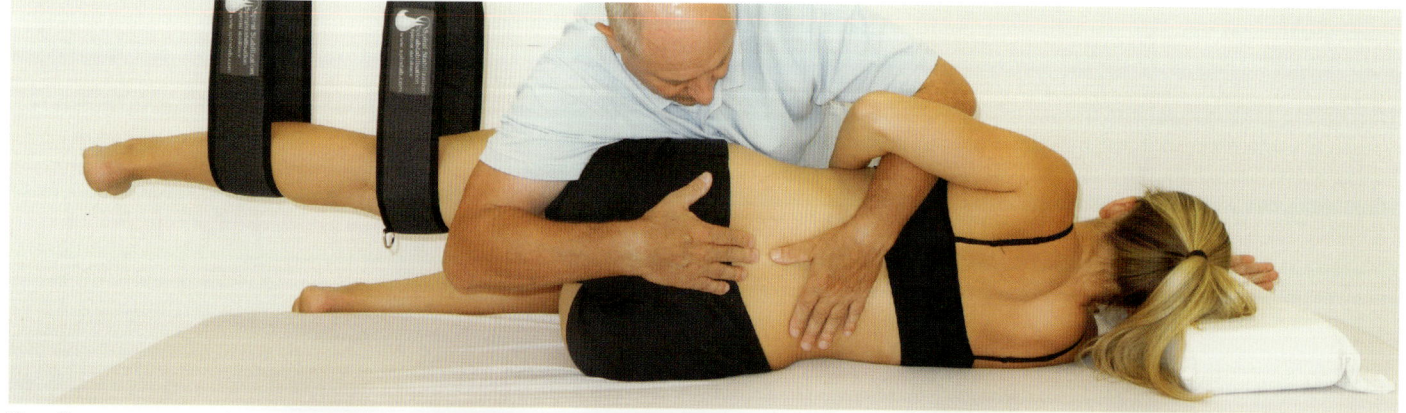

Performance
Segment L5/S1 is first stretched, then the lordosis is slightly straightened by gentle flexion.

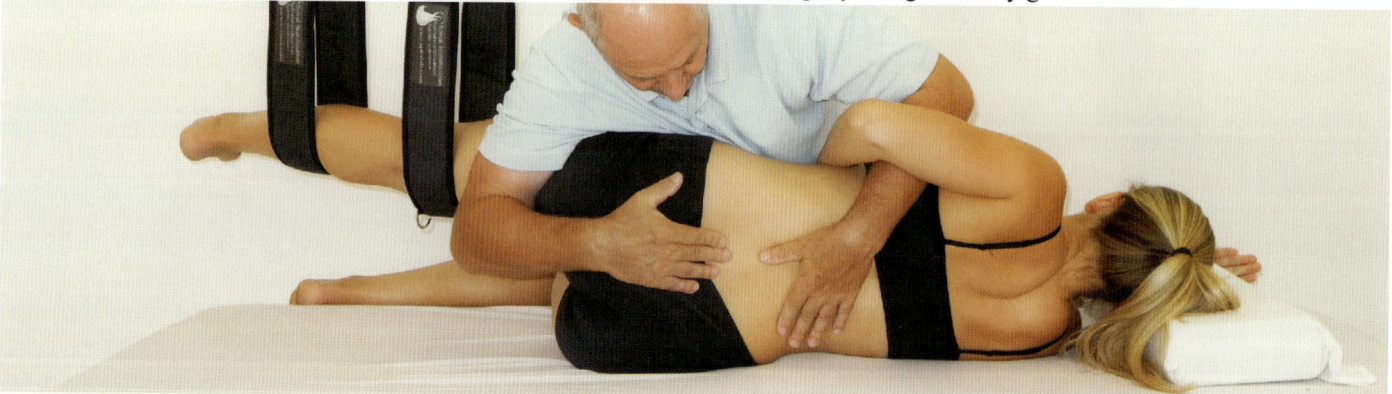

Manual techniques - lying - one limb in a hoist
M. multifidus - massage, relaxation, passive stretching

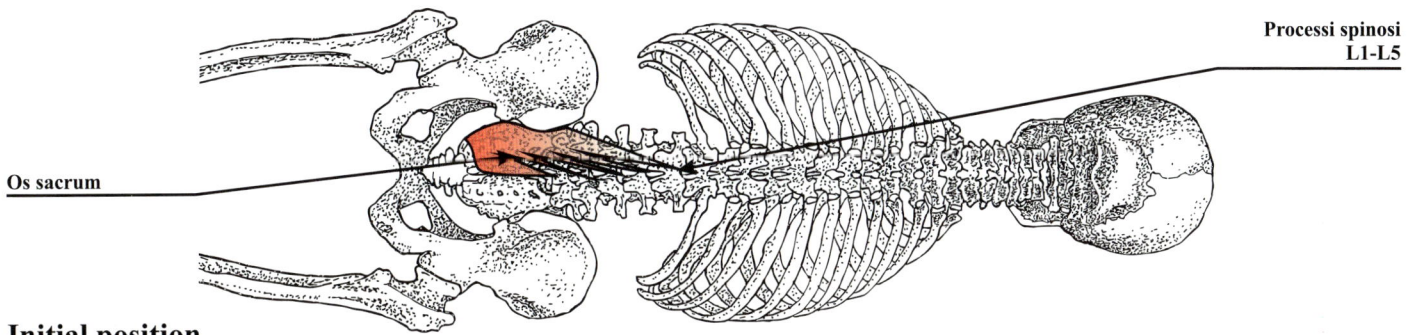

Processi spinosi L1-L5

Os sacrum

Initial position
The therapist kneels behind the patient facing the pelvis. The pelvis is stabilized from behind by the thigh and his own pelvis. The patient is straightened in the axis. The palm of the therapist's right hand stabilizes the pelvis from the front. The SIAS - spina iliaca anterior superior - is in the centre of the palm. The left hand is on the ischial tuberosity. The patient breathes in.

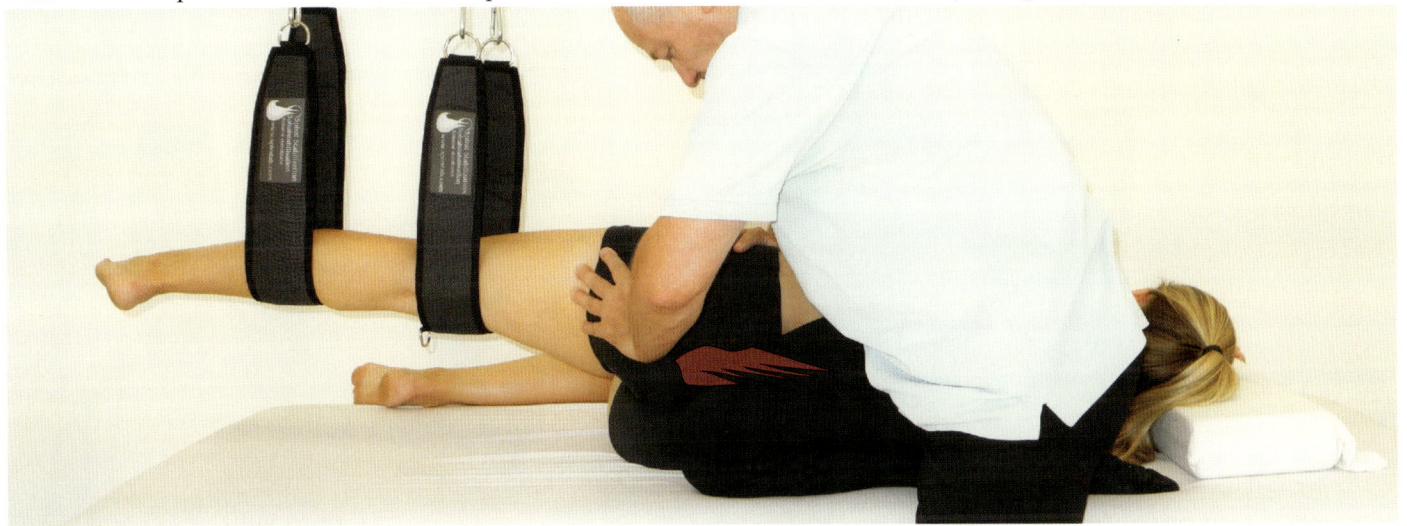

Performance
The pelvis is shifted caudally (towards the feet). The patient breathes out slowly. The pulling is slackened and the stretching is repeated 6 times. At the end of the technique the therapist pauses for about 3 seconds.

PIR. This causes a counter-pressure. While breathing out, the patient achieves further stretching. The process is repeated 3 times. This technique stretches the m. iliocostalis, m. quadratus lumborum and the lumbar spine.

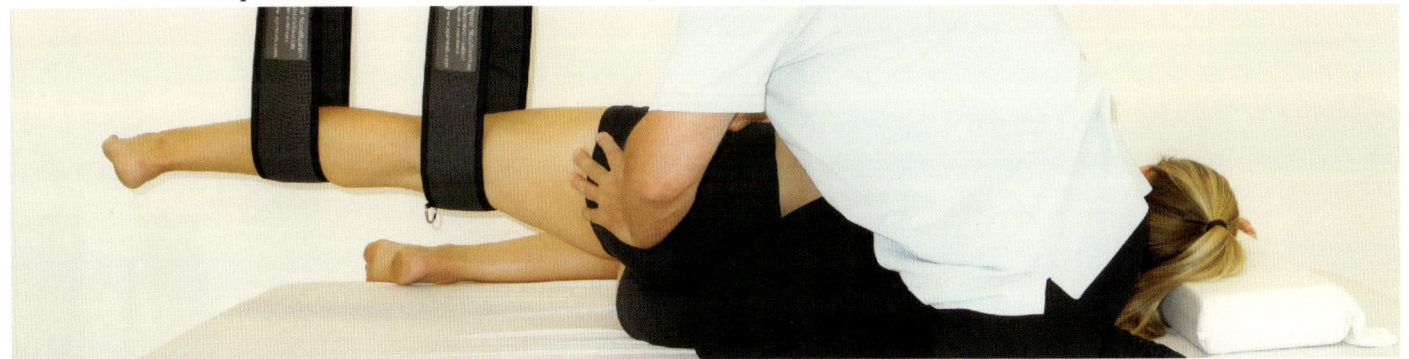

Performance
The lower part of the pelvis is rotated forwards. The axis moves in the hip joint.

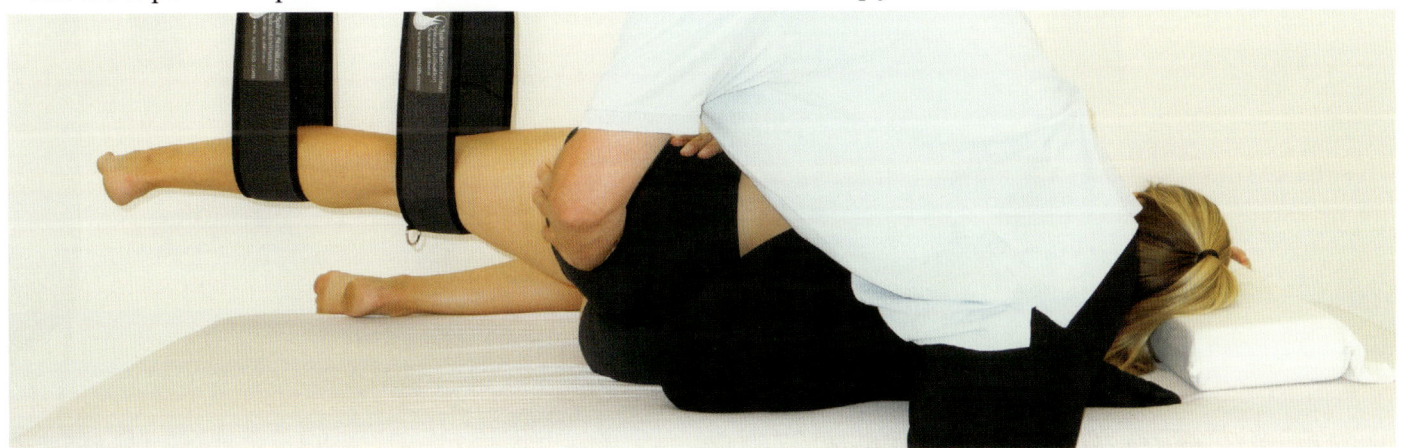

Manual techniques - lying - in a hoist
M. iliocostalis lumborum - massage, relaxation, passive stretching

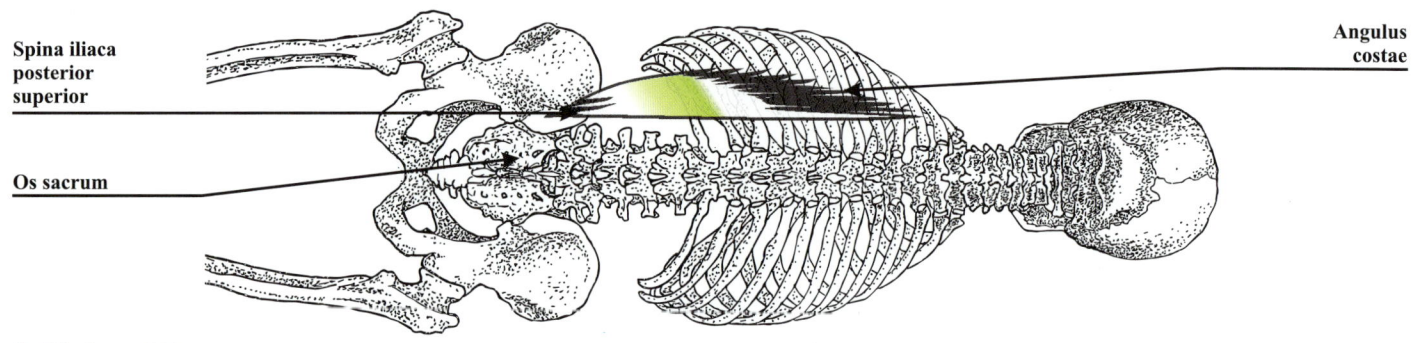

Spina iliaca posterior superior

Os sacrum

Angulus costae

Initial position

The therapist kneels behind the patient facing the head. The pelvis is stabilized from behind by the thigh and the therapist's own pelvis. The patient is in kyphosis (a long, extended forward arch).

The palm of the therapist's left hand stabilizes the lower ribs, and the fingers support the sternum.
The left thumb is placed along the 10th rib. The right hand moves along the 10th rib dorsally towards the spine.
The process of the 10th rib is in the middle of the palm. The thumb supports the rib. The patient breathes in.

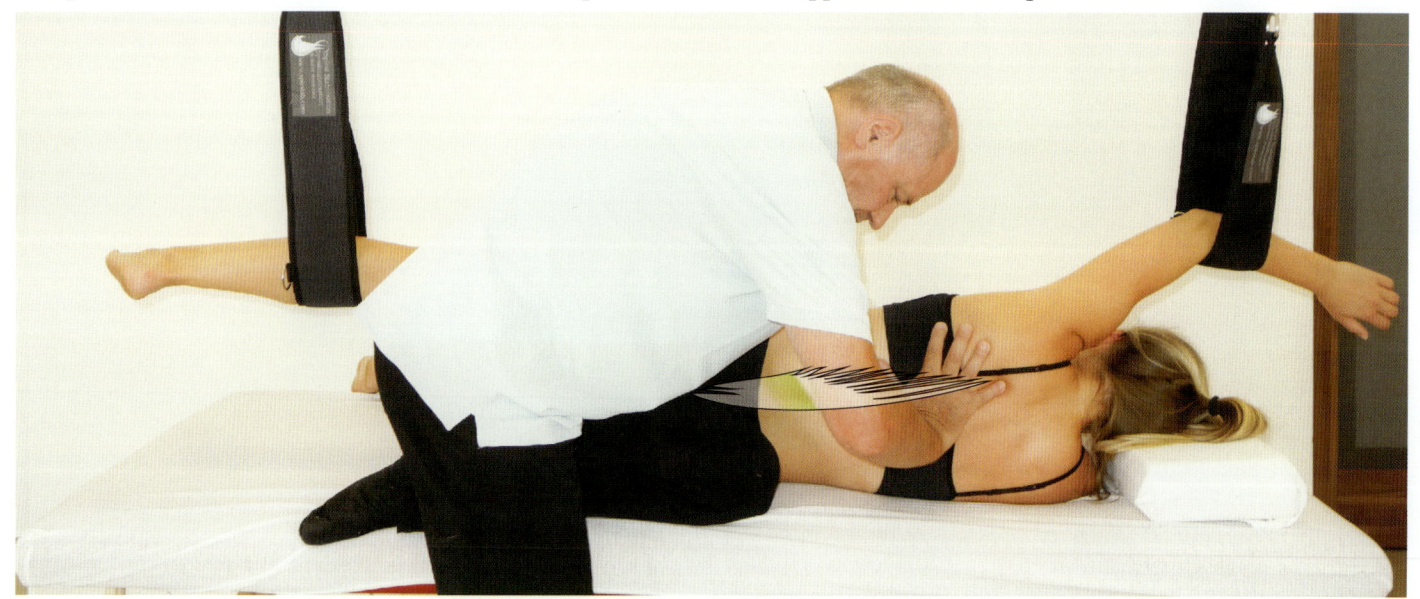

Performance

The therapist's arms and trunk lead the 10th rib first dorsally and then cranially. The patient breathes out slowly. The pulling is slackened and the stretching is repeated 6 times. At the end of the technique the therapist pauses for about 3 seconds.

PIR. The extension is held and the patient breathes in. This causes a counter-pressure. When breathing out, the patient relaxes and achieves further stretching. The process is repeated 3 times. This technique stretches the m. iliocostalis and mobilizes the ribs. The technique is repeated for all the ribs.

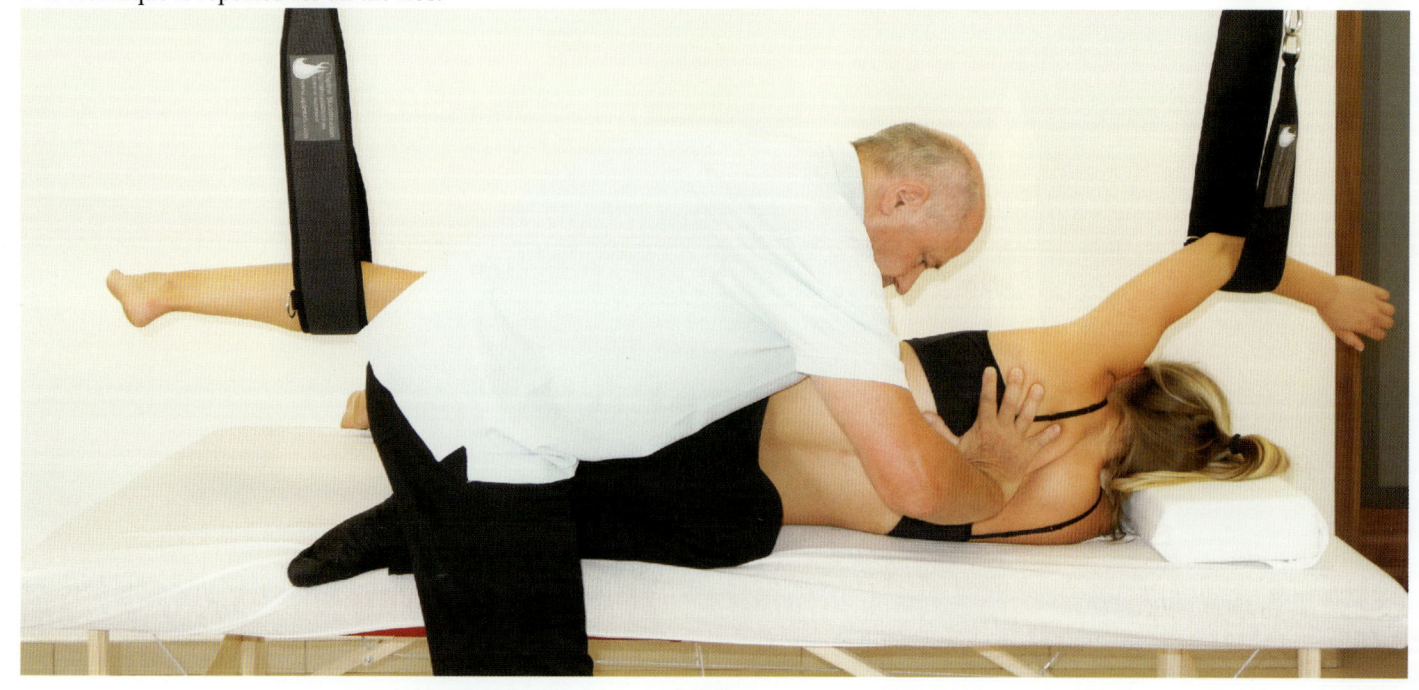

Manual techniques lying on the back in a hoist
M. erector spinae, m. quadratus lumborum, m. multifidus
- massage, relaxation, passive stretching

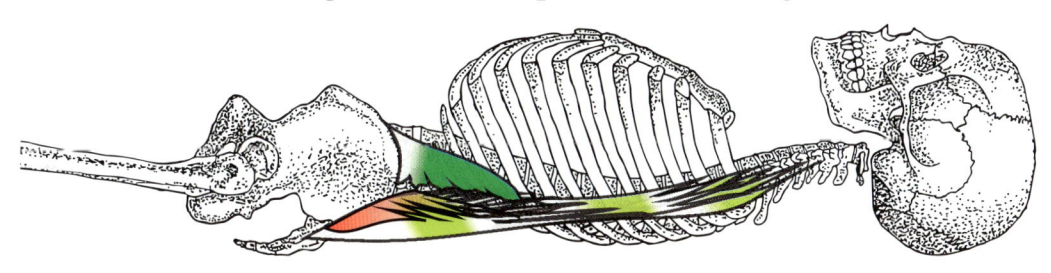

Stretching the lumbar spine in suspension
Cranial stabilization. The patient lies on her back on a mat. Punctum fixum.
Caudal stabilization. The legs are suspended at the calves and the lower part of the pelvis is suspended.
Gravity stretches the lumbar spine in the posterior pole.
Traction of the spine is improved by pulling the pelvis caudally and fixation with a rope.

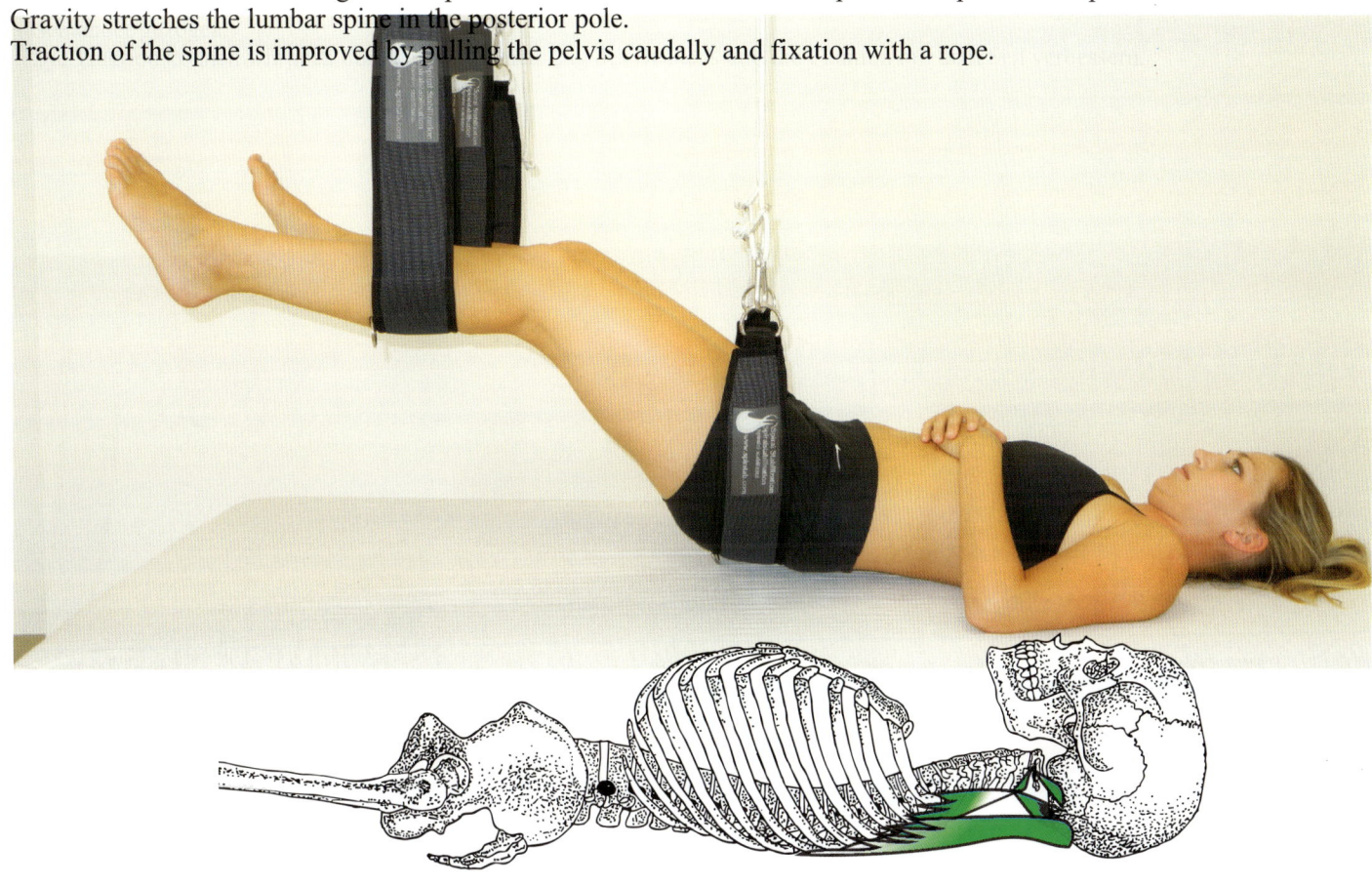

Stretching the lumbar and cervical spine in suspension
Traction of the spine is performed by pulling the pelvis caudally and fixation with a rope.
The head is suspended in a hoist and techniques for the cervical spine are performed.

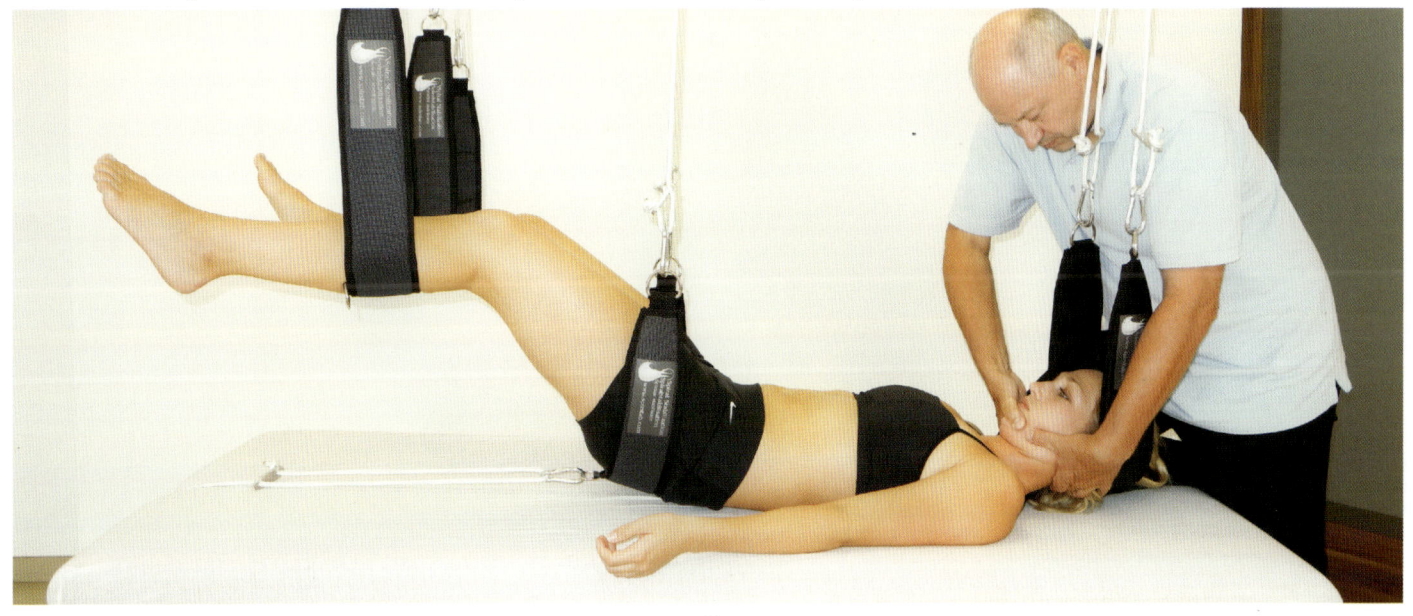

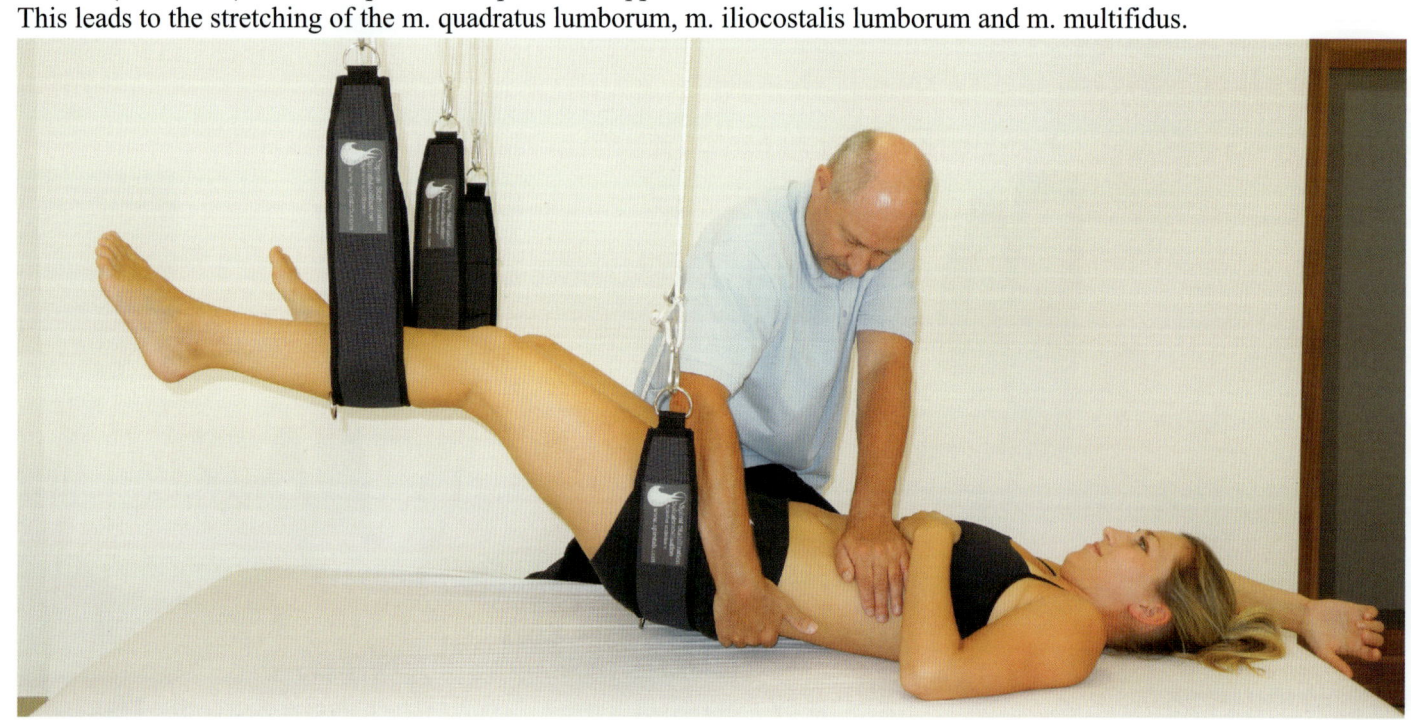

Manual techniques lying on the back in a hoist
M. quadratus lumborum - massage, relaxation, passive stretching

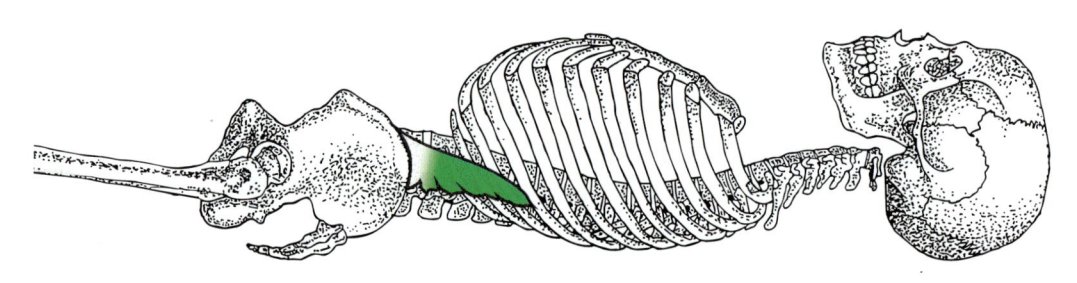

Initial position
   Cranial stabilization. The patient lies on her back on a mat. Punctum fixum.
   Caudal stabilization. The legs are suspended at the calves and the lower part of the pelvis is suspended. Gravity stretches the lumbar spine in the posterior pole. The therapist kneels and his flank rests against the patient's hip joint.
The therapist stabilizes the lower ribs with his left hand. The right hand and forearm stabilize the pelvis.

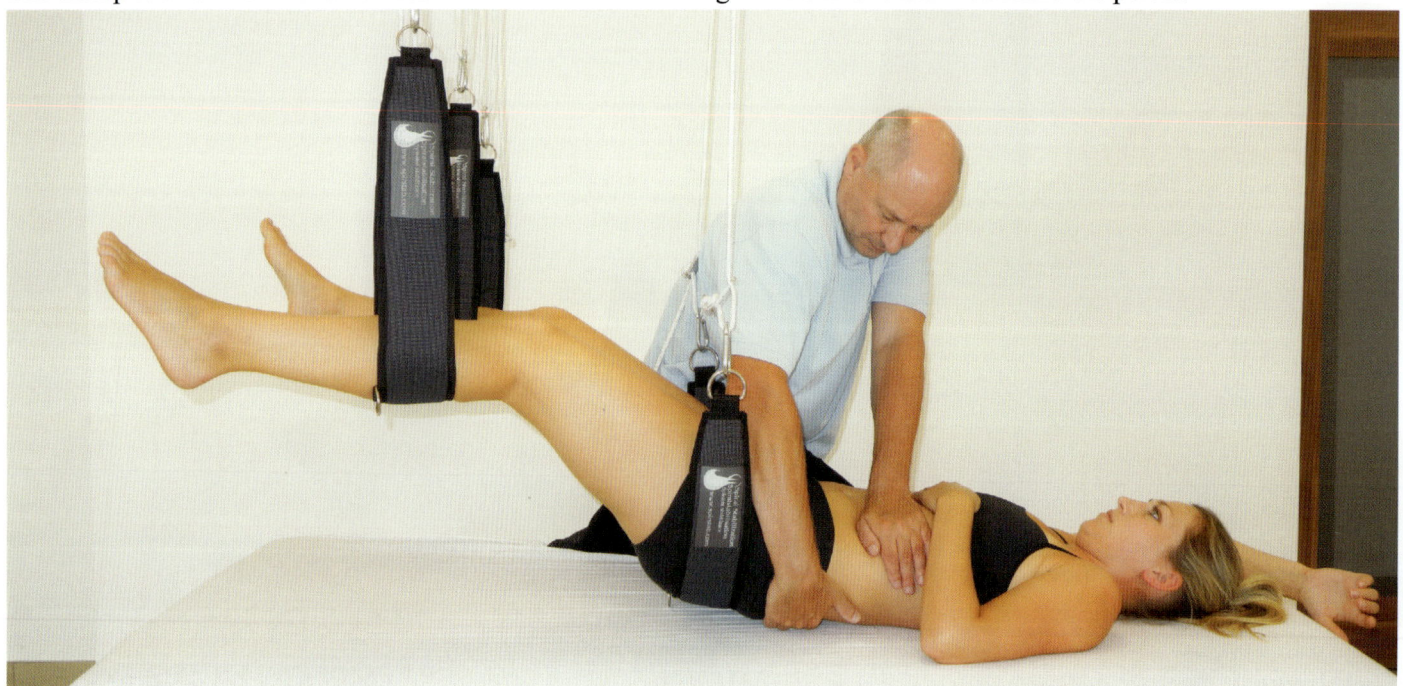

Performance
   With his right hand and forearm, the therapist pulls the pelvis caudally (downwards) and turns it laterally towards himself (to the side). The therapist's flank provides support for the movement.
This leads to the stretching of the m. quadratus lumborum, m. iliocostalis lumborum and m. multifidus.

Manual techniques in a sitting position
M. erector spinae - passive stretching, active relaxation

Exercise 1 - sitting, facing the attachment point of the elastic rope, backward pull with both arms

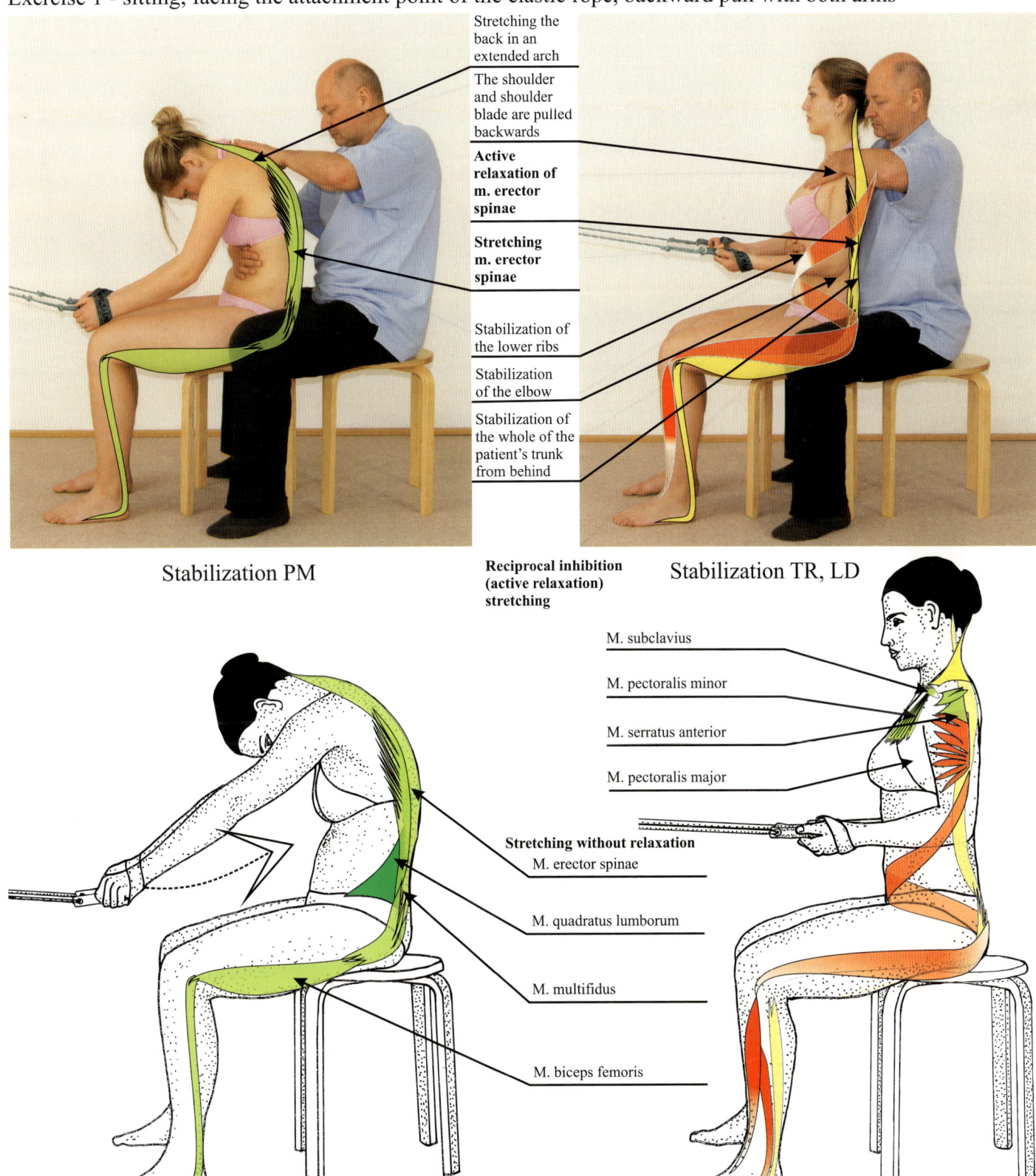

Stretching the back in an extended arch

The shoulder and shoulder blade are pulled backwards

Active relaxation of m. erector spinae

Stretching m. erector spinae

Stabilization of the lower ribs

Stabilization of the elbow

Stabilization of the whole of the patient's trunk from behind

Stabilization PM

Reciprocal inhibition (active relaxation) stretching

Stabilization TR, LD

M. subclavius
M. pectoralis minor
M. serratus anterior
M. pectoralis major

Stretching without relaxation
M. erector spinae
M. quadratus lumborum
M. multifidus
M. biceps femoris

1 - Initial position - active part of the exercise
In the initial position the back muscles are stretched:
- m. erector spinae
- m. quadratus lumborum
- m. multifidus

Then the ischiocrural muscles are stretched (muscles of the posterior side of the thigh):
- m. biceps femoris
- m. semitendinosus
- m. semimembranosus
- m. adductor magnus

2 - Performance - active part of the exercise
In the active part of the exercise the muscles of the anterior side of the shoulder girdle are stretched:
- m. subclavius
- m. pectoralis minor
- m. pectoralis major
- m. serratus anterior

The muscles of the upper side of the shoulder girdle are relaxed:
- m. trapezius pars descendens
- m. levator scapulae
- mm. scaleni
- m. semispinalis capitis, cervicis and other muscles.

Manual techniques in a sitting position
M. iliocostalis lumborum - active relaxation, massage, stretching

Exercise 6 - sitting with back to the attachment point of the elastic rope, forward circles with both arms

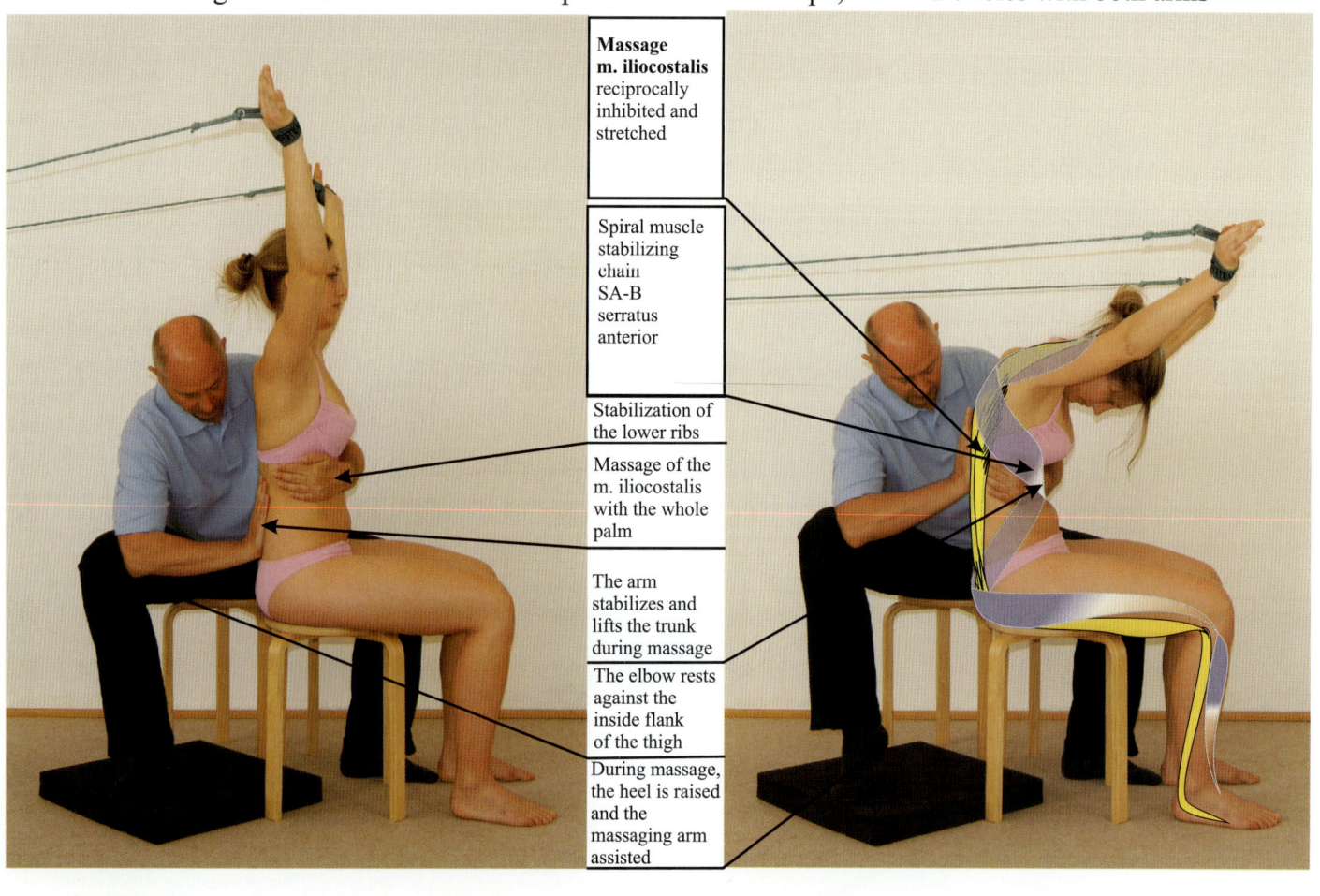

- **Massage m. iliocostalis** reciprocally inhibited and stretched
- Spiral muscle stabilizing chain SA-B serratus anterior
- Stabilization of the lower ribs
- Massage of the m. iliocostalis with the whole palm
- The arm stabilizes and lifts the trunk during massage
- The elbow rests against the inside flank of the thigh
- During massage, the heel is raised and the massaging arm assisted

M. multifidus - active relaxation, stretching

Exercise 6 - sitting with back to the attachment point of the elastic rope, forward circles with both arms

- Spiral muscle stabilizing chain SA-B serratus anterior
- Stabilization of the lower abdominal wall. The arm stabilizes and lifts the trunk.
- The elbow rests against the inside flank of the thigh
- **Stretching the m. multifidus,** reciprocally inhibited and stretched
- Stretching the pelvis downwards. The whole palm presses and the thumb moves upwards along the processes

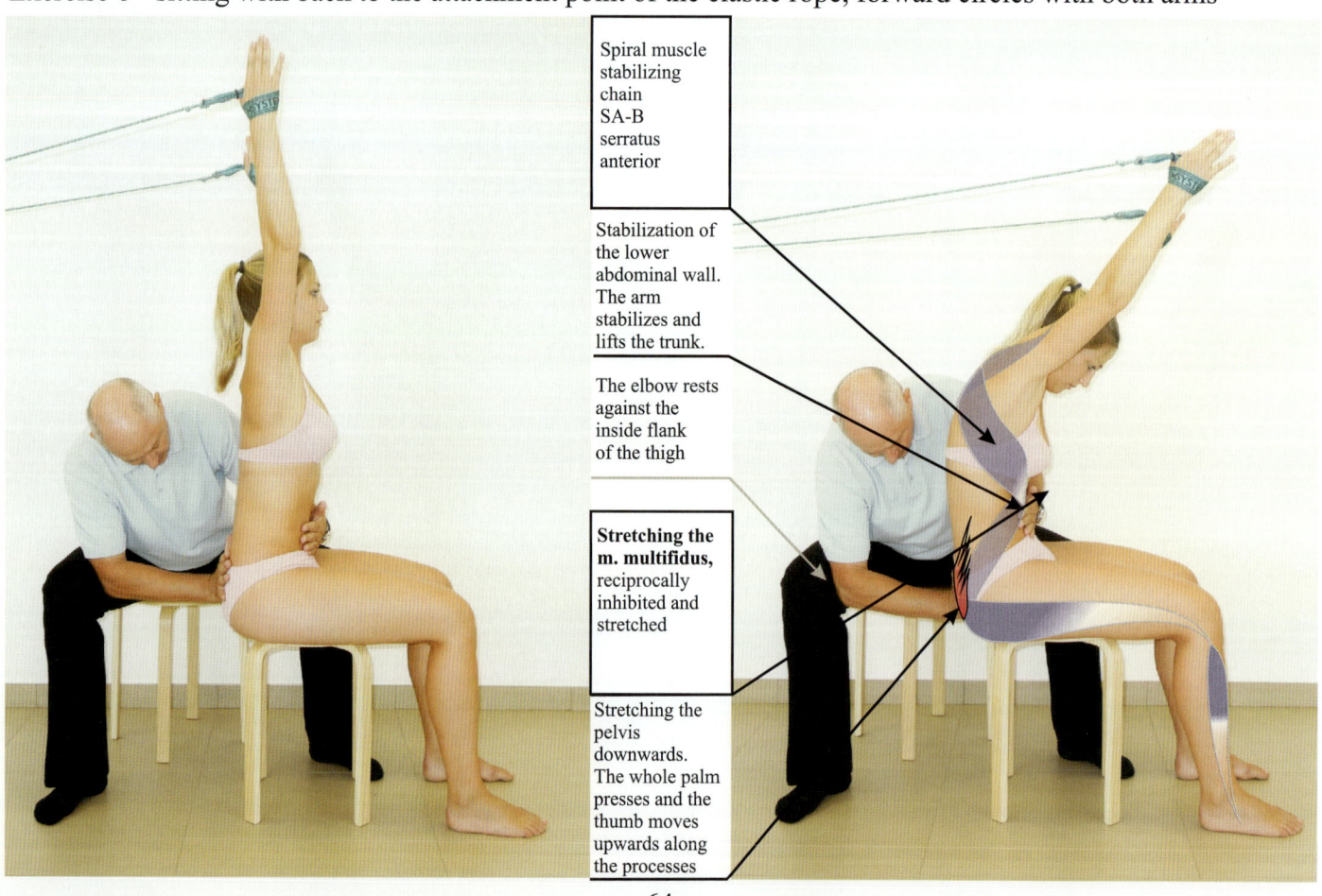

- 64 -

Exercise - stabilization, stretching

M. erector spinae, m. iliocostalis, m. longissimus thoracis, m. longissimus capitis, cervicis, m. quadratus lumborum, m. multifidus
- relaxation in reciprocal inhibition, stretching

The SA - serratus anterior and PM - pectoralis major chains are the agonists in the first part of the exercise, the LD - latissimus dorsi and TR - trapezius chains are the agonists in the second part of the exercise.

Exercise 1 - standing facing the attachment point of the elastic rope, one leg is placed forward on the mat
Backward pull with both arms, opening of the arms in outward rotation, palms turned upwards

Stabilization SA, PM   Stabilization TR, LD

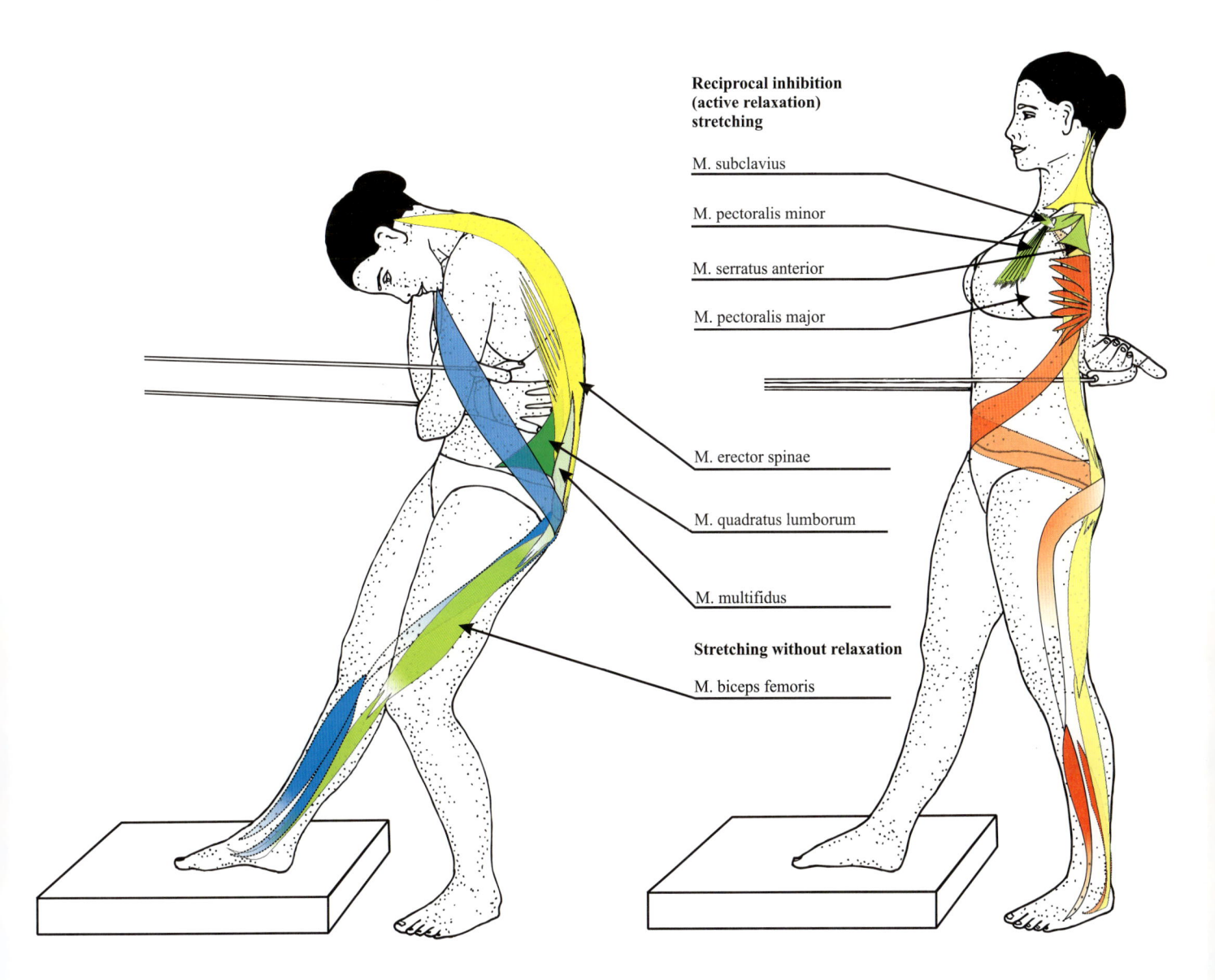

Reciprocal inhibition (active relaxation) stretching
- M. subclavius
- M. pectoralis minor
- M. serratus anterior
- M. pectoralis major
- M. erector spinae
- M. quadratus lumborum
- M. multifidus

Stretching without relaxation
- M. biceps femoris

1 - Initial position - active part of the exercise
In the initial position the back muscles are stretched:
- m. erector spinae
- m. quadratus lumborum
- m. multifidus

Then the ischiocrural muscles are stretched (muscles of the posterior side of the thigh):
- m. biceps femoris
- m. semitendinosus
- m. semimembranosus
- m. adductor magnus

2 - Performance - active part of the exercise
In the active part of the exercise the muscles of the anterior side of the shoulder girdle are stretched:
- m. subclavius
- m. pectoralis minor
- m. pectoralis major
- m. serratus anterior

The muscles of the upper side of the shoulder girdle are relaxed:
- m. trapezius, pars descendens
- m. levator scapulae
- mm. scaleni
- m. semispinalis capitis, cervicis
and other muscles.

Exercise - stabilization, stretching

M. erector spinae, m. iliocostalis, m. longissimus thoracis, m. longissimus capitis, cervicis, m. quadratus lumborum, m. multifidus
- relaxation in reciprocal inhibition, stretching

The LD - latissimus dorsi and TR - trapezius chains are the agonists in the second part of the exercise.

Exercise 2 - standing sideways on to the attachment point of the elastic rope, one leg is placed forward on the mat

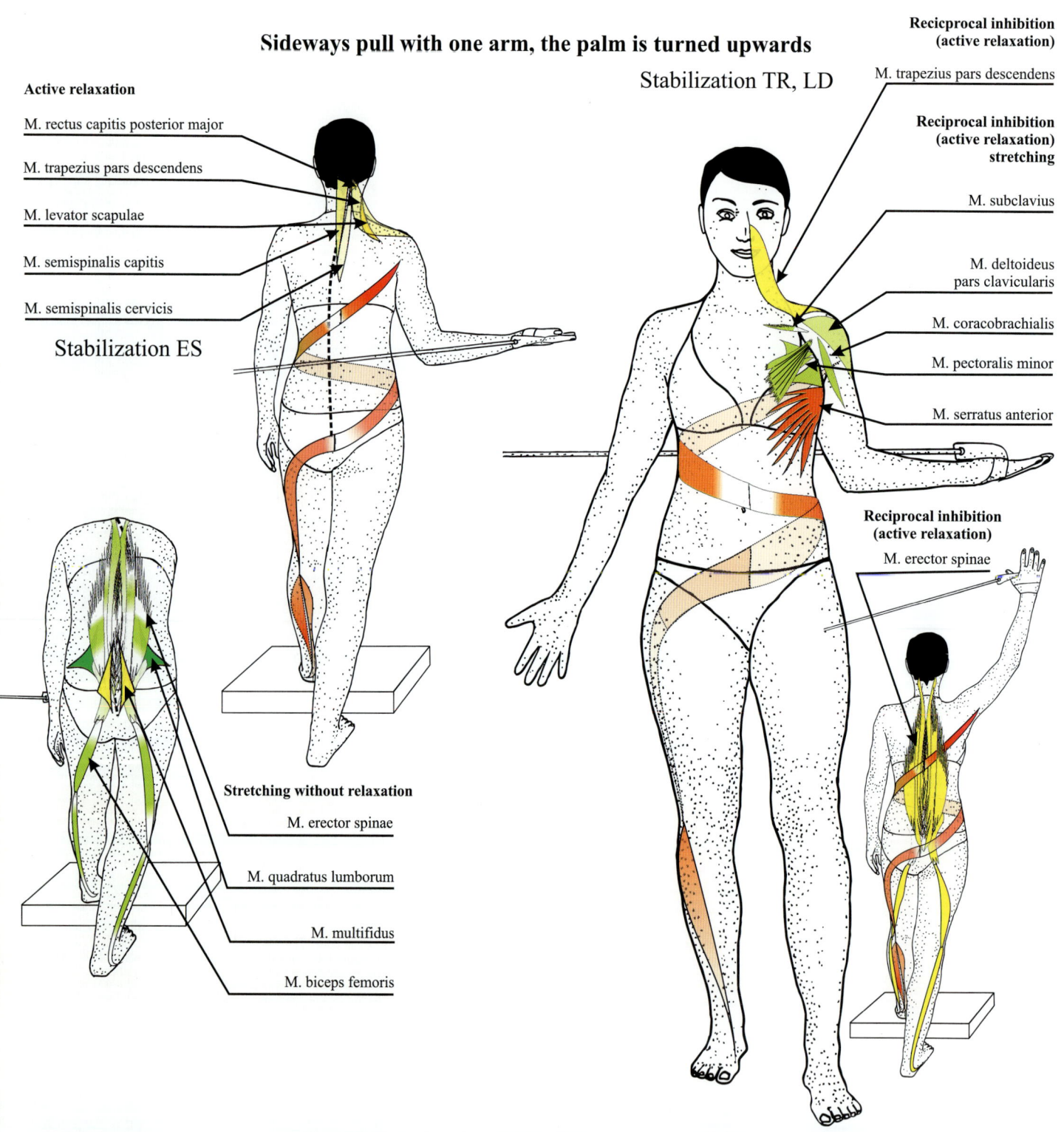

Sideways pull with one arm, the palm is turned upwards

Stabilization TR, LD

Active relaxation
- M. rectus capitis posterior major
- M. trapezius pars descendens
- M. levator scapulae
- M. semispinalis capitis
- M. semispinalis cervicis

Stabilization ES

Reciprocal inhibition (active relaxation)
- M. trapezius pars descendens

Reciprocal inhibition (active relaxation) stretching
- M. subclavius
- M. deltoideus pars clavicularis
- M. coracobrachialis
- M. pectoralis minor
- M. serratus anterior

Reciprocal inhibition (active relaxation)
- M. erector spinae

Stretching without relaxation
- M. erector spinae
- M. quadratus lumborum
- M. multifidus
- M. biceps femoris

1 - Initial position - passive part of the exercise
In the initial position these back muscles are stretched:
- m. erector spinae
- m. quadratus lumborum

2 - Performance - active part of the exercise
In the active part of the exercise the muscles in the anterior side of the shoulder girdle are stretched:
- m. subclavius
- m. pectoralis minor
- m. pectoralis major
- m. serratus anterior

2 - Performance - active part of the exercise
In the active part of the exercise the muscles in the upper part of the shoulder girdle are relaxed:
- m. trapezius pars descendens
- m. levator scapulae
- mm. scaleni
- m. semispinalis capitis, cervicis
and other muscles.

Exercise
M. erector spinae - exercise with stretching and active relaxation

Exercise 1 - standing facing the attachment point of the elastic rope with one leg on the mat, backward pull with both arms

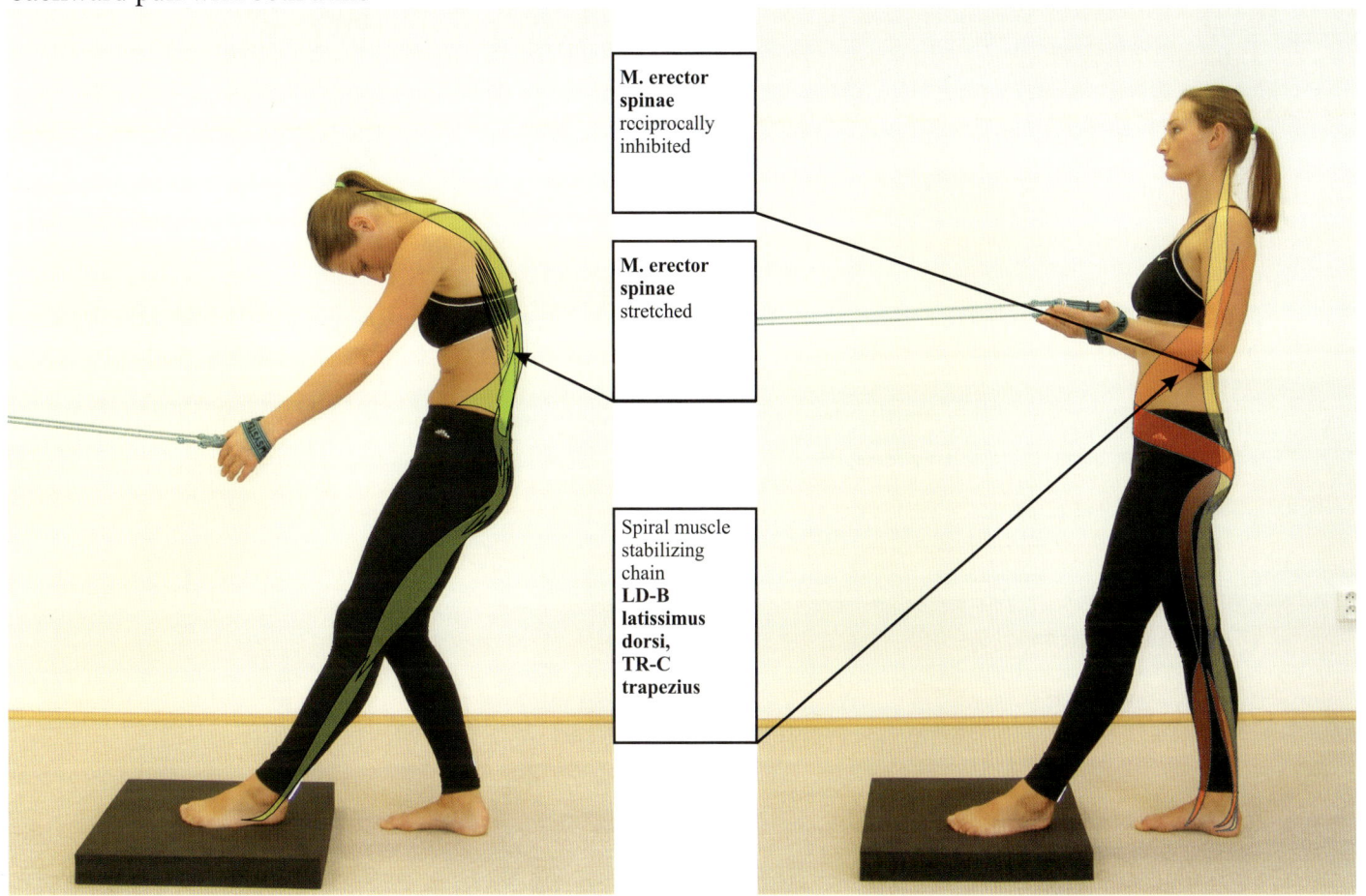

- M. erector spinae reciprocally inhibited
- M. erector spinae stretched
- Spiral muscle stabilizing chain **LD-B** latissimus dorsi, **TR-C** trapezius

M. erector spinae - exercise with stretching and active relaxation

Exercise 2 - standing sideways on to the attachment point of the elastic rope with one leg on the mat, sideways pull with one arm

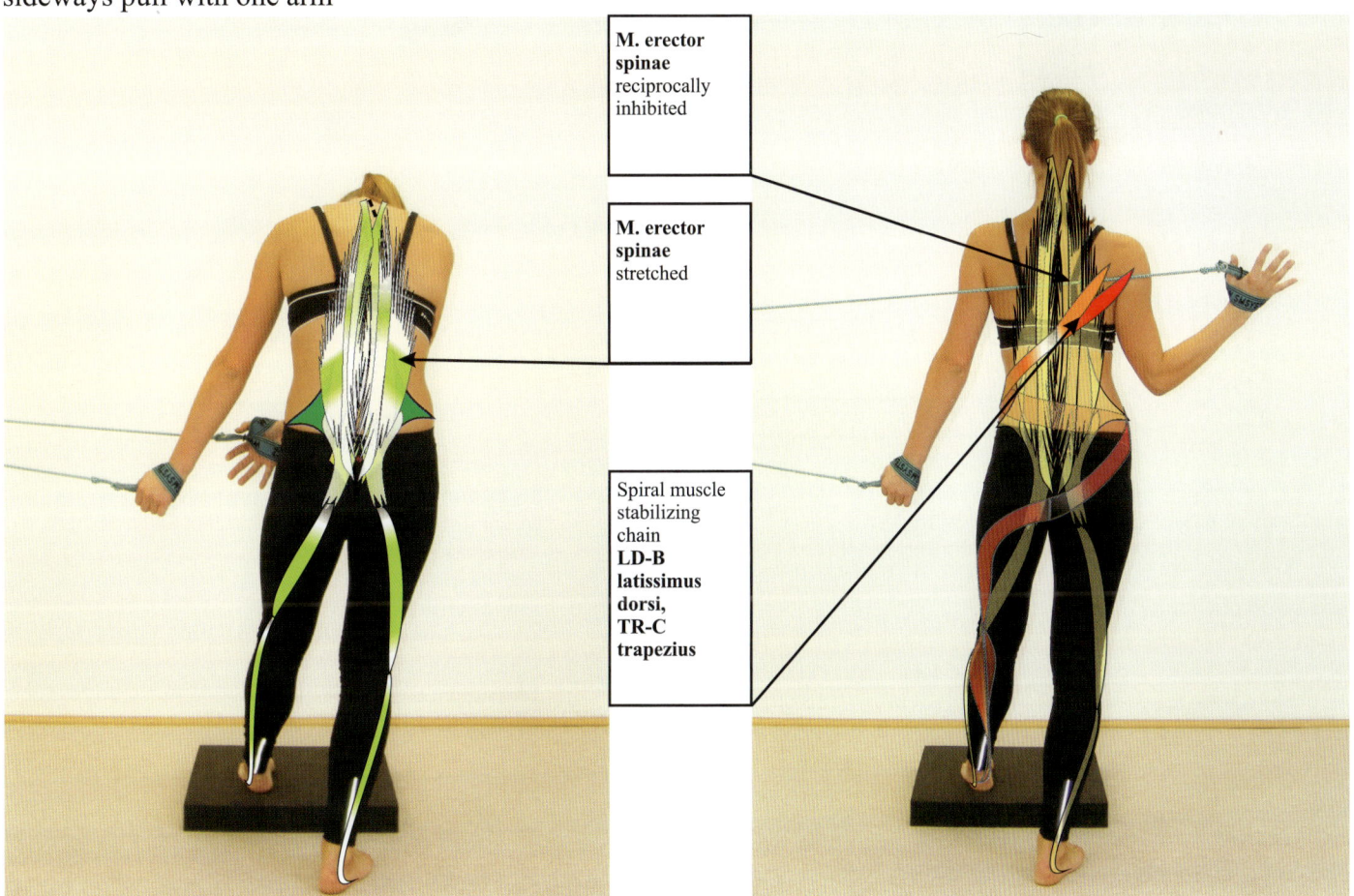

- M. erector spinae reciprocally inhibited
- M. erector spinae stretched
- Spiral muscle stabilizing chain **LD-B** latissimus dorsi, **TR-C** trapezius

Exercise - stabilization, stretching

M. erector spinae, m. iliocostalis, m. longissimus thoracis, m. longissimus capitis, cervicis, m. quadratus lumborum, m. multifidus
- relaxation in reciprocal inhibition, stretching

The PM - pectoralis major chain is the agonist in the first part of the exercise,
the LD - latissimus dorsi and TR - trapezius chains are the agonists in the second part of the exercise.

Exercise 3 - standing with back to the attachment point of the elastic rope, one leg is placed forward on the mat

Opening of the arms backwards, pulling the shoulder blades towards each other, palms turned upwards

Stabilization TR, LD   Stabilization PM

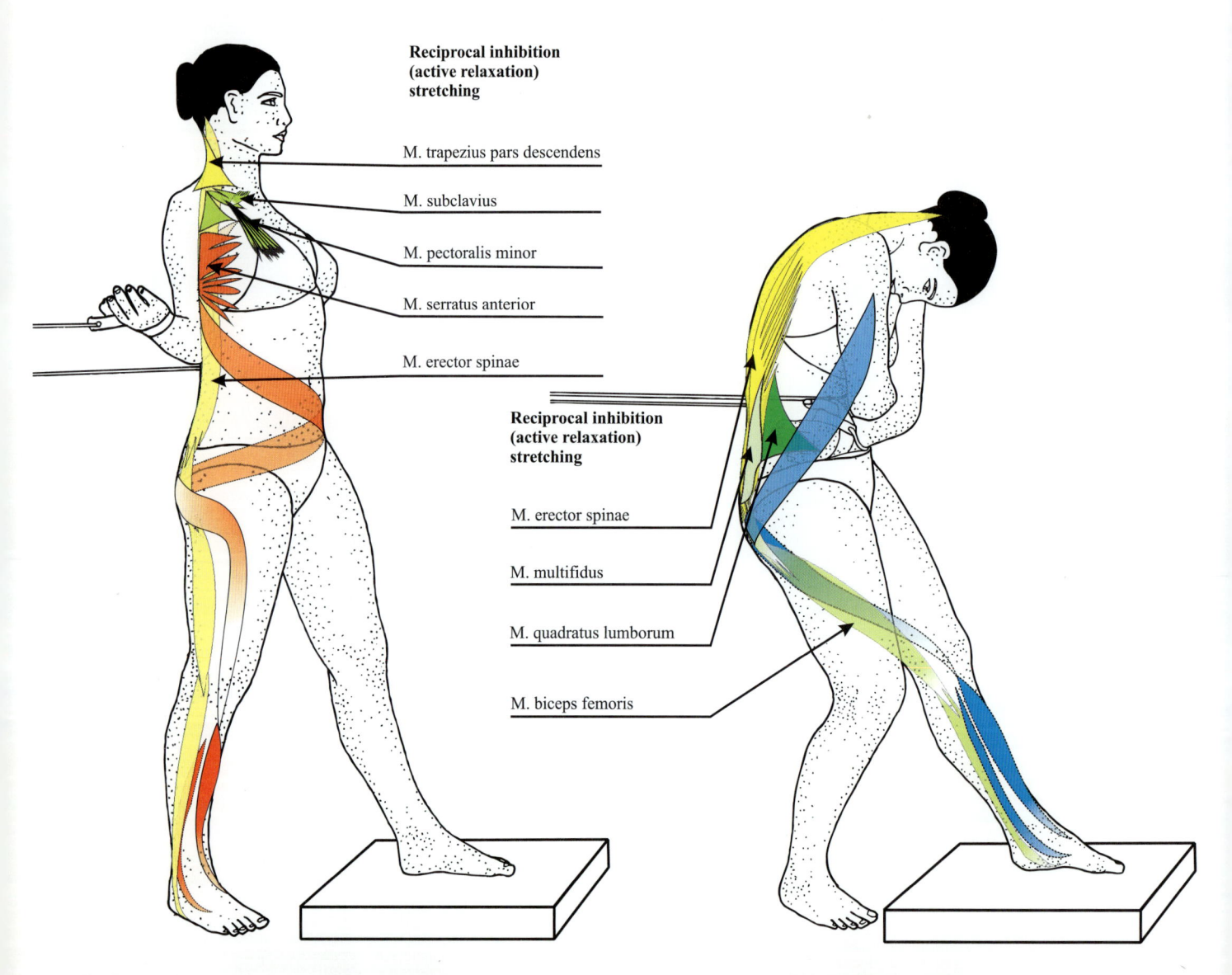

Reciprocal inhibition (active relaxation) stretching
- M. trapezius pars descendens
- M. subclavius
- M. pectoralis minor
- M. serratus anterior
- M. erector spinae

Reciprocal inhibition (active relaxation) stretching
- M. erector spinae
- M. multifidus
- M. quadratus lumborum
- M. biceps femoris

2 - Performance - active part of the exercise
In the active part of the exercise the muscles
in the anterior side of the shoulder girdle are stretched:
- m. subclavius
- m. pectoralis minor
- m. pectoralis major
- m. serratus anterior

In the upper part of the shoulder girdle the neck muscles are relaxed:
- m. trapezius pars descendens
- m. levator scapulae
- mm. scaleni
- m. semispinalis capitis, cervicis
and other muscles.

1 - Initial position - active part of the exercise
In the initial position these muscles are stretched:
- m. erector spinae
- m. quadratus lumborum
- m. multifidus
actively inhibited activity of the PM - pectoralis major chain.
Movement is stopped by tension in the ligamenta interspinalia.

Then the ischiocrural muscles are stretched
(muscles of the posterior side of the thigh):
- m. biceps femoris
- m. semitendinosus
- m. semimembranosus
- m. adductor magnus

Exercise - stabilization, stretching

M. erector spinae, m. iliocostalis, m. longissimus thoracis, m. longissimus capitis, cervicis, m. quadratus lumborum, m. multifidus
- relaxation in inhibition, stretching

The LD - latissimus dorsi and TR - trapezius chains are the agonists in the first part of the exercise, the SA - serratus anterior chain is the agonist in the second part of the exercise.

Exercise 6 - standing with back to the attachment point of the elastic rope, one leg is placed forward on the mat

Forward circles with both arms

Stabilization TR, LD   Stabilization SA

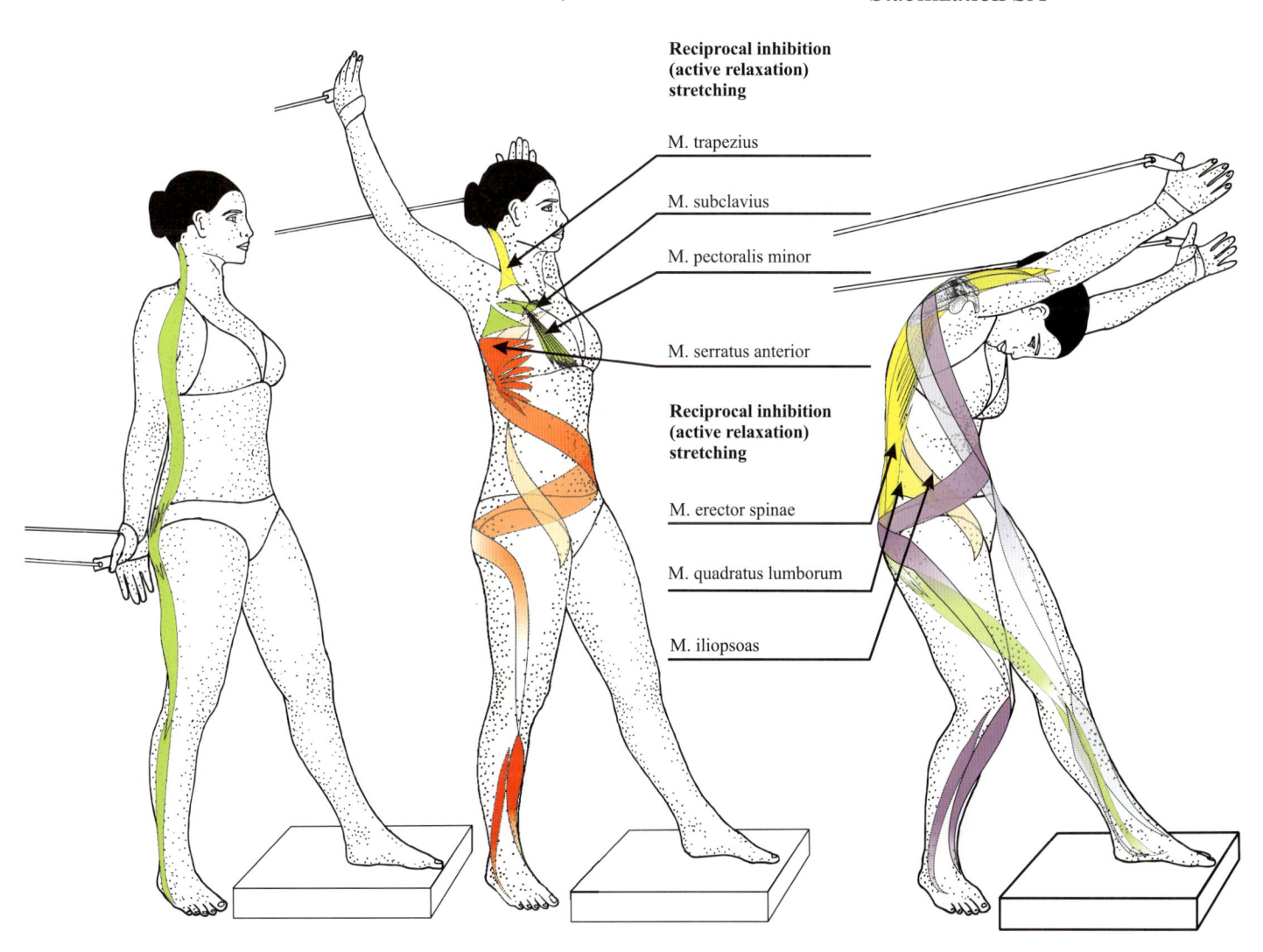

Reciprocal inhibition (active relaxation) stretching
- M. trapezius
- M. subclavius
- M. pectoralis minor
- M. serratus anterior

Reciprocal inhibition (active relaxation) stretching
- M. erector spinae
- M. quadratus lumborum
- M. iliopsoas

1 - First part of performace - active part of exercise
The muscles in the anterior side of the shoulder girdle are stretched:
- m. subclavius
- m. pectoralis minor
- m. pectoralis major
- m. serratus anterior

The muscles in the upper side of the shoulder girdle are relaxed:
- m. trapezius pars descendens
- m. levator scapulae
- mm. scaleni
- m. semispinalis capitis, cervicis etc.

2 - Performance - active part of exercise
This exercise stretches these actively inhibited back muscles:
- m. erector spinae
- m. quadratus lumborum
- m. iliopsoas

Exercise
M. erector spinae - exercise with stretching and active relaxation

Exercise 3 - standing with back to the attachment point of the elastic rope with one leg on the mat, opening of the arms backwards, shoulder blades pulled towards each other

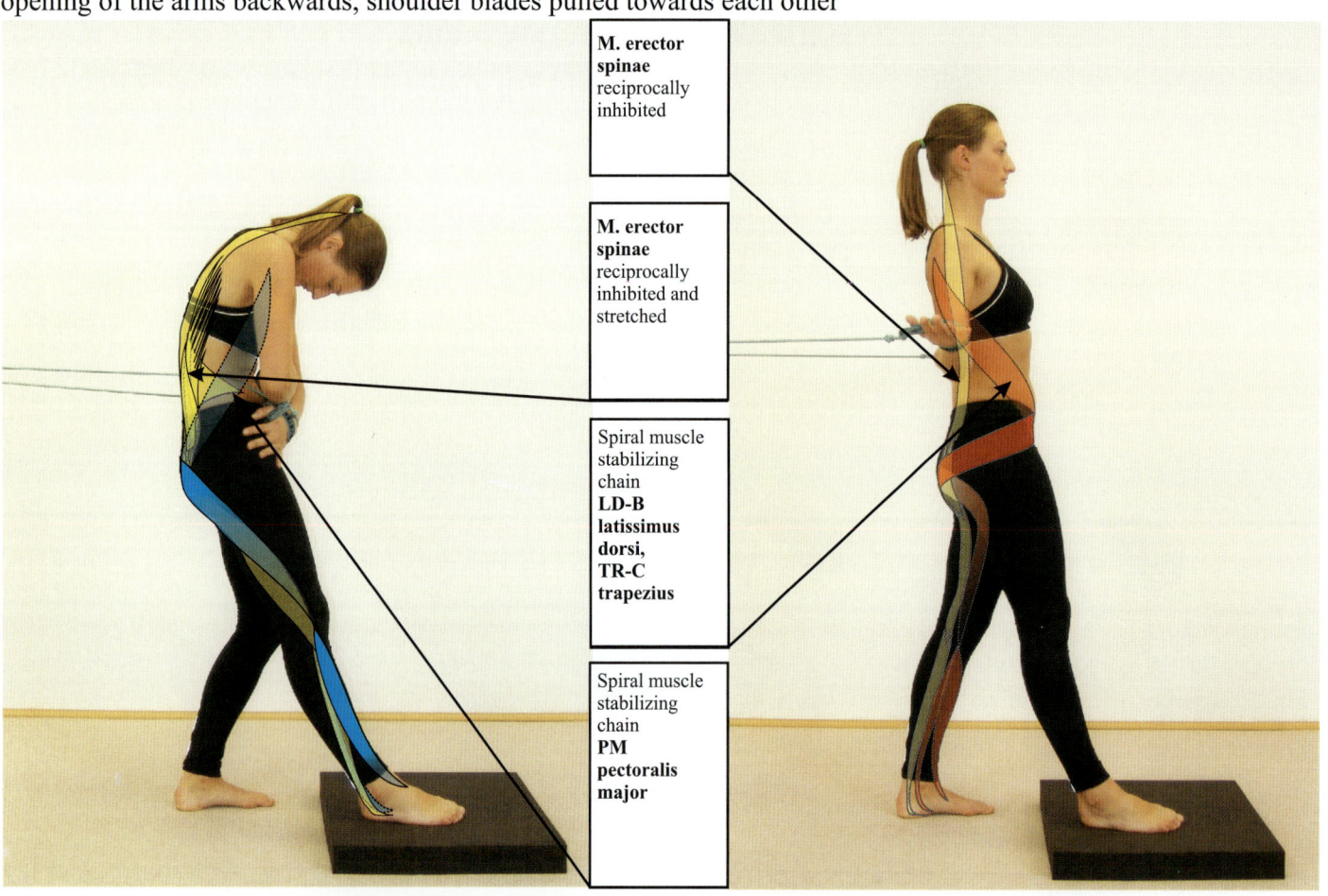

- M. erector spinae reciprocally inhibited
- M. erector spinae reciprocally inhibited and stretched
- Spiral muscle stabilizing chain **LD-B latissimus dorsi, TR-C trapezius**
- Spiral muscle stabilizing chain **PM pectoralis major**

M. erector spinae - exercise with active relaxation and stretching

Exercise 6 - standing with back to the attachment point of the elastic rope with one leg on the mat, forward circles with both arms

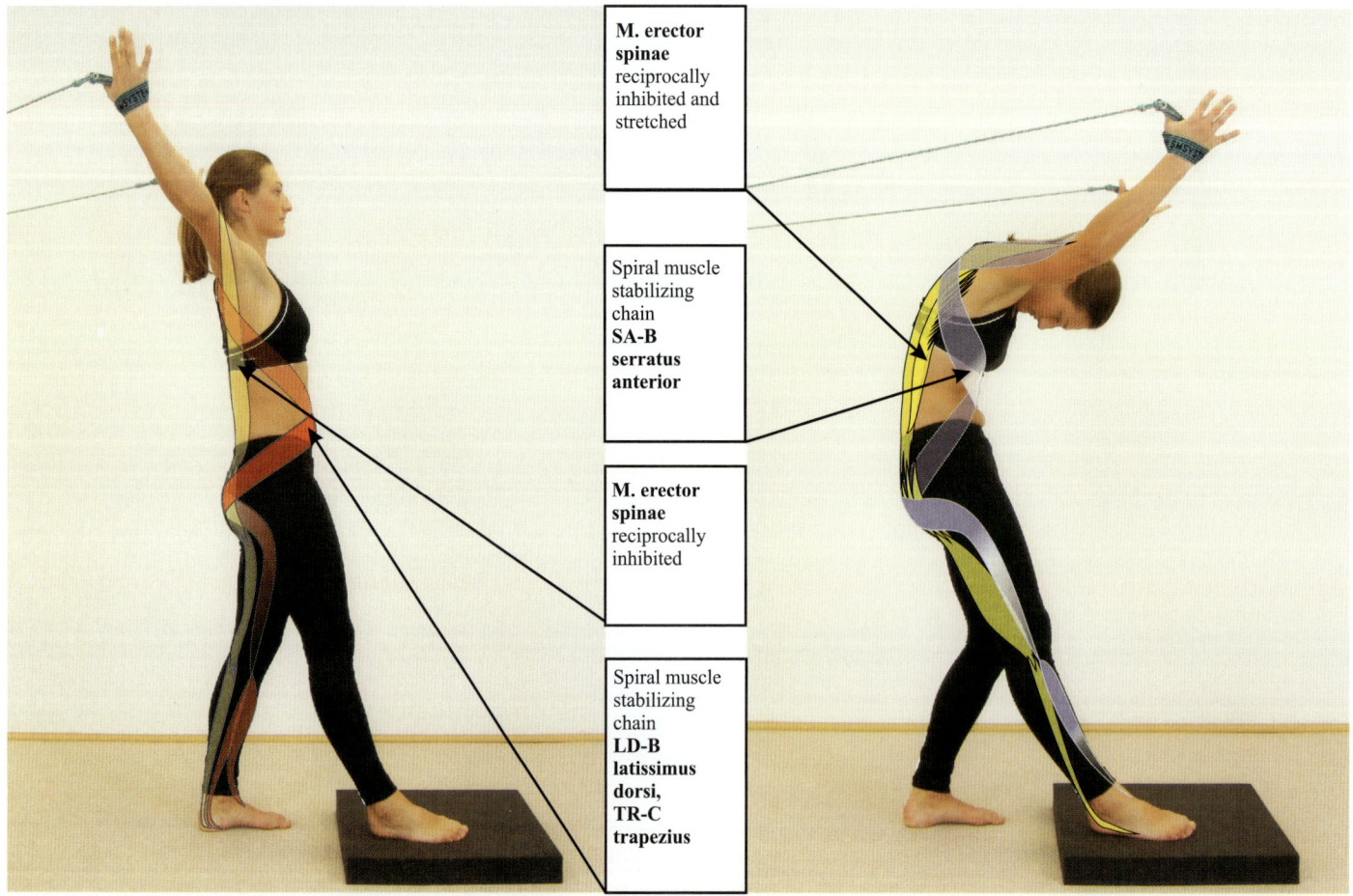

- M. erector spinae reciprocally inhibited and stretched
- Spiral muscle stabilizing chain **SA-B serratus anterior**
- M. erector spinae reciprocally inhibited
- Spiral muscle stabilizing chain **LD-B latissimus dorsi, TR-C trapezius**

Exercise - stabilization stretching

M. erector spinae, m. iliocostalis, m. longissimus thoracis, m. longissimus capitis, cervicis, m. quadratus lumborum, m. multifidus
- relaxation in reciprocal inhibition, stretching

The LD - latissimus dorsi and TR - trapezius chains are the agonists in the second part of the exercise.

Exercise 5 - kneeling facing the attachment point of the elastic rope, one leg is extended forward

Stretching the back in an extended forward arch, straightening the trunk, backward pull with both arms, palms turned upwards

Stabilization ES   Stabilization TR, LD

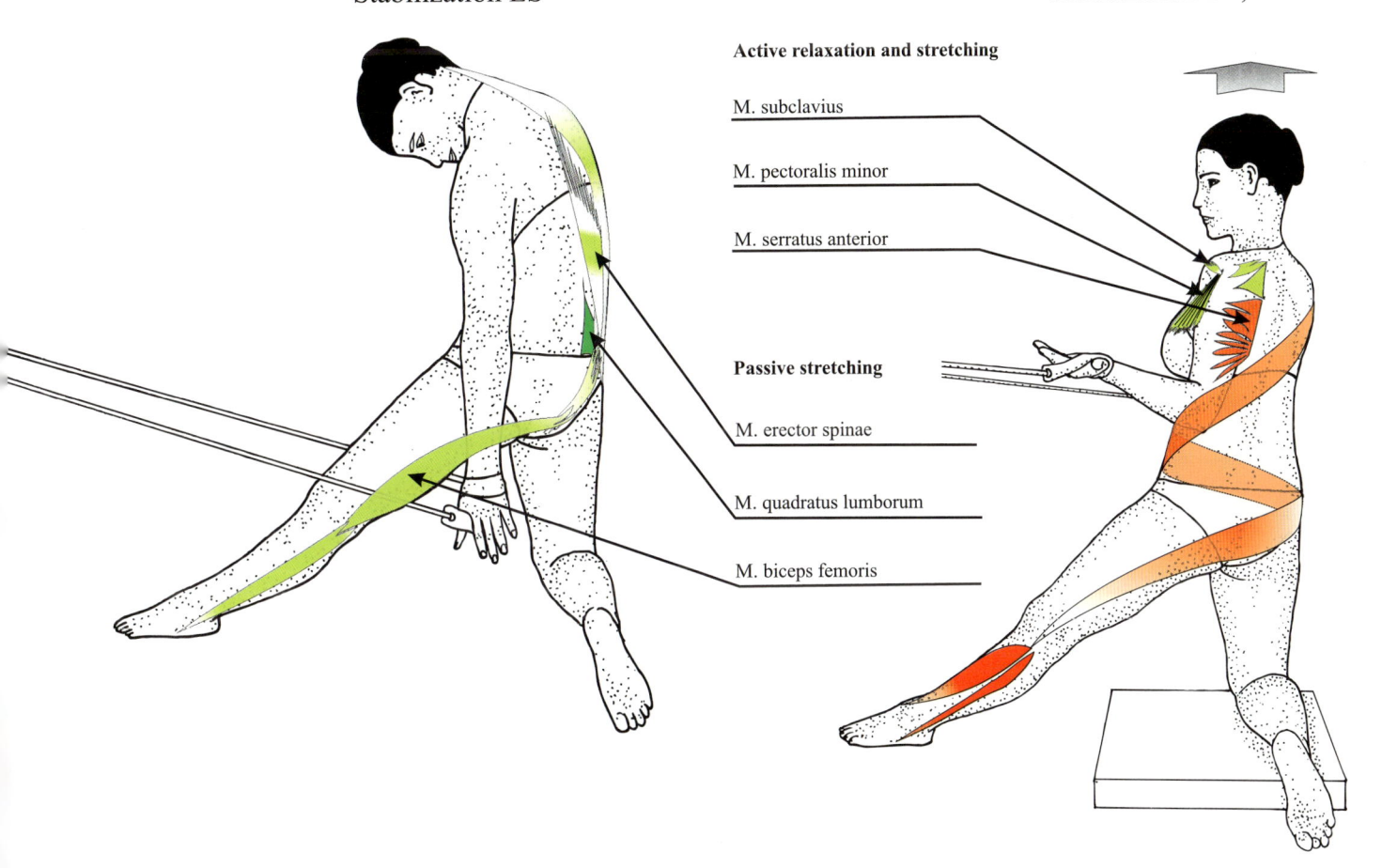

Active relaxation and stretching
M. subclavius
M. pectoralis minor
M. serratus anterior

Passive stretching
M. erector spinae
M. quadratus lumborum
M. biceps femoris

1 - Initial position - passive part of the exercise
In the initial position these back muscles are stretched:
- m. erector spinae
- m. quadratus lumborum
- m. multifidus

The ischiocrural muscles (muscles in the posterior side of the thigh) are also stretched:
- m. biceps femoris
- m. semitendinosus
- m. semimembranosus
- m. adductor magnus

2 - Performace - active part of the exercise
In the active part of the exercise the muscles in the anterior side of the shoulder girdle are stretched:
- m. subclaviuus
- m. pectoralis minor
- m. pectoralis major
- m. serratus anterior

The muscles in the upper side of the shoulder girdle are relaxed:
- m. trapezius pars descendens
- m. levator scapulae
- mm. scaleni
- m. semispinalis capitis, cervicis and other muscles.

Exercise

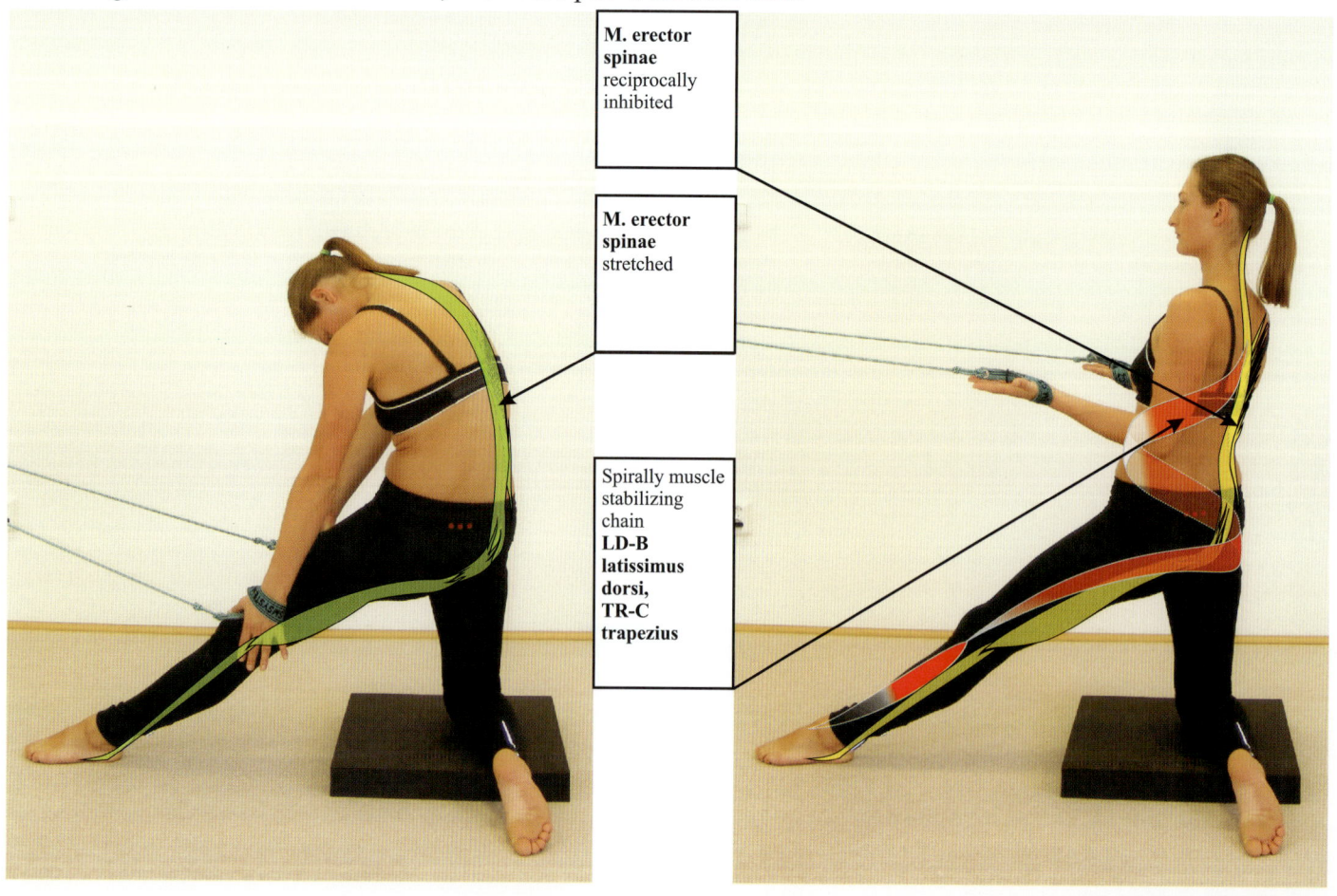

M. erector spinae - passive stretching, active relaxation

Exercise 5 - sitting facing the attachment point of the elastic rope, one leg is extended forward, stretching the back in a forward arch, backward pull with both arms

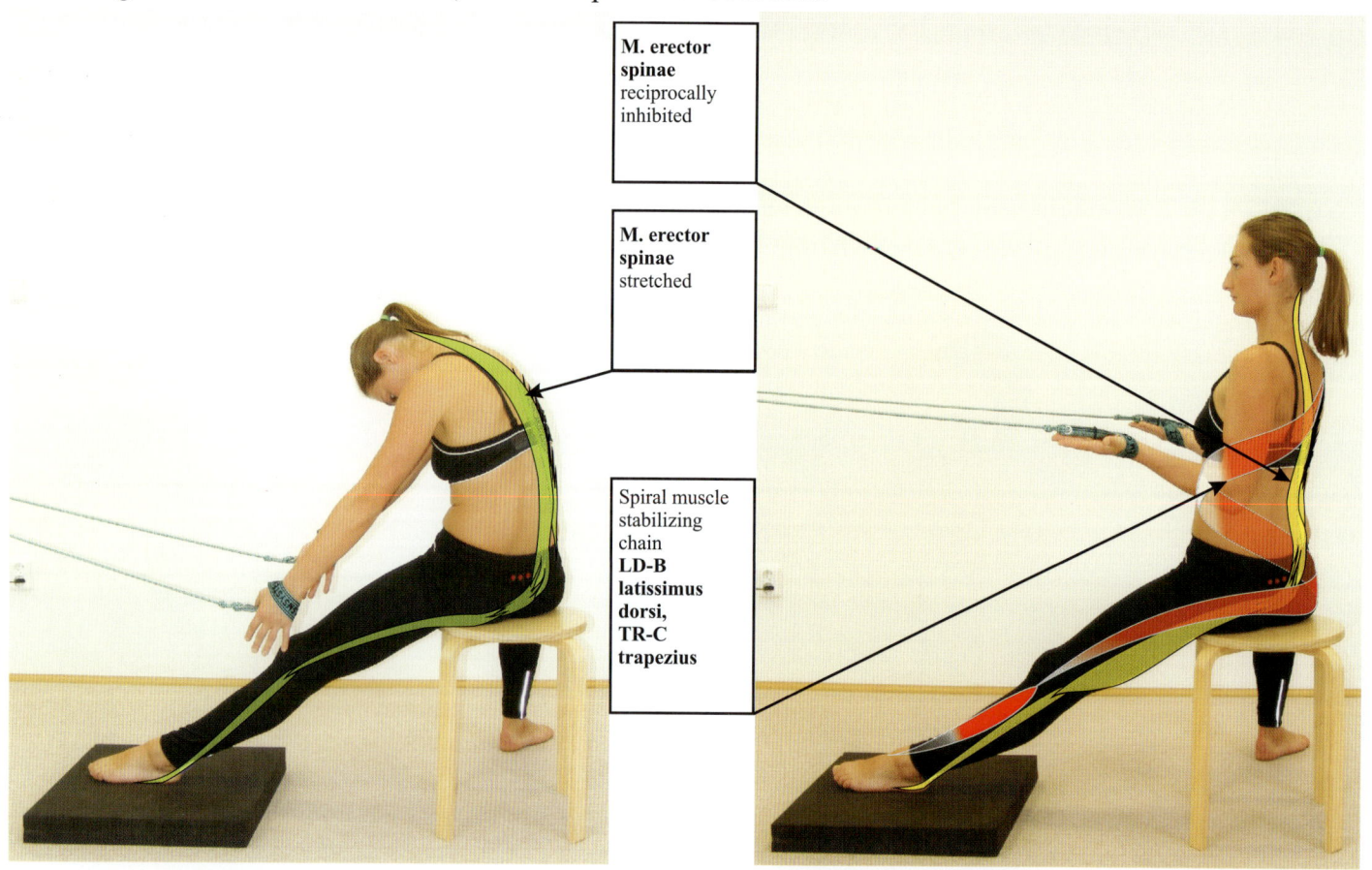

M. erector spinae reciprocally inhibited

M. erector spinae stretched

Spiral muscle stabilizing chain **LD-B** latissimus dorsi, **TR-C** trapezius

M. erector spinae - passive stretching, active relaxation

Exercise 5 - kneeling facing the attachment point of the elastic rope, one leg is extended forward, stretching the back in a forward arch, backward pull with both arms

M. erector spinae reciprocally inhibited

M. erector spinae stretched

Spirally muscle stabilizing chain **LD-B** latissimus dorsi, **TR-C** trapezius

MANUAL TECHNIQUES AND EXERCISE ACCORDING TO MUSCLE ANALYSIS

Trunk and neck
Paravertebral muscles
The posterior
upper muscle group

Muscles with a tendency towards tension and shortening:

M. semispinalis capitis
M. semispinalis cervicis
M. rectus capitis posterior major
M. rectus capitis posterior minor
M. obliquus capitis superior
M. obliquus capitis inferior

Anatomy
M. semispinalis capitis, cervicis

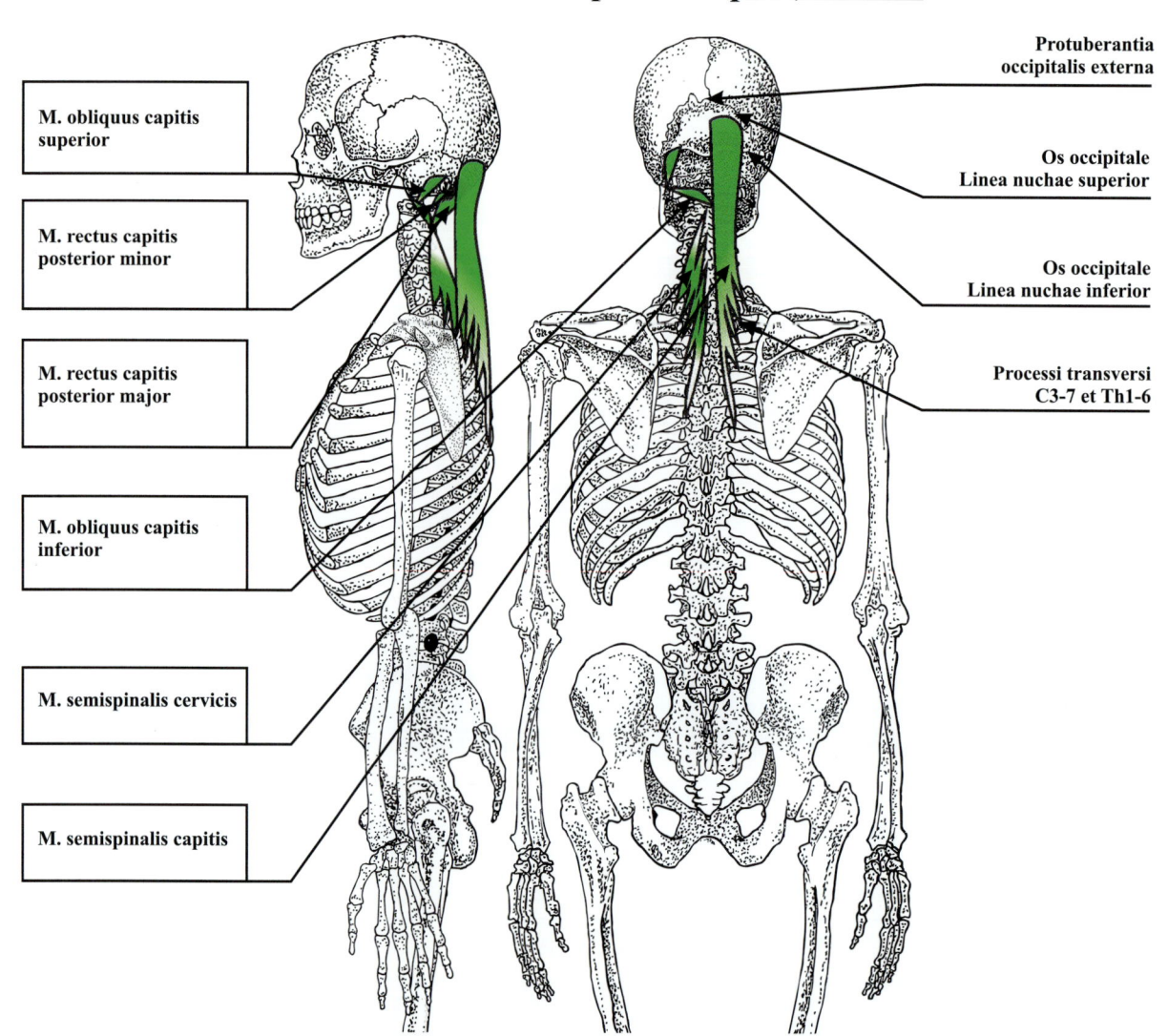

M. obliquus capitis superior

M. rectus capitis posterior minor

M. rectus capitis posterior major

M. obliquus capitis inferior

M. semispinalis cervicis

M. semispinalis capitis

Protuberantia occipitalis externa

Os occipitale Linea nuchae superior

Os occipitale Linea nuchae inferior

Processi transversi C3-7 et Th1-6

M. semispinalis cervicis
Origin:
- processi transversi Th1-6
Insertion:
- processi spinosi C2-6
Function:
   - bilateral contraction:
- extension of the neck
   - unilateral contraction:
- lateral flexion to the corresponding side
- rotation to the contralateral side
Innervation:
- rr. dorsales of the spinal nerves (C-Th transition)

M. semispinalis capitis
Origin:
- processi transversi C3-7, Th1-6
Insertion:
- processi spinosi C2-6
Function:
   - bilateral contraction:
- extension of the neck
   - unilateral contraction:
- lateral flexion to the corresponding side
- rotation to the contralateral side (head, neck, chest)
Innervation:
- rr. dorsales of the spinal nerves (C-Th transition)

M. rectus capitis posterior major
Origin:
- processus spinosus axis
Insertion:
- central third linea nuchae inferior

M. rectus capitis posterior minor
Origin:
- tuberculum posteruis atlantis
Insertion:
- inner third linea nuchae inferior
Function:
   - bilateral contraction:
- extension of the head
   - unilateral contraction:
- lateral flexion to the corresponding side
- rotation to the corresponding side
Innervation:
- ramus dorsalis C1 (n. suboccipitalis)

M. obliquus capitis superior
Origin:
- processus transversus atlantis
Insertion:
- linea nuchae inferior lateral third, above the attachment m. rectus capitis posterior major
Function:
   - bilateral contraction:
- dorsal extension of the head
   - unilateral contraction:
- lateral flexion to the corresponding side
- rotation to the opposite side
Innervation:
- ramus dorsalis C1 (n. suboccipitalis)

M. obliquus capitis inferior
Origin:
- processus spinosus axis
Insertion:
- processus transversus atlantis
Function:
   - bilateral contraction:
- dorsal extension of the head
   - unilateral contraction:
- rotation to the corresponding side
Innervation:
- ramus dorsalis C1 (n. suboccipitalis)

Muscle chains
Vertical muscle chain ES - erector spinae

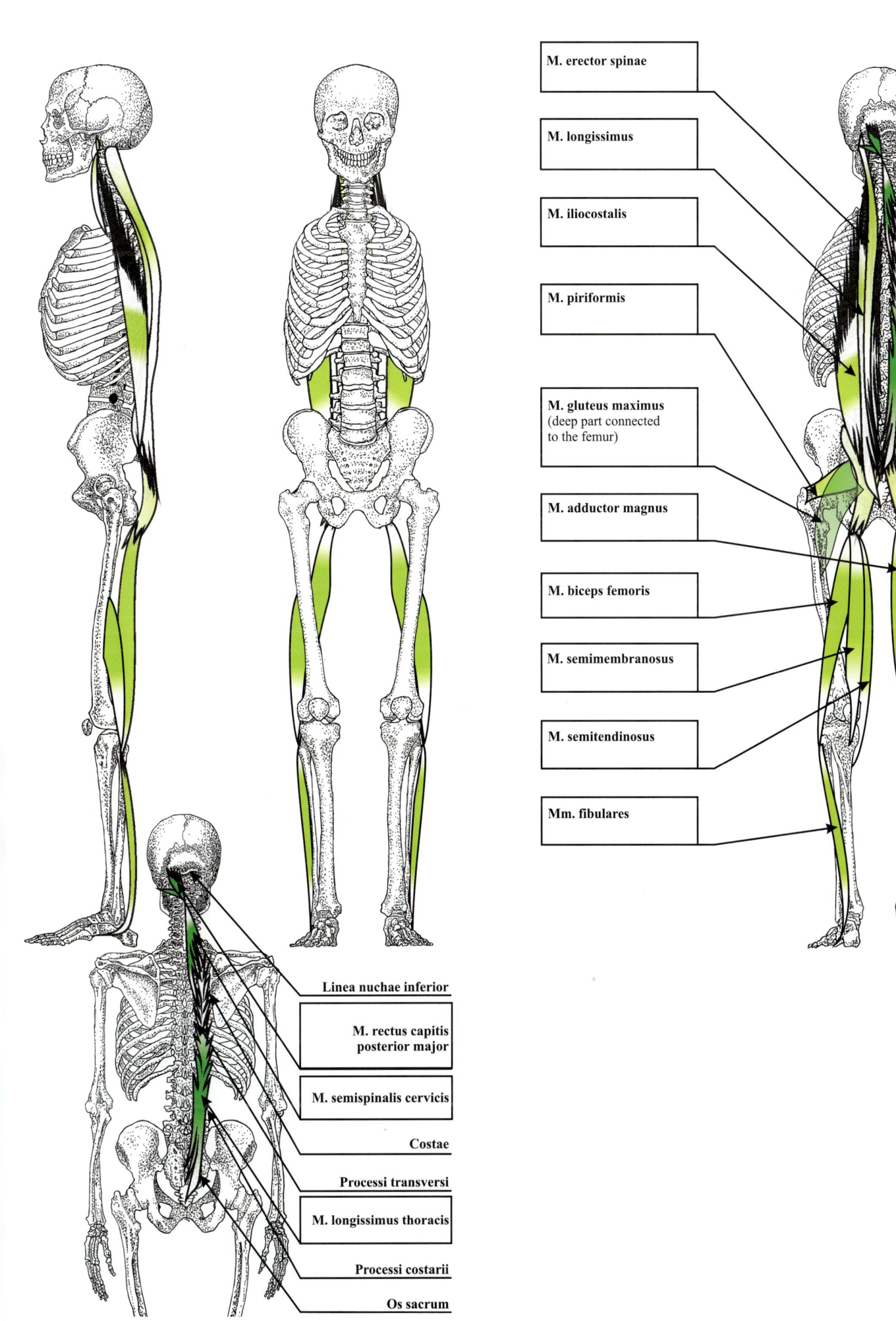

- M. erector spinae
- M. longissimus
- M. iliocostalis
- M. piriformis
- M. gluteus maximus (deep part connected to the femur)
- M. adductor magnus
- M. biceps femoris
- M. semimembranosus
- M. semitendinosus
- Mm. fibulares

- Linea nuchae inferior
- M. rectus capitis posterior major
- M. semispinalis cervicis
- Costae
- Processi transversi
- M. longissimus thoracis
- Processi costarii
- Os sacrum

- 75 -

Manual techniques lying on one side
M. semispinalis capitis, cervicis - massage with stretching

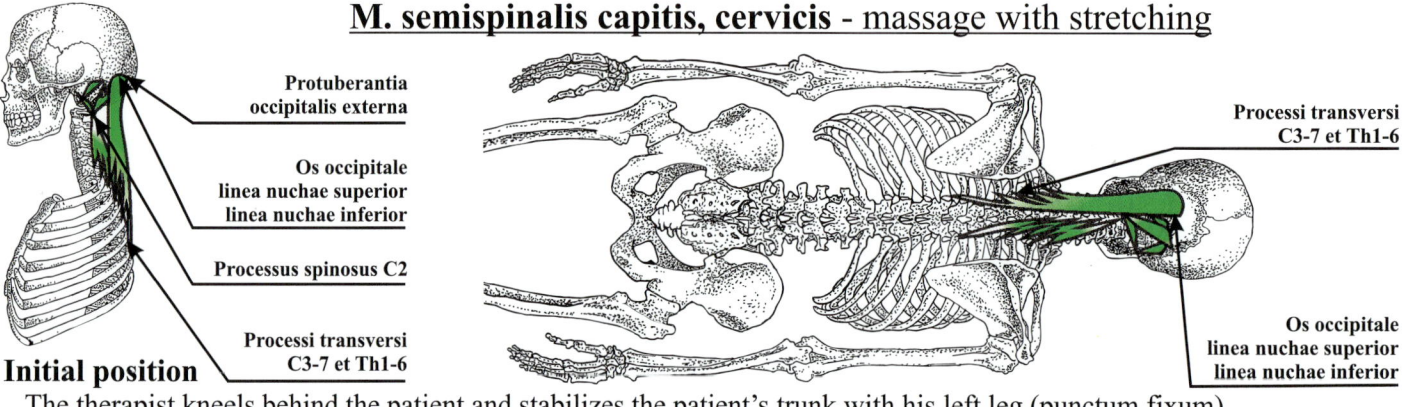

Labels (left illustration): Protuberantia occipitalis externa; Os occipitale linea nuchae superior, linea nuchae inferior; Processus spinosus C2; Processi transversi C3-7 et Th1-6

Labels (right illustration): Processi transversi C3-7 et Th1-6; Os occipitale linea nuchae superior, linea nuchae inferior

Initial position
The therapist kneels behind the patient and stabilizes the patient's trunk with his left leg (punctum fixum). The left palm rests on the shoulder and the fingers point backwards. The thenar and thumb of the right hand press next to the processes of the upper thoracic spine. The patient breathes in.

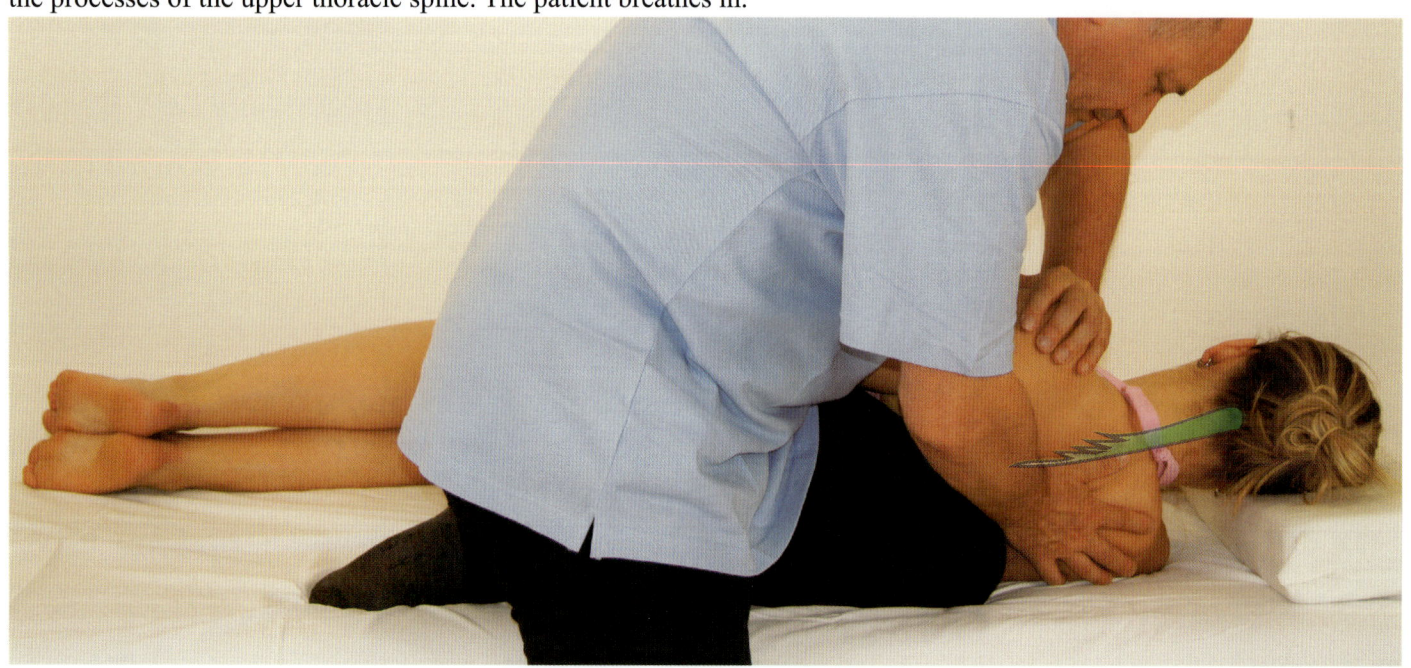

Performance
The therapist's right hand moves slowly cranially (upwards) (punctum mobile). This massages the m. semispinalis capitis and cervicis. The extension is held until the os occipitale is reached. The patient slowly breathes out. The pulling is slackened and the stretching is repeated 6 times. At the end of the technique the therapist pauses for about 3 seconds.

PIR. The extension is held and the patient breathes in. This causes a counter-pressure. When breathing out, the patient achieves further stretching. The process is repeated 3 times. This technique stretches the m. semispinalis capitis, cervicis and other neck muscles. This prepares the patient for relaxation of the neck during exercise.

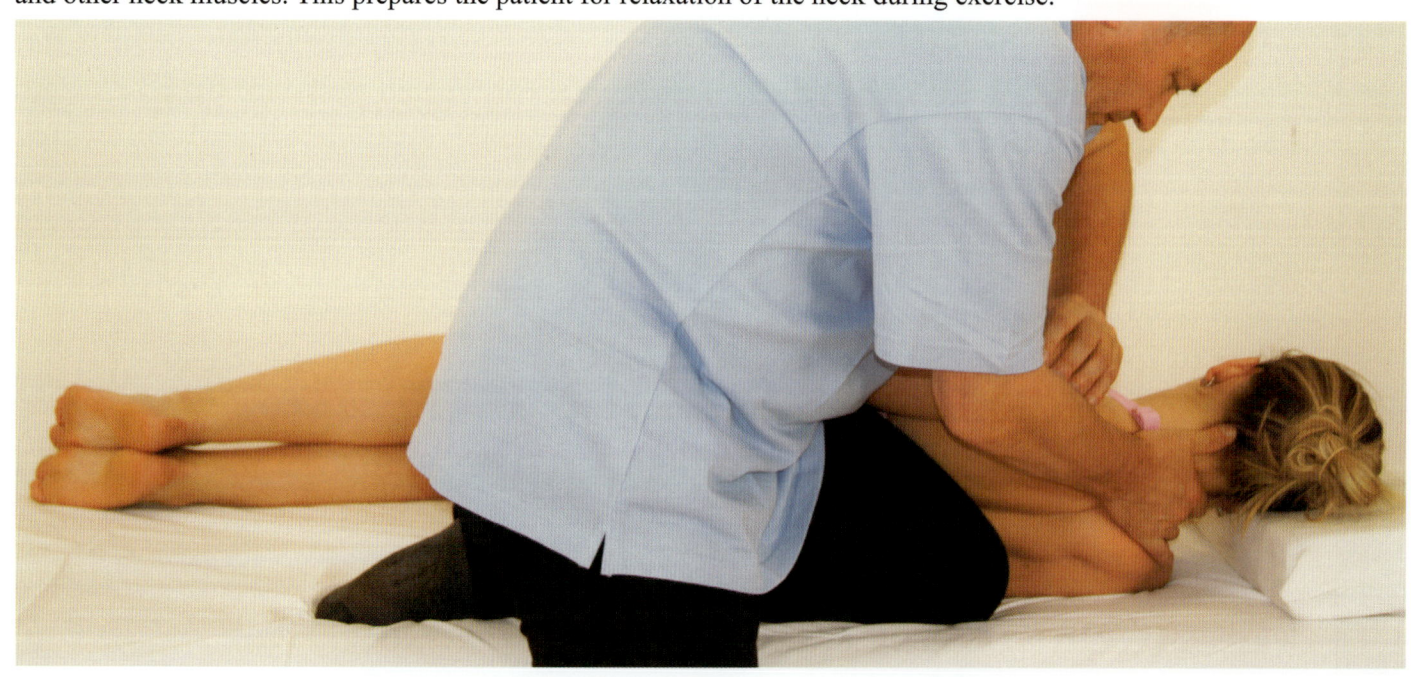

Manual techniques lying on one side
M. semispinalis capitis, cervicis - massage with stretching

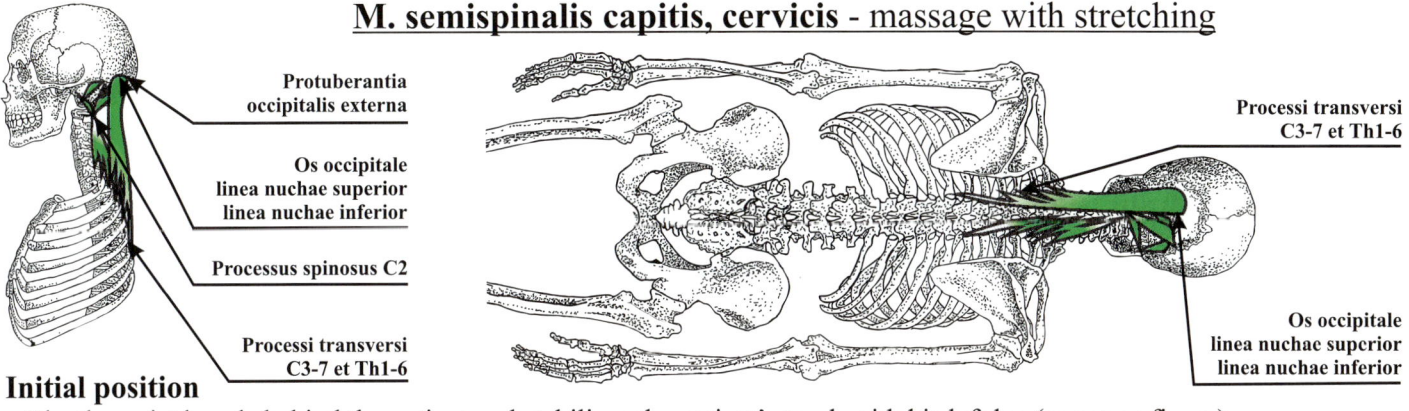

Protuberantia occipitalis externa
Os occipitale linea nuchae superior linea nuchae inferior
Processus spinosus C2
Processi transversi C3-7 et Th1-6

Processi transversi C3-7 et Th1-6
Os occipitale linea nuchae superior linea nuchae inferior

Initial position
The therapist kneels behind the patient and stabilizes the patient's trunk with his left leg (punctum fixum). The left arm changes grip and the flexor side of the forearm rests against the shoulder. Right thumb pad rests against the os occipitale and processus mastoideus. The fingers gently hold the neck from the side. The patient breathes in.

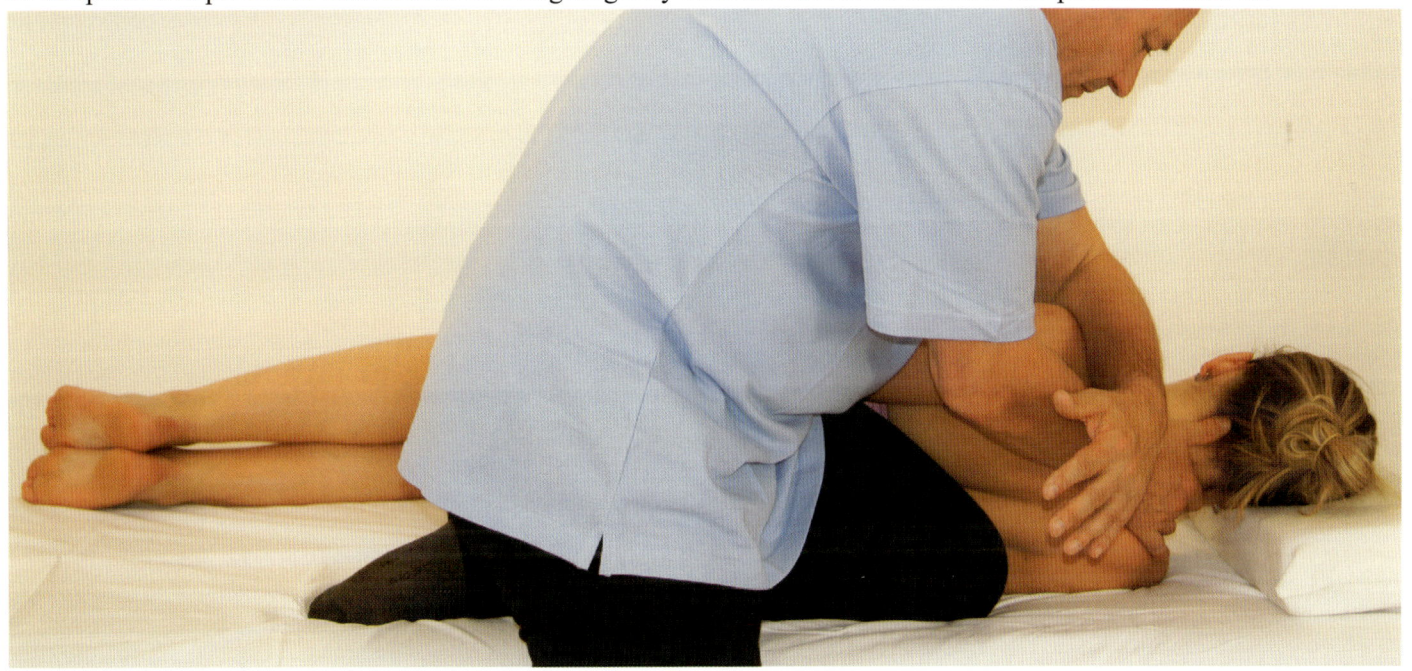

Performance
The therapist moves the whole of his body and, at the same time, moves his left forearm caudally (downwards), (punctum mobile). This stretches the m. semispinalis capitis and cervicis. The patient slowly breathes out. The pulling is slackened and the stretching is repeated 6 times. At the end of the technique the therapist pauses for about 3 seconds. The patient breathes out slowly.

PIR. The extension is held and the patient breathes in. This causes a counter-pressure. When breathing out, the patient achieves further stretching. The process is repeated 3 times. This technique stretches the m. semispinalis capitis, cervicis and other neck muscles. This prepares the patient for relaxation of the neck during exercise.

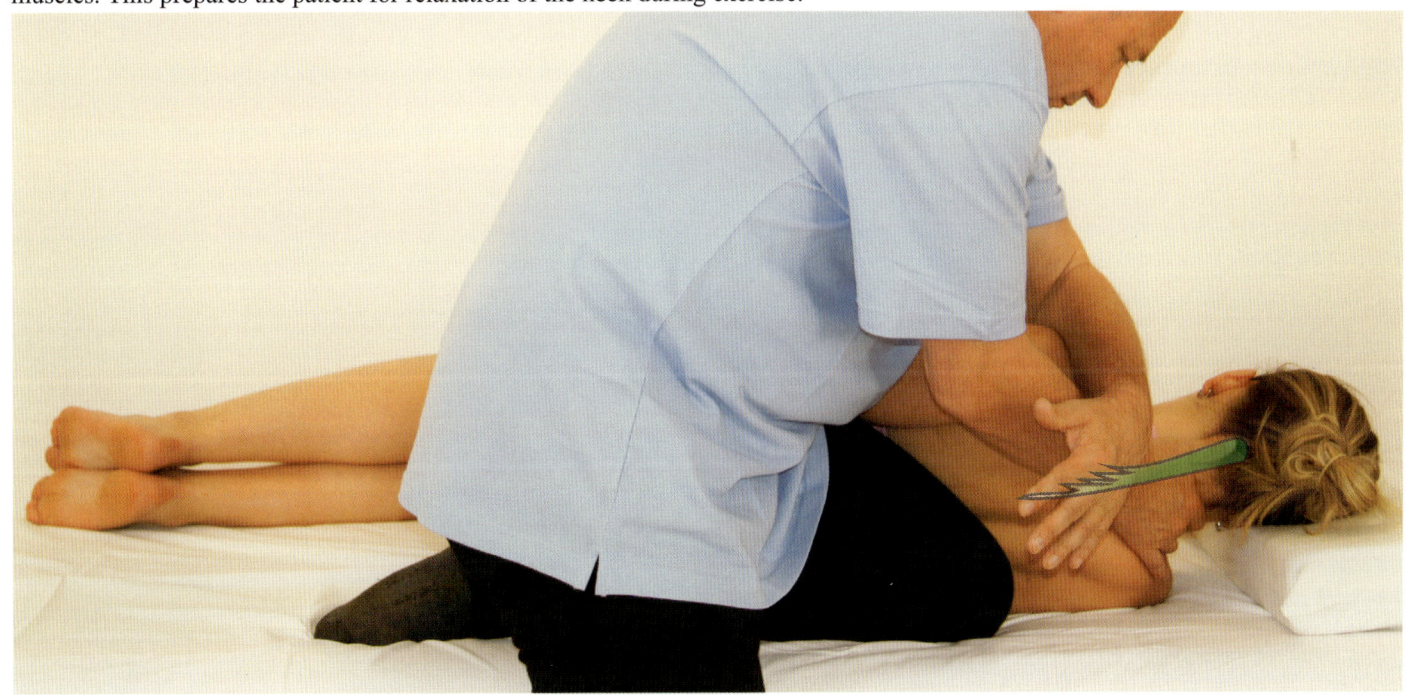

Manual techniques lying on the back in a hoist
M. semispinalis capitis, cervicis - massage with stretching

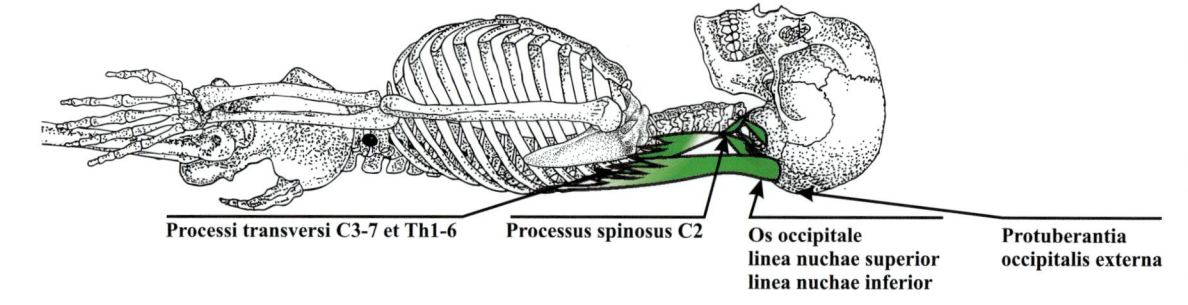

Processi transversi C3-7 et Th1-6 — Processus spinosus C2 — Os occipitale linea nuchae superior linea nuchae inferior — Protuberantia occipitalis externa

Initial position
The patient's trunk lies on the back on the bed (punctum fixum). The therapist stands behind the patient's head with one leg forward and the other behind. The therapist's fingers press on both sides of the spine towards the processi transversi. The patient breathes in.

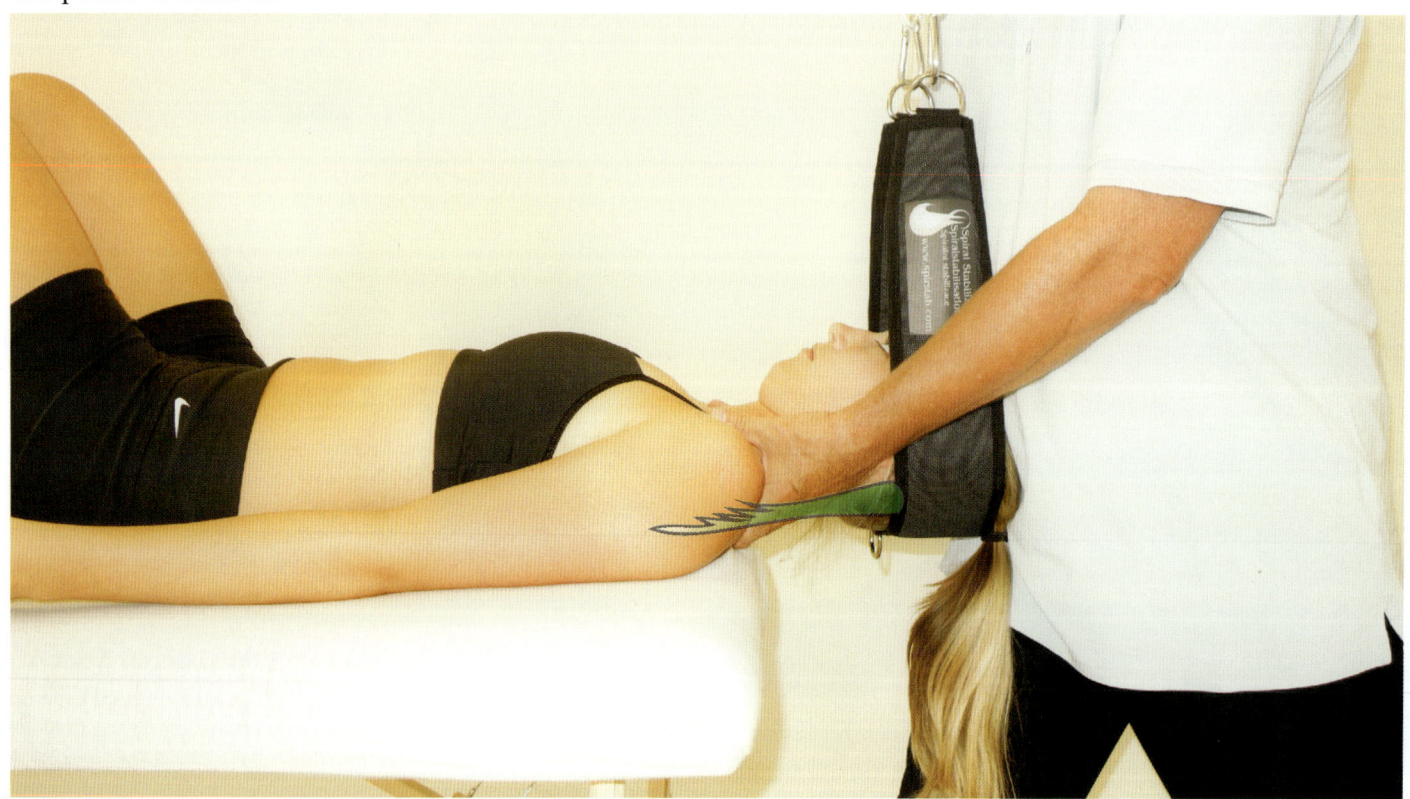

Performance
The therapist's whole body moves backwards. At the same time he moves his arms cranially (towards the head) on both sides of the spine. At the end of the movement he grasps the lower jaw and slightly rotates the head with the axis in the outer ear. This stretches m. semispinalis capitis and cervicis and the short neck extensors. The patient breathes out slowly. The pulling is slackened and the stretching is repeated 6 times. At the end of the technique the therapist pauses for about 3 seconds.

PIR. The extension is held and the patient breathes in. This causes a counter-pressure. When breathing out, the patient achieves further stretching. This process is repeated 3 times. This technique stretches the m. semispinalis capitis, cervicis and other neck muscles. This prepares the patient for relaxation of the neck during exercise.

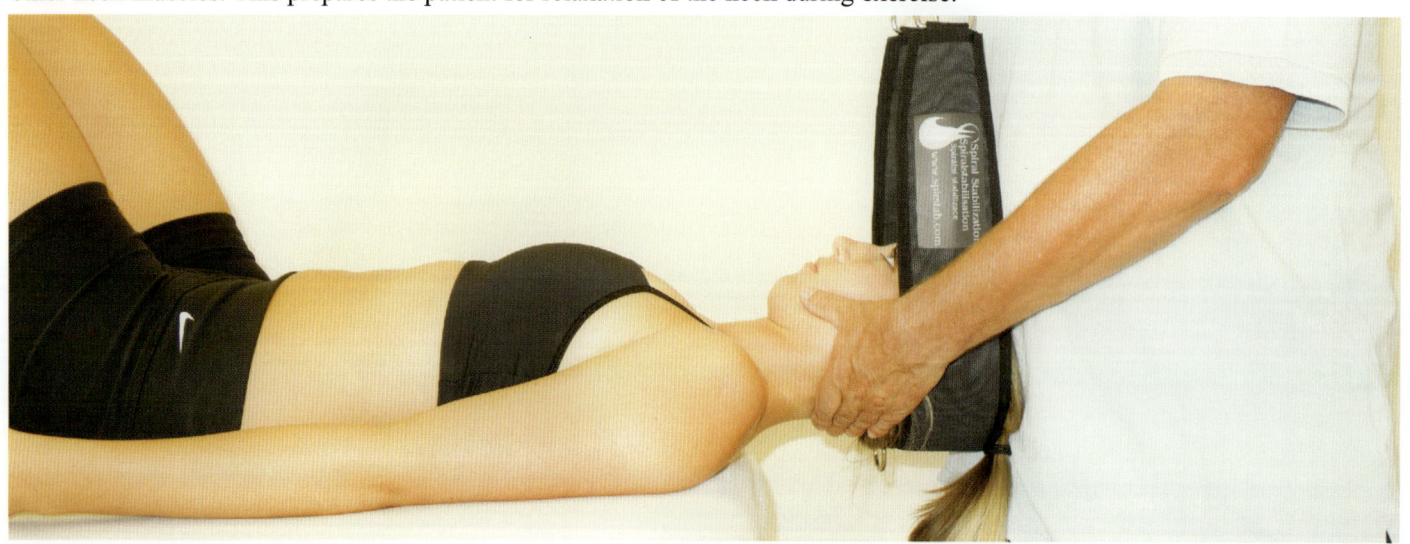

Manual techniques lying on the back in a hoist
M. rectus capitis posterior major, minor, m. obliquus capitis superior, inferior
- massage with stretching

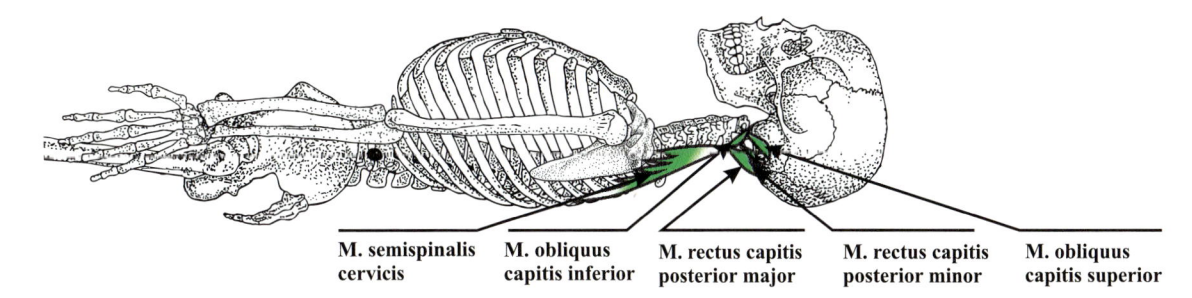

| M. semispinalis cervicis | M. obliquus capitis inferior | M. rectus capitis posterior major | M. rectus capitis posterior minor | M. obliquus capitis superior |

Initial position

The patient's lies on the back on the bed (punctum fixum). The therapist stands behinds the patient's head with one leg forward and the other behind. The therapists's right hand grasps the lower jaw from in front. His left index finger is placed between the C2 process and the os occipitale and the thumb is on the lower jaw. The patient breathes in.

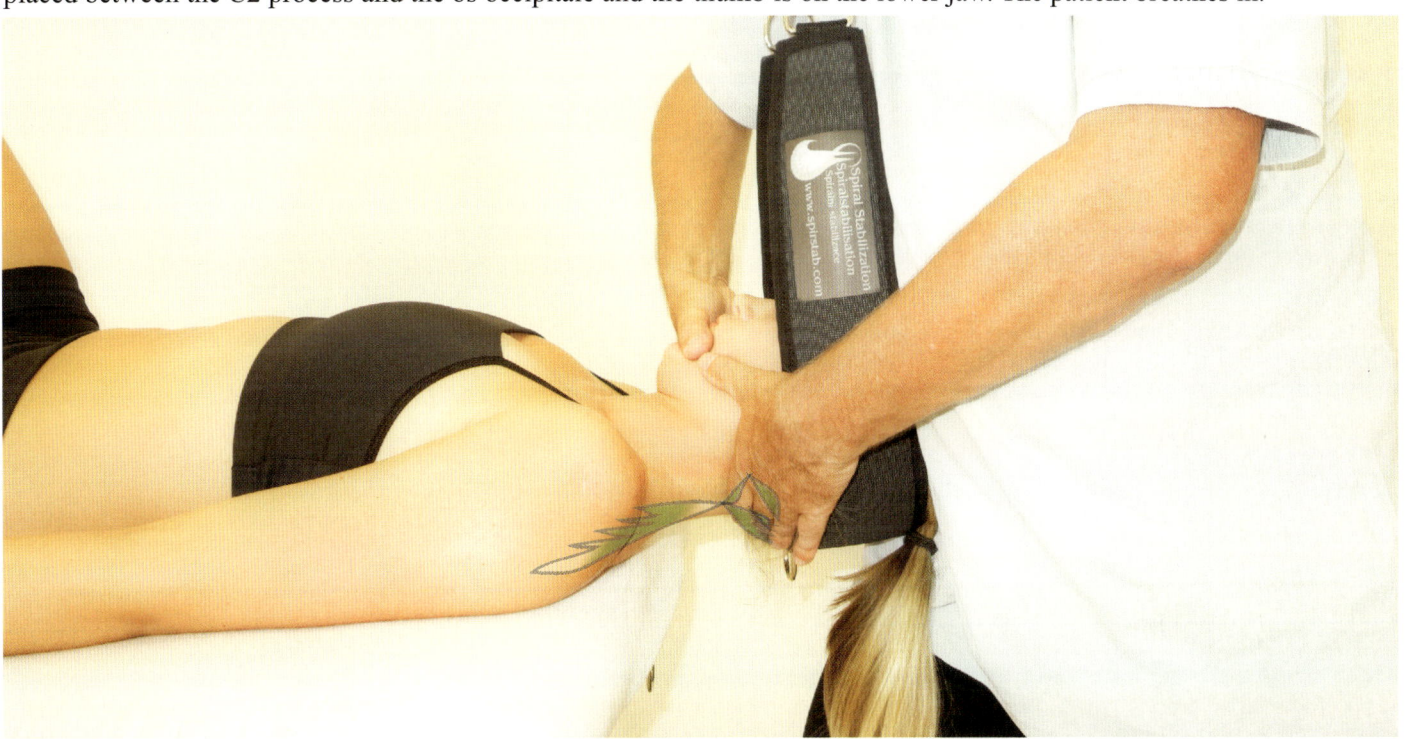

Performance

The therapist slowly and gently presses the lower jaw with his right hand obliquely and dorsally, while his left hand stretches the back of the head cranially. The head rotates in an axis passing through the outer ear. The patient breathes out slowly.
The pulling is slackened and the stretching is repeated 6 times. At the end of the technique the therapist pauses for about 3 seconds.
PIR. The extension is held and the patient breathes in. This causes a counter-pressure. When breathing out, the patient achieves further stretching. The process is repeated 3 times. This technique stretches the short neck extensors m. rectus capitis posterior major, minor, m. obliquus capitis superior, inferior and other neck muscles. This prepares the patient for relaxation of the neck during exercise.

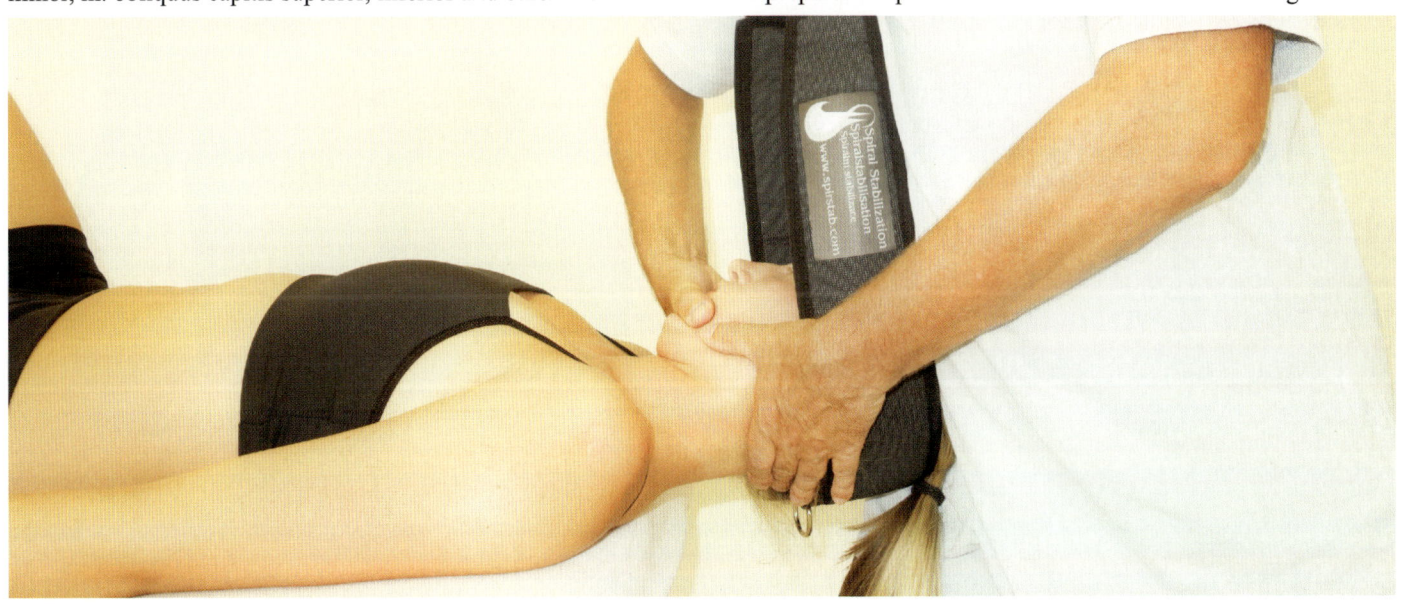

Manual techniques in a sitting position
M. semispinalis capitis, cervicis - manual stretching during exercise

Exercise 6 - sitting with back to the attachment point of the elastic rope, forward circles with both arms

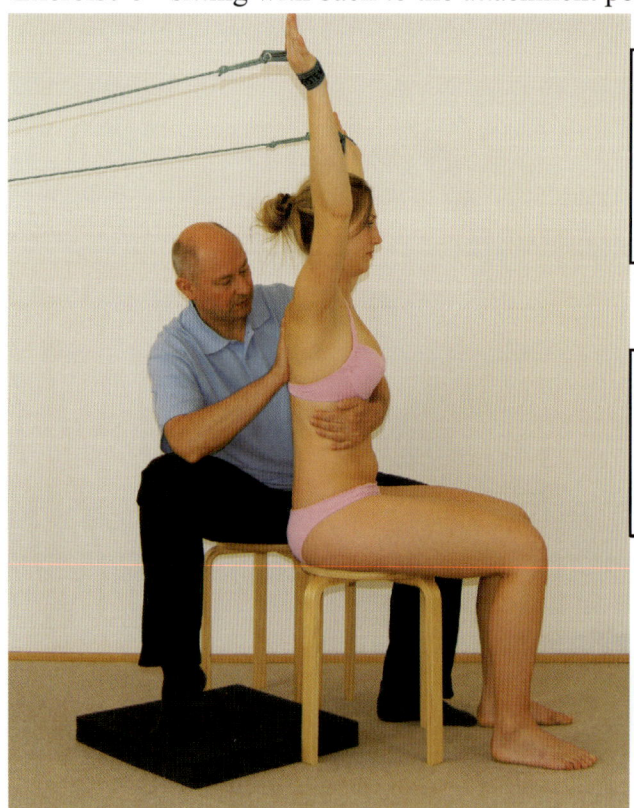

Massage of m. semispinalis capitis reciprocally inhibited and stretching

Spiral muscle stabilizing chain SA-B serratus anterior

Stabilization of the lower ribs

The stabilizing arm lifts the patient's trunk during massage

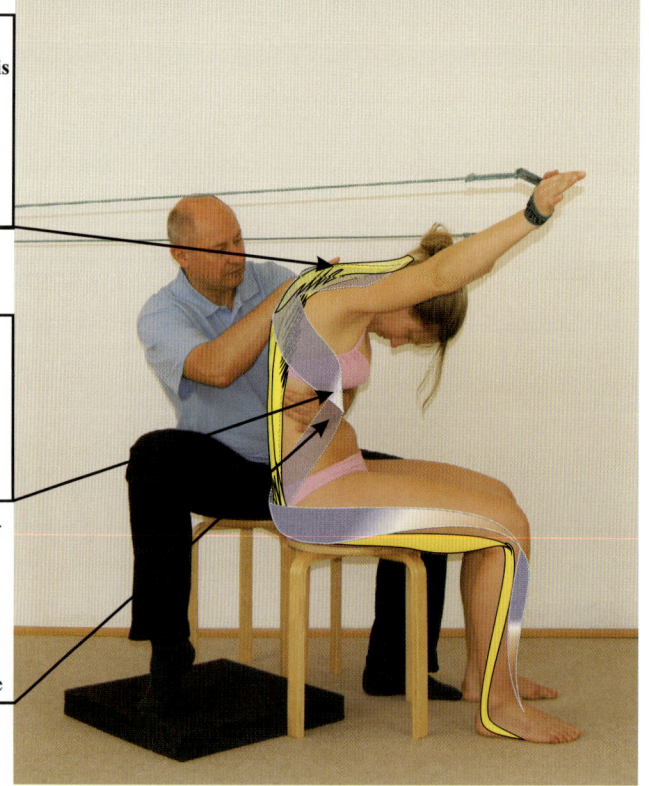

M. semispinalis capitis, cervicis - manual stretching during exercise

Exercise 2 - sitting sideways on to the attachment point of the elastic rope, sideways pull with one arm

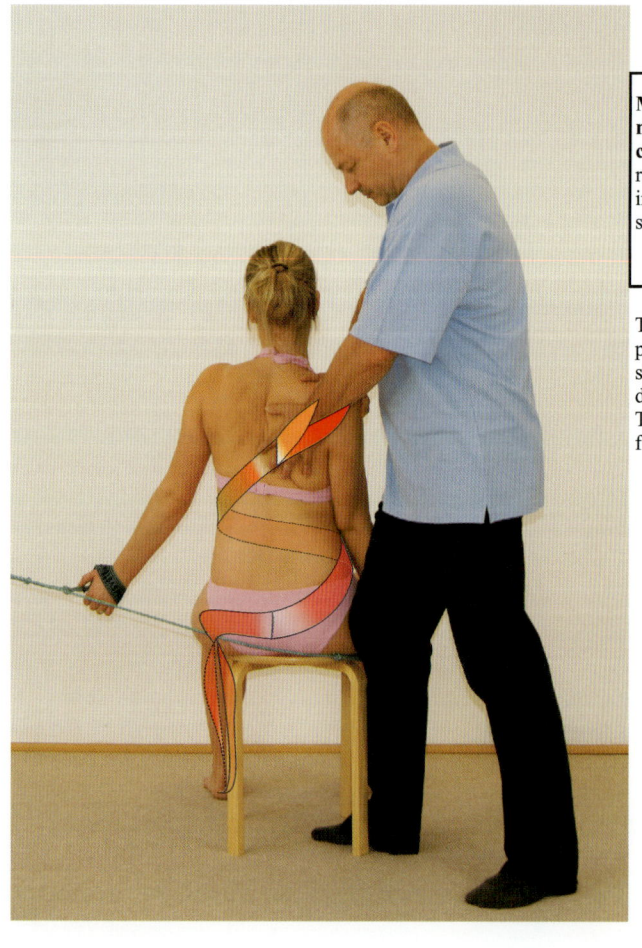

Massage of m. semispinalis capitis reciprocally inhibited and stretched

The right arm presses the shoulder blade down.
The left arm fixes the head.

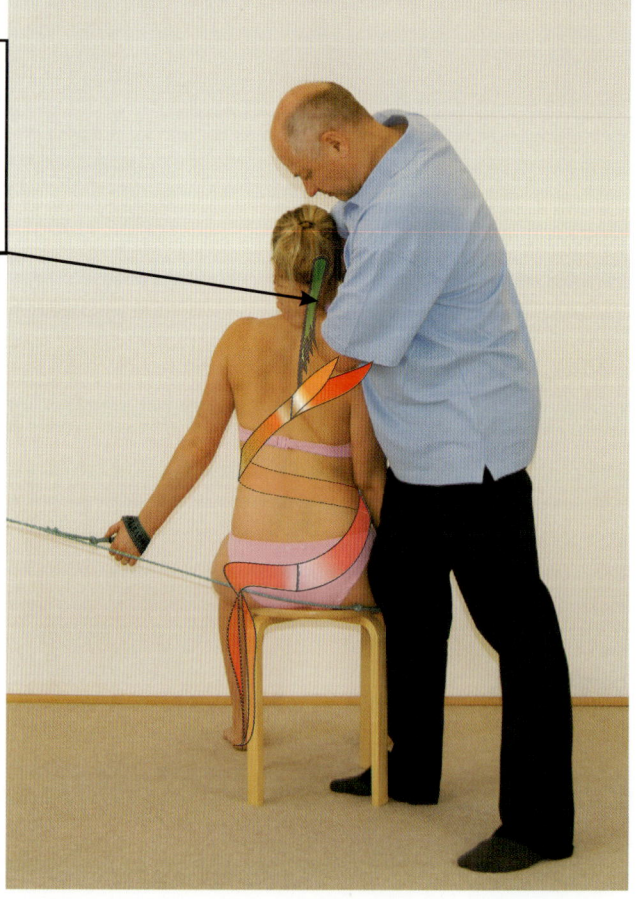

Exercise - stabilization, stretching

M. semispinalis capitis, cervicis, m. rectus capitis posterior major, minor, m. obliquus capitis superior, m. obliquus capitis inferior
- relaxation in reciprocal inhibition, stretching

The LD - latissimus dorsi and TR - trapezius chains are the agonists in the second part of the exercise.

Exercise 2 - standing sideways on the attachment point of the elastic rope, legs in the basic position

Sideways and downward pull with one arm to the hip, stretching of the neck

Active relaxation

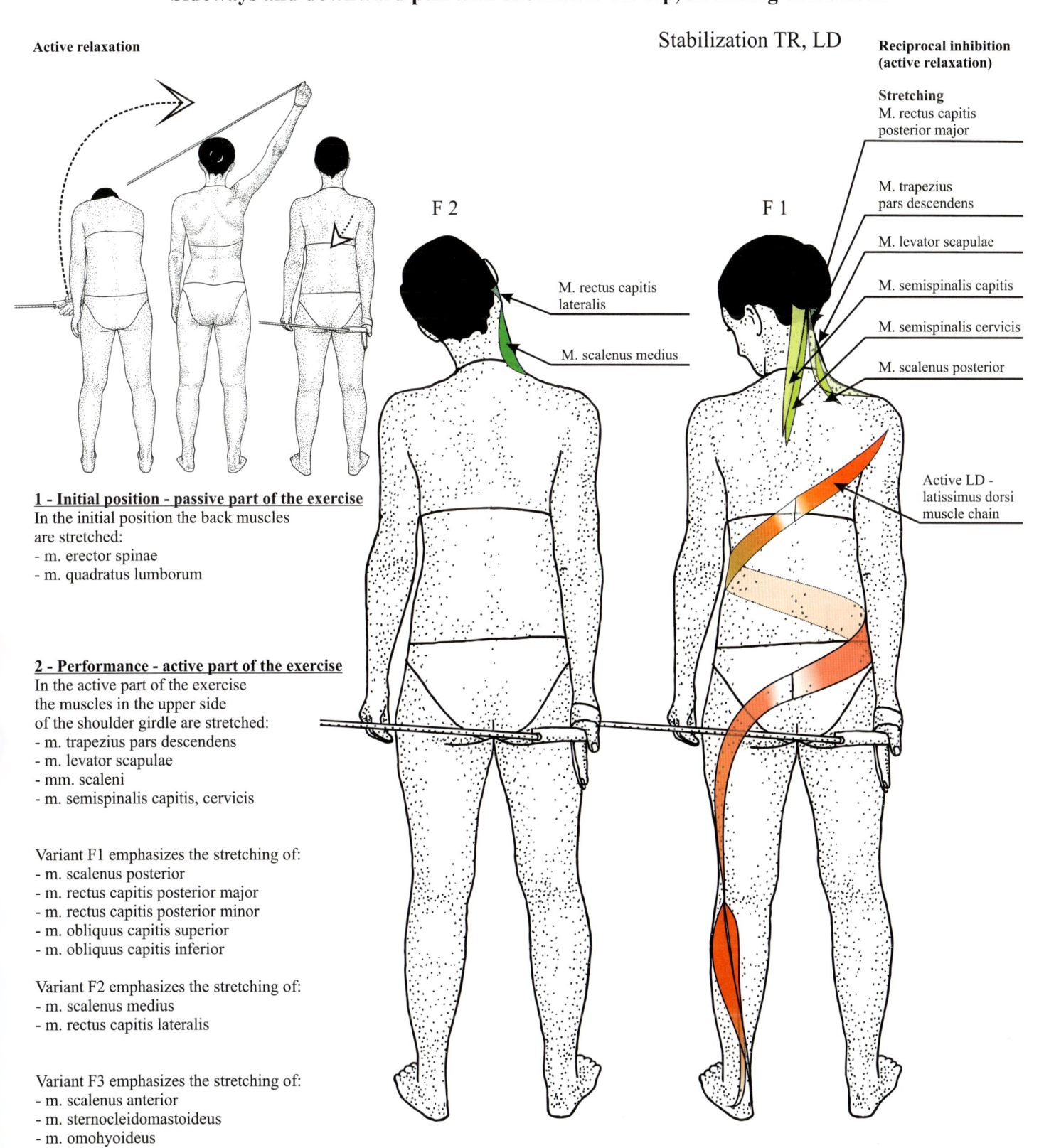

Stabilization TR, LD

Reciprocal inhibition (active relaxation)

Stretching
M. rectus capitis posterior major

M. trapezius pars descendens

M. levator scapulae

M. rectus capitis lateralis

M. scalenus medius

F 2

F 1

M. semispinalis capitis

M. semispinalis cervicis

M. scalenus posterior

Active LD - latissimus dorsi muscle chain

1 - Initial position - passive part of the exercise
In the initial position the back muscles are stretched:
- m. erector spinae
- m. quadratus lumborum

2 - Performance - active part of the exercise
In the active part of the exercise the muscles in the upper side of the shoulder girdle are stretched:
- m. trapezius pars descendens
- m. levator scapulae
- mm. scaleni
- m. semispinalis capitis, cervicis

Variant F1 emphasizes the stretching of:
- m. scalenus posterior
- m. rectus capitis posterior major
- m. rectus capitis posterior minor
- m. obliquus capitis superior
- m. obliquus capitis inferior

Variant F2 emphasizes the stretching of:
- m. scalenus medius
- m. rectus capitis lateralis

Variant F3 emphasizes the stretching of:
- m. scalenus anterior
- m. sternocleidomastoideus
- m. omohyoideus

Exercise - stabilization, stretching

M. semispinalis capitis, cervicis, m. rectus capitis posterior major, minor, m. obliquus capitis superior, m. obliquus capitis inferior - relaxation in reciprocal inhibition, stretching

The LD - latissimus dorsi and TR - trapezius chains are the agonists in the second part of the exercise.

Exercise 1 - standing facing the attachment point of the elastic rope, one leg is placed forward on the mat

Backward pull with both arms, palms turned upwards

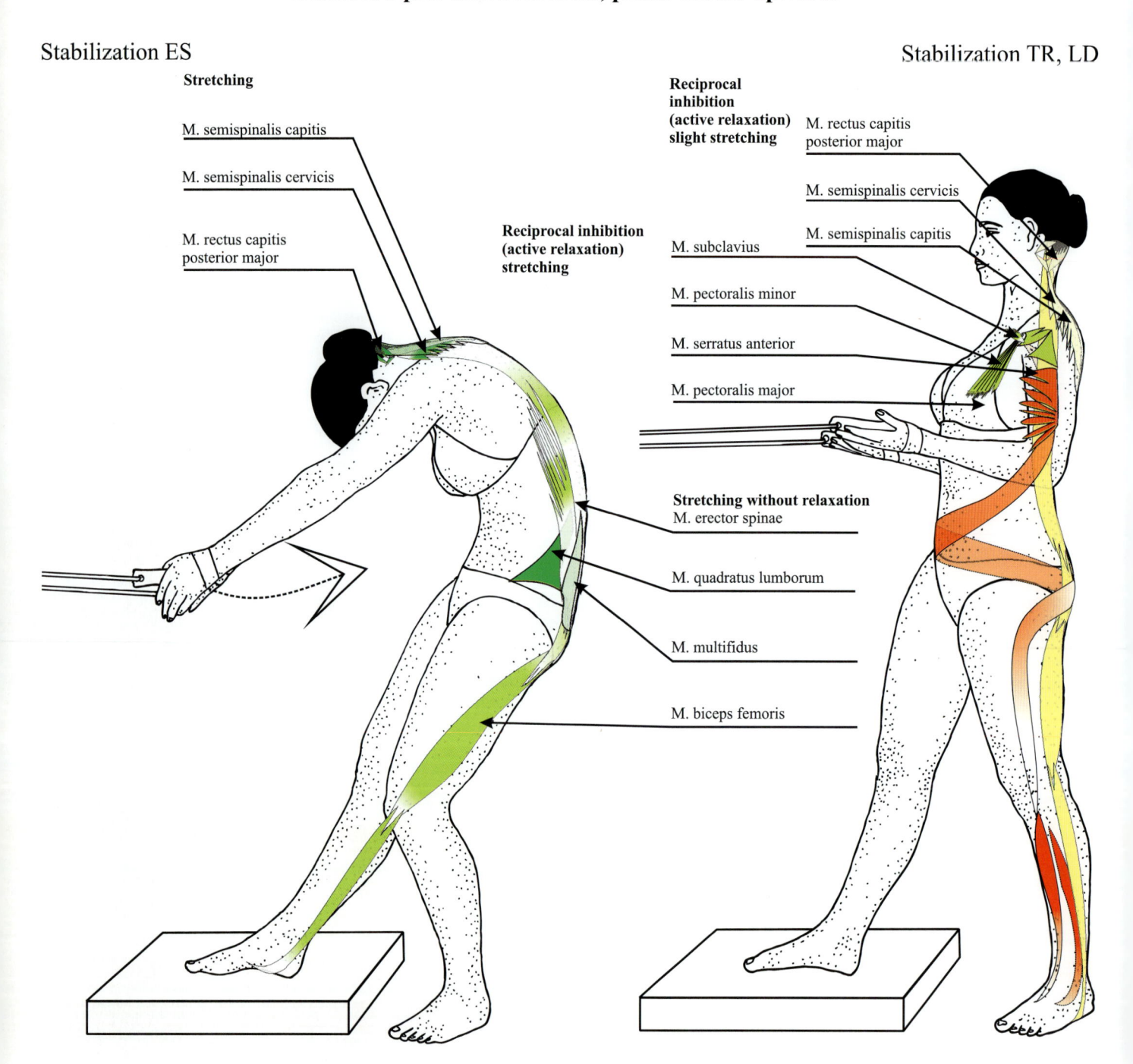

Stabilization ES — Stabilization TR, LD

Stretching:
- M. semispinalis capitis
- M. semispinalis cervicis
- M. rectus capitis posterior major

Reciprocal inhibition (active relaxation) stretching

Reciprocal inhibition (active relaxation) slight stretching:
- M. rectus capitis posterior major
- M. semispinalis cervicis
- M. semispinalis capitis
- M. subclavius
- M. pectoralis minor
- M. serratus anterior
- M. pectoralis major

Stretching without relaxation:
- M. erector spinae
- M. quadratus lumborum
- M. multifidus
- M. biceps femoris

1 - Initial position - active part of the exercise
In the initial position the back muscles are stretched:
- m. erector spinae
- m. quadratus lumborum
- m. multifidus

The ischiocrural muscles are also stretched:
- m. biceps femoris
- m. semitendinosus
- m. semimembranosus
- m. adductor magnus

2 - Performance - active part of the exercise
In the active part the muscles in the anterior part of the shoulder girdle are stretched:
- m. subclavius
- m. pectoralis minor
- m. pectoralis major
- m. serratus anterior

The muscles in the upper side of the shoulder girdle are relaxed:
- m. trapezius pars descendens
- m. levator scapulae
- mm. scaleni
- m. semispinalis capitis, cervicis and other muscles.

Exercise - stabilization, stretching

M. semispinalis capitis, cervicis, m. rectus capitis posterior major, minor, m. obliquus capitis superior, m. obliquus capitis inferior
- relaxation in reciprocal inhibition, stretching

The PM - pectoralis major chain is the agonist in the first part of the exercise,
the LD - latissimus dorsi and TR - trapezius chains are the agonists in the second part of the exercise.

Exercise 1 - standing facing the attachment point of the elastic rope, one leg is placed forward on the mat

Backward pull with both arms, opening the arms in outward rotation, palms turned upwards

Stabilization PM   Stabilization TR, LD

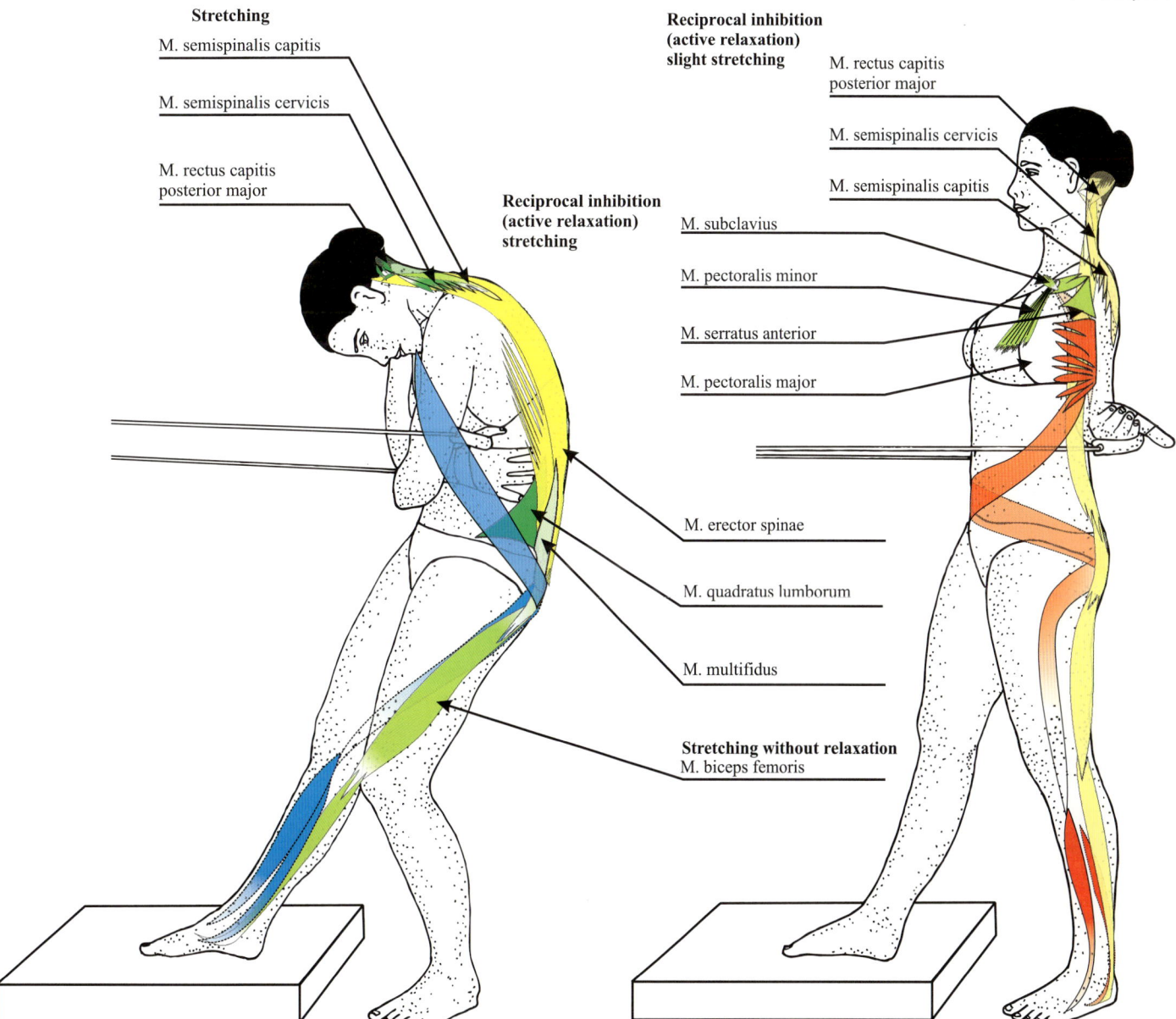

Stretching
- M. semispinalis capitis
- M. semispinalis cervicis
- M. rectus capitis posterior major

Reciprocal inhibition (active relaxation) stretching

Reciprocal inhibition (active relaxation) slight stretching
- M. rectus capitis posterior major
- M. semispinalis cervicis
- M. semispinalis capitis
- M. subclavius
- M. pectoralis minor
- M. serratus anterior
- M. pectoralis major
- M. erector spinae
- M. quadratus lumborum
- M. multifidus

Stretching without relaxation
M. biceps femoris

1 - Initial position - active part of the exercise
In the initial position the back muscles are stretched:
- m. erector spinae
- m. quadratus lumborum
- m. multifidus

The ischiocrural muscles are also stretched:
- m. biceps femoris
- m. semitendinosus
- m. semimembranosus
- m. adductor magnus

2 - Performance - active part of the exercise
In the active part of the exercise the muscles in the anterior side of the shoulder girdle are stretched:
- m. subclavius
- m. pectoralis minor
- m. pectoralis major
- m. serratus anterior

The muscles in the upper side of the shoulder girdle are relaxed:
- m. trapezius, pars descendens
- m. levator scapulae
- mm. scaleni
- m. semispinalis capitis, cervicis
- m. rectus capitis posterior major
- m. rectus capitis posterior minor
- m. obliquus capitis superior
- m. obliquus capitis inferior

Exercise - stabilization, stretching

M. semispinalis capitis, cervicis, m. rectus capitis posterior major, minor, m. obliquus capitis superior, m. obliquus capitis inferior - relaxation in reciprocal inhibition, stretching

The LD - latissimus dorsi and TR - trapezius chains are the agonists in the first part of the exercise, the SA - serratus anterior chain is the agonist in the second part of the exercise.

Exercise 6 - standing with back to the attachment point of the elastic rope, the legs are in the basic position

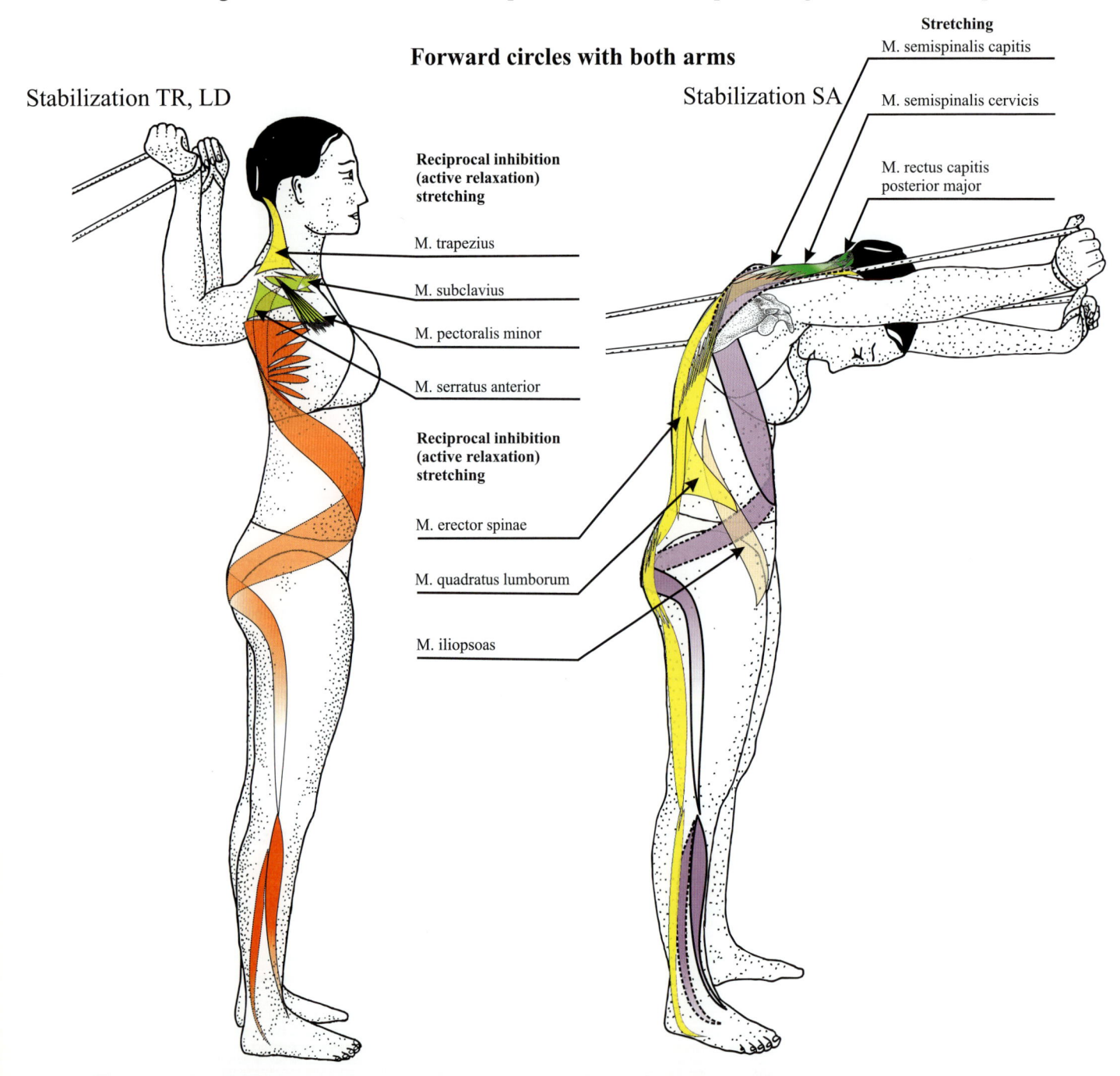

Forward circles with both arms

Stabilization TR, LD

Stabilization SA

Stretching
- M. semispinalis capitis
- M. semispinalis cervicis
- M. rectus capitis posterior major

Reciprocal inhibition (active relaxation) stretching
- M. trapezius
- M. subclavius
- M. pectoralis minor
- M. serratus anterior

Reciprocal inhibition (active relaxation) stretching
- M. erector spinae
- M. quadratus lumborum
- M. iliopsoas

1 - The first part of performance - active part of the exercise
The muscles in the anterior side of the shoulder girdle are stretched:
- m. subclavius
- m. pectoralis minor
- m. pectoralis major
- m. serratus anterior

The muscles in the upper side of the shoulder girdle are relaxed:
- m. trapezius pars descendens
- m. levator scapulae
- mm. scaleni
- m. semispinalis capitis, cervicis etc.

2 - Performance - active part of the exercise
During the performance of the exercise the actively inhibited back muscles are stretched:
- m. erector spinae
- m. quadratus lumborum
- m. iliopsoas
- m. rectus capitis posterior major
- m. rectus capitis posterior minor
- m. obliquus capitis superior
- m. obliquus capitis inferior

Exercise - stabilization, stretching

M. semispinalis capitis, cervicis, m. rectus capitis posterior major, minor, m. obliquus capitis superior, m. obliquus capitis inferior - relaxation in reciprocal inhibition, stretching

The LD - latissimus dorsi and TR - trapezius chains are the agonists in the first part of the exercise, the SA - serratus anterior chain is the agonist in the second part of the exercise.

Exercise 6 - standing with back to the attachment point of the elastic rope, one leg is placed forward on the mat

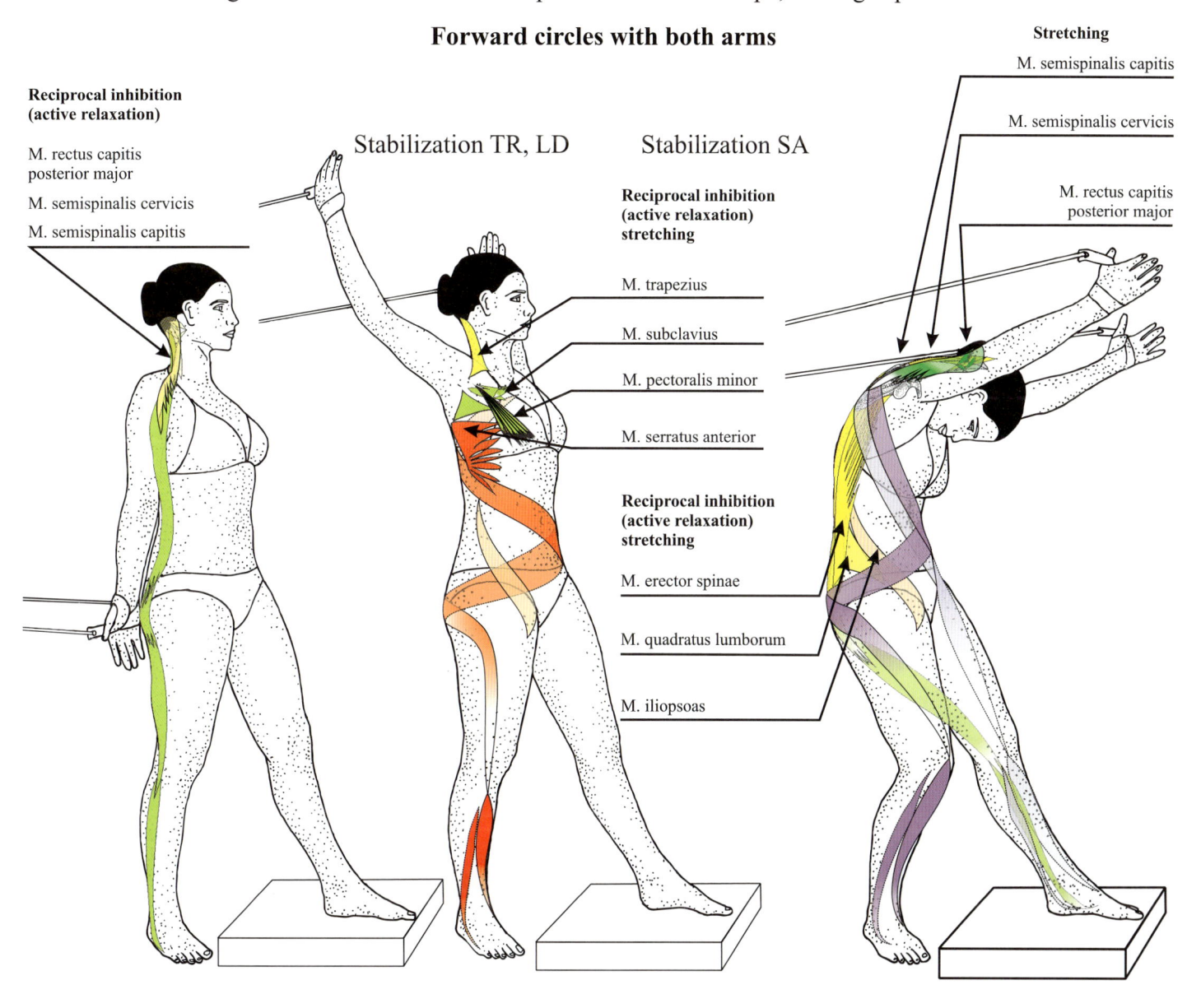

Forward circles with both arms   **Stretching**

Reciprocal inhibition (active relaxation)
M. rectus capitis posterior major
M. semispinalis cervicis
M. semispinalis capitis

Stabilization TR, LD   Stabilization SA

Reciprocal inhibition (active relaxation) stretching
M. trapezius
M. subclavius
M. pectoralis minor
M. serratus anterior

Reciprocal inhibition (active relaxation) stretching
M. erector spinae
M. quadratus lumborum
M. iliopsoas

Stretching
M. semispinalis capitis
M. semispinalis cervicis
M. rectus capitis posterior major

1 - The first part of performance - active part of the exercise
The muscles in the anterior side of the shoulder girdle are stretched:
- m. subclavius
- m. pectoralis minor
- m. pectoralis major
- m. serratus anterior

The muscles in the upper side of the shoulder girdle are relaxed:
- m. trapezius pars descendens
- m. levator scapulae
- mm. scaleni
- m. semispinalis capitis, cervicis etc.

2 - Performance - active part of the exercise
During the performance of the exercise the actively inhibited back muscles are stretched:
- m. erector spinae
- m. quadratus lumborum
- m. iliopsoas
- m. rectus capitis posterior major
- m. rectus capitis posterior minor
- m. obliquus capitis superior
- m. obliquus capitis inferior

Exercise - stabilization, stretching
M. semispinalis capitis, cervicis, m. rectus capitis posterior major, minor, m. obliquus capitis superior, m. obliquus capitis inferior - relaxation in reciprocal inhibition, stretching

The LD - latissimus dorsi and TR - trapezius chains are the agonists in the second part of the exercise.

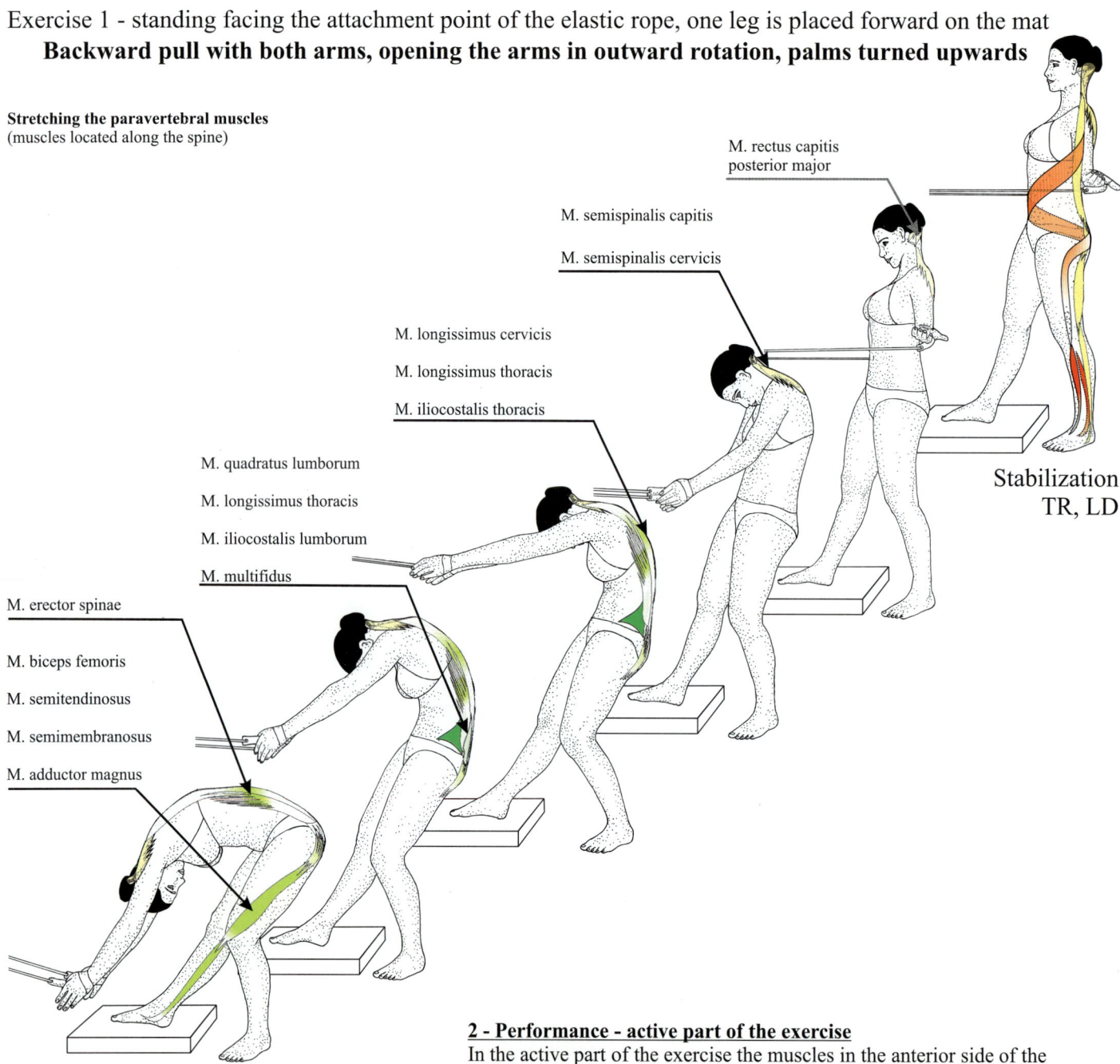

Exercise 1 - standing facing the attachment point of the elastic rope, one leg is placed forward on the mat
Backward pull with both arms, opening the arms in outward rotation, palms turned upwards

Stretching the paravertebral muscles
(muscles located along the spine)

M. rectus capitis posterior major
M. semispinalis capitis
M. semispinalis cervicis
M. longissimus cervicis
M. longissimus thoracis
M. iliocostalis thoracis
M. quadratus lumborum
M. longissimus thoracis
M. iliocostalis lumborum
M. multifidus
M. erector spinae
M. biceps femoris
M. semitendinosus
M. semimembranosus
M. adductor magnus

Stabilization TR, LD

1 - Initial position - active part of the exercise
In the initial position the back muscles are stretched:
- m. erector spinae
- m. quadratus lumborum
- m. multifidus

The ischiocrural muscles are also stretched:
- m. biceps femoris
- m. semitendinosus
- m. semimembranosus
- m. adductor magnus

2 - Performance - active part of the exercise
In the active part of the exercise the muscles in the anterior side of the shoulder girdle are stretched:
- m. subclavius
- m. pectoralis minor
- m. pectoralis major
- m. serratus anterior

The muscles in the upper side of the shoulder girdle are relaxed:
- m. trapezius, pars descendens
- m. levator scapulae
- mm. scaleni
- m. semispinalis capitis, cervicis
- m. rectus capitis posterior major
- m. rectus capitis posterior minor
- m. obliquus capitis superior
- m. obliquus capitis inferior

Exercise - stabilization, stretching

M. semispinalis capitis, cervicis, m. rectus capitis posterior major, minor, m. obliquus capitis superior, m. obliquus capitis inferior
- relaxation in reciprocal inhibition, stretching

The PM - pectoralis major chain is the agonist in the first part of the exercise,
LD - latissimus dorsi and TR - trapezius chains are the agonists in the second part of the exercise.

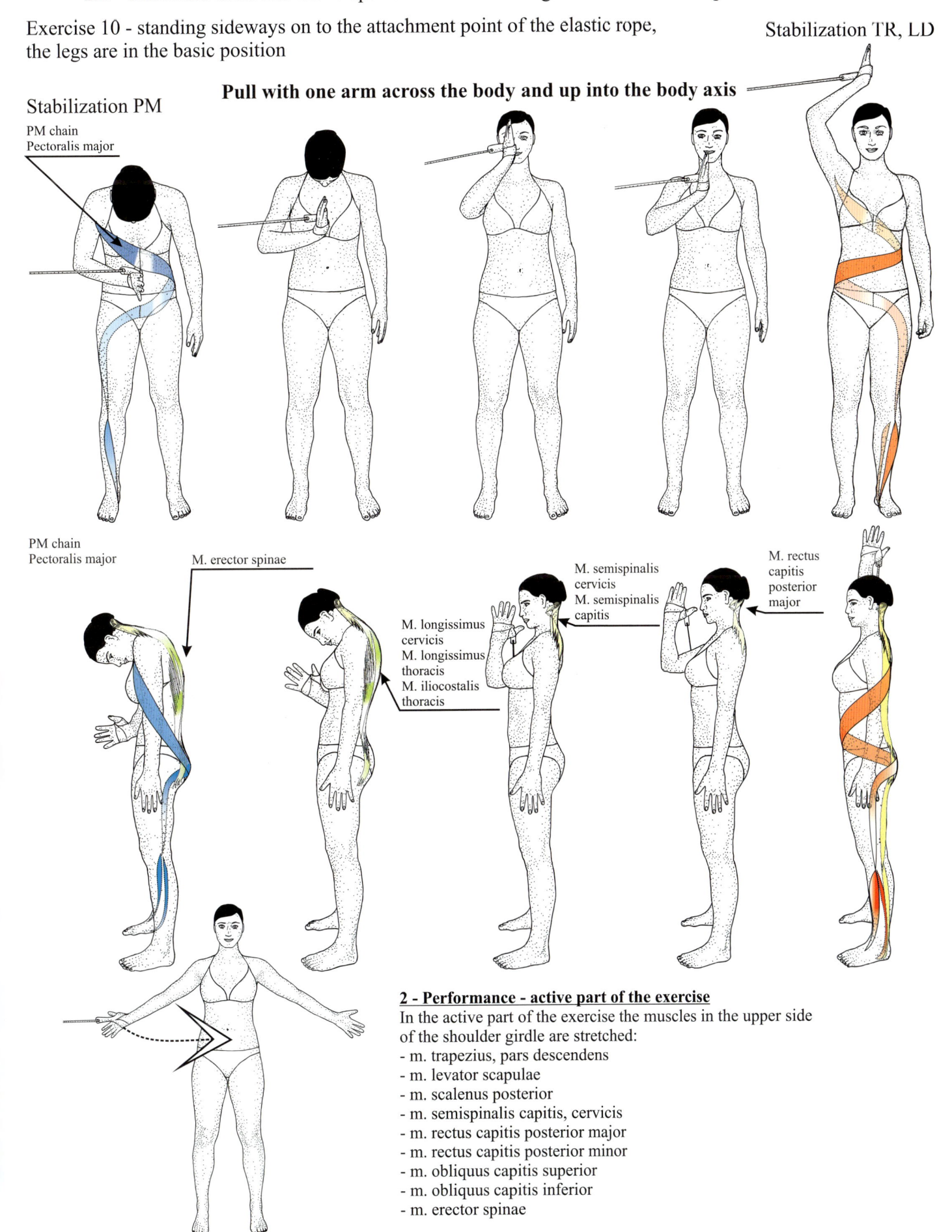

Exercise 10 - standing sideways on to the attachment point of the elastic rope, the legs are in the basic position

Stabilization PM
PM chain
Pectoralis major

Stabilization TR, LD

Pull with one arm across the body and up into the body axis

PM chain
Pectoralis major

M. erector spinae

M. longissimus cervicis
M. longissimus thoracis
M. iliocostalis thoracis

M. semispinalis cervicis
M. semispinalis capitis

M. rectus capitis posterior major

2 - Performance - active part of the exercise
In the active part of the exercise the muscles in the upper side of the shoulder girdle are stretched:
- m. trapezius, pars descendens
- m. levator scapulae
- m. scalenus posterior
- m. semispinalis capitis, cervicis
- m. rectus capitis posterior major
- m. rectus capitis posterior minor
- m. obliquus capitis superior
- m. obliquus capitis inferior
- m. erector spinae

Exercise
M. semispinalis capitis, cervicis - exercises with stretching

Exercise 2 - standing sideways on to the attachment point of the elastic rope, one leg is placed forward on the mat

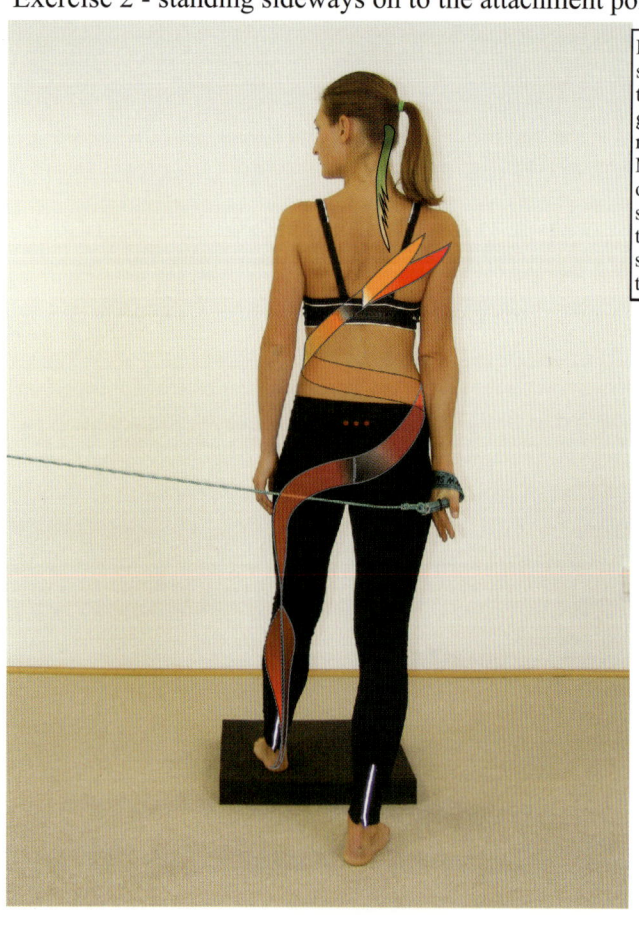

Relaxation and stretching of the posterior group of neck muscles. Mobilization of the cervical spine. The trunk is spirally stabilized by the LD and TR.

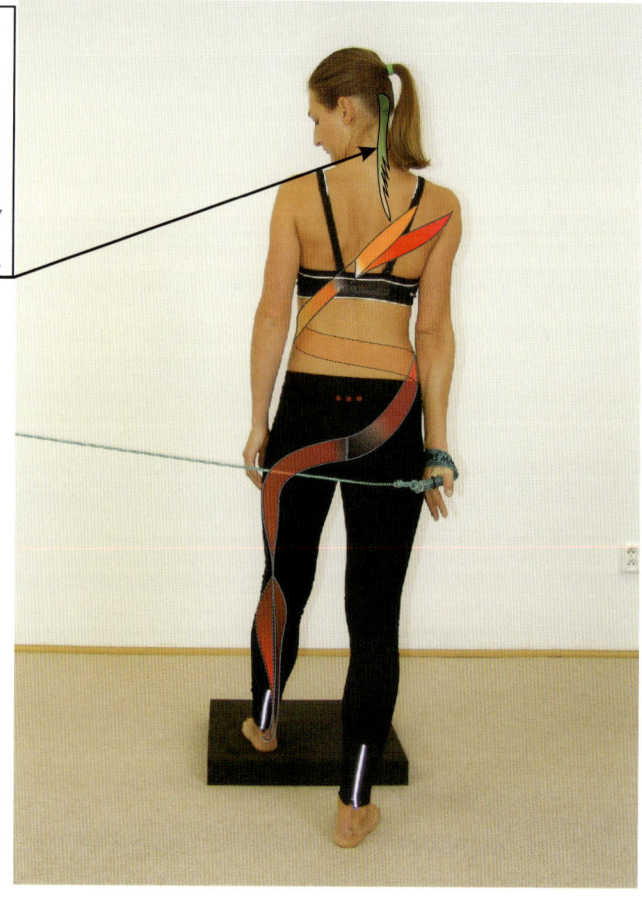

M. semispinalis capitis, cervicis - exercises with stretching

Exercise 11 - standing facing the attachment point of the elastic rope, crossed movement pattern, extension of the arm in the shoulder girdle and extension of the opposite leg in the pelvic girdle

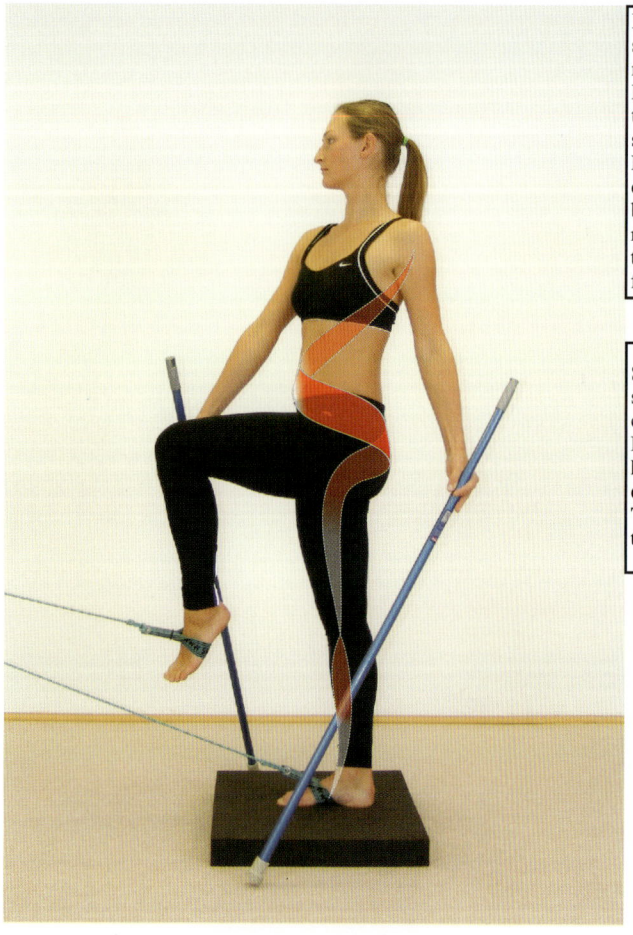

Relaxation and stretching of the neck muscles. Mobilization of the cervical spine. Mobilization comes from below and rotates the trunk under a fixed head.

Spiral muscle stabilizing chain
**LD-B latissimus dorsi,
TR-C trapezius**

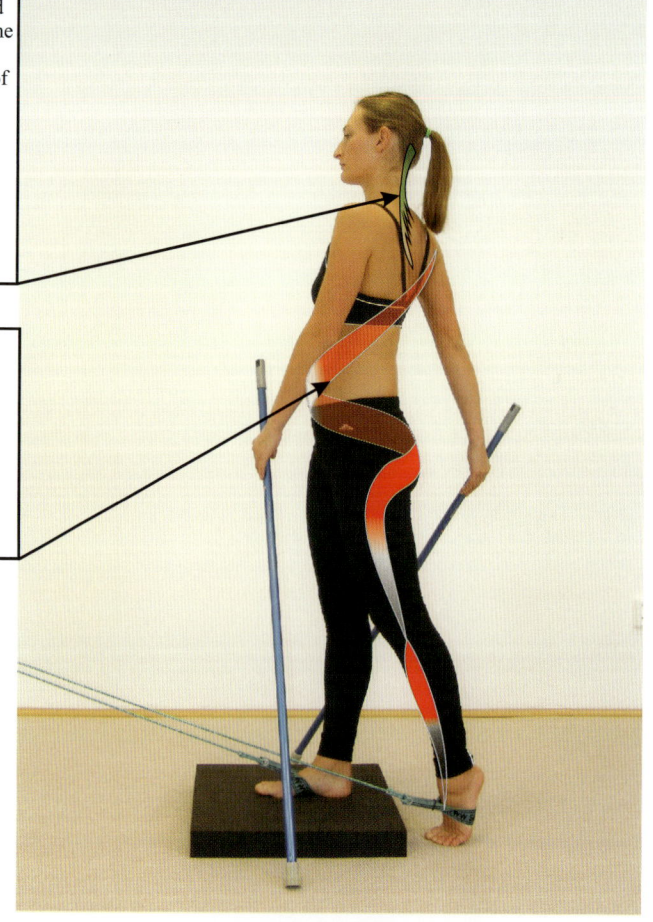

Exercise
M. semispinalis capitis, cervicis - exercises with stretching

Exercise 5 - kneeling facing the attachment point of the elastic rope, one leg is extended forward

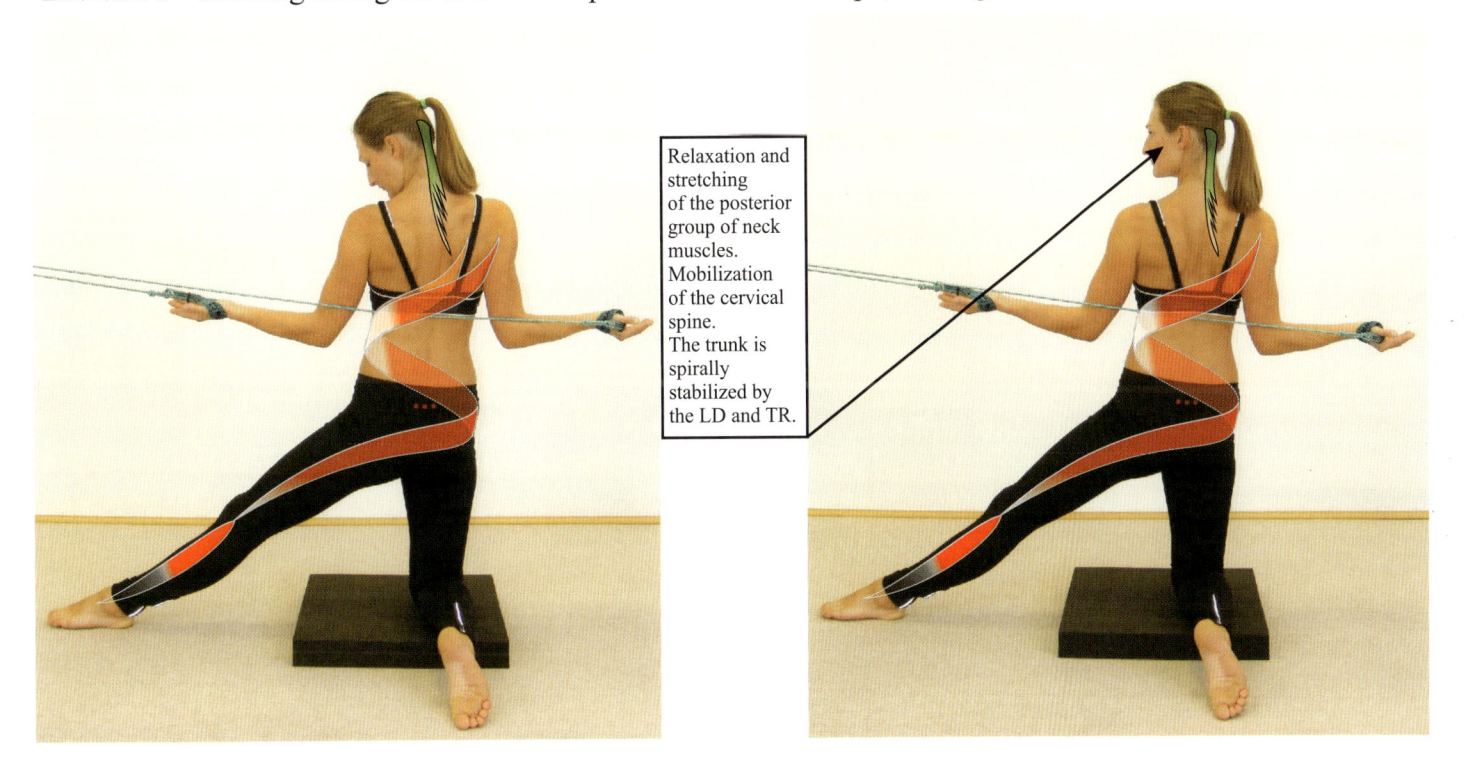

Relaxation and stretching of the posterior group of neck muscles. Mobilization of the cervical spine. The trunk is spirally stabilized by the LD and TR.

M. semispinalis capitis, cervicis - exercises with stretching

Exercise 1 - standing facing the attachment point of the elastic rope, one leg is placed forward on the mat

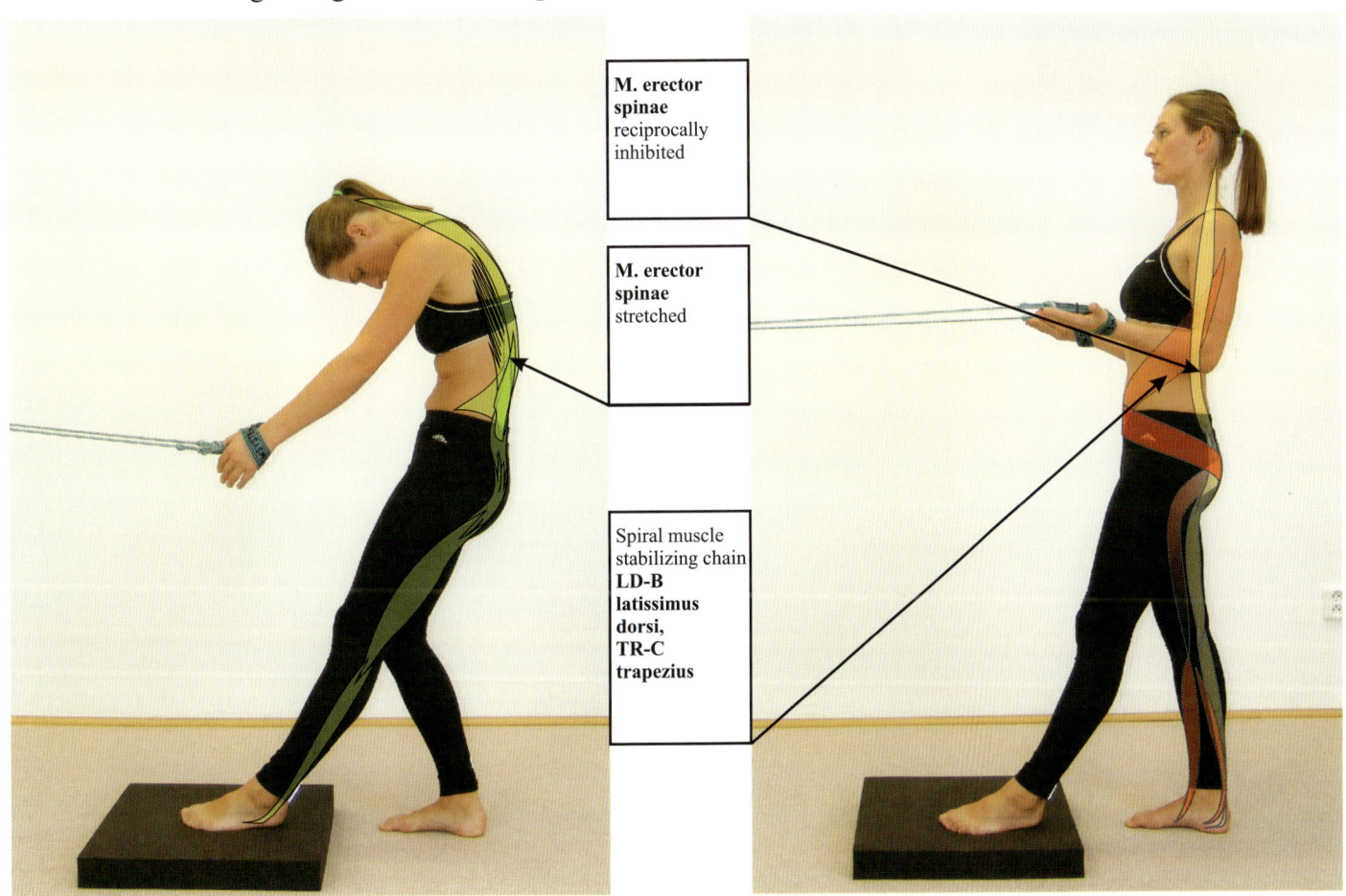

M. erector spinae reciprocally inhibited

M. erector spinae stretched

Spiral muscle stabilizing chain **LD-B** latissimus dorsi, **TR-C** trapezius

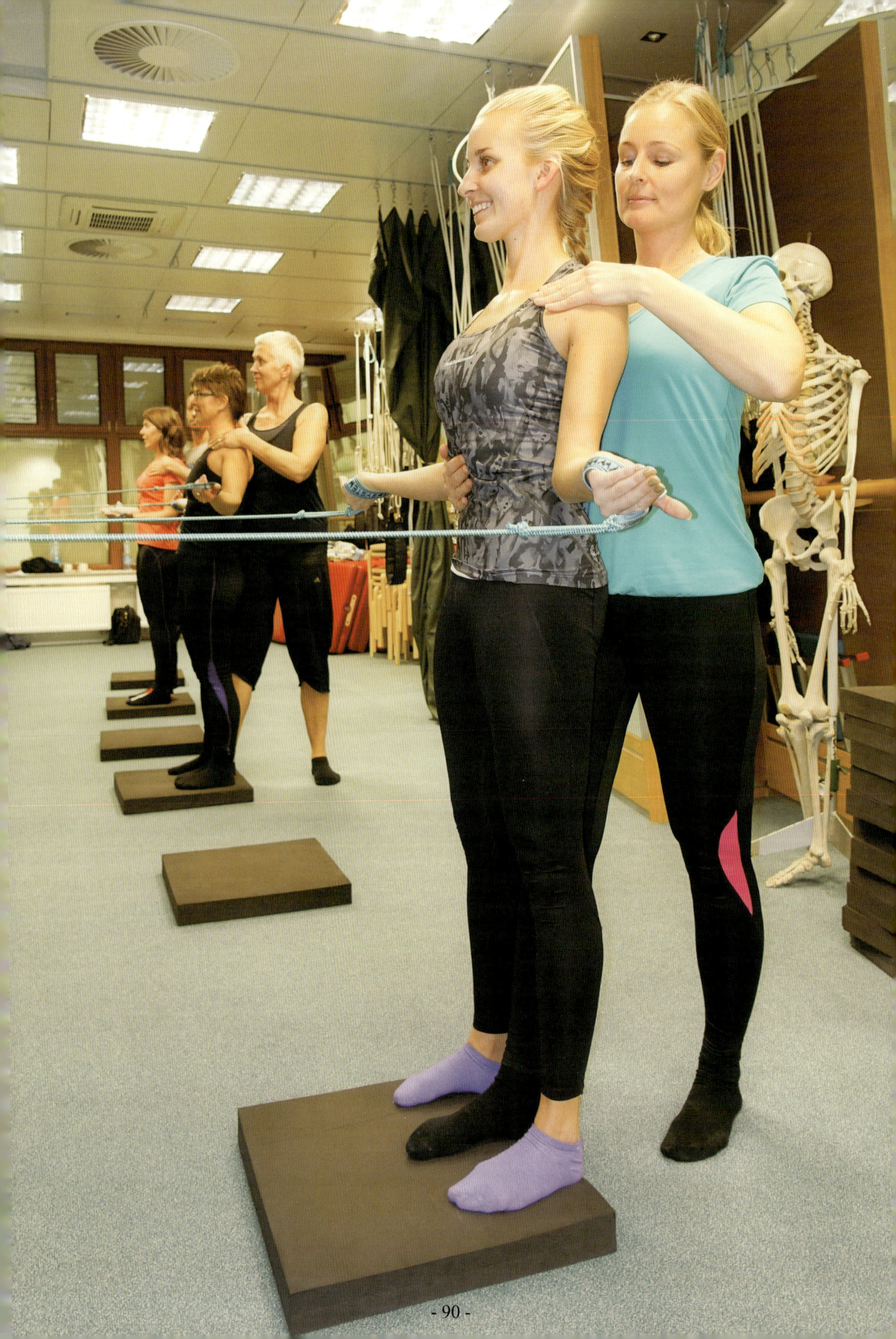

MANUAL TECHNIQUES AND EXERCISE ACCORDING TO MUSCLE ANALYSIS

Shoulder girdle
The anterior muscle group

Muscles with a tendency towards tension and shortening:

M. subclavius
M. pectoralis minor
M. serratus anterior
M. pectoralis major pars clavicularis

Anatomy

M. subclavius

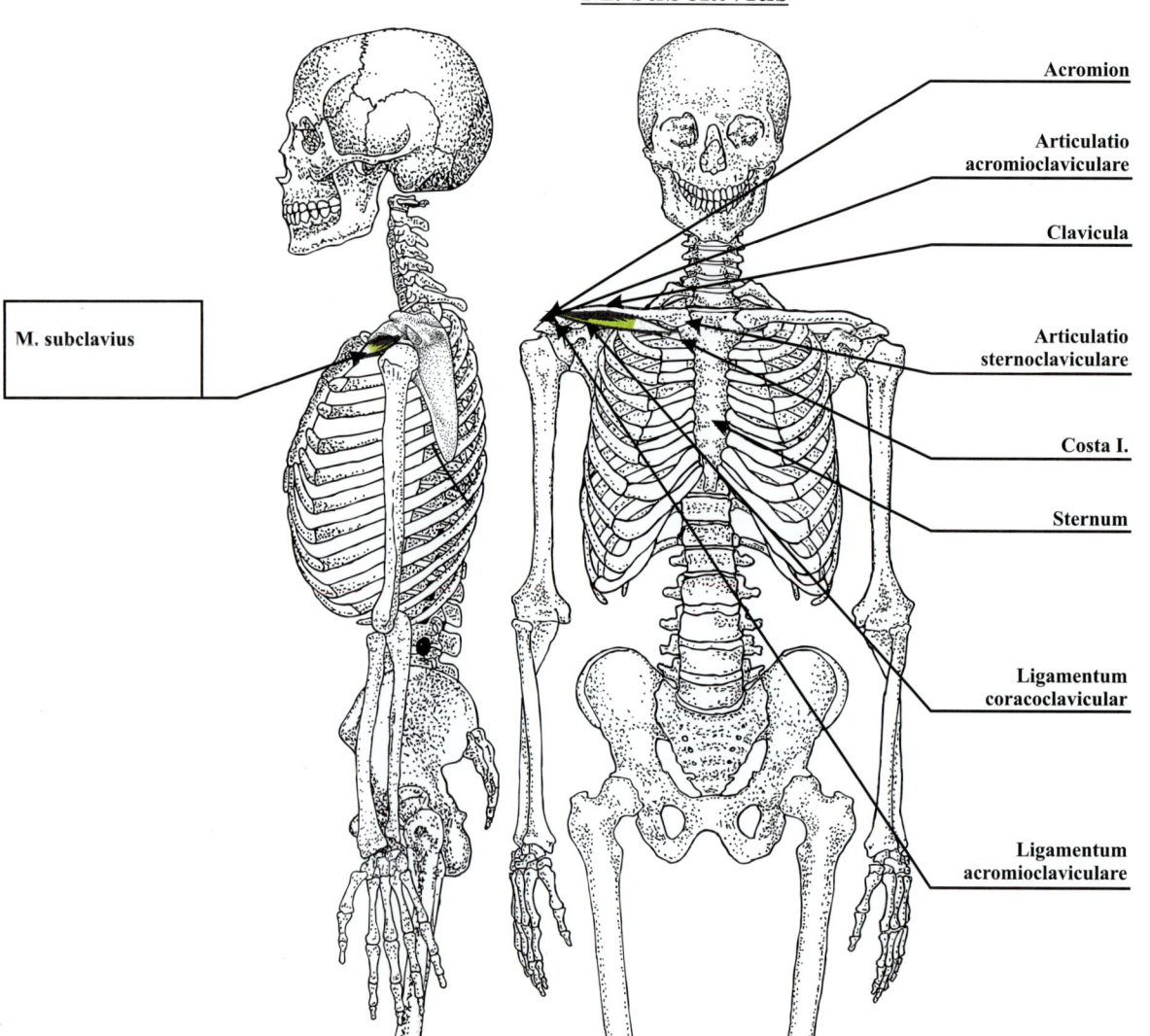

Labels: Acromion, Articulatio acromioclaviculare, Clavicula, Articulatio sternoclaviculare, Costa I., Sternum, Ligamentum coracoclaviculare, Ligamentum acromioclaviculare, M. subclavius

Muscles with a tendency **towards tension and shortening** These muscles must be **relaxed and stretched**

Relaxation

Stretching

Strengthening

Stabilization

M. subclavius
Origin:
- 1st rib at the transition of the bony and cartilaginous parts
Insertion:
- lower part of the clavicle (collar bone), lateral third
Function:
- fixation of the clavicle in the sternoclavicular joint
Innervation:
- n. subclavius (C6-Th1)

Manual techniques lying down
M. subclavius - massage, relaxation, passive stretching

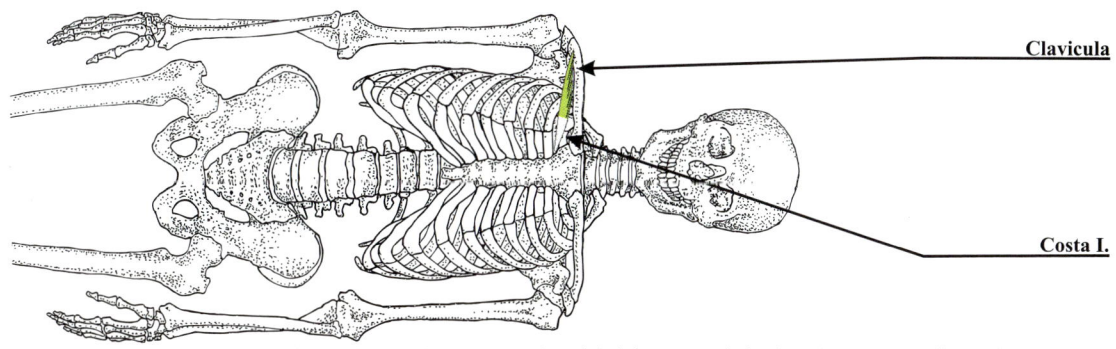

Clavicula

Costa I.

Initial position
The therapist kneels behind the patient and stabilizes the patient's trunk with his own right leg (punctum fixum). The whole of the left middle finger is placed under the clavicle (collar bone). The tip of the finger is at the sternum, while the palm rests on the shoulder. The fingers must not bend. The right palm rests against the left arm in the area of the patient's shoulder (not the chest). The patient breathes in.

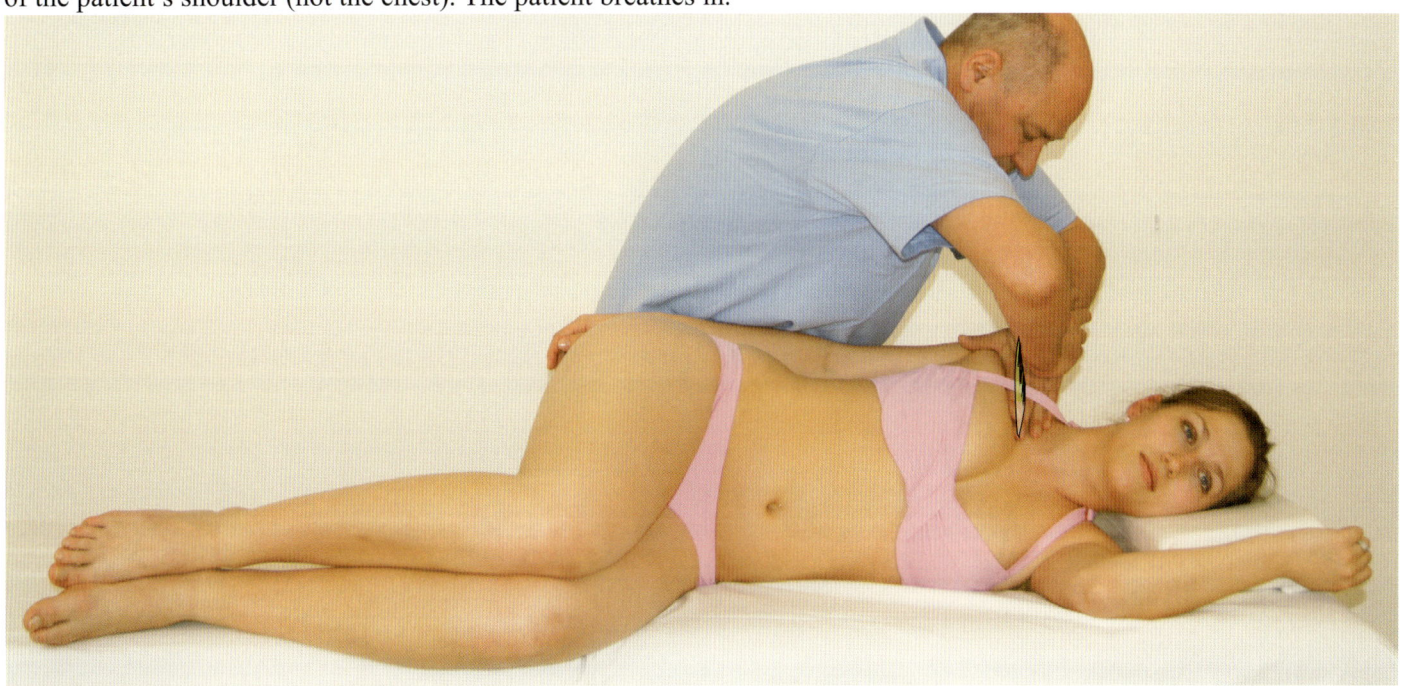

Performance
The therapist shifts the weight of the body to the left arm and shifts the shoulder blade dorsally (backwards), (punctum mobile). This stretches the m. subscapularis. The position of the hand on the shoulder does not change. The patient breathes out slowly. The pulling is slackened and the stretching is repeated 6 times. At the end of the technique the therapist pauses for about 3 seconds.

PIR. The extension is held and the patient breathes in. This causes a counter-pressure. When breathing out, the patient achieves further stretching. The process is repeated 3 times. This technique stretches the m. subclavius and other muscles of the anterior side of the shoulder girdle. This prepares the patient for the correct extent of the movement of the shoulder blade backwards during exercise.

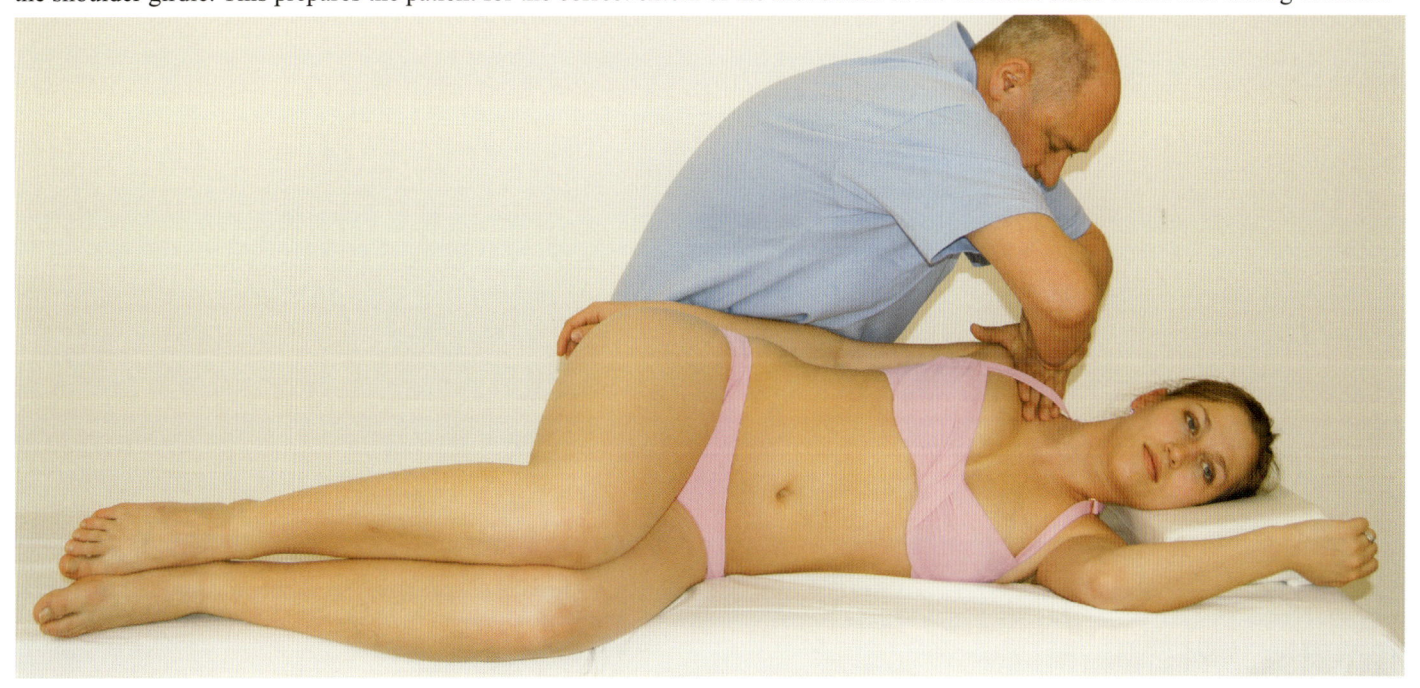

Anatomy
M. pectoralis minor

Processus coracoideus scapulae

Clavicula

Costa II.

Costa V.

M. pectoralis minor

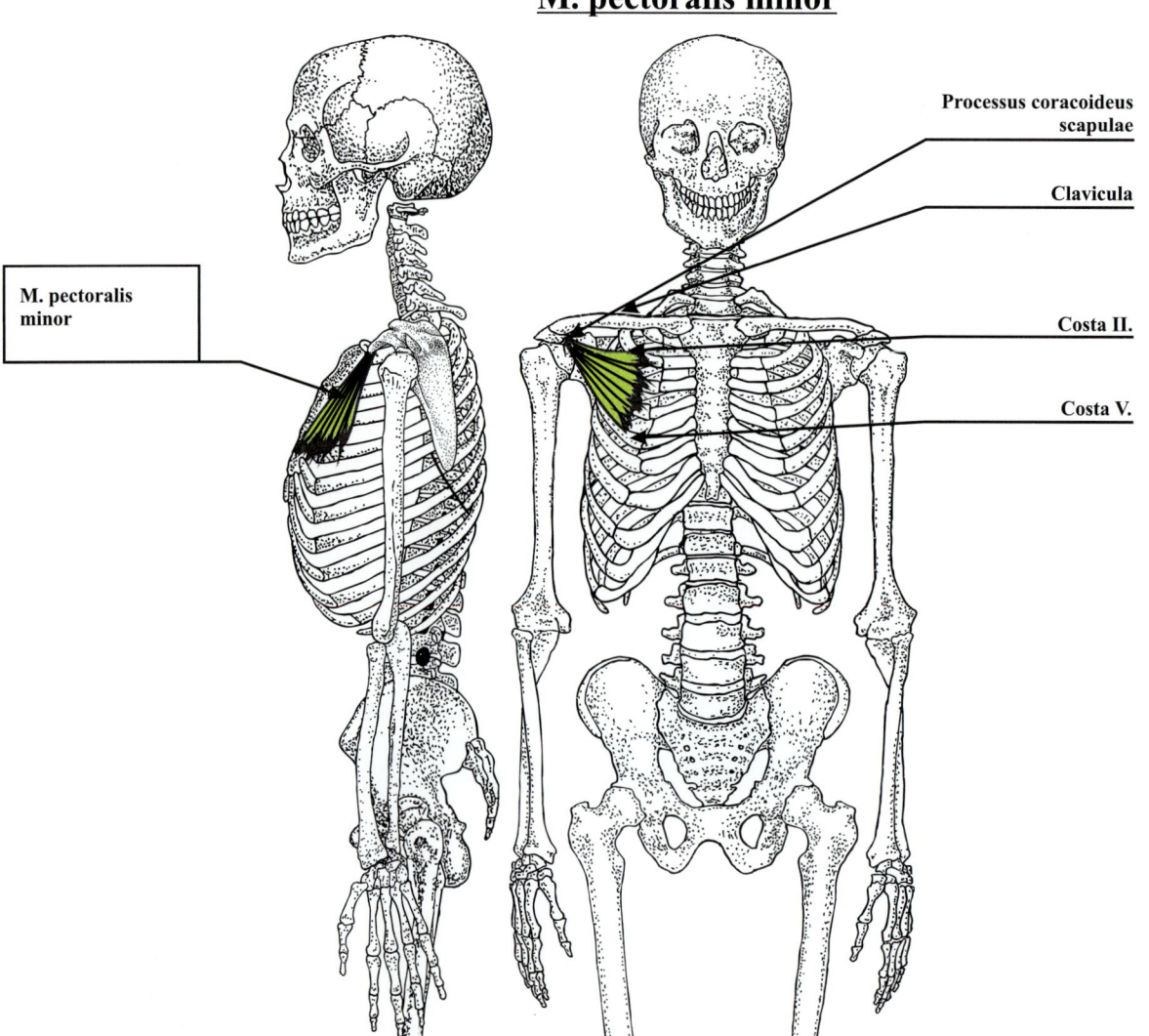

Muscles with a tendency towards **tension** and **shortening**. These muscles must be **relaxed** and **stretched**

Relaxation

Stretching

Strengthening

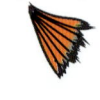

Stabilization

M. pectoralis minor
Origin:
- 3rd-5th rib
Insertion:
- processus coracoideus scapulae
Function:
- pulls the shoulder blade ventromedially
- auxiliary respiratory muscle - inspiration (breathing in)
Innervation:
- nn. pectorales mediales et laterales (C6-Th1)

Manual techniques lying down
M. pectoralis minor - massage, relaxation and passive stretching

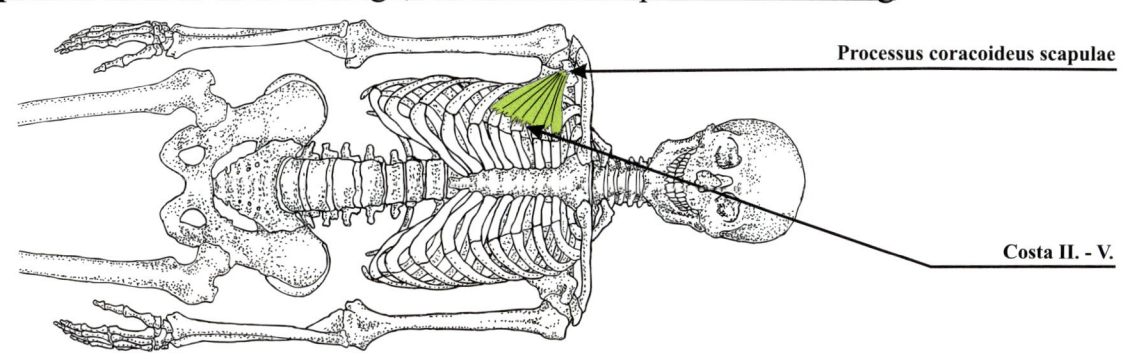

Processus coracoideus scapulae

Costa II. - V.

Initial position
The therapist kneels behind the patient and stabilizes the patient's trunk with his own right leg (punctum fixum).
The fingers of the left hand are placed on the chest pointing towards the 2nd rib. The palm rests on the shoulder. The fingers must not bend. The right palm rests against the left arm in the area of the patient's shoulder (not the chest). The patient breathes in.

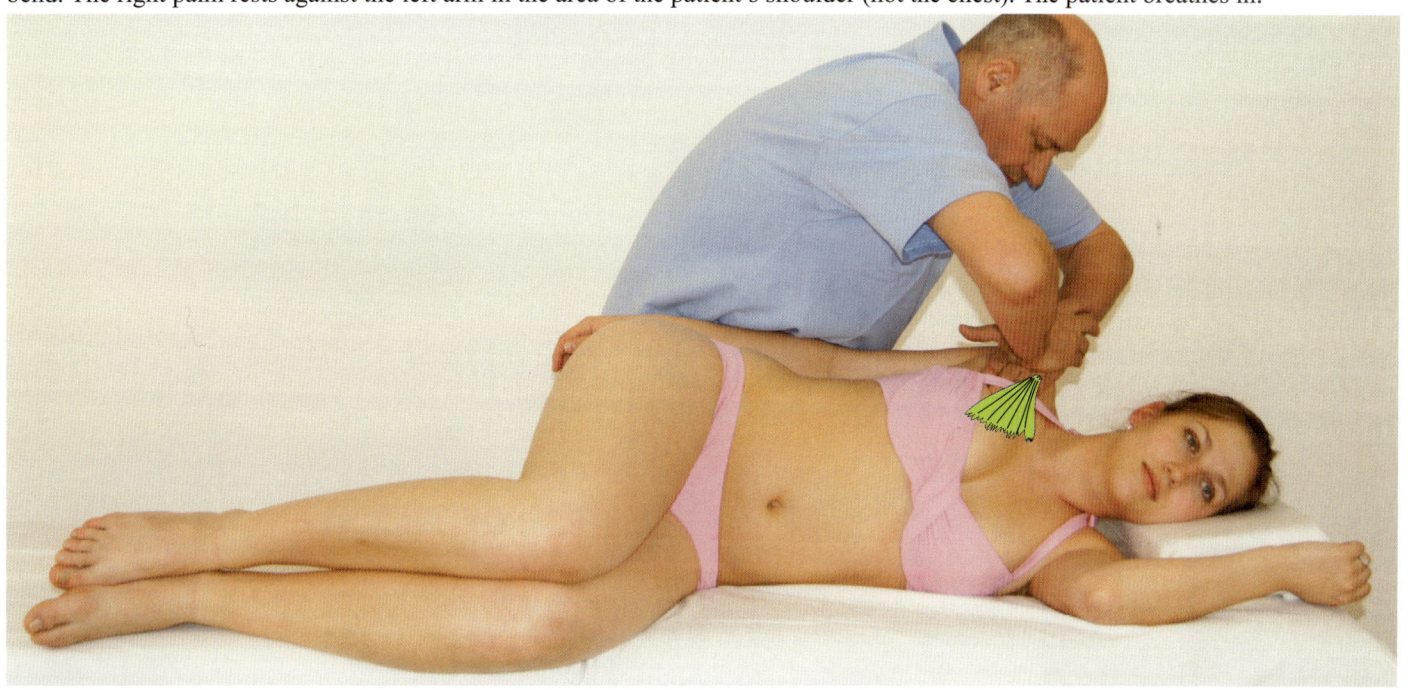

Performance
The therapist shifts the weight of the body to the left arm and shifts the shoulder blade backwards (punctum mobile). This stretches the m. pectoralis minor. The position of the hand on the shoulder does not change. The patient breathes out slowly. The pulling is slackened and the stretching is repeated 6 times. At the end of the technique the therapist pauses for about 3 seconds.
PIR. The extension is held and the patient breathes in. This causes a counter-pressure. When breathing out, the patient achieves further stretching. The processes is repeated 3 times. In the same way, the technique is performed in the direction of the 3rd, 4th and 5th ribs. This technique stretches the m. pectoralis minor and other muscles of the anterior side of the shoulder girdle.
This prepares the patient for the correct extent of the movement of the shoulder blade backwards during exercise.

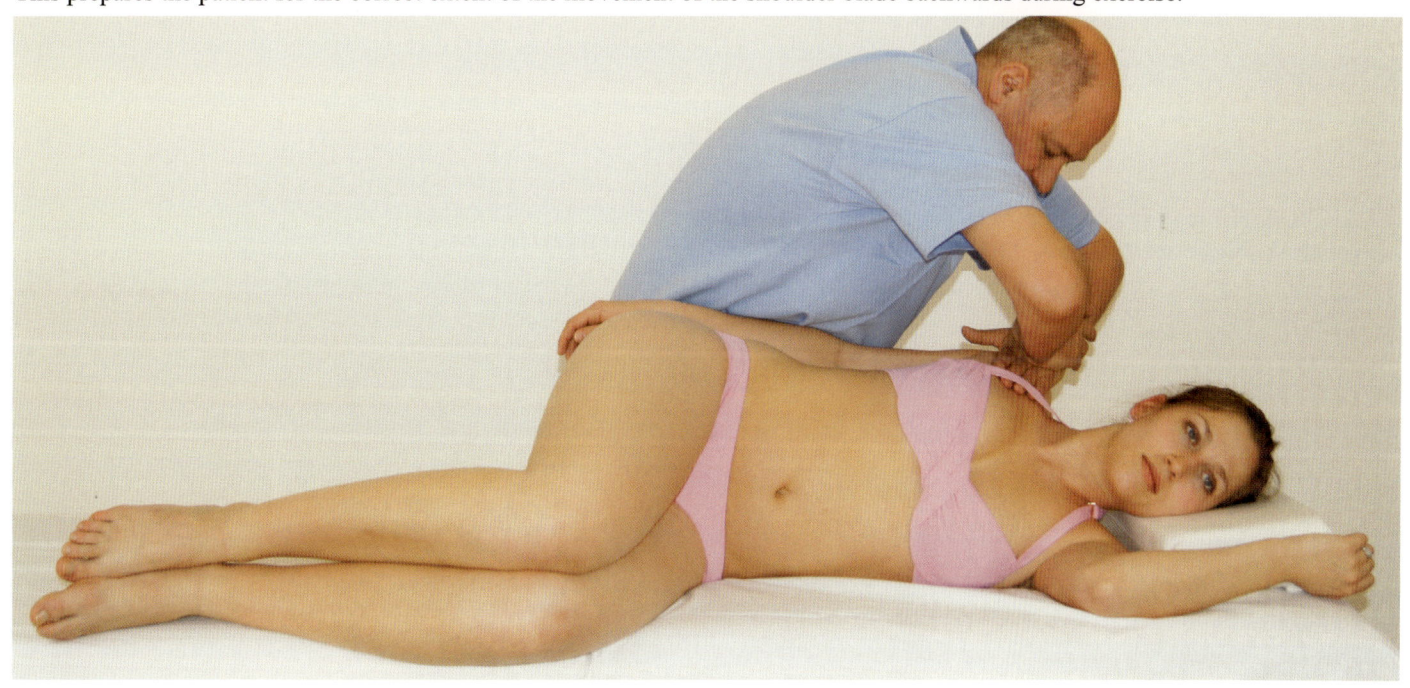

Manual techniques - sitting - one limb in a hoist
M. pectoralis minor - *massage, relaxation and passive stretching*
M. subclavius - *massage, relaxation, passive stretching*

Initial position

The therapist kneels behind the patient and rests the patient's trunk against himself (punctum fixum). The whole of the fingers of the right hand are placed on the chest pointing towards the 1st, 2nd, 3rd, 4th and 5th ribs, while the index finger rests on the clavicle and the middle finger on the m. subclavius just below the clavicle. The palm rests on the shoulder. The fingers must not bend.

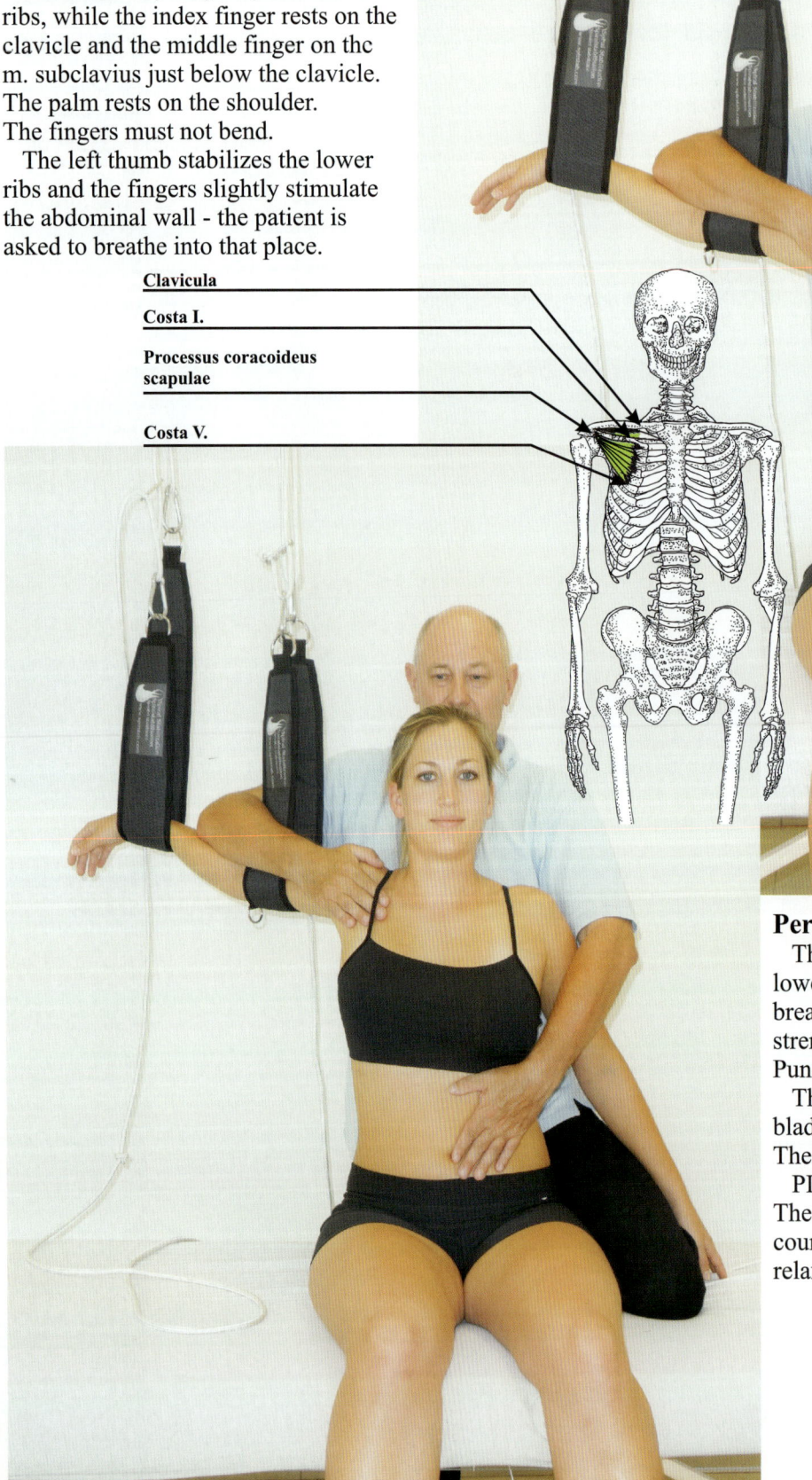

The left thumb stabilizes the lower ribs and the fingers slightly stimulate the abdominal wall - the patient is asked to breathe into that place.

Clavicula
Costa I.
Processus coracoideus scapulae
Costa V.

Performance

The therapist's left hand stimulates the lower abdomen, and the patient is asked to breathe into that place. The left thumb strengthens the stabilization of the lower ribs. Punctum fixum.

The right hand slowly pulls the shoulder blade backwards and slightly downwards. The patient actively assists in this movement.

PIR. This stretched position is held. The patient breathes in, causing a slight counter-pressure, then breathes out and relaxes.

Manual techniques in a sitting position

M. subclavius, m. pectoralis minor - massage, active relaxation, stretching

Exercise 2 - sitting, sideways pull with one arm, fixation of the lower ribs, stretching the shoulder backwards, correction of the axis of the trunk and head, massage

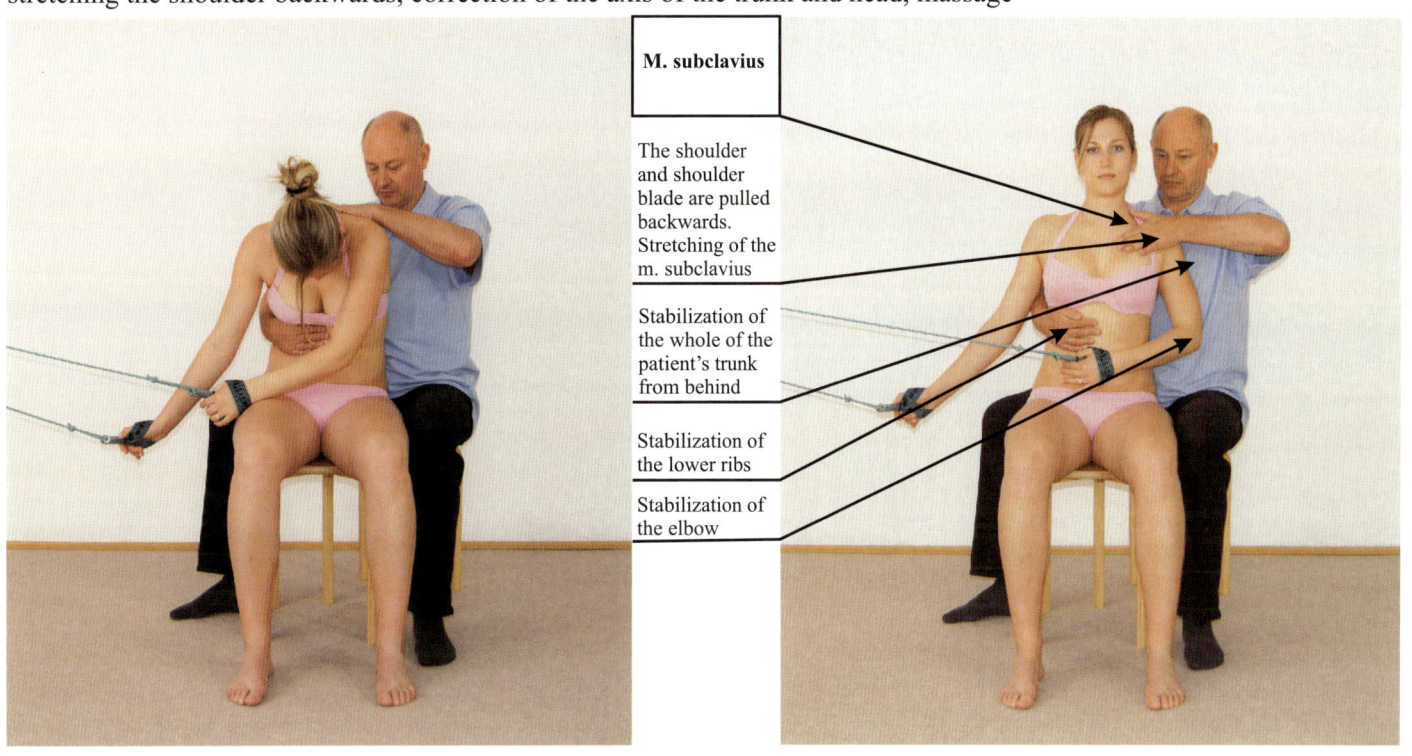

M. subclavius

The shoulder and shoulder blade are pulled backwards. Stretching of the m. subclavius

Stabilization of the whole of the patient's trunk from behind

Stabilization of the lower ribs

Stabilization of the elbow

M. subclavius, m. pectoralis minor - active relaxation, stretching

Exercise 2 - sitting, sideways pull with one arm, fixation of the lower ribs, stretching of the shoulder backwards, correction of the axis of the trunk and head, massage

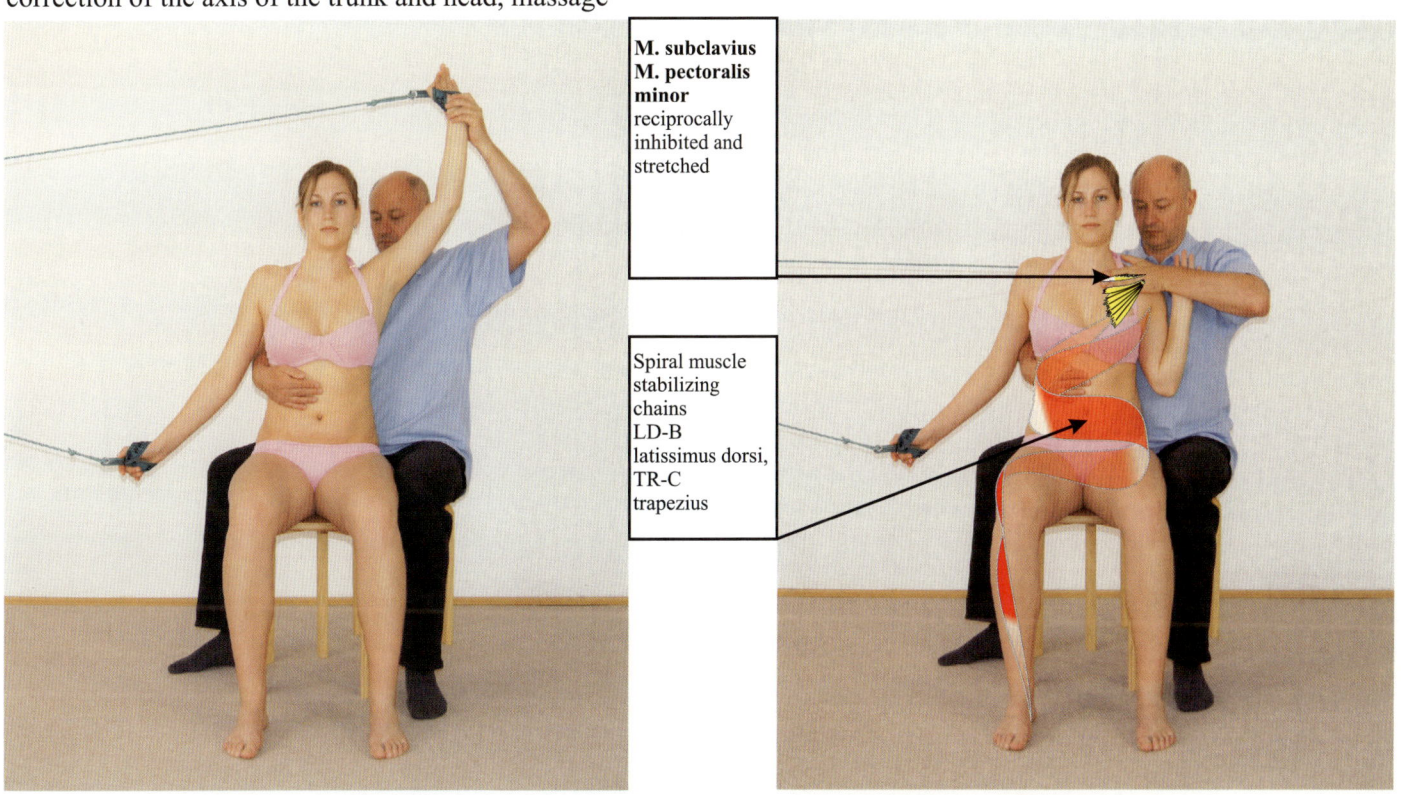

M. subclavius
M. pectoralis minor
reciprocally inhibited and stretched

Spiral muscle stabilizing chains LD-B latissimus dorsi, TR-C trapezius

Stretching of the m. subclavius and pectoralis minor inhibited in reciprocal inhibition.
The agonists are the spirals TR and LD, which stabilize the body.
The M. subclavius and m. pectoralis minor are reciprocally inhibited and stretched at the same time.

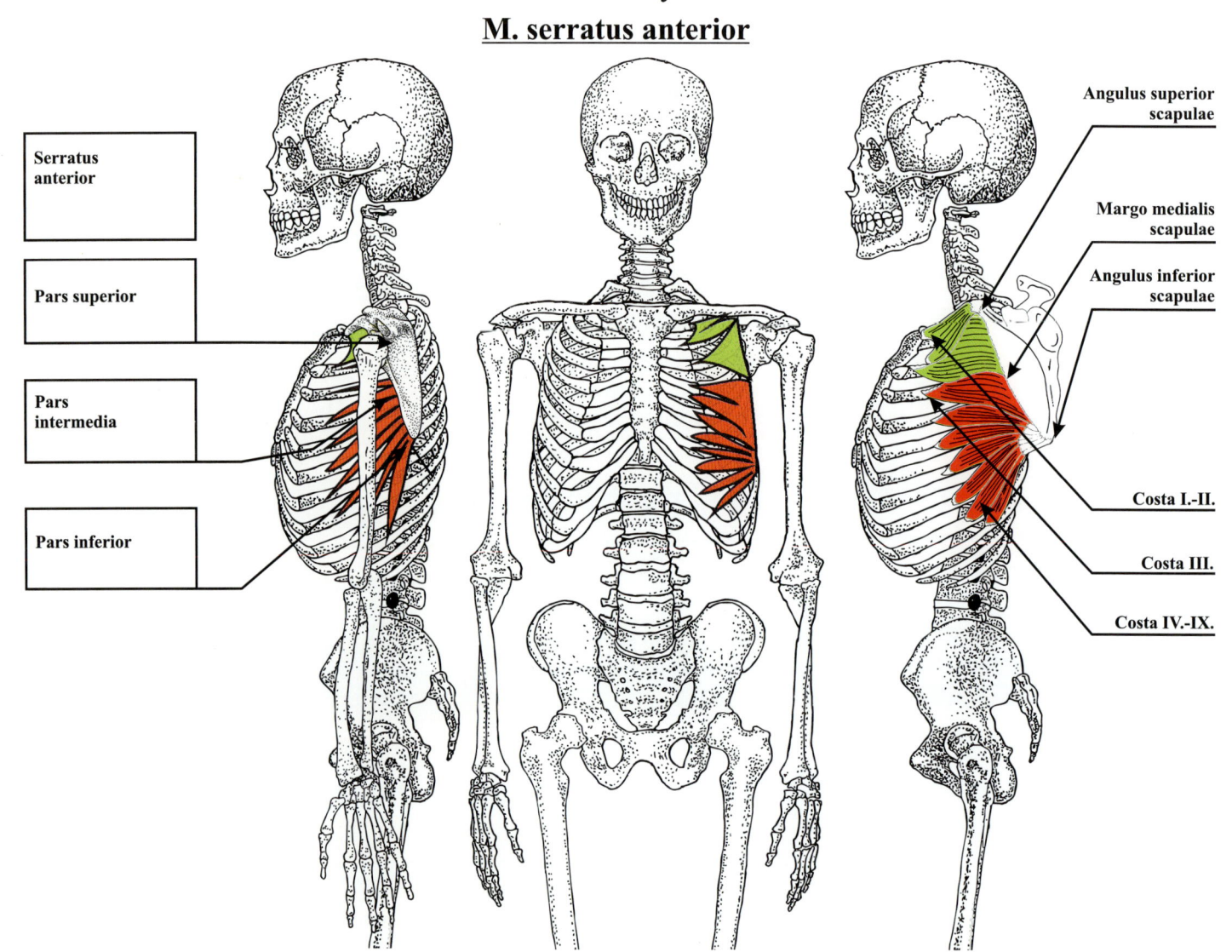

Anatomy
M. serratus anterior

| Serratus anterior |
| Pars superior |
| Pars intermedia |
| Pars inferior |

Angulus superior scapulae
Margo medialis scapulae
Angulus inferior scapulae
Costa I.-II.
Costa III.
Costa IV.-IX.

M. serratus anterior
Origin: - pars superior
- 1st and 2nd rib
        - pars intermedia
- 3rd rib
        - pars inferior
- 4th - 9th rib
Insertion: scapula
        - pars superior
- angulus superior
        - pars intermedia
- margo medialis
        - pars inferior
- angulus inferior
Function:
- moves the shoulder blade laterally and ventrally (whole muscle)
- acts as auxiliary respiratory muscle when the shoulder girdle is fixed
- pars inferior:
  - rotation of the shoulder blade, turning of the angulus inferior laterally and ventrally (enables elevation of the arm above 90°)
- pars superior:
  - return of the elevated arm (functions antagonistically against the pars inferior)
Innervation:
- n. thoracicus longus (C5-7)

Muscles with a tendency **towards internal muscle imbalance**

Muscle fibres with a tendency **towards weakening** These fibres must be **strengthened**

Muscle fibres with a tendency towards **tension and shortening** These fibres must be **relaxed and stretched**

The spiral part of the m. serratus anterior has a tendency towards weakening

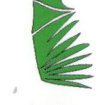

Relaxation
Stretching
Strengthening
Stabilization

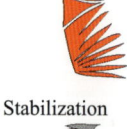

Manual techniques lying down
M. serratus anterior - massage, relaxation, passive stretching

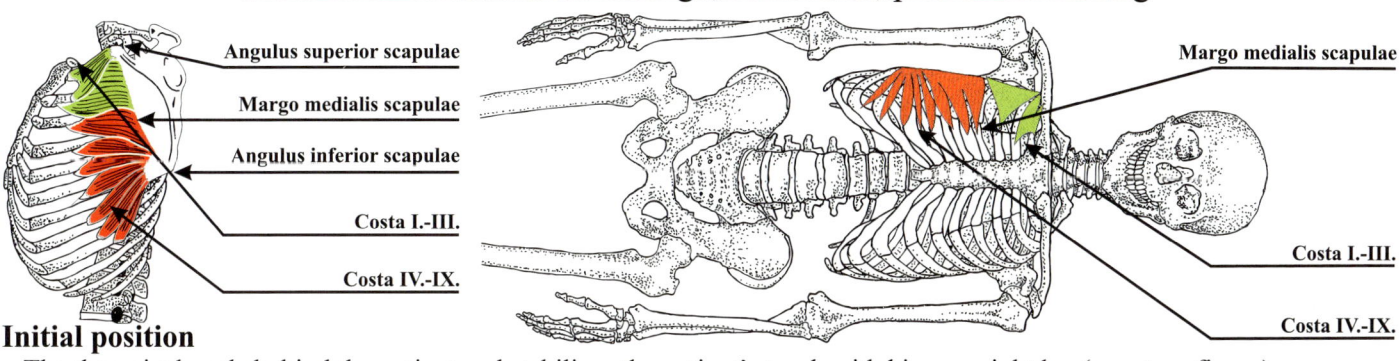

Angulus superior scapulae
Margo medialis scapulae
Angulus inferior scapulae
Costa I.-III.
Costa IV.-IX.

Margo medialis scapulae
Costa I.-III.
Costa IV.-IX.

Initial position
   The therapist kneels behind the patient and stabilizes the patient's trunk with his own right leg (punctum fixum). The right palm is placed on the shoulder with the fingers pointing dorsally (backwards). The palm and fingers of the left hand rest against the shoulder blade from behind. The patient breathes in.

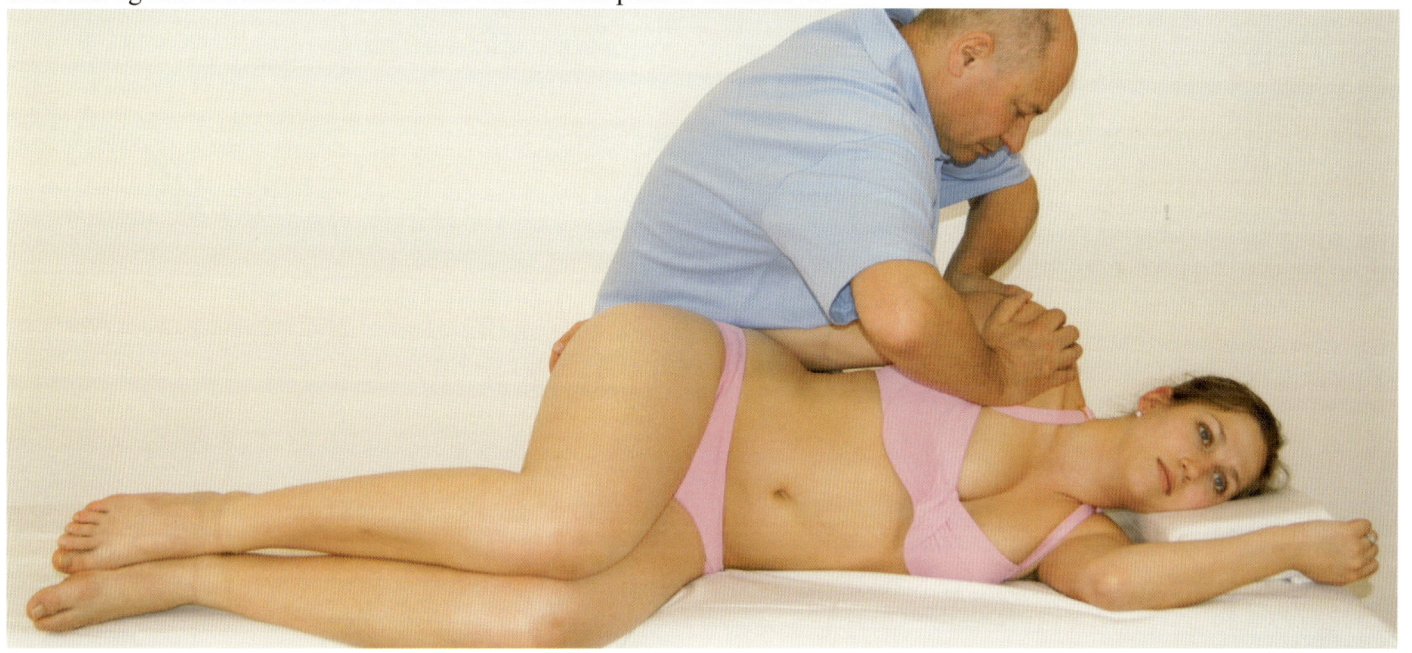

Performance
   The therapist shifts the weight of the body to the right arm and shifts the shoulder blade dorsally (backwards), (punctum mobile). This stretches the m. serratus anterior to the full extent. This initiates the massage of the m. serratus anterior and m. subscapularis. The patient slowly breathes out. The pulling is slackened and the stretching is repeated 6 times. At the end of the technique the therapist pauses for about 3 seconds.
   PIR. The extension is held and the patient breathes in. When breathing out the patient achieves further stretching. The process is repeated 3 times. In the same way, the technique is performed towards the 3rd, 4th and 5th ribs. This technique stretches the m. serratus anterior and other muscles of the anterior side of the shoulder girdle. This prepares the patient for the correct extent of backward movement of the shoulder blade during exercise.

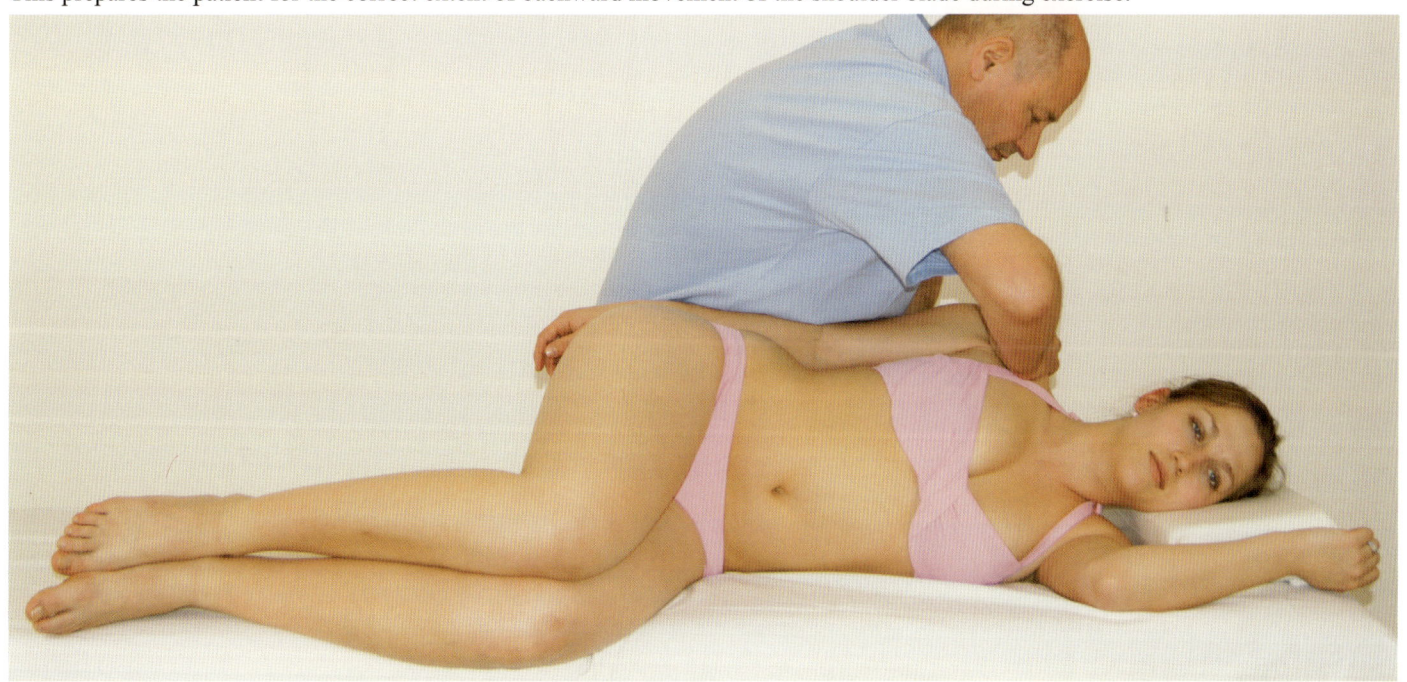

Exercise - stabilization, stretching
M. subclavius, m. pectoralis minor, m. serratus anterior
- relaxation in reciprocal inhibition, stretching

The LD - latissimus dorsi and TR - trapezius chains are the agonists in the second part of the exercise.

Exercise 1 - standing facing the attachment point of the elastic rope, the legs are in the basic position

Backward pull with both arms

Stabilization TR, LD

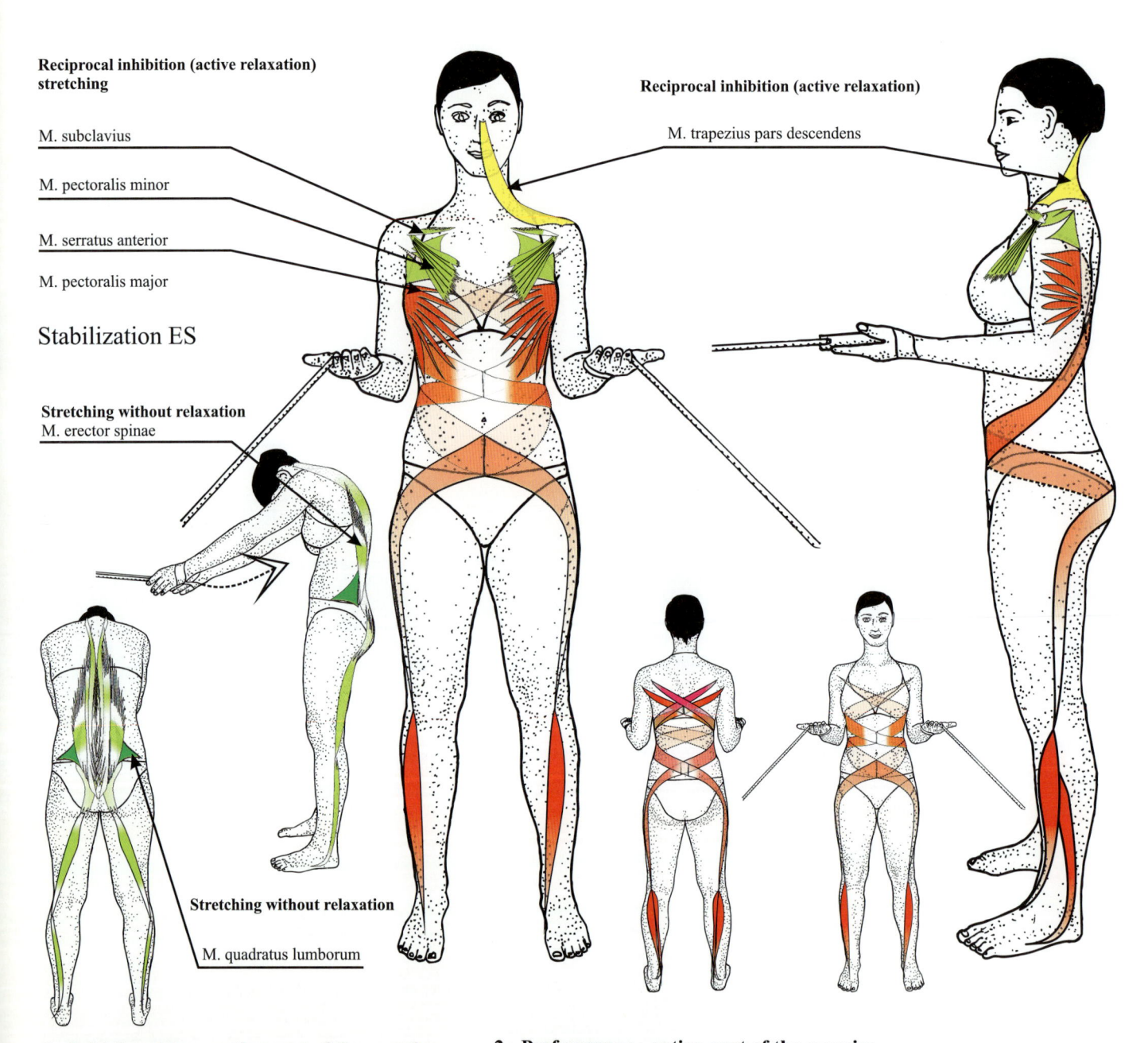

Reciprocal inhibition (active relaxation) stretching
M. subclavius
M. pectoralis minor
M. serratus anterior
M. pectoralis major

Stabilization ES

Stretching without relaxation
M. erector spinae

Reciprocal inhibition (active relaxation)
M. trapezius pars descendens

Stretching without relaxation
M. quadratus lumborum

1 - Initial position - active part of the exercise
In the initial position the back muscles are stretched:
- m. erector spinae
- m. quadratus lumborum

2 - Performance - active part of the exercise
In the active part of the exercise the muscles in the anterior side of the shoulder girdle are stretched:
- m. subclavius
- m. pectoralis minor
- m. pectoralis major
- m. serratus anterior

The muscles in the upper side of the shoulder girdle are relaxed:
- m. trapezius, pars descendens
- m. levator scapulae
- mm. scaleni
- m. semispinalis capitis, cervicis and other muscles.

Exercise - stabilization, stretching
M. subclavius, m. pectoralis minor, m. serratus anterior
- relaxation in reciprocal inhibition, stretching

The LD - latissimus dorsi and TR - trapezius chains are the agonists in the second part of the exercise.

Exercise 2 - standing sideways on to the attachment point of the elastic rope, the legs are in the basic position

Sideways pull with one arm

Stabilization TR, LD

Reciprocal inhibition (active relaxation)

M. trapezius pars descendens

Reciprocal inhibition (active relaxation) stretching

M. subclavius

M. deltoideus pars clavicularis

M. coracobrachialis

M. pectoralis minor

M. serratus anterior

Active relaxation

M. rectus capitis posterior major

M. trapezius pars descendens

M. levator scapulae

M. semispinalis capitis

M. semispinalis cervicis

Stabilization ES

Stretching without relaxation
M. quadratus lumborum

M. erector spinae

1 - Initial position
- passive part
of the exercise
In the initial position the back muscles are stretched:
- m. erector spinae
- m. quadratus lumborum

2 - Performance
- active part of the exercise
In the active part of the exercise the muscles in the anterior side of the shoulder girdle are stretched:
- m. subclavius
- m. pectoralis minor
- m. pectoralis major

2 - Performance
- active part of the exercise
In the active part of the exercise the muscles in the upper side of the shoulder girdle are relaxed:
- m. trapezius pars descendens
- m. levator scapulae
- mm. scaleni
- m. semispinalis capitis, cervicis
and other muscles.

Exercise - stabilization, stretching

M. subclavius, m. pectoralis minor, m. serratus anterior
- relaxation in reciprocal inhibition, stretching

The PM - pectoralis major chain is agonist in the first part of the exercise,
the LD - latissimus dorsi and TR - trapezius chains are the agonists in the second part of the exercise.

Exercise 3 - standing with back to the attachment point of the elastic rope, the legs are in the basic position

Opening the arms backwards, pulling the shoulder blades towards each other

Stabilization TR, LD   Stabilization PM

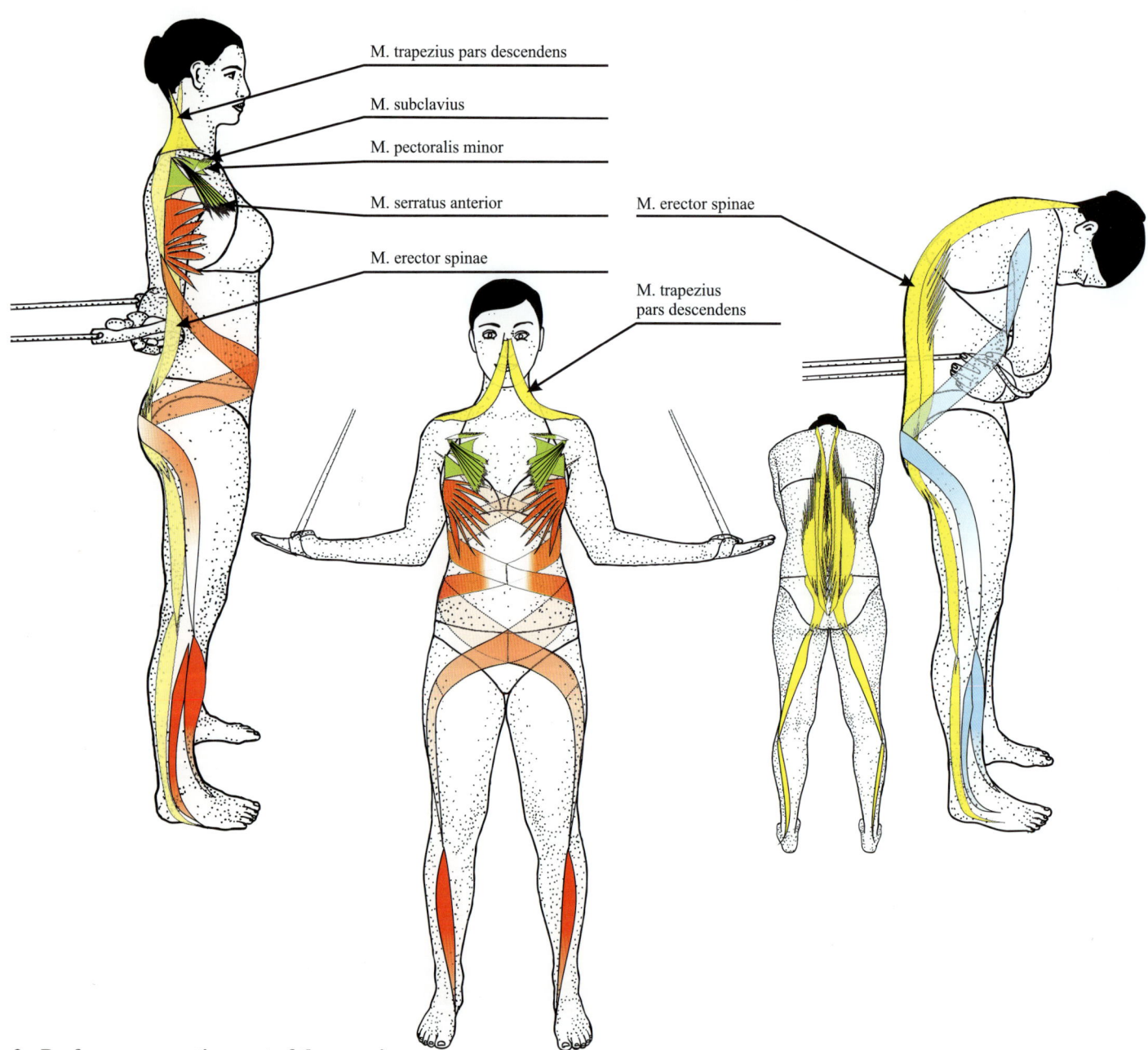

Labels:
- M. trapezius pars descendens
- M. subclavius
- M. pectoralis minor
- M. serratus anterior
- M. erector spinae
- M. erector spinae
- M. trapezius pars descendens

2 - Performance - active part of the exercise
In the active part of the exercise the muscles in the anterior side of the shoulder girdle are stretched:
- m. subclavius
- m. pectoralis minor
- m. pectoralis major
- m. serratus anterior

In the upper part of the shoulder girdle, the neck muscles are stretched:
- m. trapezius pars descendens
- m. levator scapulae
- mm. scaleni
- m. semispinalis capitis, cervicis
and other muscles.

1 - Initial position - active part of the exercise
In the initial position the m. erector spinae, actively inhibited by the activity of the PM - pectoralis major chain, is stretched.
The movement is stopped by the tension in the ligamenta interspinalia.

Exercise

M. subclavius, m. pectoralis minor, m. serratus anterior - active relaxation and stretching

Exercise 2 - sitting sideways on to the attachment point of the elastic rope, sideways pull with the shoulder blade

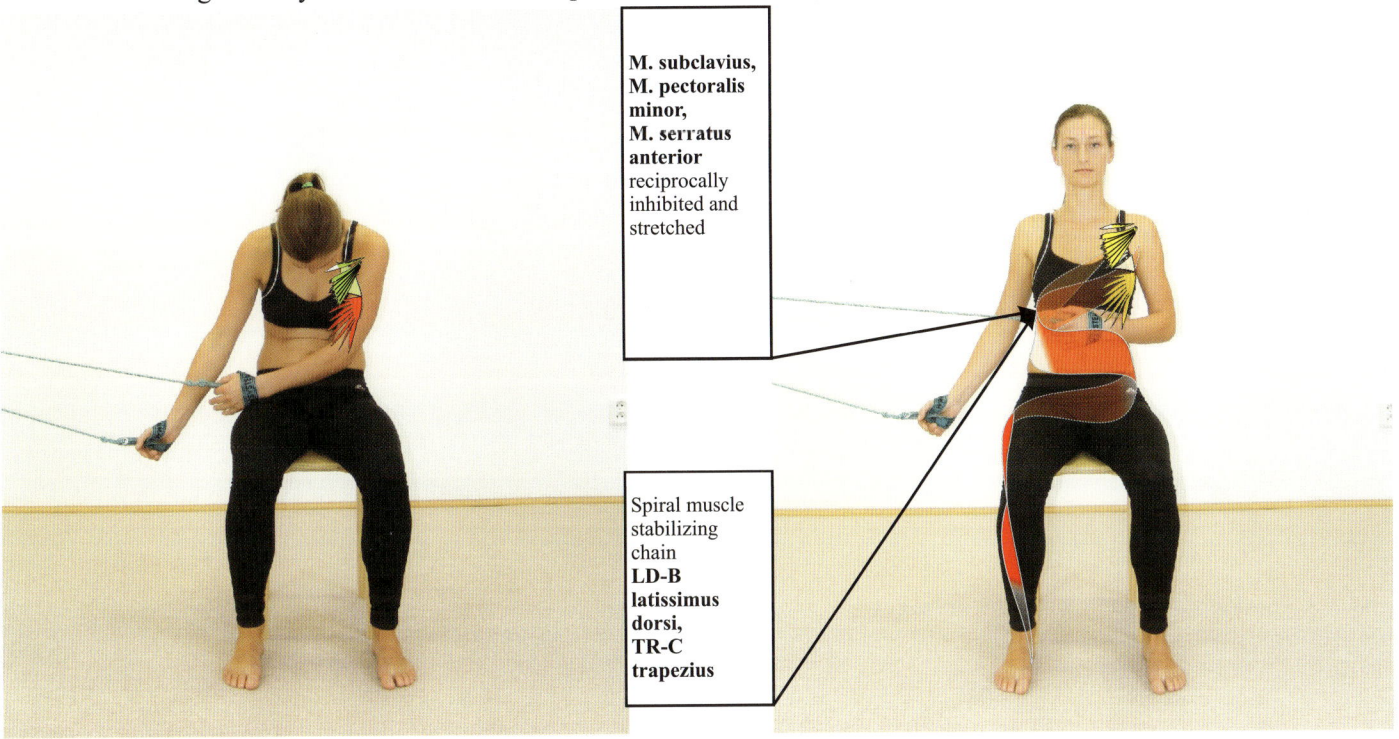

M. subclavius, M. pectoralis minor, M. serratus anterior reciprocally inhibited and stretched

Spiral muscle stabilizing chain **LD-B** latissimus dorsi, **TR-C** trapezius

M. subclavius, m. pectoralis minor, m. serratus anterior - active relaxation and stretching

Exercise 2 - sitting sideways on to the attachment point of the elastic rope, sideways pull with one arms

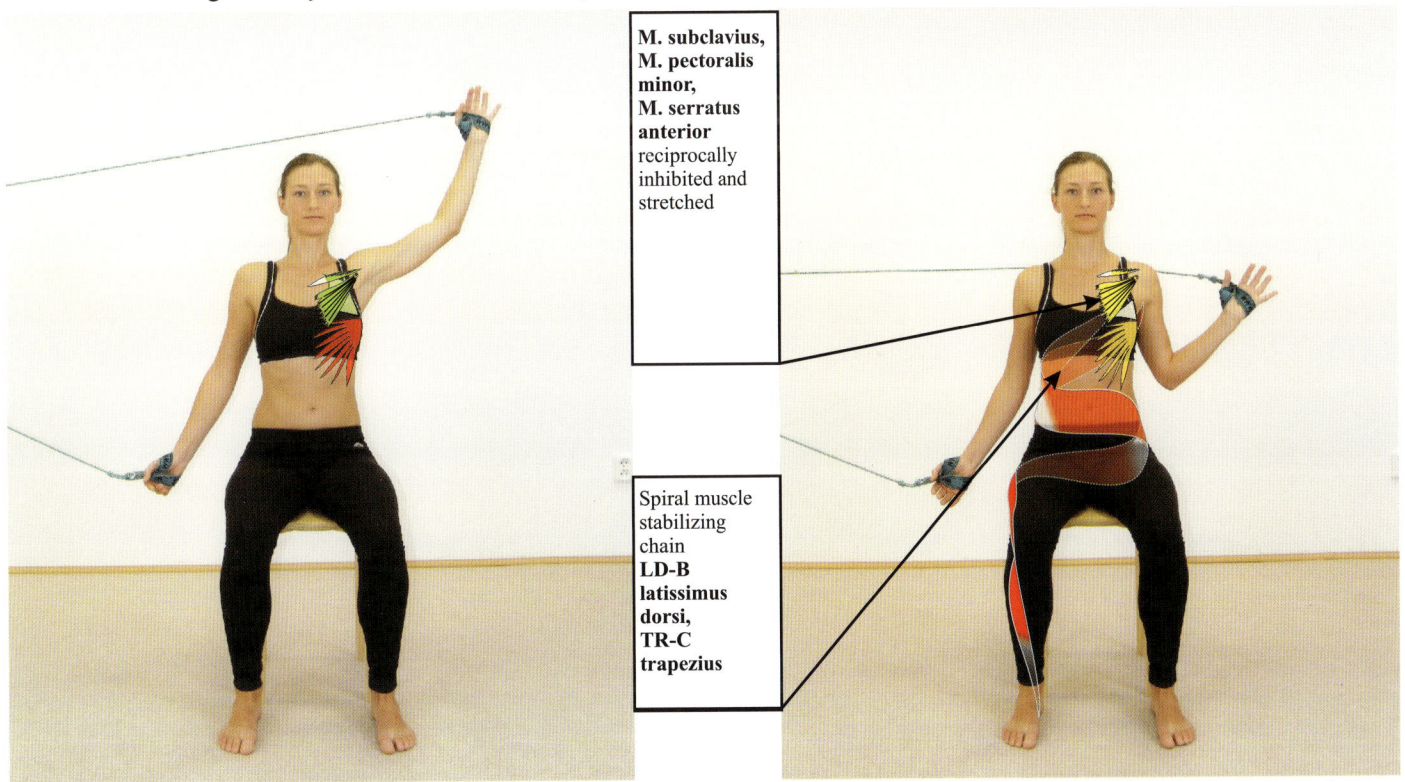

M. subclavius, M. pectoralis minor, M. serratus anterior reciprocally inhibited and stretched

Spiral muscle stabilizing chain **LD-B** latissimus dorsi, **TR-C** trapezius

Stretching the m. subclavius, m. pectoralis minor, m. serratus anterior, m. pectoralis major inhibited in reciprocal inhibition.
The agonist is the LD and TR spirals, which stabilize the body. The M. subclavius, m. pectoralis minor, m. serratus anterior, m. pectoralis major are reciprocally inhibited and stretched at the same time.

Exercise
M. subclavius, m. pectoralis minor, m. serratus anterior - active relaxation and stretching

Exercise 2 - standing sideways on to the attachment point of the elastic rope, sideways pull with the shoulder blade

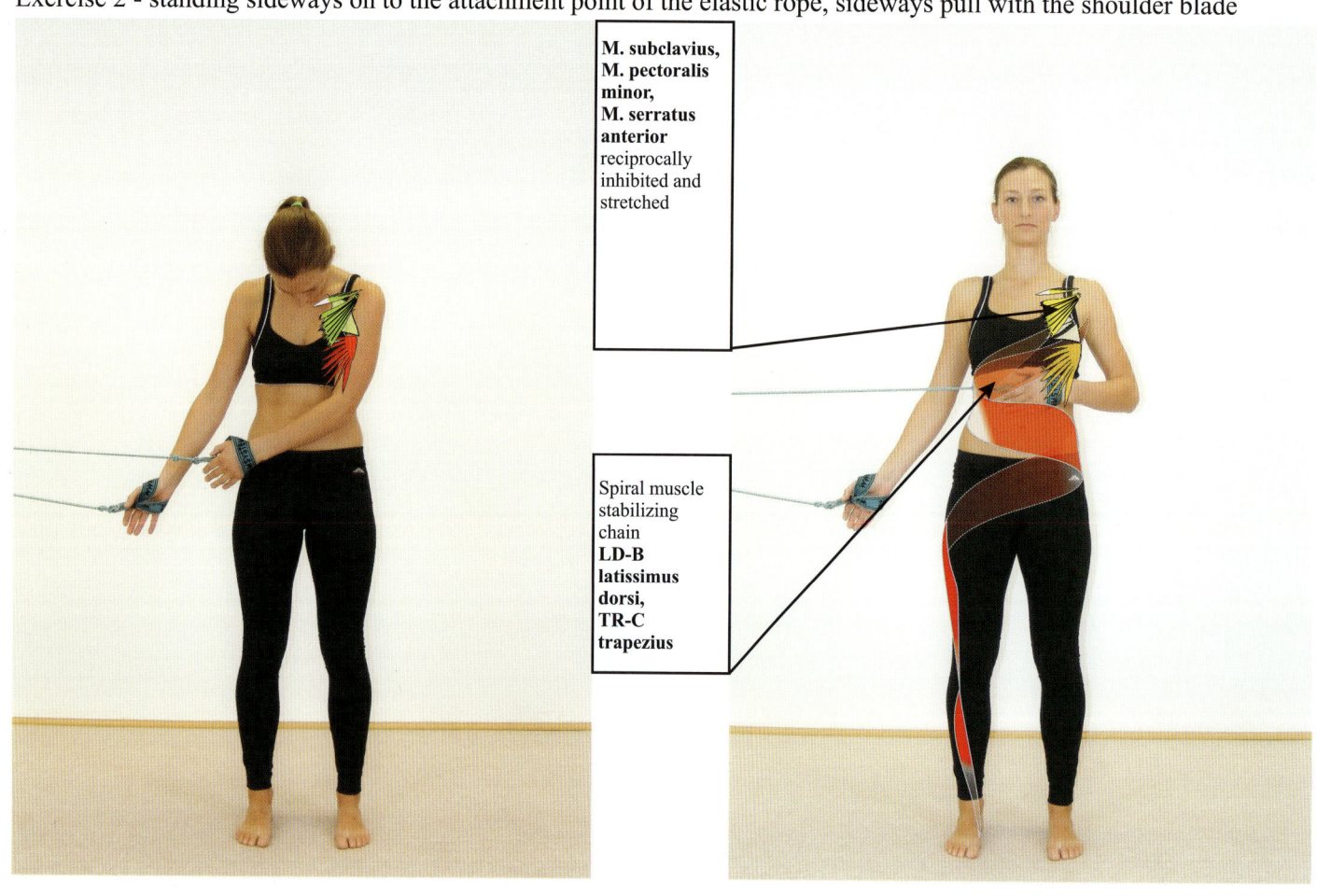

M. subclavius, M. pectoralis minor, M. serratus anterior reciprocally inhibited and stretched

Spiral muscle stabilizing chain **LD-B latissimus dorsi, TR-C trapezius**

M. subclavius, m. pectoralis minor, m. serratus anterior - active relaxation and stretching

Exercise 2 - standing sideways on to the attachment point of the elastic rope, sideways pull with one arm

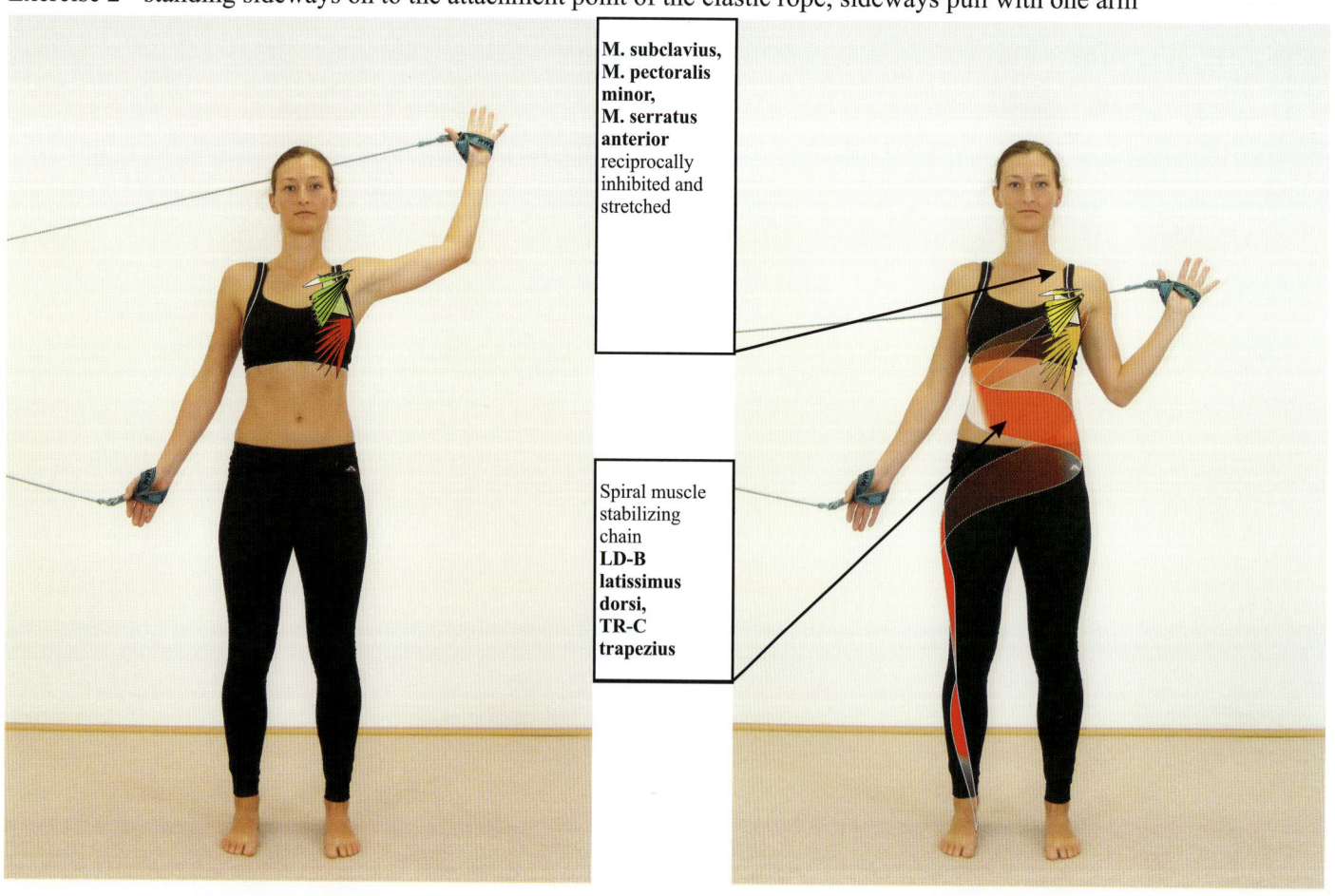

M. subclavius, M. pectoralis minor, M. serratus anterior reciprocally inhibited and stretched

Spiral muscle stabilizing chain **LD-B latissimus dorsi, TR-C trapezius**

Exercise
M. subclavius, m. pectoralis minor, m. serratus anterior - active relaxation and stretching

Exercise 1 - standing facing the attachment point of the elastic rope with one leg on the mat, backward pull with both arms

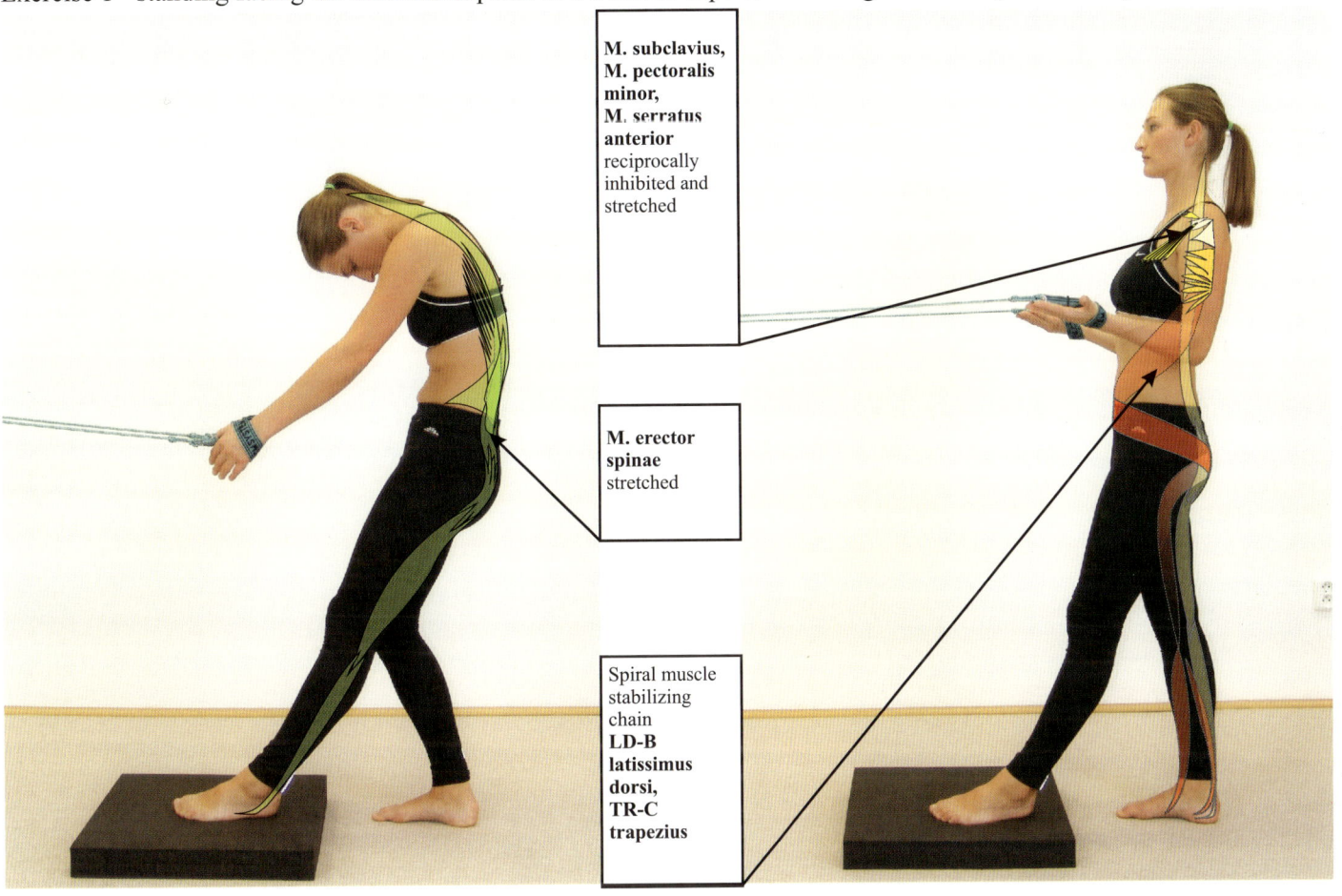

M. subclavius, M. pectoralis minor, M. serratus anterior reciprocally inhibited and stretched

M. erector spinae stretched

Spiral muscle stabilizing chain **LD-B latissimus dorsi, TR-C trapezius**

M. subclavius, m. pectoralis minor, m. serratus anterior - active relaxation and stretching

Exercise 3 - standing with back to the attachment of the elastic rope, one leg on the mat, backward pull with both arms

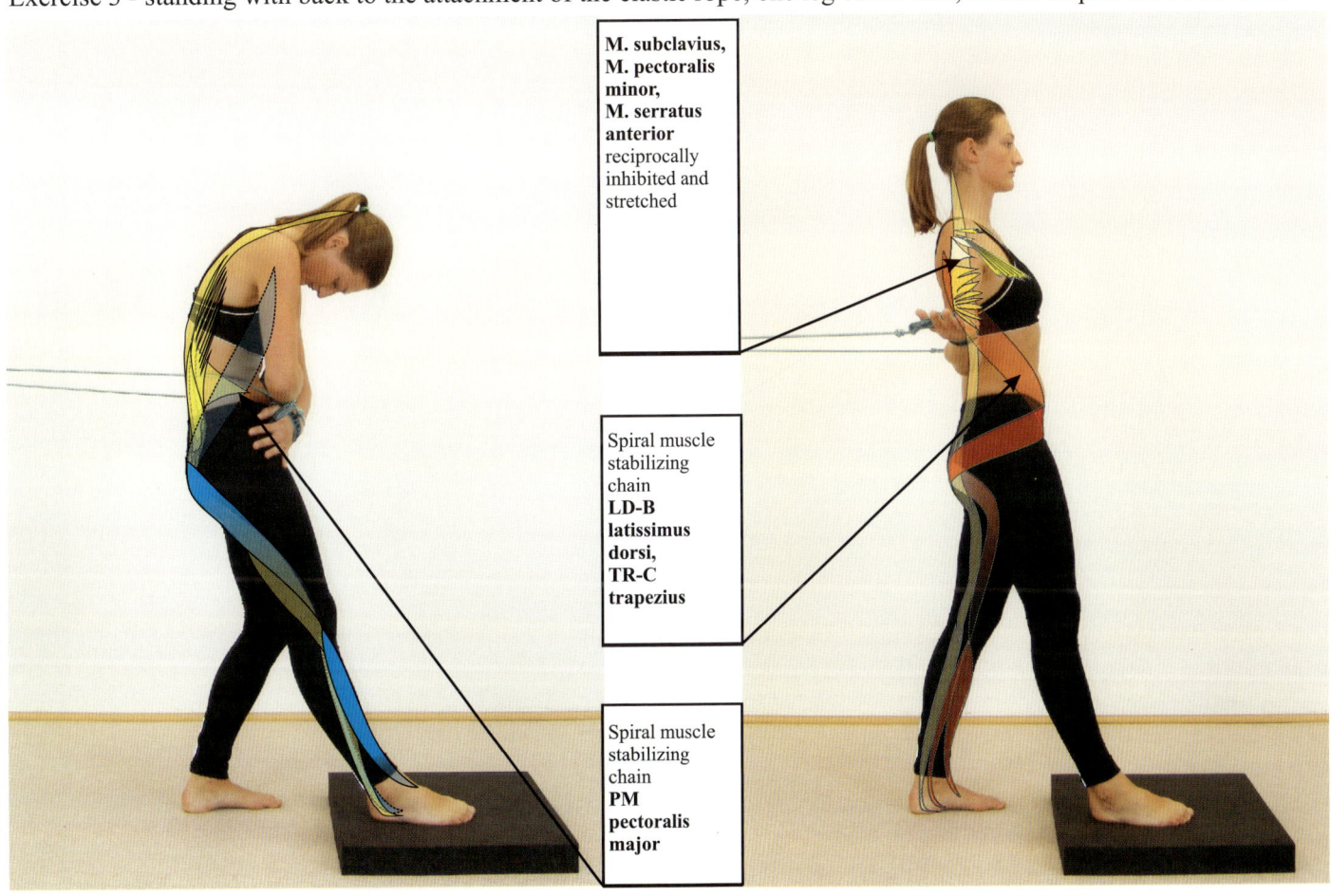

M. subclavius, M. pectoralis minor, M. serratus anterior reciprocally inhibited and stretched

Spiral muscle stabilizing chain **LD-B latissimus dorsi, TR-C trapezius**

Spiral muscle stabilizing chain **PM pectoralis major**

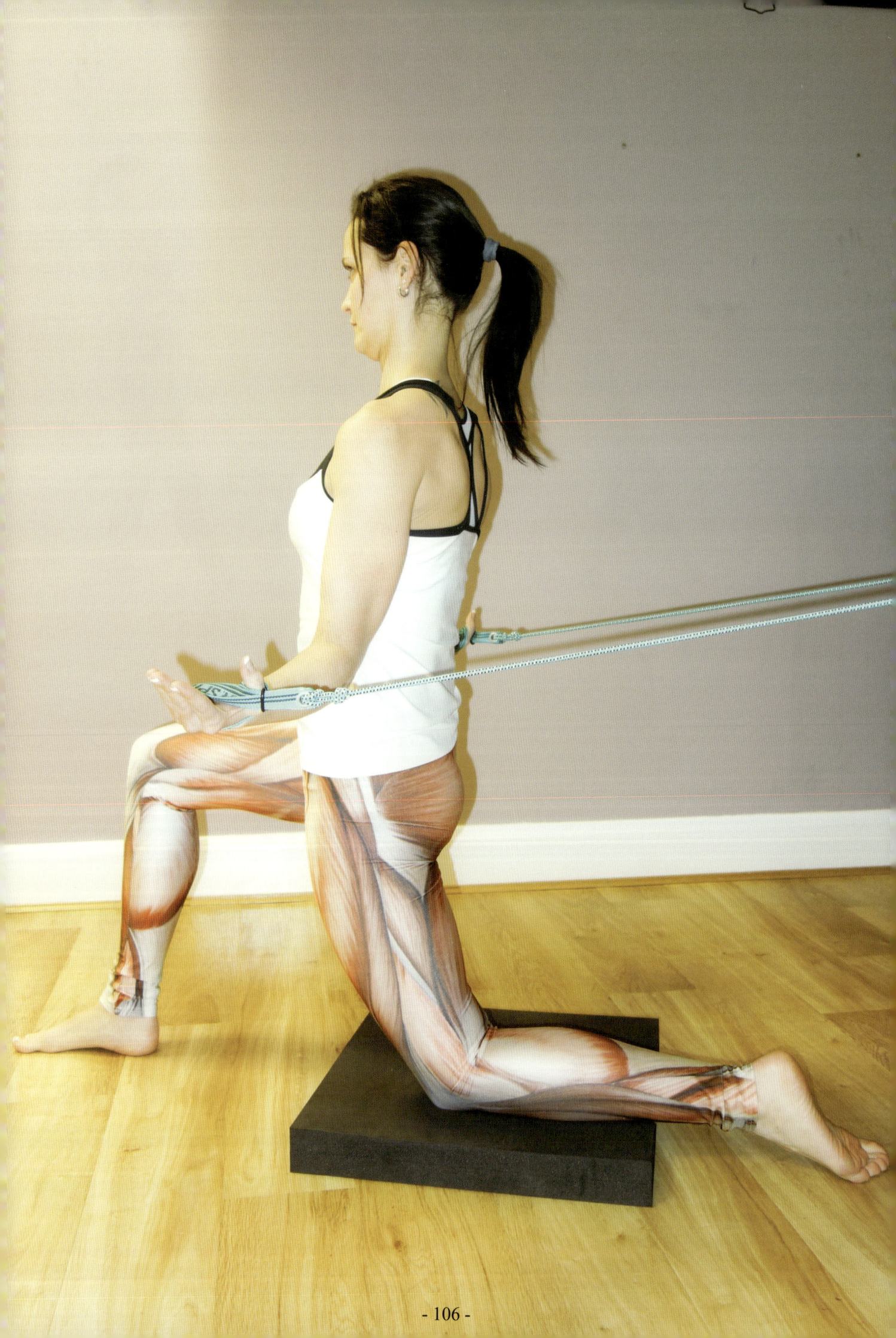

MANUAL TECHNIQUES AND EXERCISE ACCORDING TO MUSCLE ANALYSIS

Pelvic girdle
The anterior muscle group
Muscles with a tendency towards tension and shortening:

M. rectus femoris
M. tensor fasciae latae
M. gluteus medius
M. iliopsoas
M. psoas major
M. psoas minor
M. iliacus

Paravertebral muscles
The anterior lower muscle group
with a tendency towards tension and shortening:

M. psoas major
M. psoas minor

Paravertebral muscles
The anterior upper muscle group
Muscles with a tendency towards tension and shortening:

M. longus capitis
M. longus cervicis

Anatomy
M. rectus femoris, m. tensor fasciae latae, m. gluteus medius

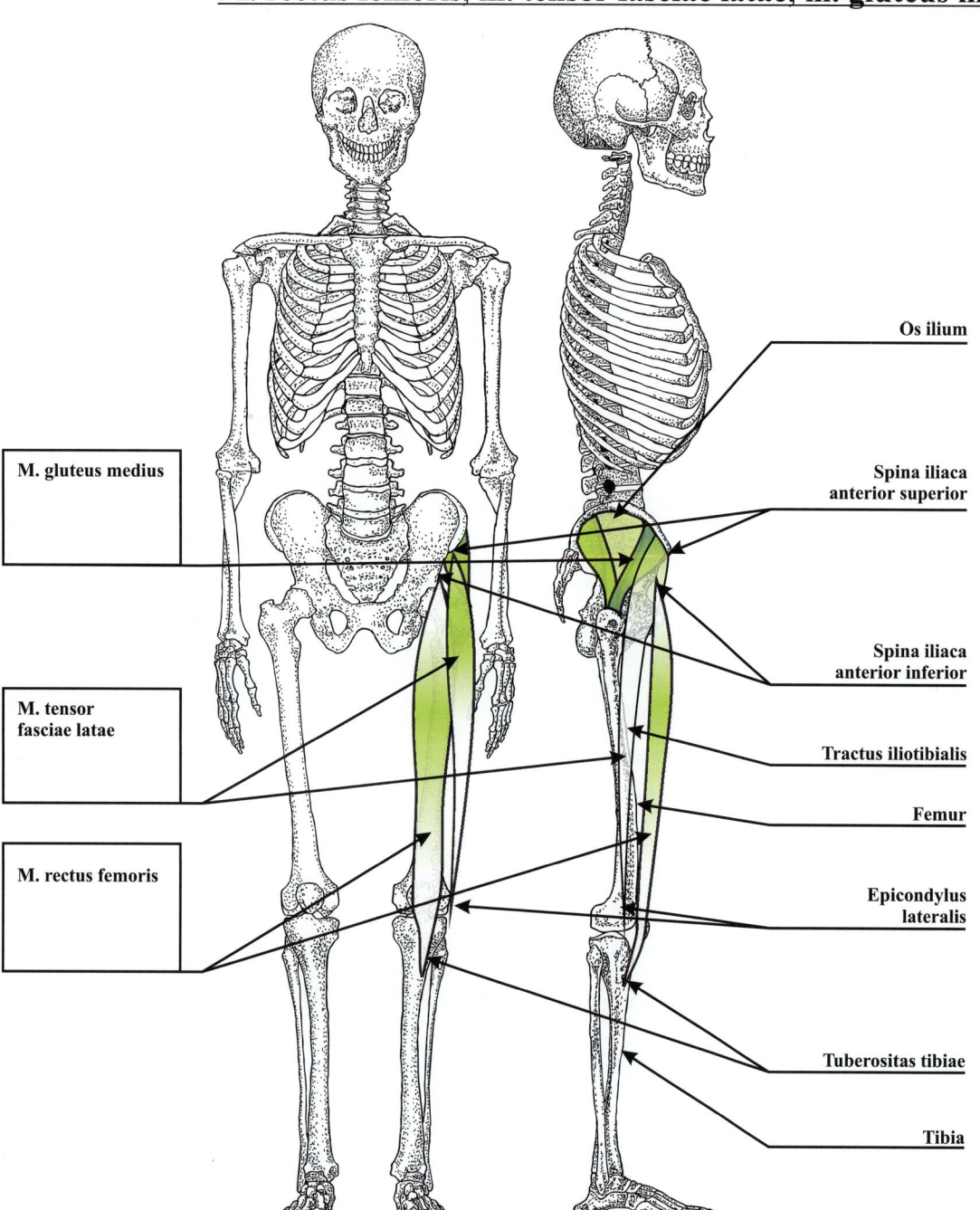

Muscles with a tendency towards tension and shortening These muscles must be **relaxed and stretched**

Relaxation

Stretching

Stretching

Stabilization

M. gluteus medius

M. tensor fasciae latae

M. rectus femoris

Os ilium

Spina iliaca anterior superior

Spina iliaca anterior inferior

Tractus iliotibialis

Femur

Epicondylus lateralis

Tuberositas tibiae

Tibia

M. rectus femoris
Origin:
- spina iliaca anterior inferior
- os ilium, above the acetabulum
Insertion:
- tuberositas tibiae
Function: - hip joint:
- flexion (bending)
  - knee joint:
- extension (stretching)
Innervation:
- n. femoralis (L2-4)

M. gluteus medius
Origin:
- crista iliaca labium externum
- ala ossi ilii
Insertion:
- trochanter major
Function: - hip joint:
- flexion (bending) anterior part
- extension (stretching) posterior part
- abduction (sideways movement) whole muscle
Innervation:
- n. femoralis (L2-4)

M. tensor fasciae latae
Origin:
- spina iliaca anterior superior
- ala osis ilii
Insertion:
- fascia lata
- tractus iliotibialis
- epicondylus lateralis
Function: - hip:
- flexion (bending) of the hip joint
- abduction (pulling away) of the thigh
- inward rotation of the thigh
  - knee:
- extension (stretching)
- outward rotation
Innervation:
- n. gluteus superior (L4-S1)

- 108 -

Manual techniques lying on one side
M. rectus femoris - stretching

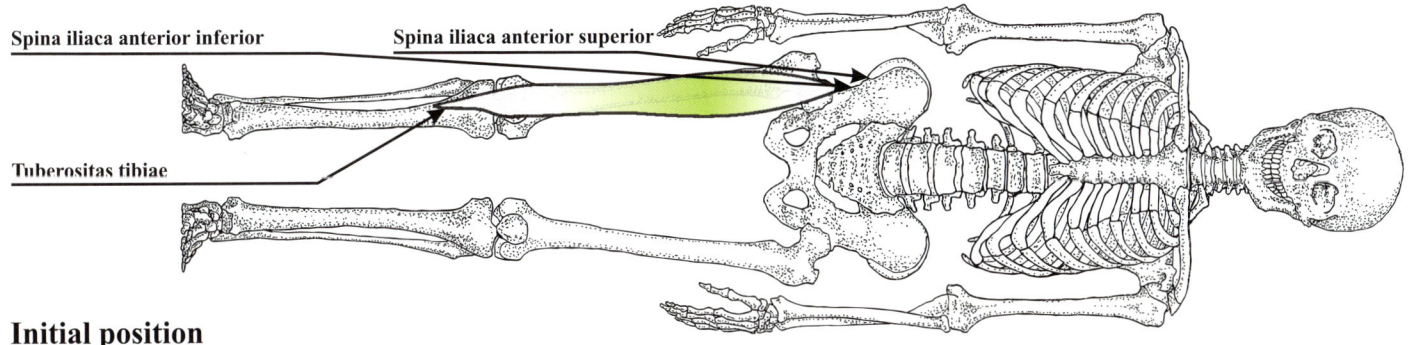

Spina iliaca anterior inferior   Spina iliaca anterior superior

Tuberositas tibiae

Initial position
The therapist kneels behind the patient facing the pelvis. He stabilizes the patient's trunk and pelvis with his left leg (punctum fixum). The left palm is placed on the - SIAS spina iliaca anterior superior. The fingers must not bend but are gently spread over the largest possible area. The right hand grasps the patient's knee. The patient's lower leg lies on the forearm. The leg is placed horizontally. The patient breathes in.

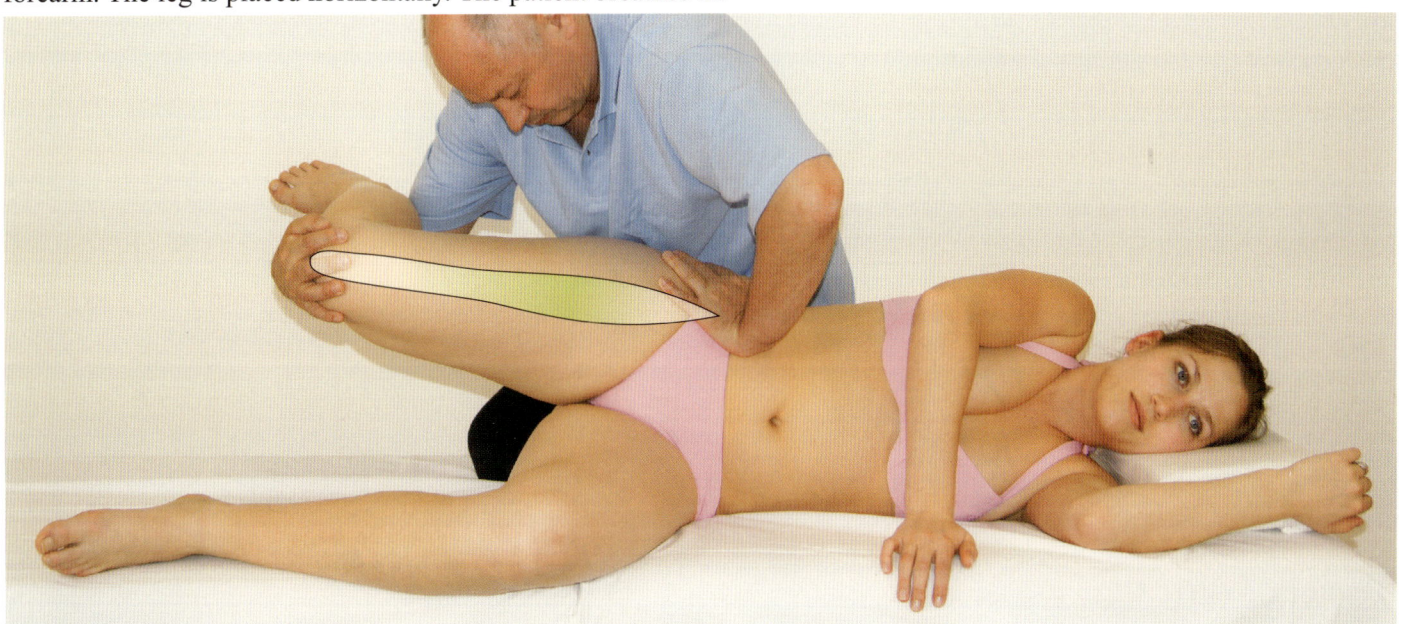

Performance
The therapist shifts the weight of the body to the left arm and stabilizes the pelvis from in front (punctum fixum). The patient's thigh is pulled backwards with the right arm. This stretches the m. rectus femoris. The patient slowly breathes out. The pulling is slackened and the stretching is repeated 6 times. At the end of the tecnhique the therapist pauses for about 3 seconds.
  PIR. The extension is held and the patient breathes in. This causes a counter-pressure. When breathing out, the patient achieves further stretching. The process is repeated 3 times.
  Reciprocal inhibition. At the end of the passive stretching, the patient is asked to engage the buttocks and make an active backward movement (step backwards). The extension in the hip increases by 5 to 10 cm. The M. gluteus maximus is the agonist here, while the inhibited m. rectus femoris is the antagonist. This technique stretches the m. rectus femoris and other muscles of the anterior side of the pelvic girdle. This prepares the patient for the correct extent of backward movement of the leg during exercise.

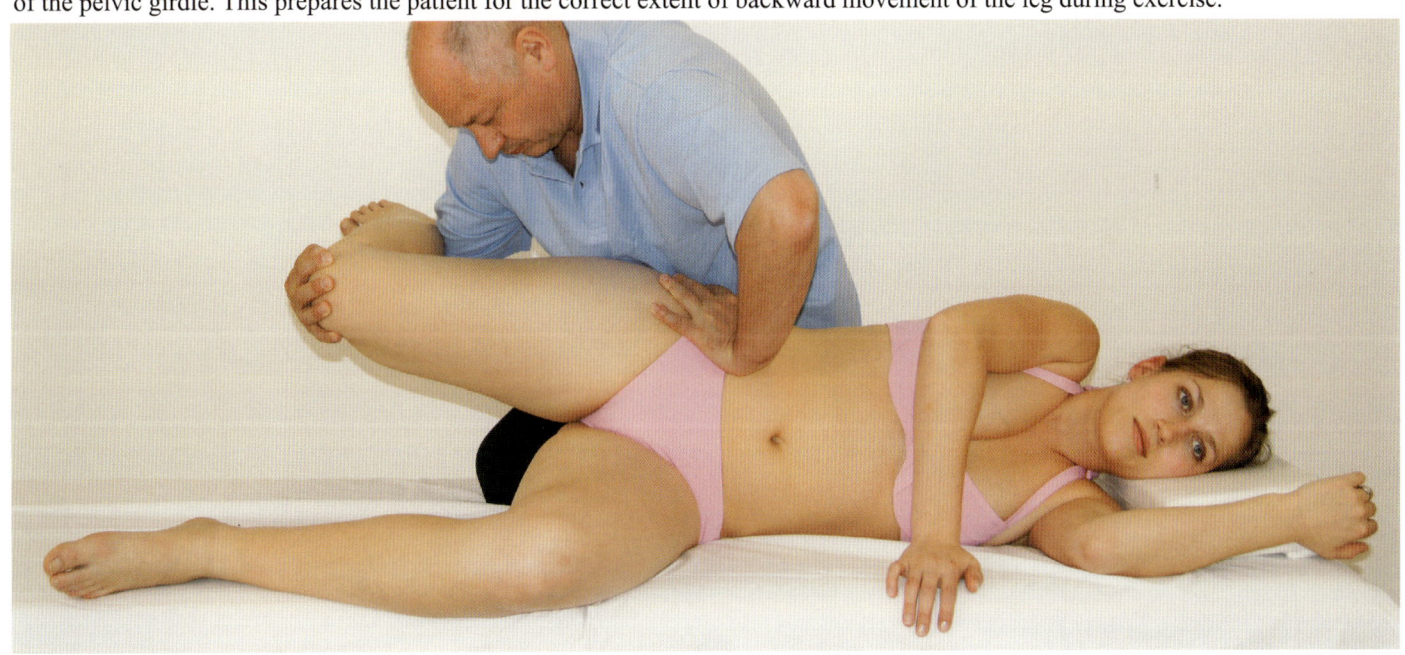

Manual techniques lying on one side
M. tensor fasciae latae, m. gluteus medius - stretching

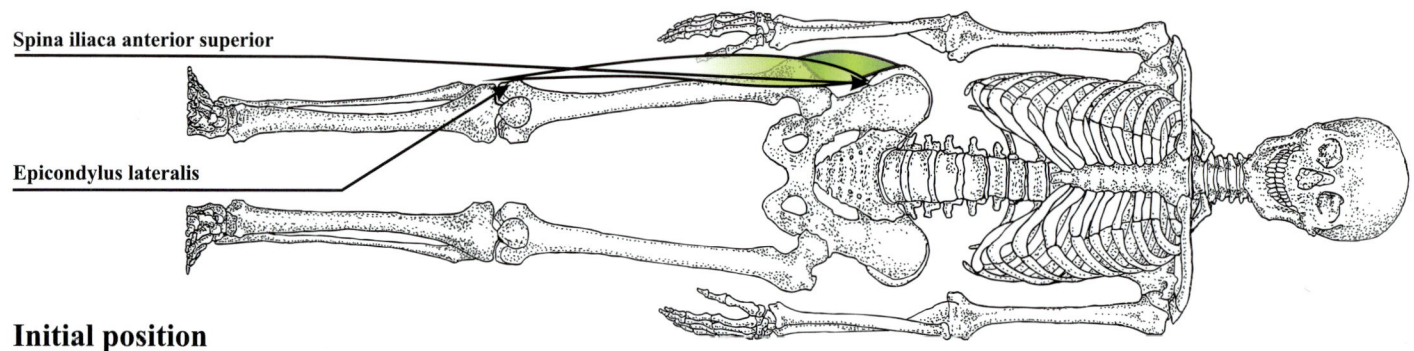

Spina iliaca anterior superior

Epicondylus lateralis

Initial position
The therapist kneels behind the patient facing the pelvis. The patient stabilizes the patient's trunk and pelvis with his left leg (punctum fixum). The left palm is placed on the SIAS - spina iliaca anterior superior.
The fingers must not bend but are gently spread over the largest possible area. The right hand grasps the patient's knee. The patient's lower leg lies on the forearm. The leg is placed obliquely downwards (medially). The patient breathes in.

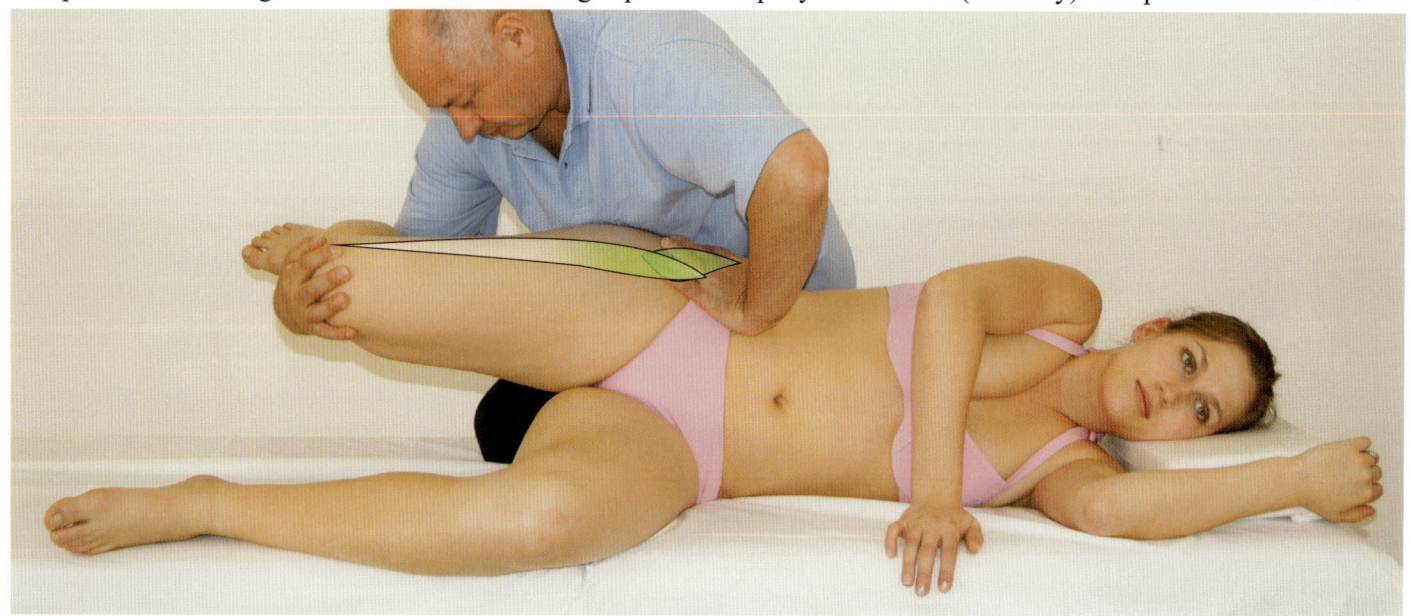

Performance
The therapist shifts the weight of the body to the left arm and stabilizes the pelvis from in front (punctum fixum). The patient's thigh is pulled backwards and downwards (medially) with the right arm. This stretches the m. tensor fasciae latae and anterior part of the m. gluteus medius. The patient breathes out slowly. The pulling is slackened and the stretching is repeated 6 times. At the end of the technique the therapist pauses for about 3 seconds.

PIR. The extension is held and the patient breathes in. This causes a counter-pressure. When breathing out, the patient achieves further stretching. The process is repeated 3 times.

Reciprocal inhibition. At the end of the passive stretching the patient is asked to engage the buttocks and make an active backward movement (step backwards) The extension in the hip increases by 5 to 10 cm. The M. gluteus maximus is the agonist here, while the inhibited m. tensor fasciae latae is the antagonist. This technique stretches the m. tensor fasciae latae and other muscles of the anterior side of the pelvic girdle. This prepares the patient for the correct extent of backward movement of the leg during exercise and walking.

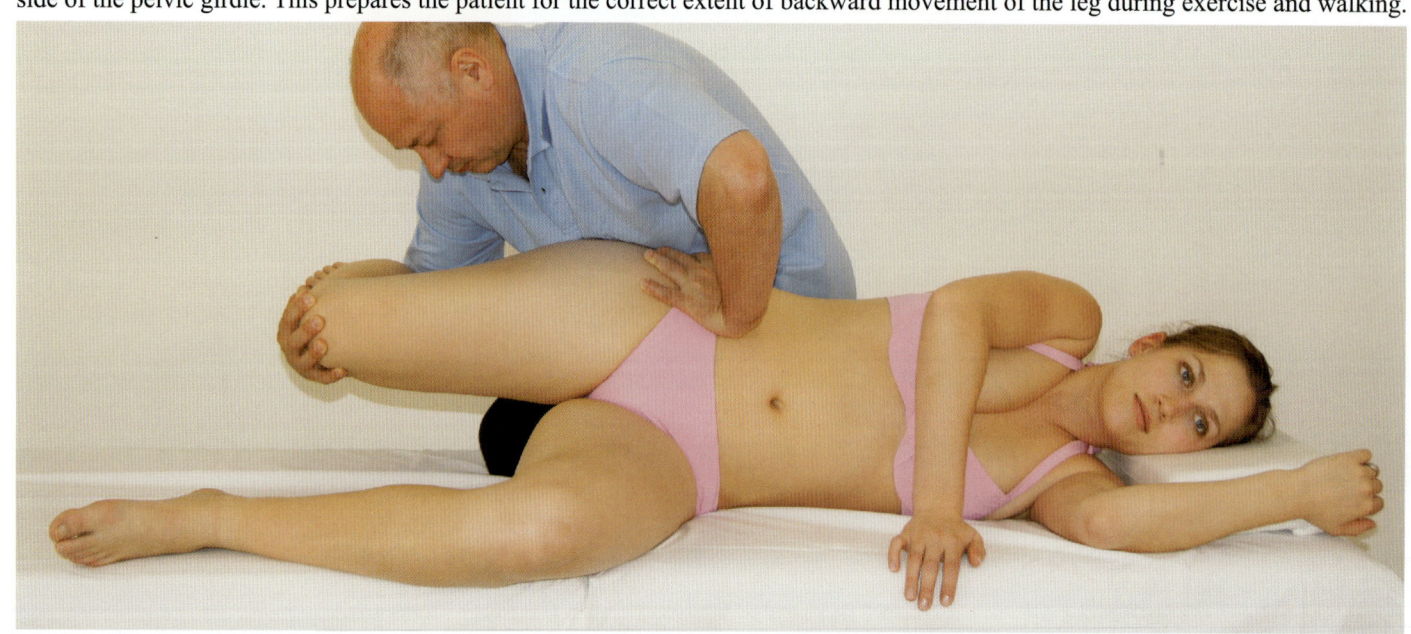

Manual techniques - lying - one limb in a hoist
M. rectus femoris - stretching

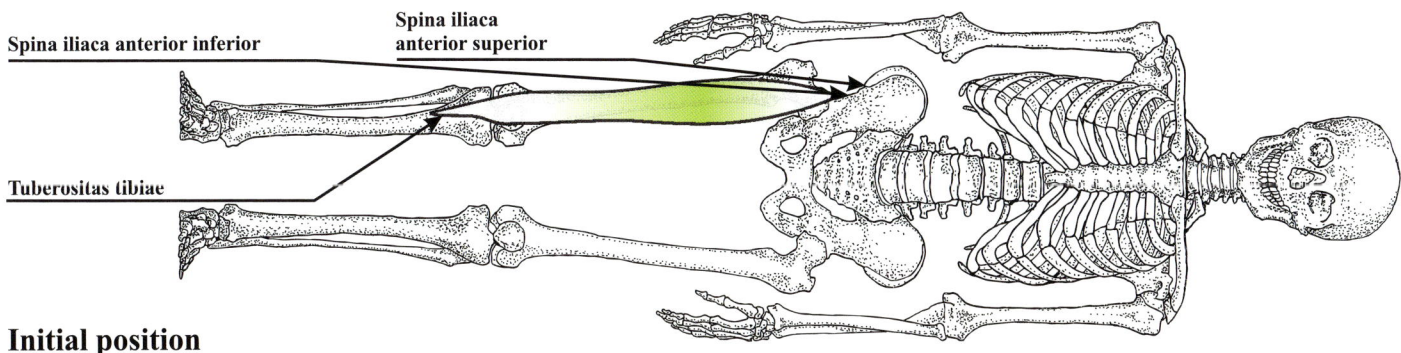

Spina iliaca anterior inferior
Spina iliaca anterior superior
Tuberositas tibiae

Initial position
The therapist kneels behind the patient facing the pelvis. He stabilizes the patient's trunk and pelvis with his left leg (punctum fixum). The left palm is placed on the SIAS - spina iliaca anterior superior.
The fingers must not bend but are gently spread over the largest possible area. The right hand grasps the patient's knee. The patient's lower leg lies on the forearm. The leg is placed horizontally. The patient breathes in.

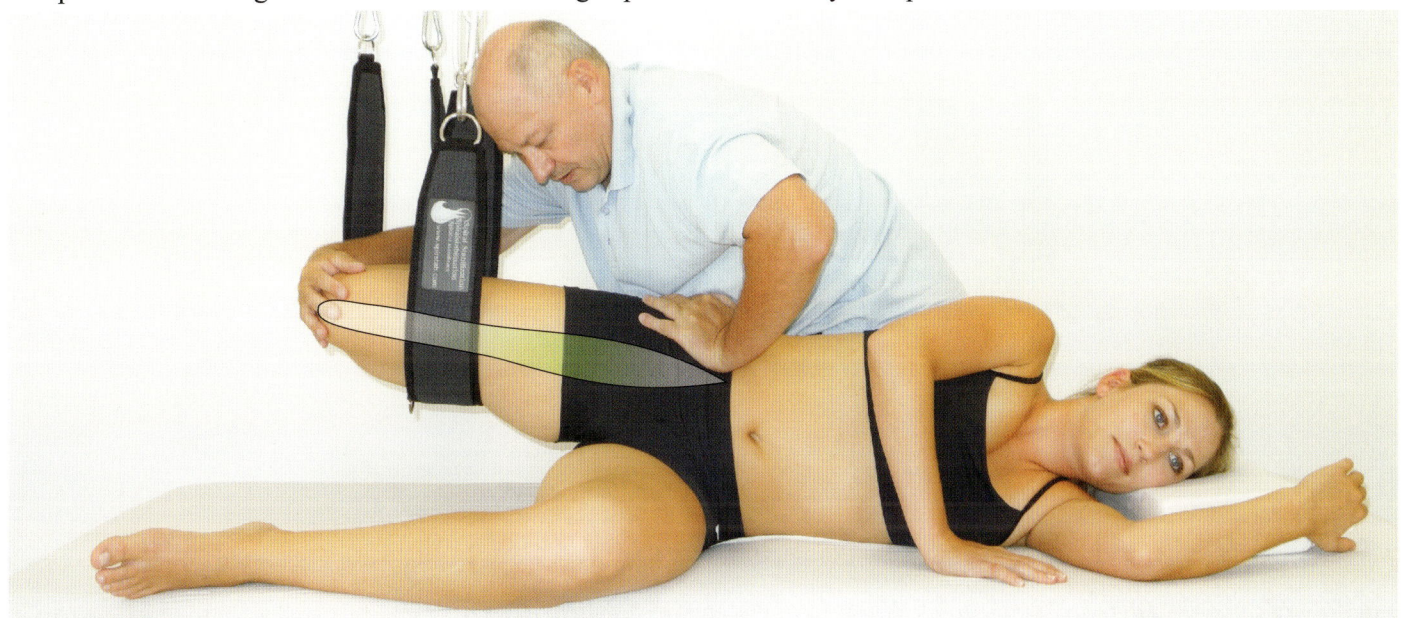

Performance
The therapist shifts the weight of the body to the left arm and stabilizes the pelvis from in front (punctum fixum).
The patient's thigh is pulled backwards with the right arm. This stretches the m. rectus femoris.
The patient breathes out slowly. The pulling is slackened and the stretching is repeated 6 times.
At the end of the technique the therapist pauses for about 3 seconds.
  PIR. The extension is held and the patient breathes in. This causes a counter-pressure.
When breathing out, the patient achieves further stretching. The process is repeated 3 times.
  Reciprocal inhibition. At the end of the passive stretching, the patient is asked to engage the buttocks and make an active backward movement (step backwards). The extension in the hip increases by 5 to 10 cm. The M. gluteus maximus is the agonist here, while the inhibited m. rectus femoris is the antagonist. This technique stretches the m. rectus femoris and other muscles of the anterior side of the pelvic girdle. This prepares the patient for the correct extent of backward movement of the leg during exercise.

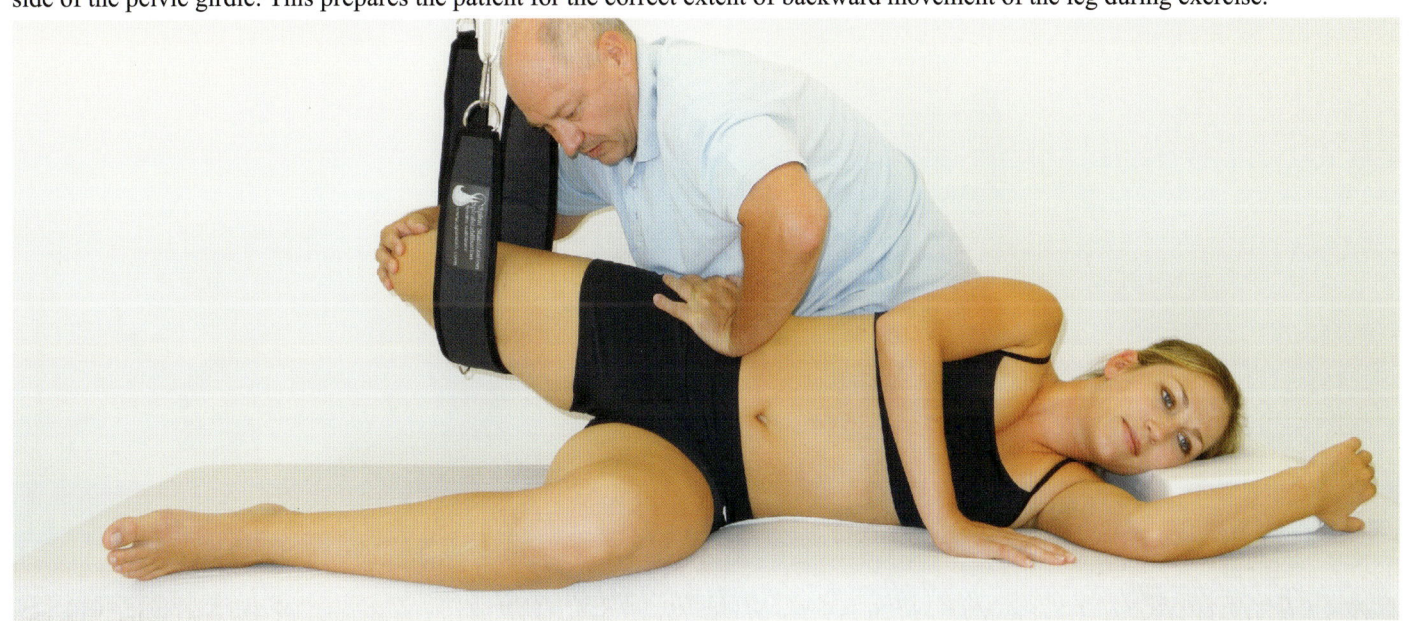

Manual techniques - lying - one limb in a hoist
M. tensor fasciae latae, m. gluteus medius - stretching

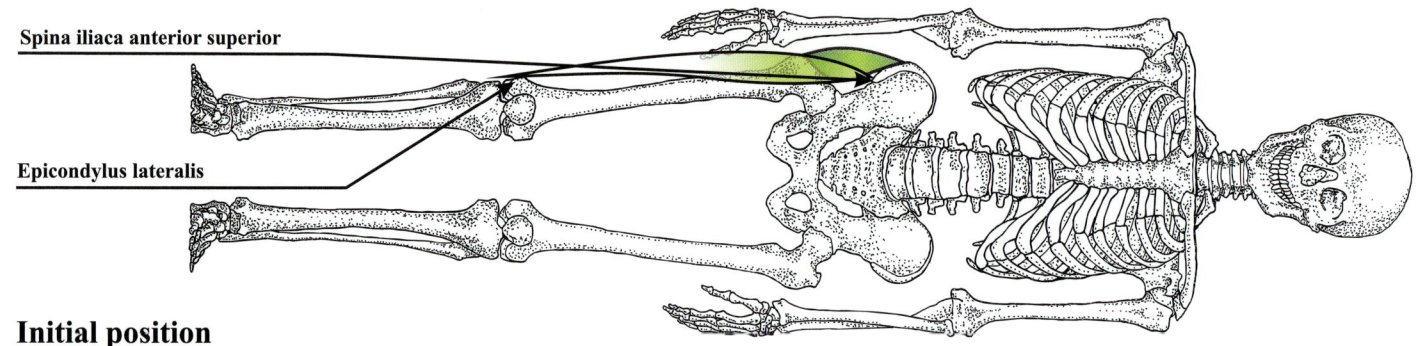

Spina iliaca anterior superior

Epicondylus lateralis

Initial position

The therapist kneels behind the patient facing the pelvis. He stabilizes the patient's trunk and pelvis with his own left leg (punctum fixum). The left palm is placed on the SIAS - spina iliaca anterior superior.
The fingers must not bend but are gently spread over the largest possible area. The right hand grasps the patient's knee. The patient's lower leg lies on the forearm. The leg is placed obliquely downwards (medially). The patient breathes in.

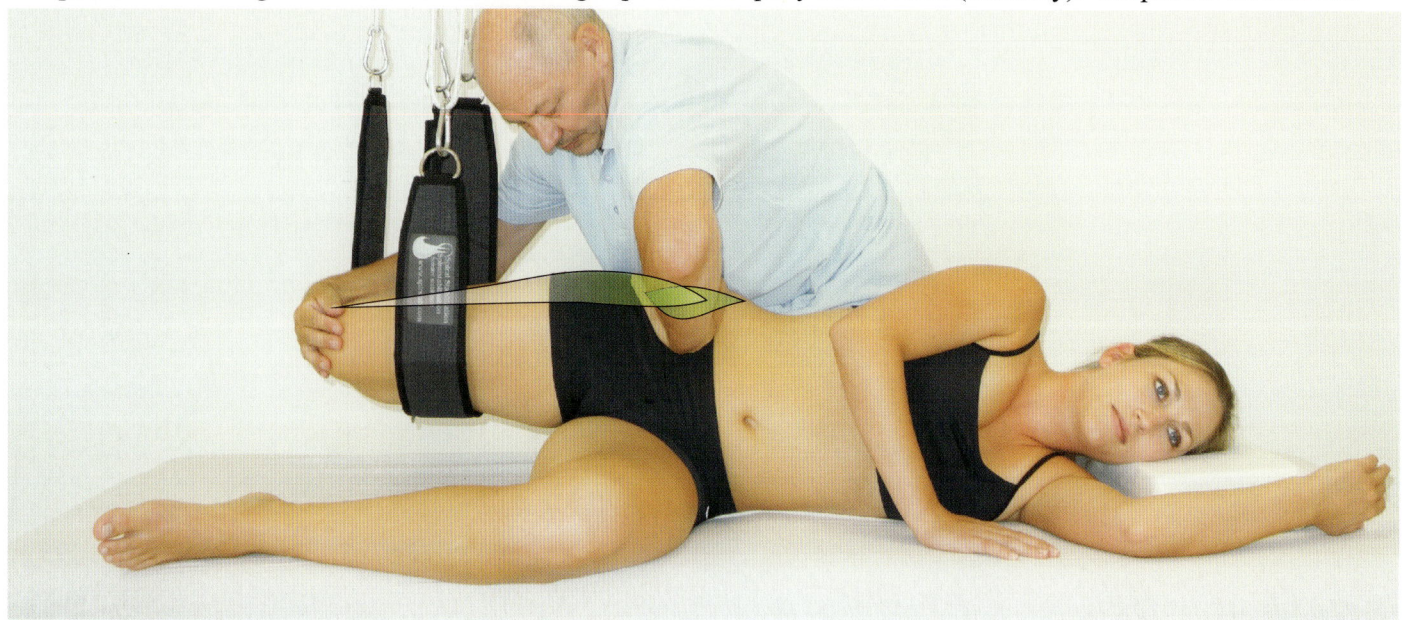

Performance

The therapist shifts the weight of the body to the left arm and stabilizes the pelvis from in front (punctum fixum).
The patient's thigh is pulled backwards and downwards (medially) with the right arm. This stretches the m. tensor fasciae latae and anterior part of the m. gluteus medius. The patient breathes out slowly. The pulling is slackened and the stretching is repeated 6 times. At the end of the technique the therapist pauses for 3 seconds.

PIR. The extension is held and the patient breathes in. This causes a counter-pressure. When breathing out, the patient achieves further stretching. The process is repeated 3 times.

Reciprocal inhibition. At the end of the passive stretching the patient is asked to engage the buttocks and make and active backward movement (step backwards). The extension in the hip increases by 5 to 10 cm. The M. gluteus maximus is the agonist here, while the inhibited m. tensor fasciae latae is the antagonist. This technique stretches the m. tensor fasciae latae and other muscles of the anterior side of the pelvis girdle. This prepares the patient for the correct extent of backward movement of the leg during exercise and walking.

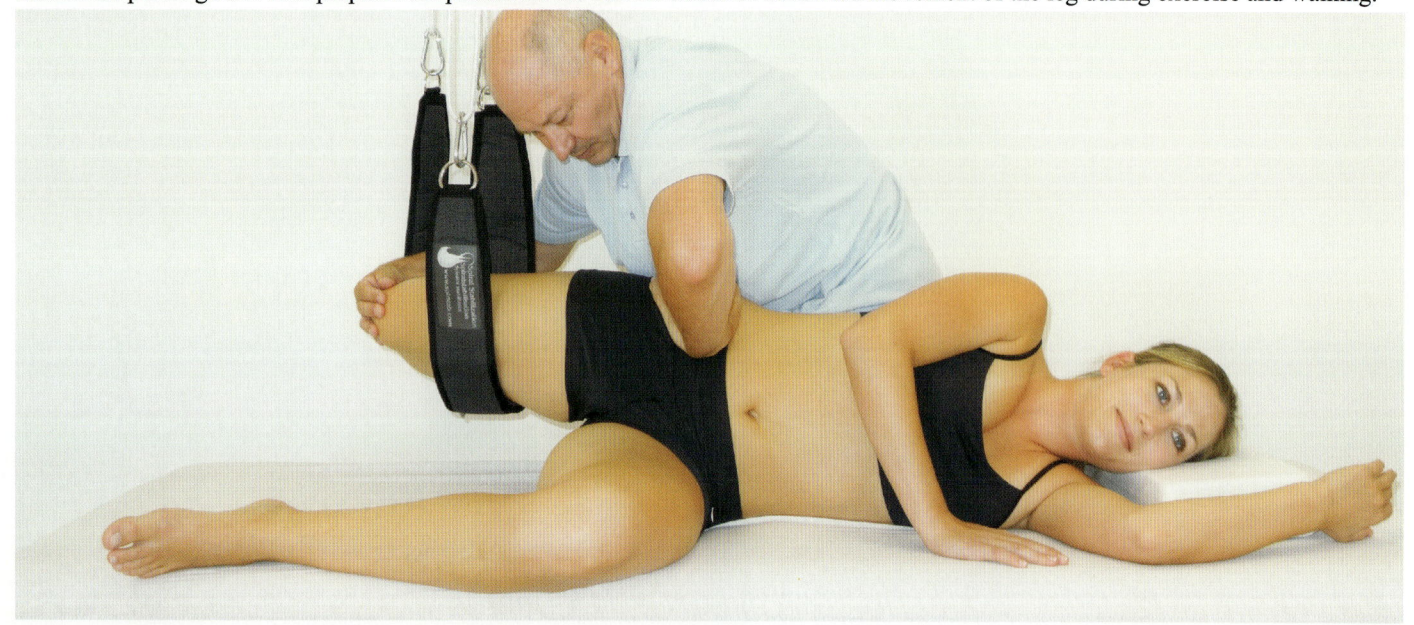

Exercise - stabilization, stretching
M. rectus femoris, m. tensor fasciae latae, m. iliopsoas, m. gluteus medius
- relaxation in reciprocal inhibition, stretching

The PM - pectoralis major chain is agonist in the first part of the exercise,
the LD - latissimus dorsi and TR - trapezius chains are the agonists in the second part of the exercise.

Exercise 4 - kneeling on both knees with back to the attachment point of the elastic rope

Opening the arms backwards, pulling the shoulder blades towards each other, pushing the pelvis forward

Stabilization PM

Stabilization TR, LD

- M. erector spinae
- M. quadratus lumborum

- M. trapezius
- M. subclavius
- M. pectoralis minor
- M. serratus anterior
- M. erector spinae
- M. iliopsoas
- M. gluteus medius (anterior part)
- M. tensor fasciae latae
- M. rectus femoris

1 - Initial position - active part of the exercise
In the initial position the back muscles are stretched:
- m. erector spinae
- m. quadratus lumborum

2 - Performance - active part of the exercise
In the active part of the exercise the muscles in the anterior side of the pelvic girdle are stretched:
- m. iliopsoas
- m. gluteus medius
- m. tensor fasciae latae
- m. rectus femoris

The muscles in the anterior side of the shoulder girdle are stretched:
- m. subclavius
- m. pectoralis minor
- m. pectoralis major
- m. serratus anterior

The muscles in the upper side of the shoulder girdle are relaxed:
- m. trapezius, pars descendens
- m. levator scapulae
- mm. scaleni
- m. semispinalis capitis, cervicis
and other muscles.

Exercise - stabilization, stretching
M. rectus femoris, m. tensor fasciae latae, m. iliopsoas, m. gluteus medius
m. psoas major, m. psoas minor, m. iliacus
- relaxation in reciprocal inhibition, stretching

The LD - latissimus dorsi and TR - trapezius chains are the agonists in the second part of the exercise.

Exercise 4 - kneeling on one knee with back to the attachment point of the elastic rope

Opening the arms backwards, pulling the shoulder blades towards each other, pushing the pelvis forward

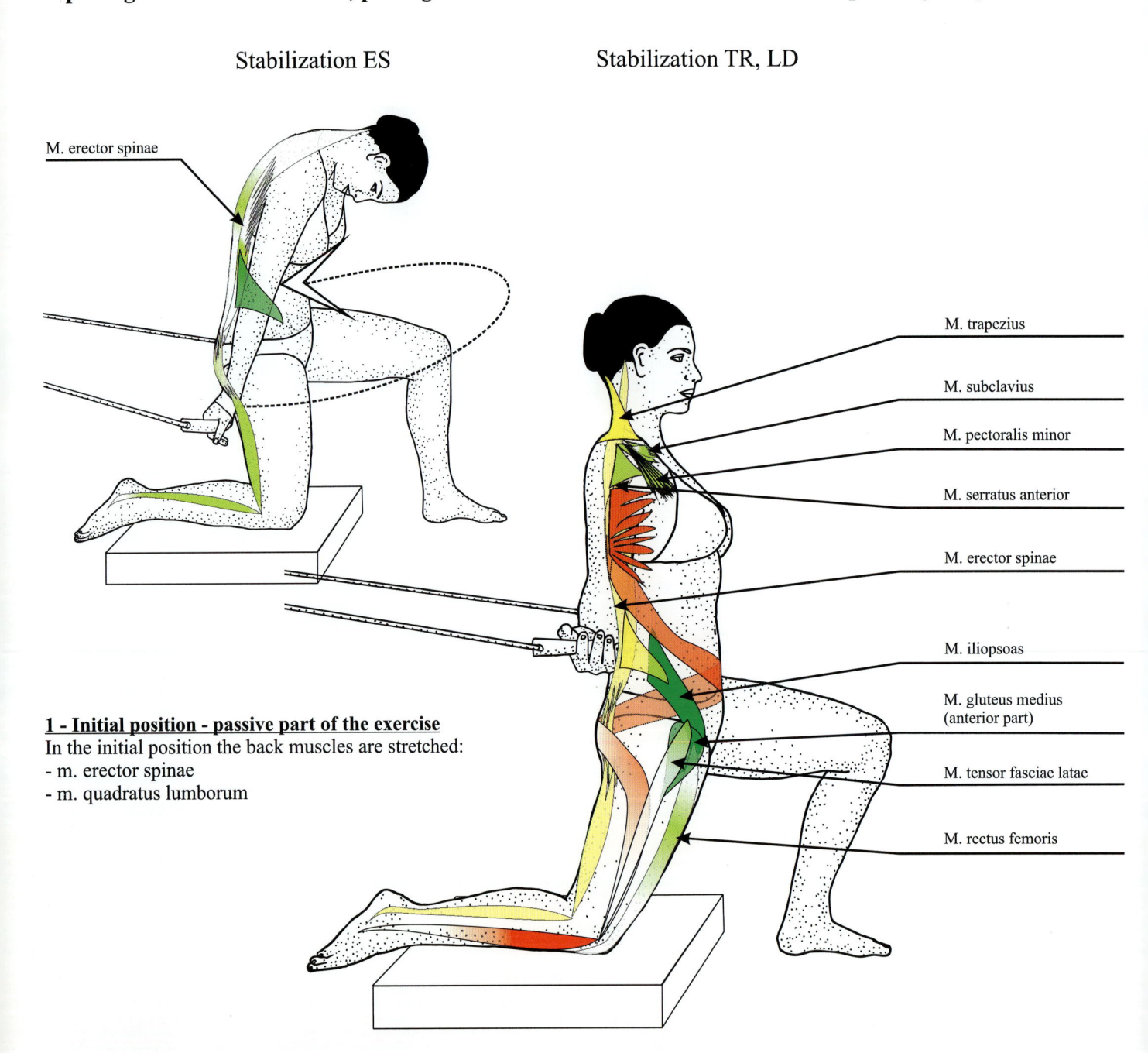

Stabilization ES   Stabilization TR, LD

M. erector spinae

M. trapezius
M. subclavius
M. pectoralis minor
M. serratus anterior
M. erector spinae
M. iliopsoas
M. gluteus medius (anterior part)
M. tensor fasciae latae
M. rectus femoris

1 - Initial position - passive part of the exercise
In the initial position the back muscles are stretched:
- m. erector spinae
- m. quadratus lumborum

2 - Performance - active part of the exercise
In the active part of the exercise the muscles in the anterior part of the pelvic girdle are stretched:
- m. iliopsoas
- m. gluteus medius (anterior part)
- m. tensor fasciae latae
- m. rectus femoris

The muscles in the anterior part of the shoulder girdle are stretched:
- m. subclavius
- m. pectoralis minor
- m. pectoralis major
- m. serratus anterior

The muscles in the upper side of the shoulder girdle are relaxed:
- m. trapezius pars descendens
- m. levator scapulae
- mm. scaleni
- m. semispinalis capitis, cervicis etc.

Exercise - stabilization, stretching
M. rectus femoris, m. tensor fasciae latae, m. iliopsoas, m. gluteus medius
m. psoas major, m. psoas minor, m. iliacus
- relaxation in reciprocal inhibition, stretching

The LD - latissimus dorsi and TR - trapezius chains are the agonists in the second part of the exercise.

Exercise 11 - balanced, stabilized standing position facing the attachment point of the elastic rope, supported by two poles

Extension (stretching) of the leg at the hip

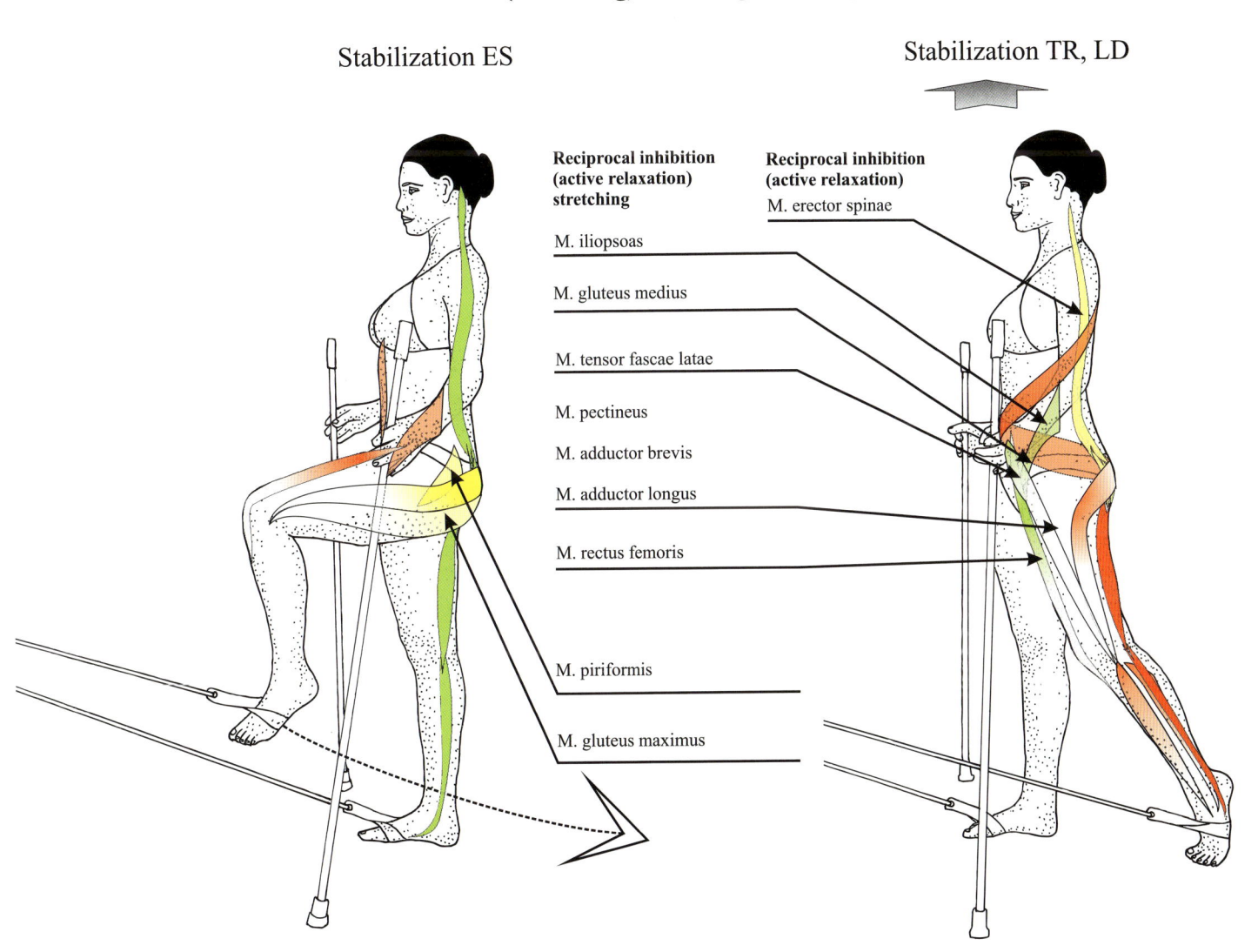

Stabilization ES   Stabilization TR, LD

Reciprocal inhibition (active relaxation) stretching
- M. iliopsoas
- M. gluteus medius
- M. tensor fascae latae
- M. pectineus
- M. adductor brevis
- M. adductor longus
- M. rectus femoris
- M. piriformis
- M. gluteus maximus

Reciprocal inhibition (active relaxation)
- M. erector spinae

1 - Initial postion - passive part of the exercise
In the initial position the muscles in the posterior part of the pelvic girdle are stretched:
- m. gluteus maximus
- m. piriformis

2 - Performance - active part of the exercise
In the active part of the exercise the muscles in the anterior part of the pelvic girdle are stretched:
- m. iliopsoas
- m. gluteus medius (anterior part)
- m. tensor fasciae latae
- m. rectus femoris
- m. pectineus
- m. adductor brevis
- m. adductor longus

Exercise - stabilization, stretching
M. rectus femoris, m. tensor fasciae latae, m. iliopsoas, m. gluteus medius
m. psoas major, m. psoas minor, m. iliacus
- relaxation in reciprocal inhibition, stretching

The SA - serratus anterior and PM - pectoralis major chains are agonists in the first part of the exercise, the LD - latissimus dorsi and TR - trapezius chains are the agonists in the second part of the exercise.

Exercise 11 - balanced, stabilized standing position facing the attachment point of the elastic rope, firm support from the barre

Double crossed extension - stretching the arm at the shoulder and the opposing leg at the hip

Stabilization SA, PM   Stabilization TR, LD

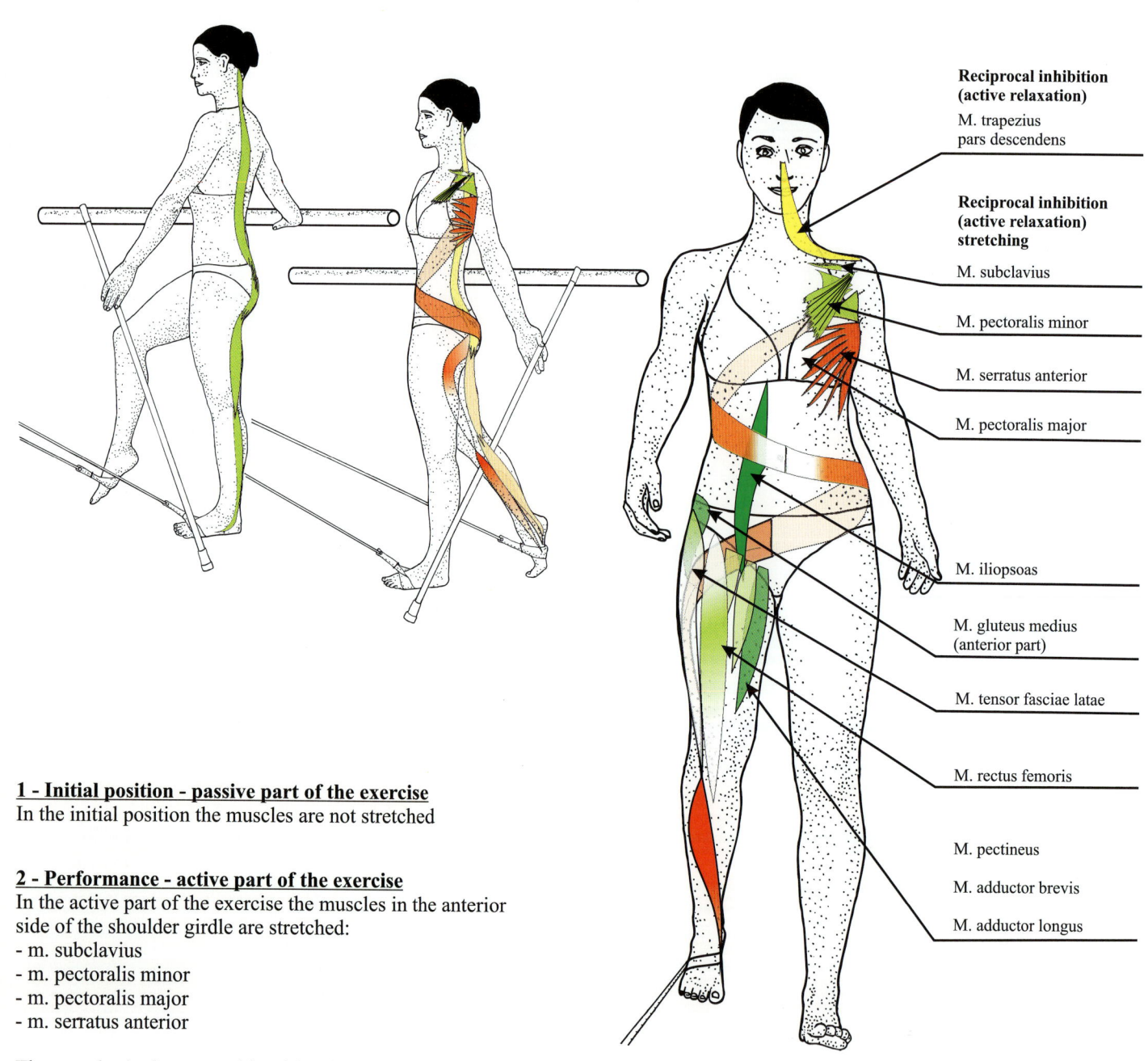

Reciprocal inhibition (active relaxation)
M. trapezius pars descendens

Reciprocal inhibition (active relaxation) stretching
M. subclavius
M. pectoralis minor
M. serratus anterior
M. pectoralis major
M. iliopsoas
M. gluteus medius (anterior part)
M. tensor fasciae latae
M. rectus femoris
M. pectineus
M. adductor brevis
M. adductor longus

1 - Initial position - passive part of the exercise
In the initial position the muscles are not stretched

2 - Performance - active part of the exercise
In the active part of the exercise the muscles in the anterior side of the shoulder girdle are stretched:
- m. subclavius
- m. pectoralis minor
- m. pectoralis major
- m. serratus anterior

The muscles in the upper side of the shoulder girdle are relaxed:
- m. trapezius, pars descendens
- m. levator scapulae
- mm. scaleni
- m. semispinalis capitis, cervicis and other muscles.

2 - Performance - active part of the exercise
In the active part of the active the muscles in the anterior part of the pelvic girdle are stretched:
- m. iliopsoas
- m. gluteus medius (anterior part)
- m. tensor fasciae latae
- m. rectus femoris
- m. pectineus
- m. adductor brevis
- m. adductor longus

Exercise - stabilization, stretching
M. rectus femoris, m. tensor fasciae latae, m. iliopsoas, m. gluteus medius
m. psoas major, m. psoas minor, m. iliacus
- relaxation in reciprocal inhibition, stretching

The SA - serratus anterior and PM - pectoralis major chains are agonists in the first part of the exercise, the LD - latissimus dorsi and TR - trapezius chains are the agonists in the second part of the exercise.

Exercise 11 - balanced, stabilized standing position facing the attachment point of the elastic rope, supported by two poles

Double crossed extension - stretching the arm at the shoulder and the opposing leg at the hip

Stabilization SA, PM   Stabilization TR, LD

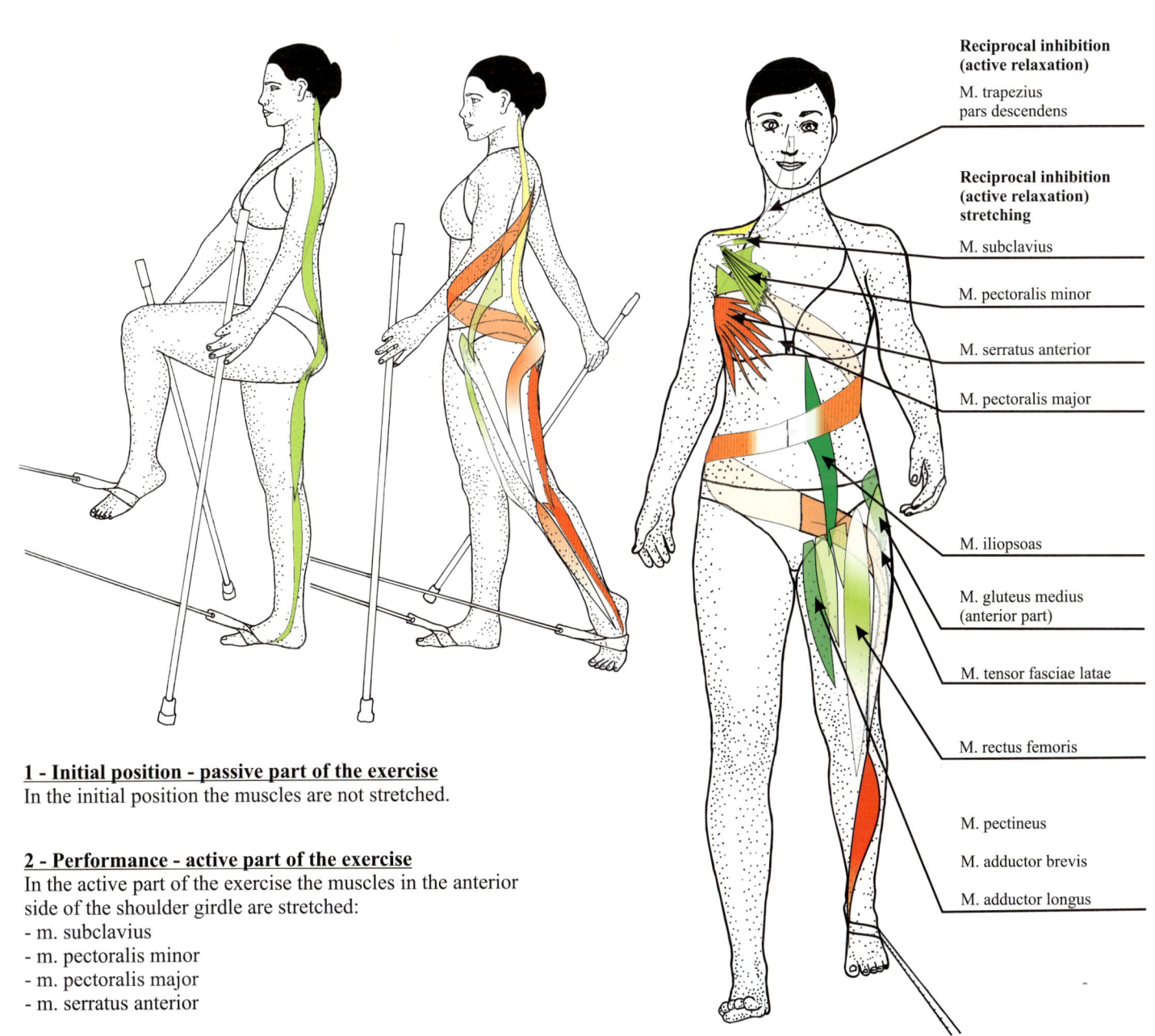

Reciprocal inhibition (active relaxation)
M. trapezius pars descendens

Reciprocal inhibition (active relaxation) stretching
M. subclavius
M. pectoralis minor
M. serratus anterior
M. pectoralis major
M. iliopsoas
M. gluteus medius (anterior part)
M. tensor fasciae latae
M. rectus femoris
M. pectineus
M. adductor brevis
M. adductor longus

1 - Initial position - passive part of the exercise
In the initial position the muscles are not stretched.

2 - Performance - active part of the exercise
In the active part of the exercise the muscles in the anterior side of the shoulder girdle are stretched:
- m. subclavius
- m. pectoralis minor
- m. pectoralis major
- m. serratus anterior

The muscles in the upper side of the shoulder girdle are relaxed:
- m. trapezius, pars descendens
- m. levator scapulae
- mm. scaleni
- m. semispinalis capitis, cervicis and other muscles.

2 - Performance - active part of the exercise
In the active part of the exercise the muscles in the anterior side of the pelvic girdle are stretched:
- m. iliopsoas
- m. gluteus medius (anterior part)
- m. tensor fasciae latae
- m. rectus femoris
- m. pectineus
- m. adductor brevis
- m. adductor longus

Exercise - stabilization, stretching
M. pectineus, m. adductor brevis, m. adductor longus, m. adductor magnus - relaxation in reciprocal inhibition, stretching

The TR - trapezius, LD - latissimus dorsi, SA - serratus anterior and PM - Pectoralis major chains are the agonists in both part of the exercise.

Exercise 13 - balanced, stabilized standing position sideways on to the attachment of the elastic rope, optional support from two poles

Abduction at the hip, sideways pull with one leg, counter-movement of the arms
Stabilization TR, LD, SA, PM

LD-B1 latissimus dorsi

LD-A latissimus dorsi
LD-A2 latissimus dorsi
LD-B2 latissimus dorsi
LD-G latissimus dorsi

M. piriformis
M. tensor fasciae latae

M. pectineus
M. adductor brevis
M. adductor longus
M. adductor magnus

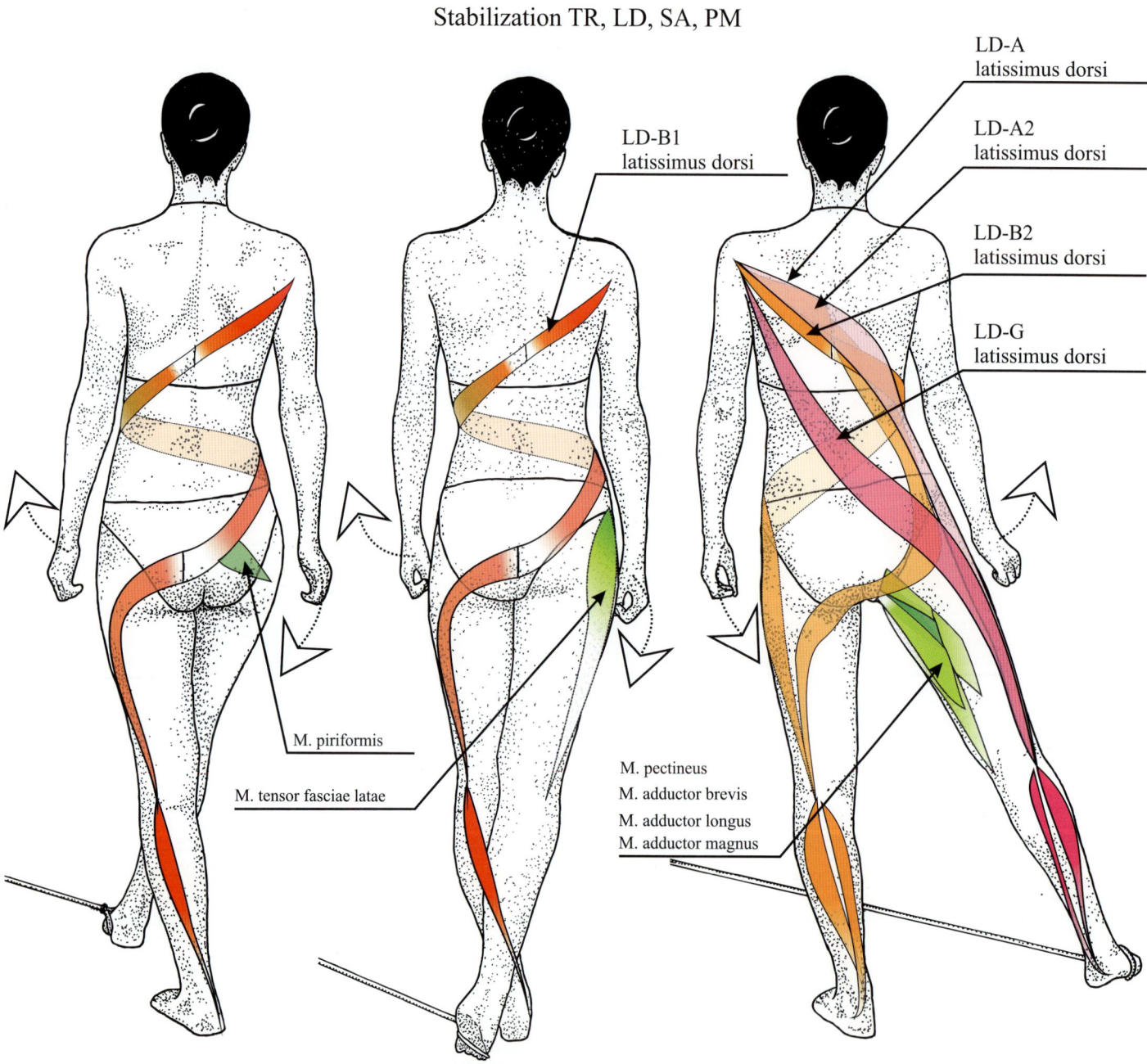

1 - Initial position - active part of the exercise
The initial position is actively stabilized by the LD-B - latissimus dorsi spiral muscle chain.

2 - Performance - active part of the exercise
The exercise is performed on the opposing standing leg.
The active part of the exercise is stabilized by the spiral muscle chains:
LD-A, LD-A2, LD-B2 and LD-G
- latissimus dorsi.
The ES erector spinae vertical muscle chain is relaxed.
At the same time, these chains contribute to active stabilization:
SA - serratus anterior
PM - pectoralis major.

2 - Performance - active part of the exercise
In the active part of the exercise the muscles in the inner side of the thigh are stretched:
- m. adductor brevis, longus
- m. pectineus
- m. adductor magnus

In the initial position with the leg extended forward, the m. piriformis is stretched

In the initial position with the leg behind, the m. tensor fasciae latae is stretched.

Anatomy
M. iliopsoas
M. psoas major, m. psoas minor, m. iliacus

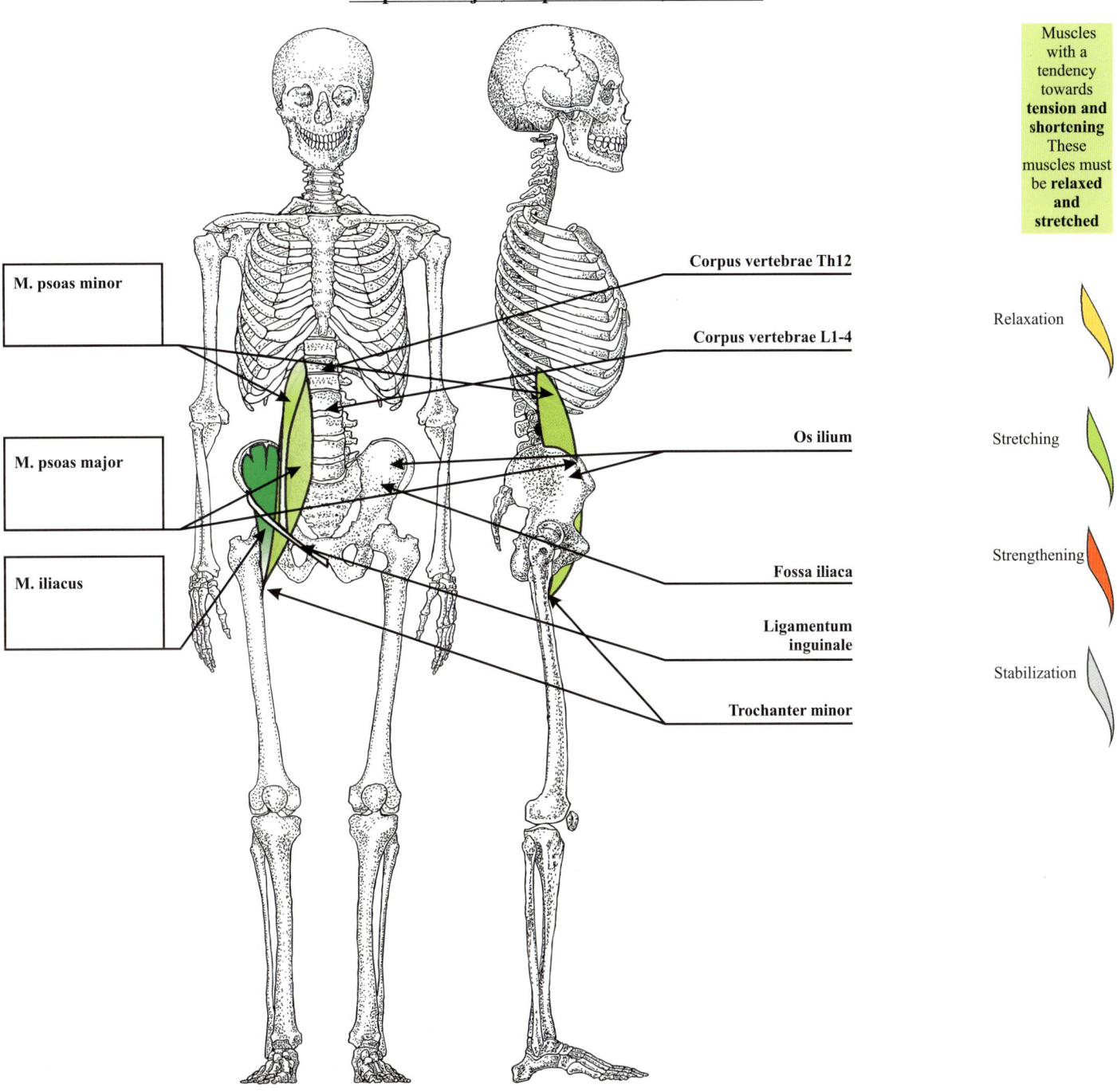

Muscles with a tendency towards tension and shortening — These muscles must be **relaxed and stretched**

M. psoas minor

M. psoas major

M. iliacus

Corpus vertebrae Th12
Corpus vertebrae L1-4
Os ilium
Fossa iliaca
Ligamentum inguinale
Trochanter minor

Relaxation
Stretching
Strengthening
Stabilization

M. iliopsoas

M. psoas major
Origin: - superficial layer
- lateral part of the vertebral bodies Th12, L1-4, disci intervertebrales
        - deep layer
- processus costarii L1-5
Insertion:
- trochanter minor osis femoris
Function: - hip joint:
- flexion and outward rotation
        - lumbar spine - unilaterally:
- lateroflexion of the trunk towards the ipsilateral side
        - lumbar spine bilaterally:
- flexion of the lumbar spine
- lifting the trunk from a lying position
Innervation:
- n. femoralis (Th1-L4), plexus lumbalis

M. psoas minor
Origin:
- lateral part of the vertebral bodies Th12, L1
Insertion:
- ligamentum inguimale
Function:
        - lumbar spine - unilaterally:
- lateroflexion of the trunk towards the ipsilateral side
        - lumbar spine bilaterally:
- flexion of the lumbar spine
- lifting the trunk from a lying position
Innervation:
- n. femoralis (Th12 - L4), plexus lumbalis

M. iliacus
Origin:
- fossa iliaca
Insertion:
- trochanter minor
Function: - hip:
- flexion (bending) of the hip joint
- outward rotation of the thigh
- bends the spine in flexion
- creates hyperlordosis when there is an attempt to straighten up
- straightening the trunk from lying on the back
Innervation:
- n. femoralis (L 2 - 4)
- direct branches of the plexus lumbalis

Muscle chains
Vertical muscle chain **IP - iliopsoas**
M. psoas major, m. psoas minor, m. iliacus
Ventral (anterior) deep vertical

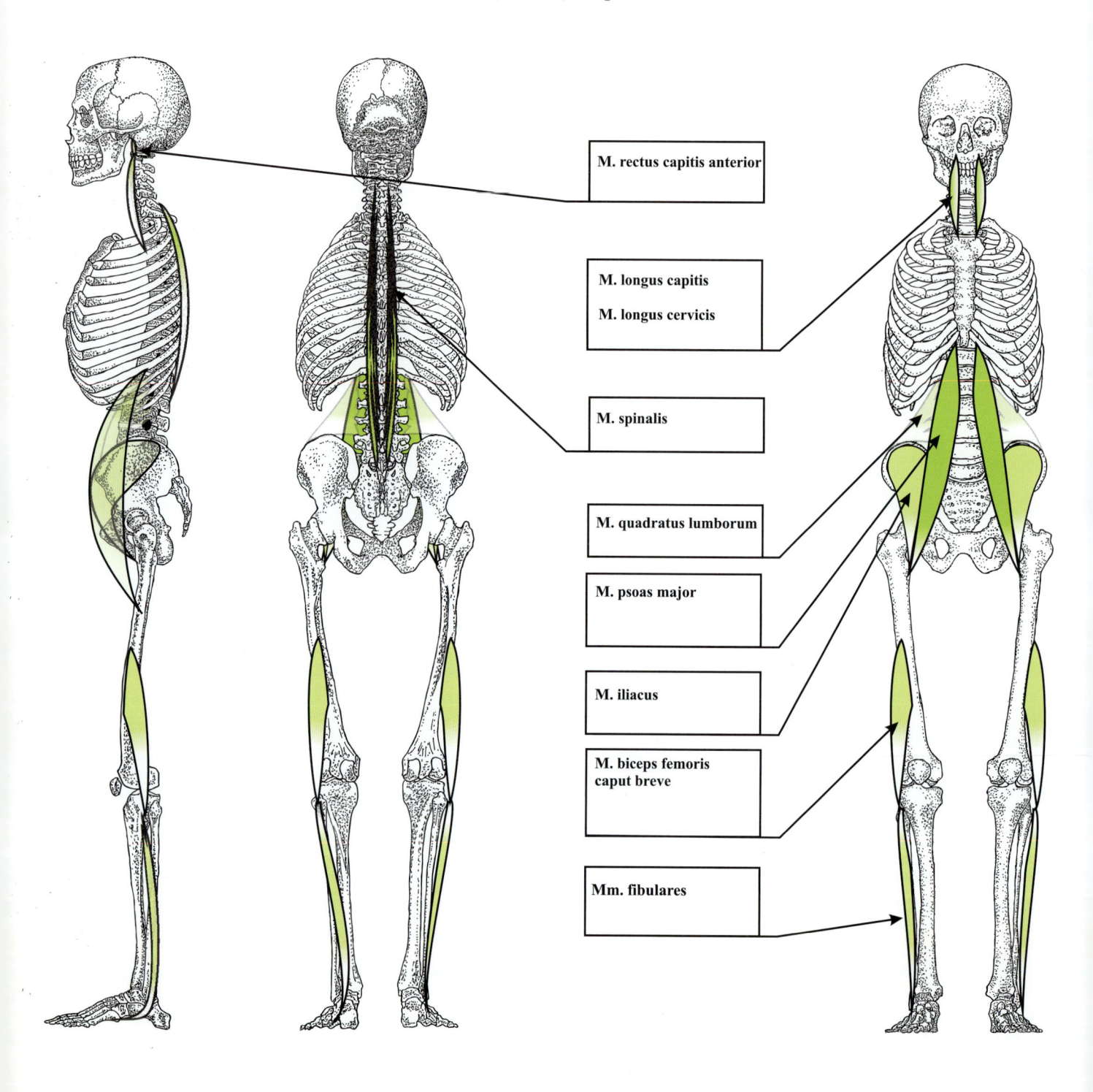

- M. rectus capitis anterior
- M. longus capitis
- M. longus cervicis
- M. spinalis
- M. quadratus lumborum
- M. psoas major
- M. iliacus
- M. biceps femoris caput breve
- Mm. fibulares

Anatomy
M. pectineus, m. adductor brevis, m. adductor longus

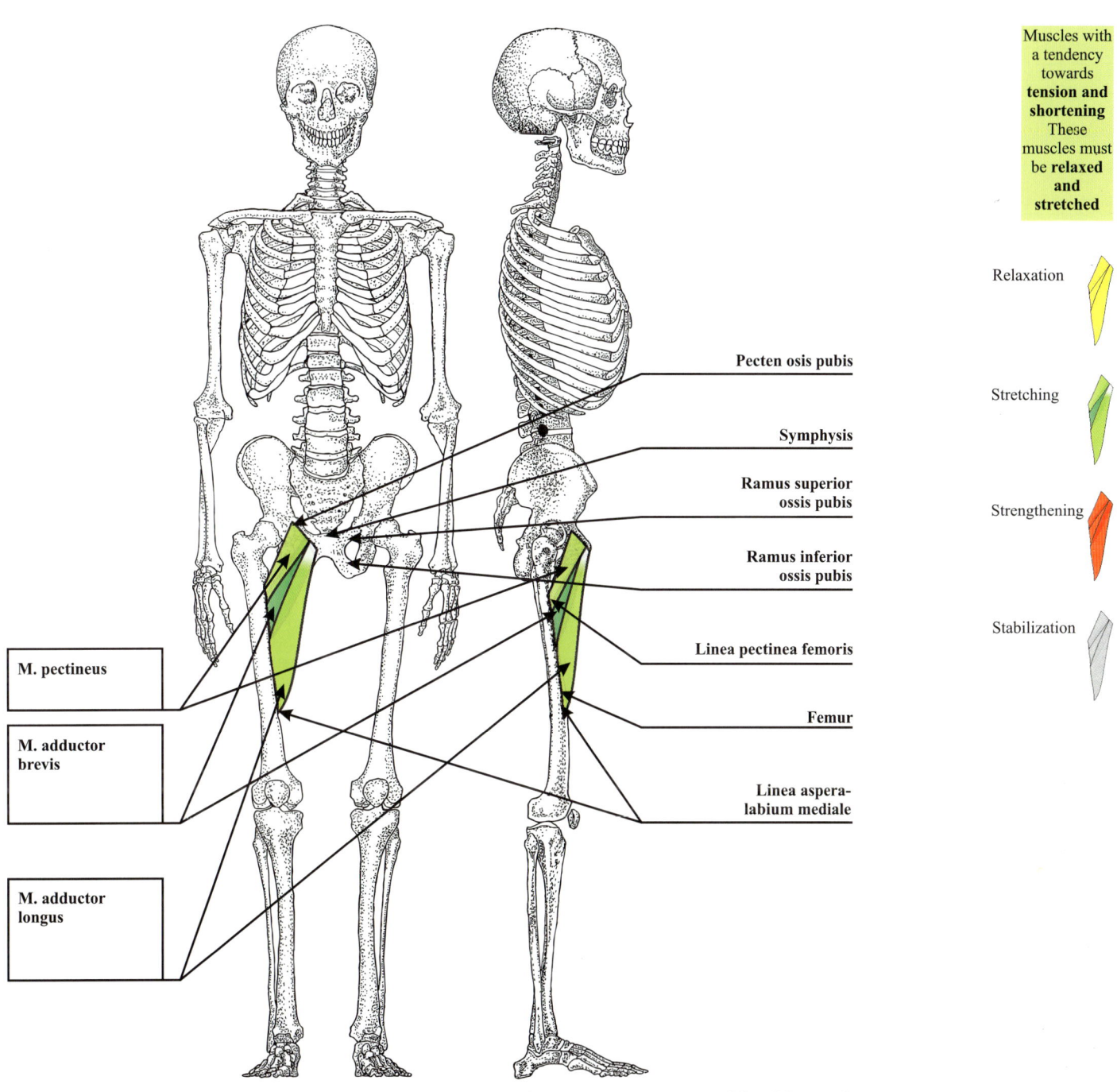

*Muscles with a tendency towards **tension and shortening**. These muscles must be **relaxed and stretched***

Relaxation

Stretching

Strengthening

Stabilization

Labels: Pecten osis pubis, Symphysis, Ramus superior ossis pubis, Ramus inferior ossis pubis, Linea pectinea femoris, Femur, Linea aspera - labium mediale

M. pectineus
Origin:
- pecten ossis pubis
Insertion:
- femur, linea pectinea, proximal part, linea aspera - labium mediale
Function: - hip joint:
- adduction (pulling in)
- flexion (bending)
- outward rotation
- stabilization of the pelvic in the frontal and sagittal planes
Innervation:
- n. femoralis
- n. obturatorius (L2-4)

M. adductor brevis
Origin:
- ramus inferior ossis pubis
Insertion:
- femur, linea aspera - labium mediale, upper third of the femur
Function: - hip joing:
- adduction (pulling in)
- flexion to 70° (bending)
- outward rotation
   - pelvis:
- stabilization of the pelvis in the frontal and sagittal planes
Innervation:
- n. obturatorius (L2-4)

M. adductor longus
Origin:
- ramus superior ossis pubis and anterior part of the symphysis
Insertion:
- femur, linea aspera - labium mediale, central third of the femur
Function: - hip joint:
- adduction (pulling in)
- flexion to 70° (bending)
- outward rotation
   - pelvis:
- stabilization of the pelvis in the frontal and sagittal planes
Innervation:
- n. obturatorius (L2-4)

Muscle chains
Spiral muscle chain **LD-D - latissimus dorsi**

The LD muscle chain is activated by a backward movement of the arm - extension.
The LD-D participates in flexion of the leg during walking.

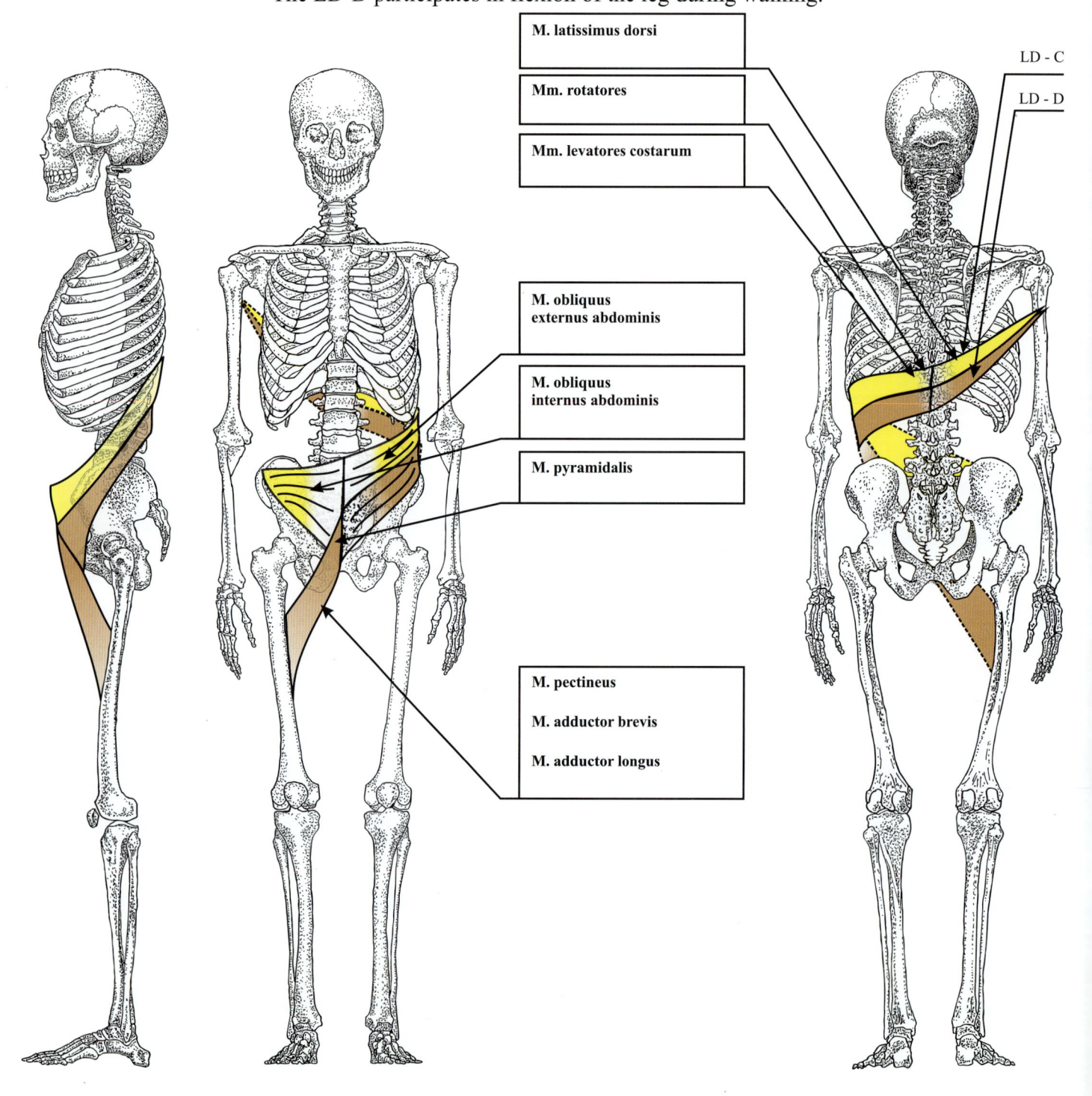

- M. latissimus dorsi
- Mm. rotatores
- Mm. levatores costarum
- M. obliquus externus abdominis
- M. obliquus internus abdominis
- M. pyramidalis
- M. pectineus
- M. adductor brevis
- M. adductor longus

LD - C
LD - D

Anatomy - muscle chains

M. pectineus, m. adductor brevis, m. adductor longus

Vertical stabilization chain RA - rectus abdominis
Ventral (anterior) superficial vertical

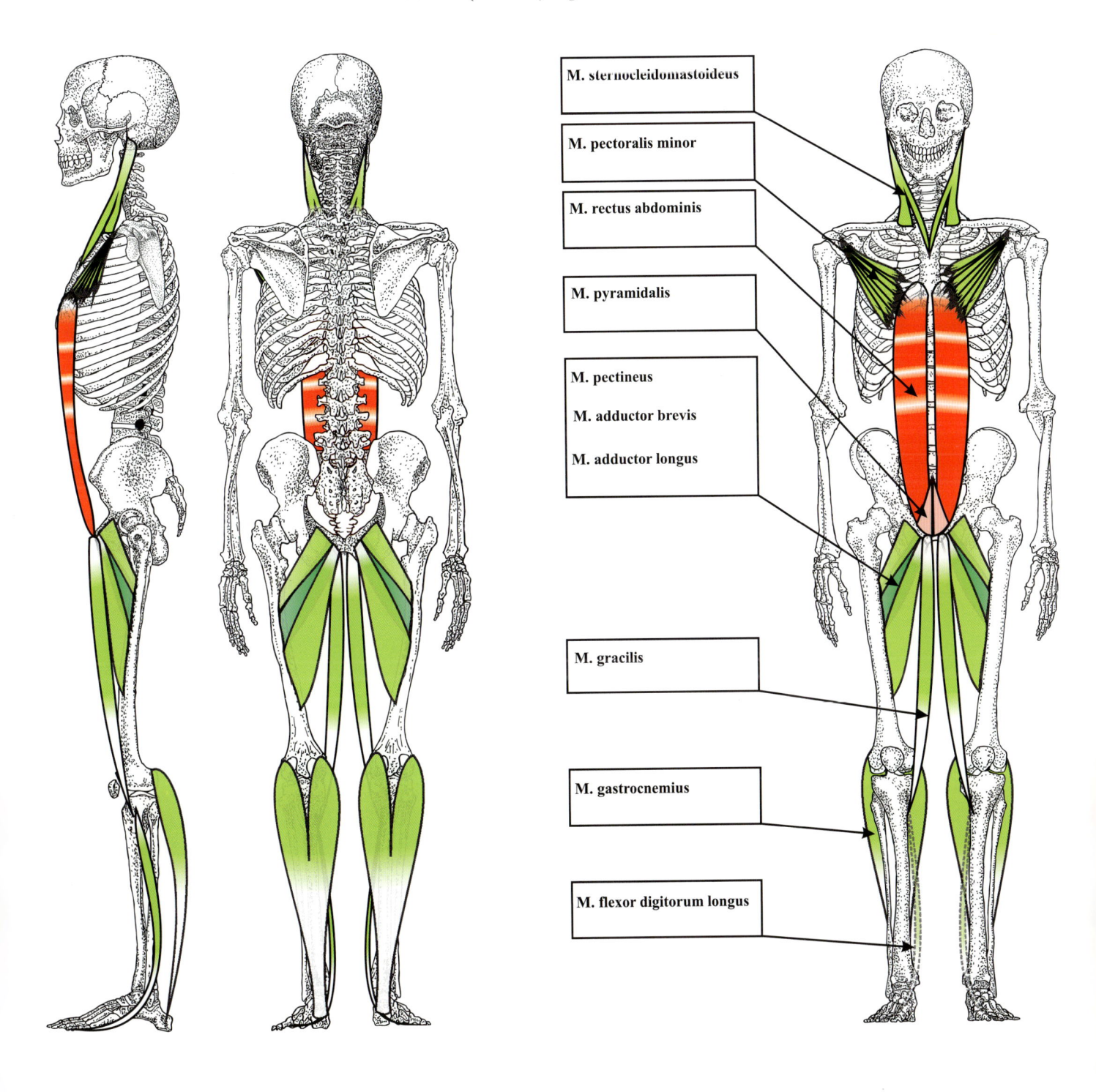

- M. sternocleidomastoideus
- M. pectoralis minor
- M. rectus abdominis
- M. pyramidalis
- M. pectineus
- M. adductor brevis
- M. adductor longus
- M. gracilis
- M. gastrocnemius
- M. flexor digitorum longus

Manual techniques lying on one side
M. iliopsoas major, m. pectineus, m. adductor brevis, m. adductor longus

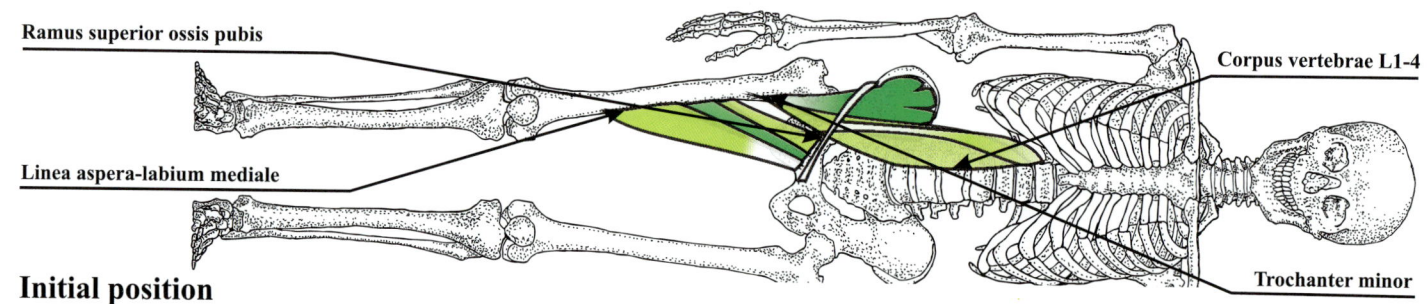

Ramus superior ossis pubis

Linea aspera-labium mediale

Corpus vertebrae L1-4

Trochanter minor

Initial position
The therapist kneels behind the patient facing the pelvis. He stabilizes the patient's trunk and pelvis with his left leg (punctum fixum). The left palm is placed on the SIAS - spina iliaca anterior superior.
The fingers must not bend, but are gently spread over the largest possible area. The right hand grasps the patient's knee. The patient's lower leg lies on the forearm. The leg is placed obliquely upwards (laterally). The patient breathes in.

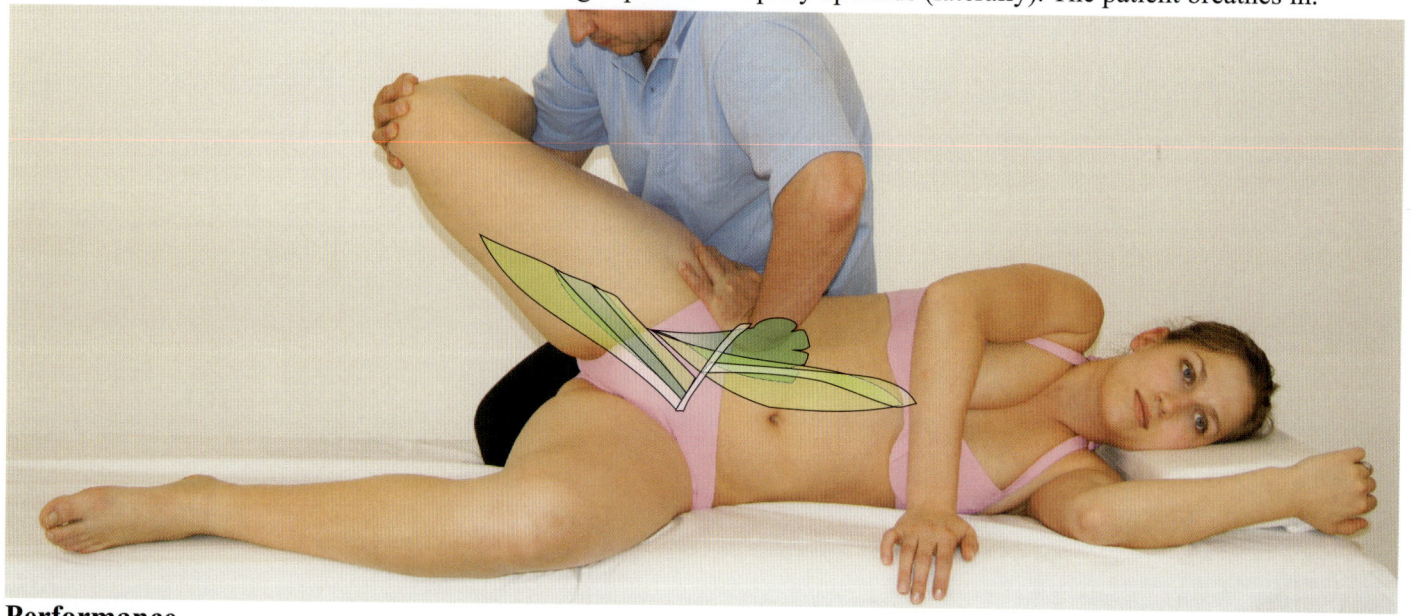

Performance
The therapist shifts the weight of the body to the left arm and stabilizes the pelvis from in front (punctum fixum).
The patient's thigh is pulled backwards and upwards (laterally) with the right arm. This stretches the m. ilopsoas and adductors. The patient breathes out slowly. The pulling is slackened and the stretching is repeated 6 times. At the end of the technique the therapist pauses for 3 seconds.
  PIR. The extension is held and the patient breathes in. This causes a counter-pressure. When breathing out, the patient achieves further stretching. The process is repeated 3 times.
  Reciprocal inhibition. At the end of the passive stretching the patient is asked to engage the buttocks and make an active backward movement (step backwards). The extension in the hip increases by 5 to 10 cm. The m. gluteus maximus is the agonist here, while the inhibited m. iliopsoas is the antagonist. This technique stretches the m. ilopsoas and other muscles of the anterior side of the pelvic girdle. This prepares the patient for the correct extent of backward movement of the leg during exercise and walking.

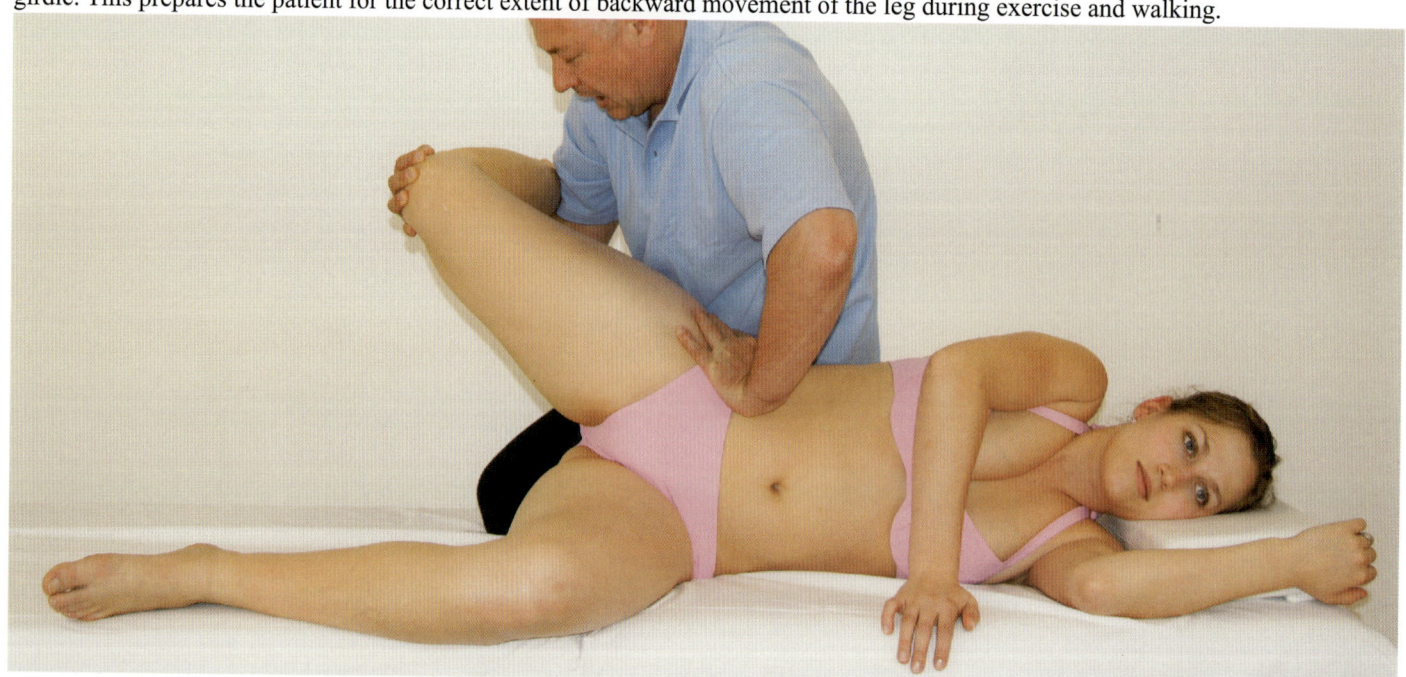

Manual techniques - lying - one limb in a hoist
M. iliopsoas, m. pectineus, m. adductor brevis, m. adductor longus

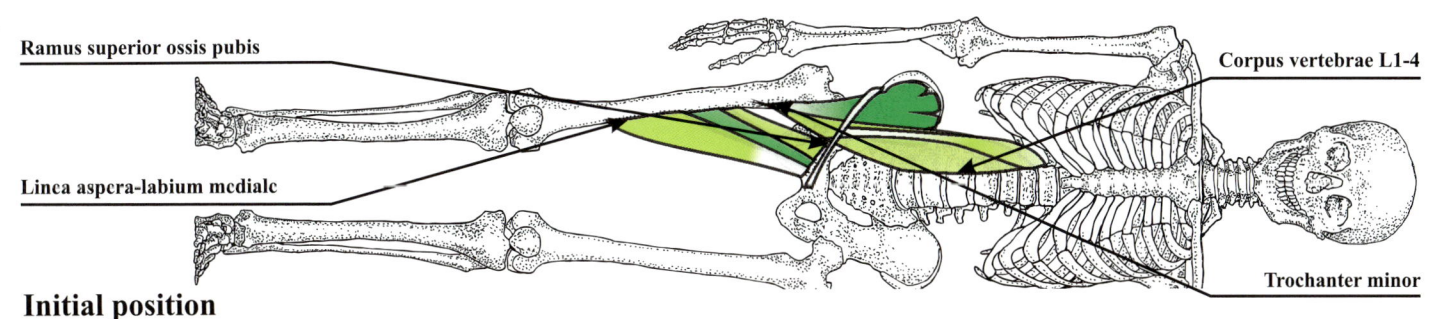

Ramus superior ossis pubis
Linea aspera-labium mediale
Corpus vertebrae L1-4
Trochanter minor

Initial position
The therapist kneels behind the patient facing the pelvis. He stabilizes the patient's trunk and pelvis with his left leg (punctum fixum). The left palm is placed on the SIAS - spina iliaca anterior superior.
The fingers must not bend but are spread gently over the largest possible area. The right hand grasps the patient's knee. The patient's lower leg lies on the forearm. The leg is placed obliquely upwards (laterally). The patient breathes in.

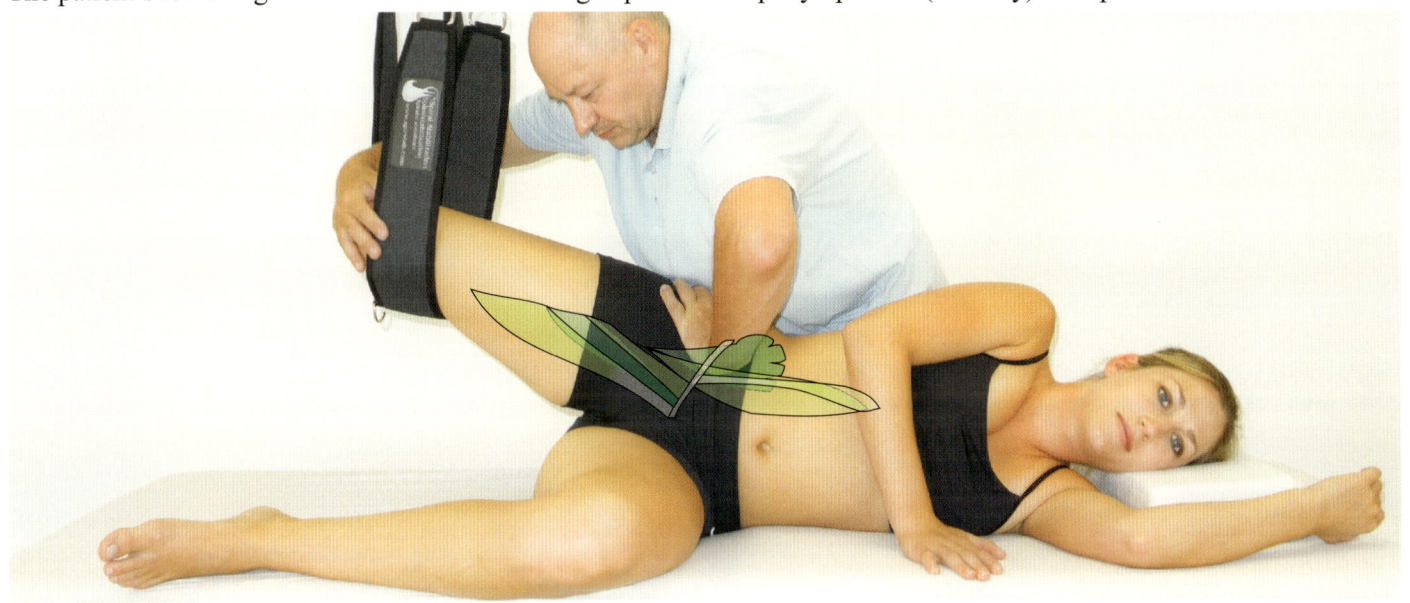

Performance
The therapist shifts the weight of the body to the left arm and stabilizes the pelvis from front (punctum fixum). The patient's thigh is pulled backwards and upwards (laterally) with the right arm. This stretches the m. ilopsoas and adductors. The patient breathes out slowly. The pulling is slackened and the stretching is repeated 6 times. At the end of the technique the therapist pauses for about 3 seconds.
PIR. The extension is held and the patient breathes in. This causes a counter-pressure. When breathing out, the patient achieves further stretching. The process is repeated 3 times.
Reciprocal inhibition. At the end of the passive stretching the patient is asked to engage the buttocks and make an active backward movement (step backwards). The extension in the hip increases by 5 to 10 cm. The m. gluteus maximus is the agonist here, while the inhibited m. iliopsoas is the antagonist. This technique stretches the m. iliopsoas and other muscles of the anterior side of the pelvic girdle. This prepares the patient for the correct extent of backward movement of the leg during exercise and walking.

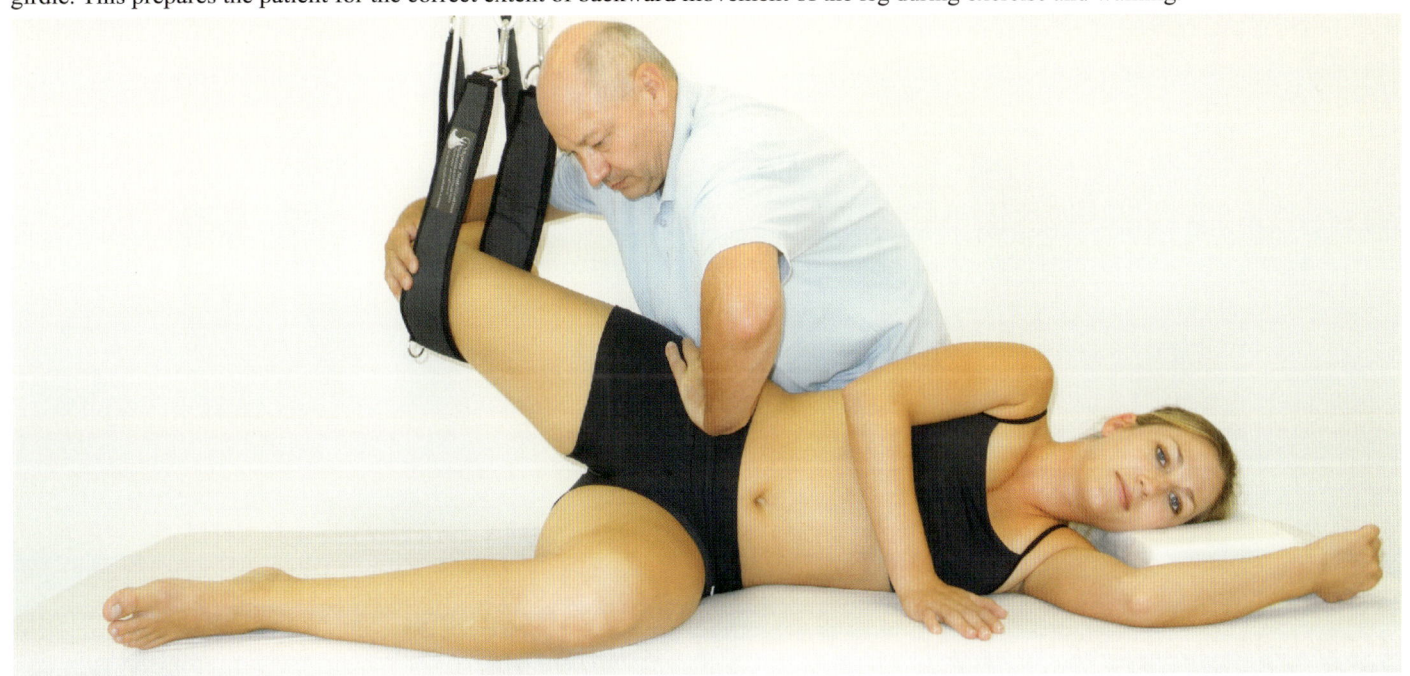

Manual techniques kneeling, standing

M. iliopsoas, m. rectus femoris - active relaxation and stretching

Exercise 4 - kneeling on one knee with back to the attachment of the elastic rope, opening of the arms backward, pulling the shoulder blades towards each other, pushing the pelvis forward

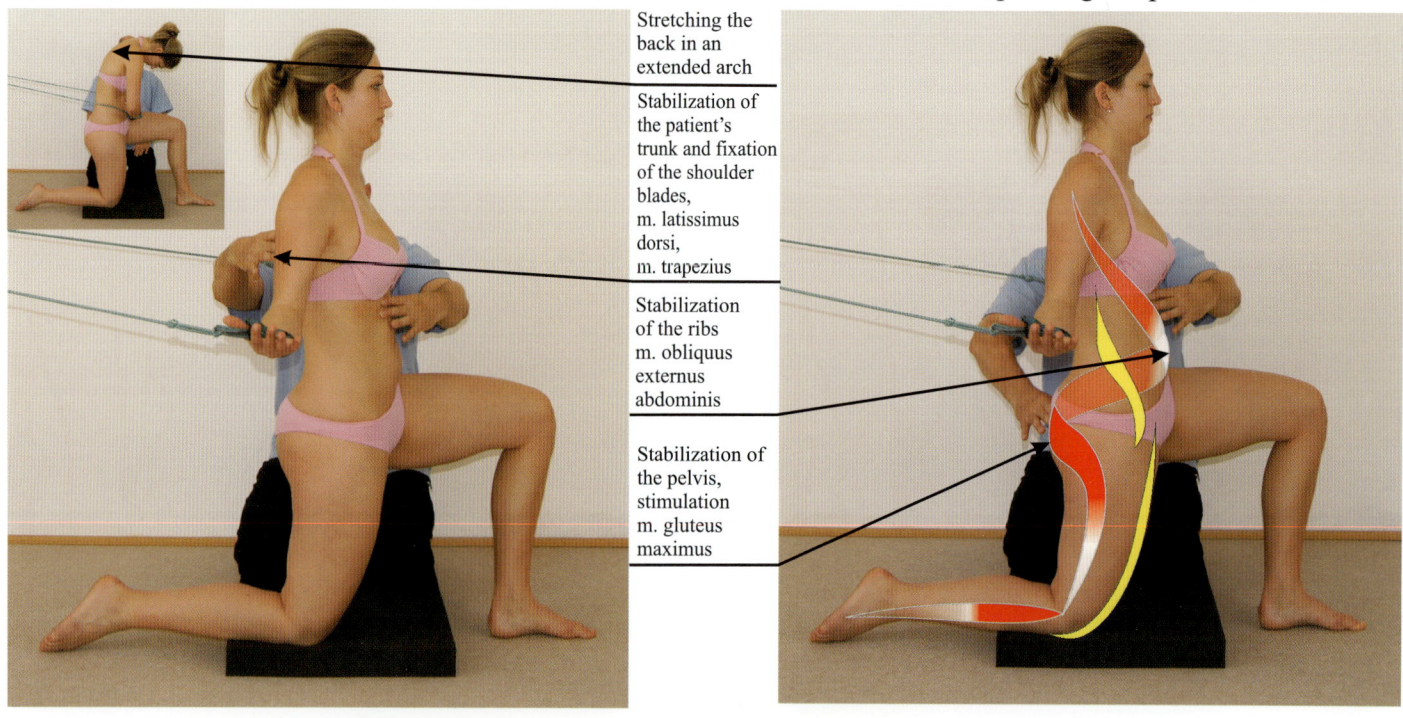

- Stretching the back in an extended arch
- Stabilization of the patient's trunk and fixation of the shoulder blades, m. latissimus dorsi, m. trapezius
- Stabilization of the ribs m. obliquus externus abdominis
- Stabilization of the pelvis, stimulation m. gluteus maximus

Exercise 11 - balanced, stabilized standing position facing the attachment point of the elastic, support from two poles, double crossed extension - stretching the arms at the shoulder, and the opposite legs at the hip, stabilization of the lower ribs, stretching the shoulder backwards

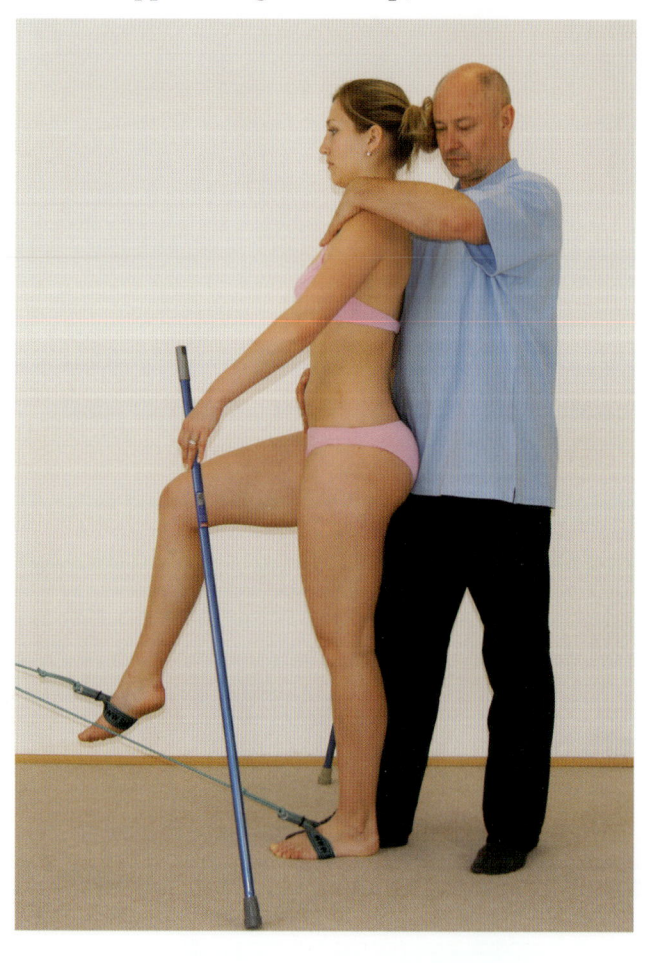

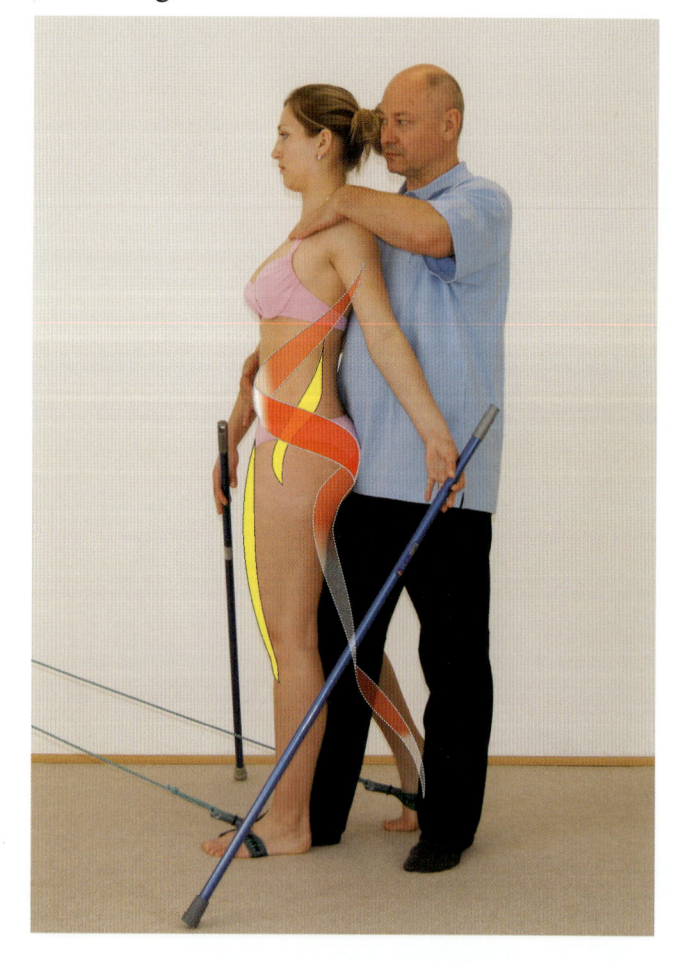

Exercise

M. rectus femoris, m. tensor fasciae latae, m. iliopsoas, m. gluteus medius, short adductors - active relaxation and stretching

Exercise 4 - sitting with back to the attachment of the elastic rope, one leg is stretched backwards, opening of the arms backwards, pulling the shoulder blades towards each other, pushing the pelvis forward

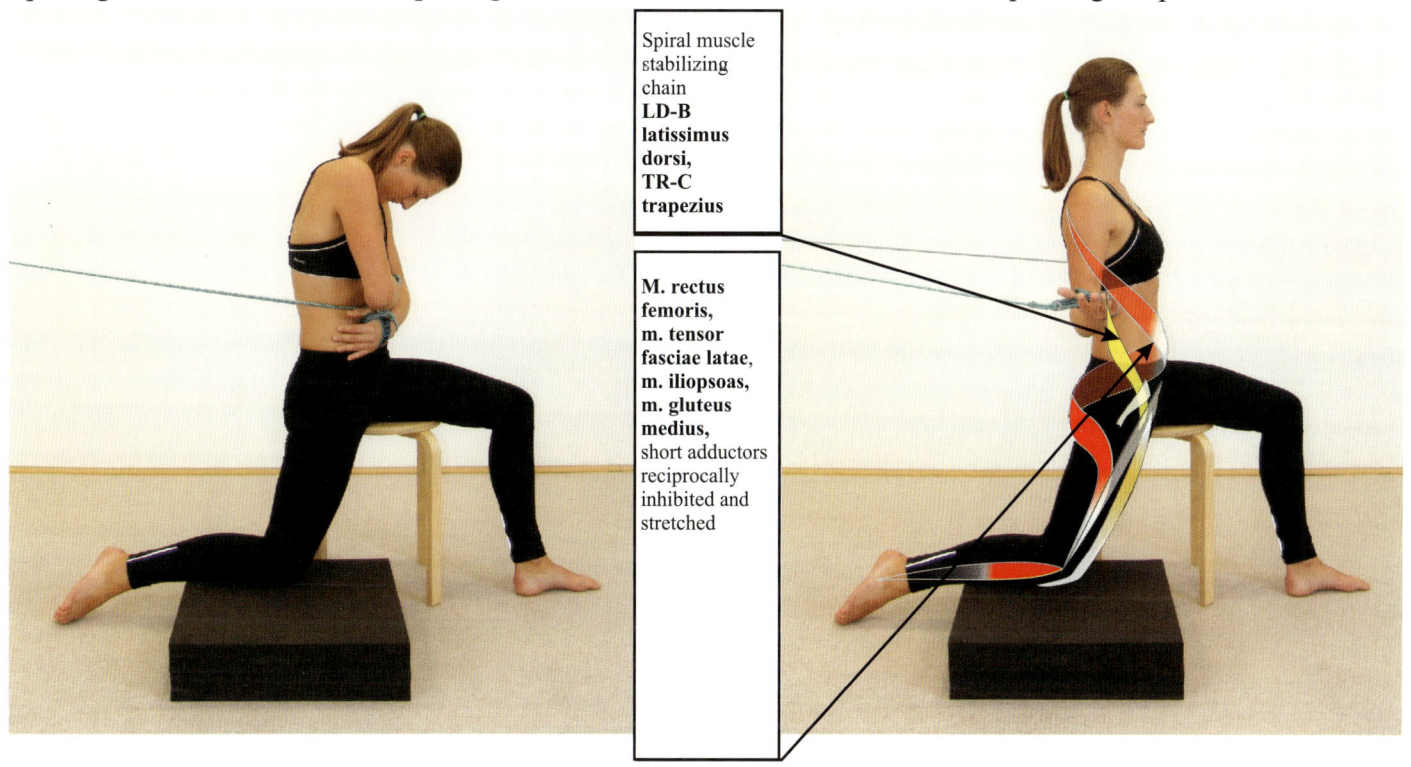

Spiral muscle stabilizing chain **LD-B** latissimus dorsi, **TR-C** trapezius

M. rectus femoris, m. tensor fasciae latae, m. iliopsoas, m. gluteus medius, short adductors reciprocally inhibited and stretched

M. rectus femoris, m. tensor fasciae latae, m. iliopsoas, m. gluteus medius, short adductors - active relaxation and stretching

Exercise 4 - kneeling on one knee with back to the attachment of the elastic rope, opening the arms backwards, pulling the shoulder blades towards each other, pushing the pelvis forward

Spiral stabilizing muscle chain **LD-B** latissimus dorsi, **TR-C** trapezius

M. rectus femoris, m. tensor fasciae latae, m. iliopsoas, m. gluteus medius, short adductors reciprocally inhibited and stretched

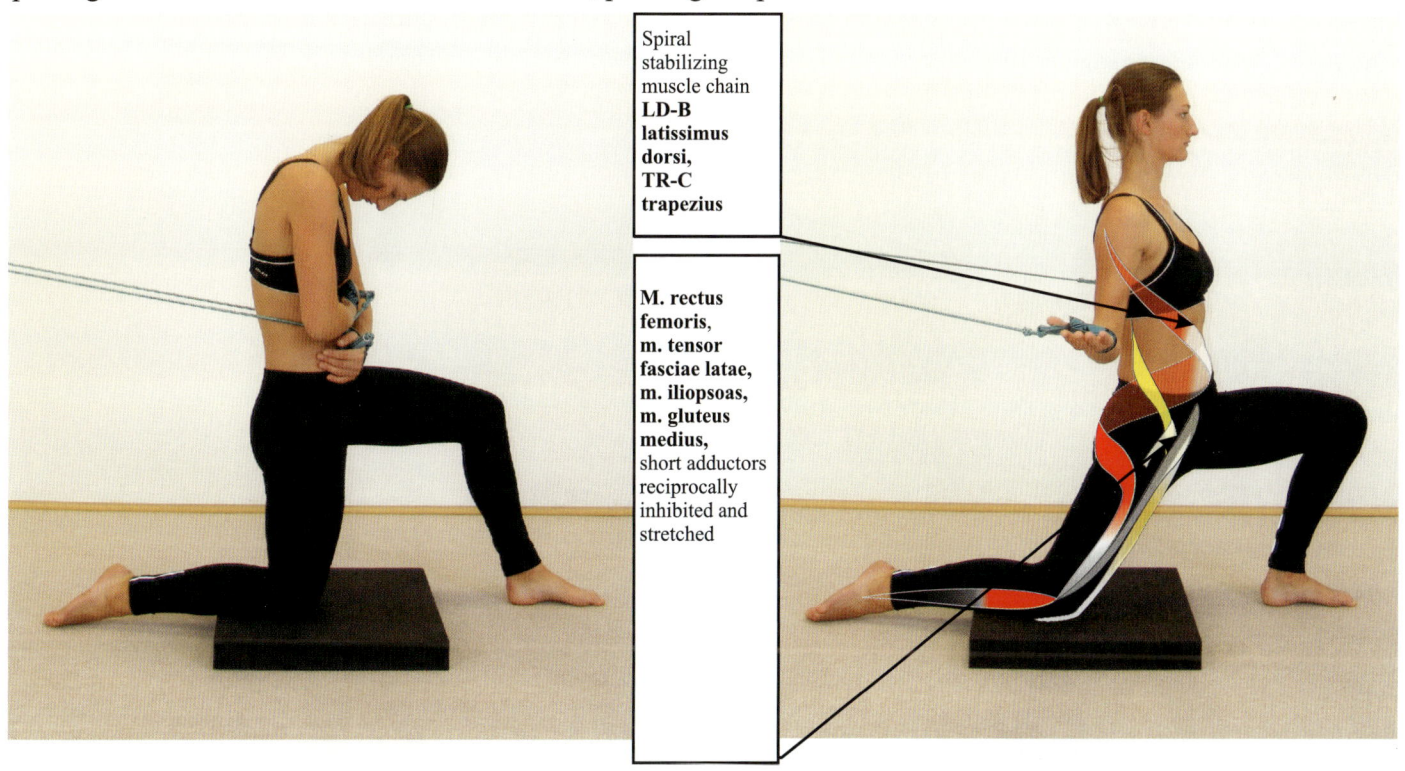

Stretching of the m. rectus femoris, m. tensor fasciae latae, m. iliopsoas, m. gluteus medius, m. pectineus, m. adductor brevis, m. adductor longus, inhibited in reciprocal inhibition.
The agonist is the LD and TR spirals, which stabilize the body.
The hip flexors are reciprocally inhibited and stretched at the same time.

Exercise

M. rectus femoris, m. tensor fasciae latae, m. iliopsoas, m. gluteus medius, short adductors - active relaxation and stretching

Exercise 4 - kneeling on both knees with back to the attachment point of the elastic rope, opening the arms backwards, pulling the shoulder blades towards each other, pushing the pelvis forward

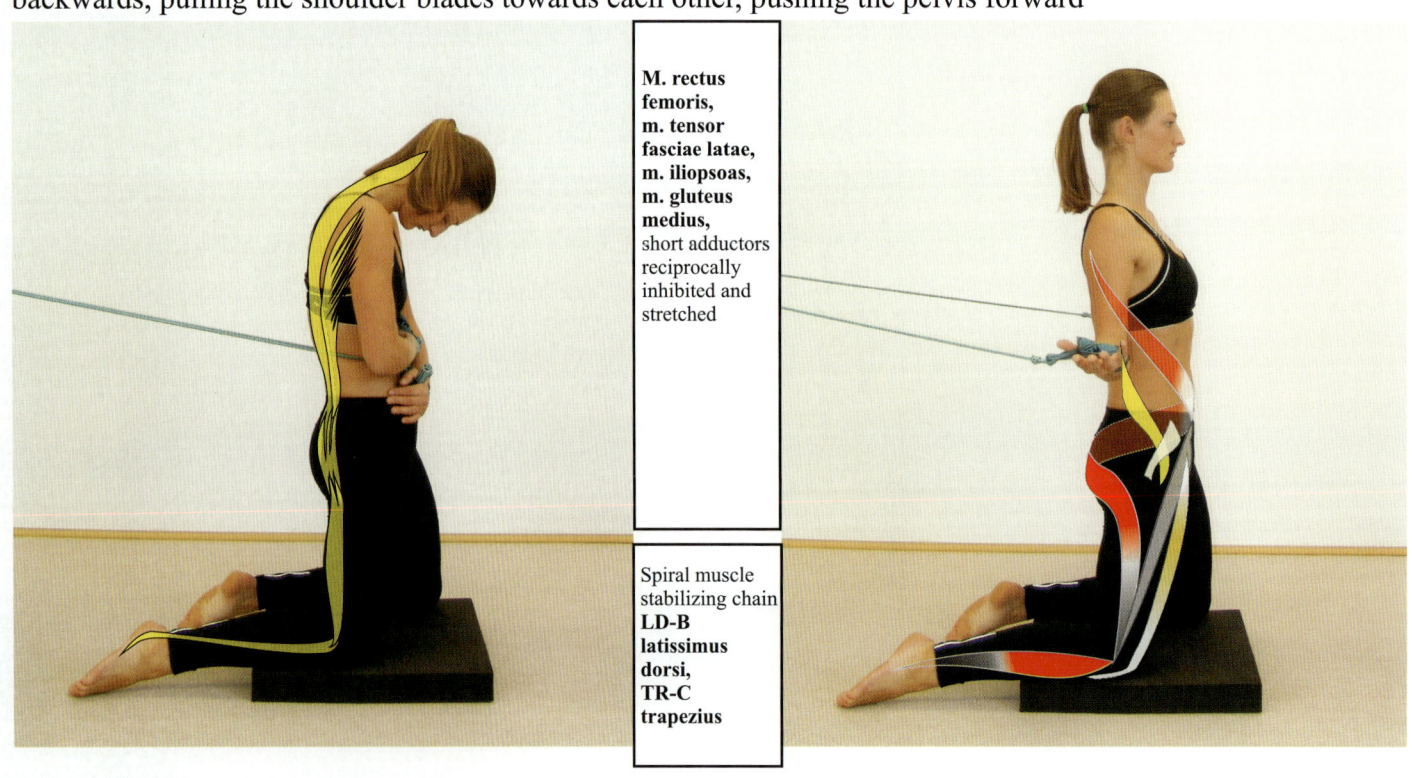

M. rectus femoris, m. tensor fasciae latae, m. iliopsoas, m. gluteus medius, short adductors reciprocally inhibited and stretched

Spiral muscle stabilizing chain LD-B latissimus dorsi, TR-C trapezius

M. rectus femoris, m. tensor fasciae latae, m. iliopsoas, m. gluteus medius, short adductors - active relaxation and stretching

Exercise 3 - standing with back to the attachment point of the elastic rope with one leg on the mat, opening the arms backwards, pulling the shoulder blades towards each other, shifting the weight to the front leg

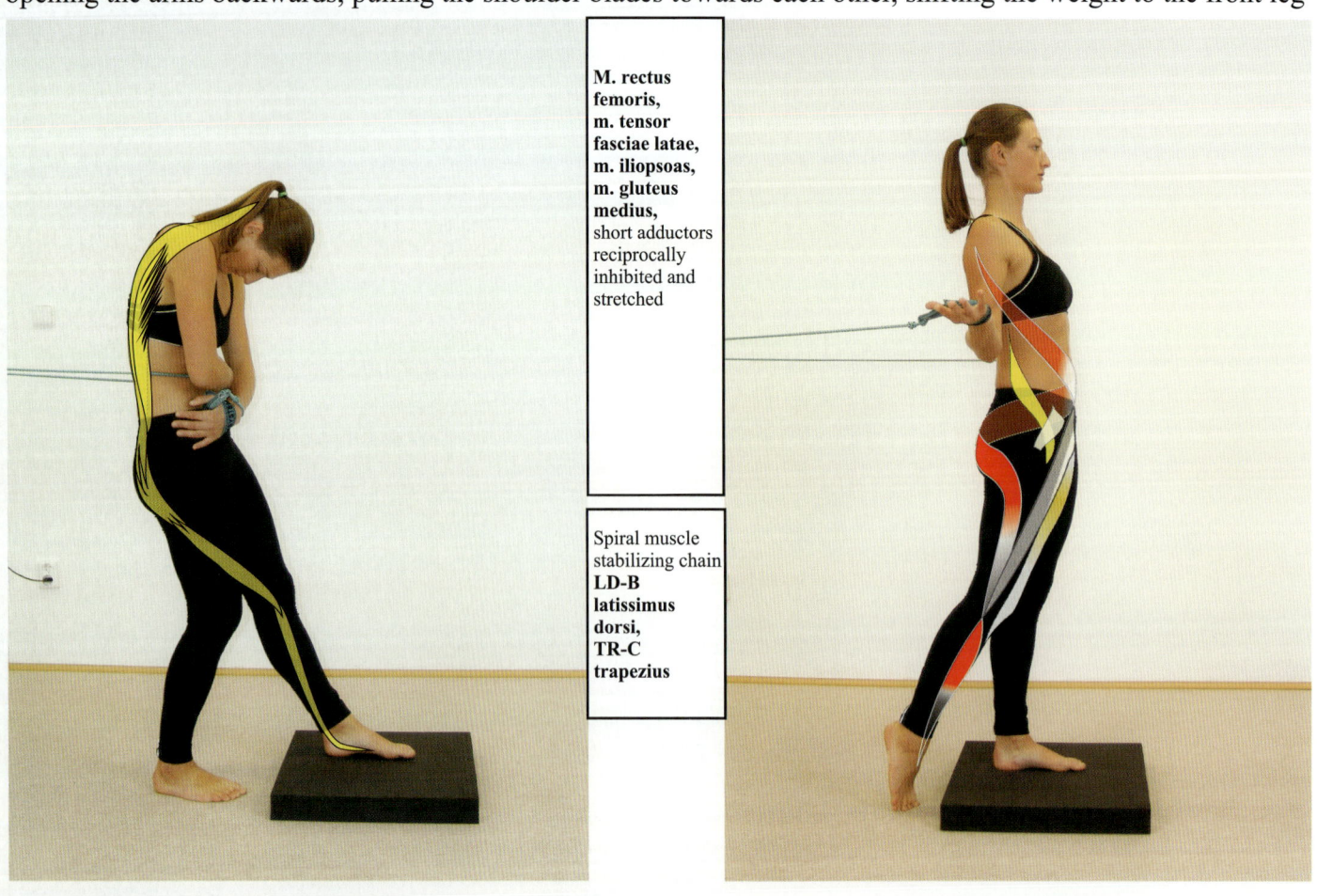

M. rectus femoris, m. tensor fasciae latae, m. iliopsoas, m. gluteus medius, short adductors reciprocally inhibited and stretched

Spiral muscle stabilizing chain LD-B latissimus dorsi, TR-C trapezius

Exercise
M. rectus femoris, m. tensor fasciae latae, m. iliopsoas
m. gluteus medius, short adductors - active relaxation and stretching

Exercise 11 - balanced, stabilized standing position facing the attachment of the elastic rope, support from two poles, double crossed extension - stretching the arms at the shoulder and the opposite legs at the hip

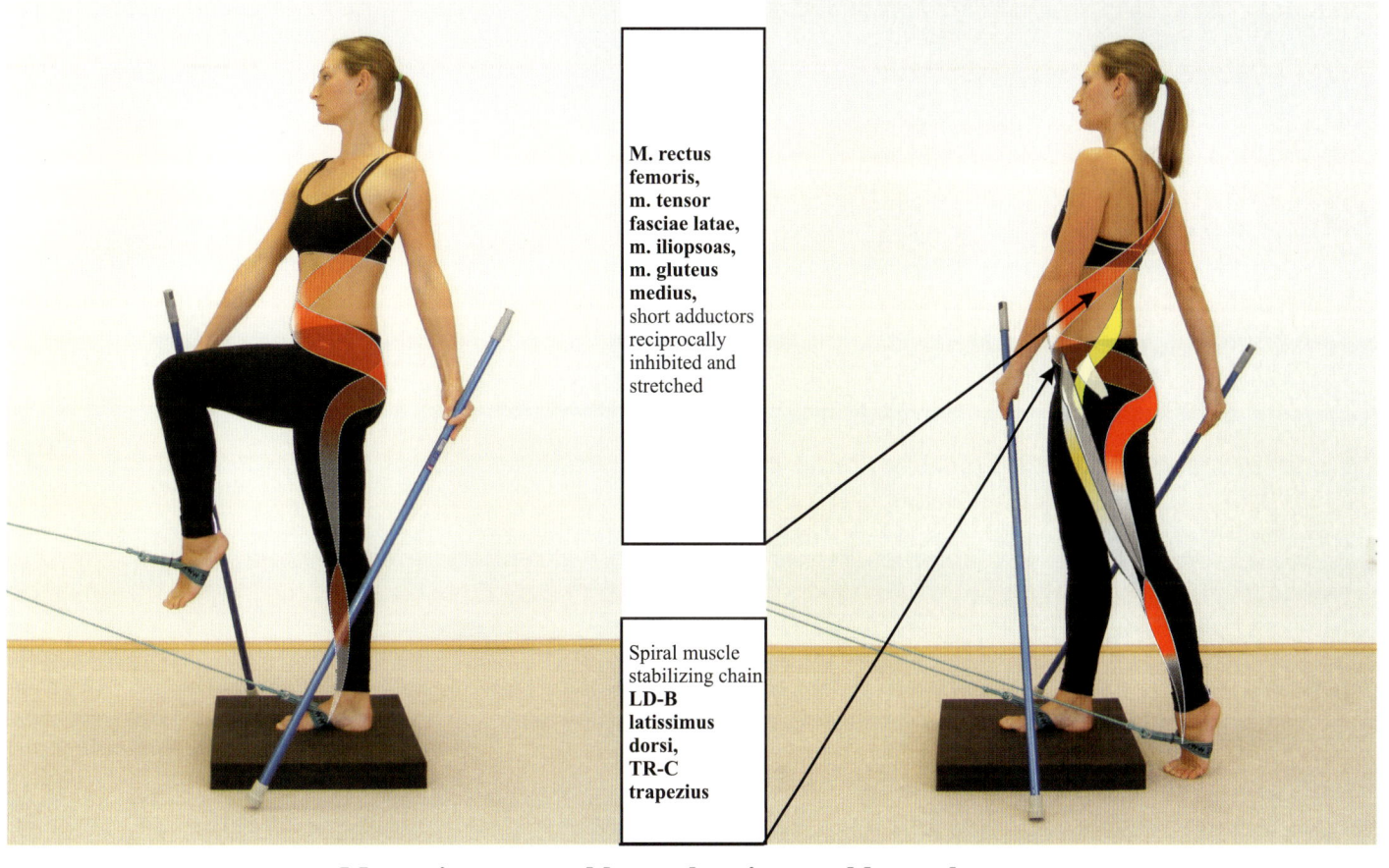

M. rectus femoris, m. tensor fasciae latae, m. iliopsoas, m. gluteus medius, short adductors reciprocally inhibited and stretched

Spiral muscle stabilizing chain **LD-B** latissimus dorsi, **TR-C** trapezius

M. pectineus, m. adductor brevis, m. adductor longus
- active relaxation and stretching

Exercise 13 - balanced, stabilized standing position sideways on to the attachment of the elastic rope, optional support from two poles, abduction in the hip, sideways pull with one leg, counter-movement of the arms

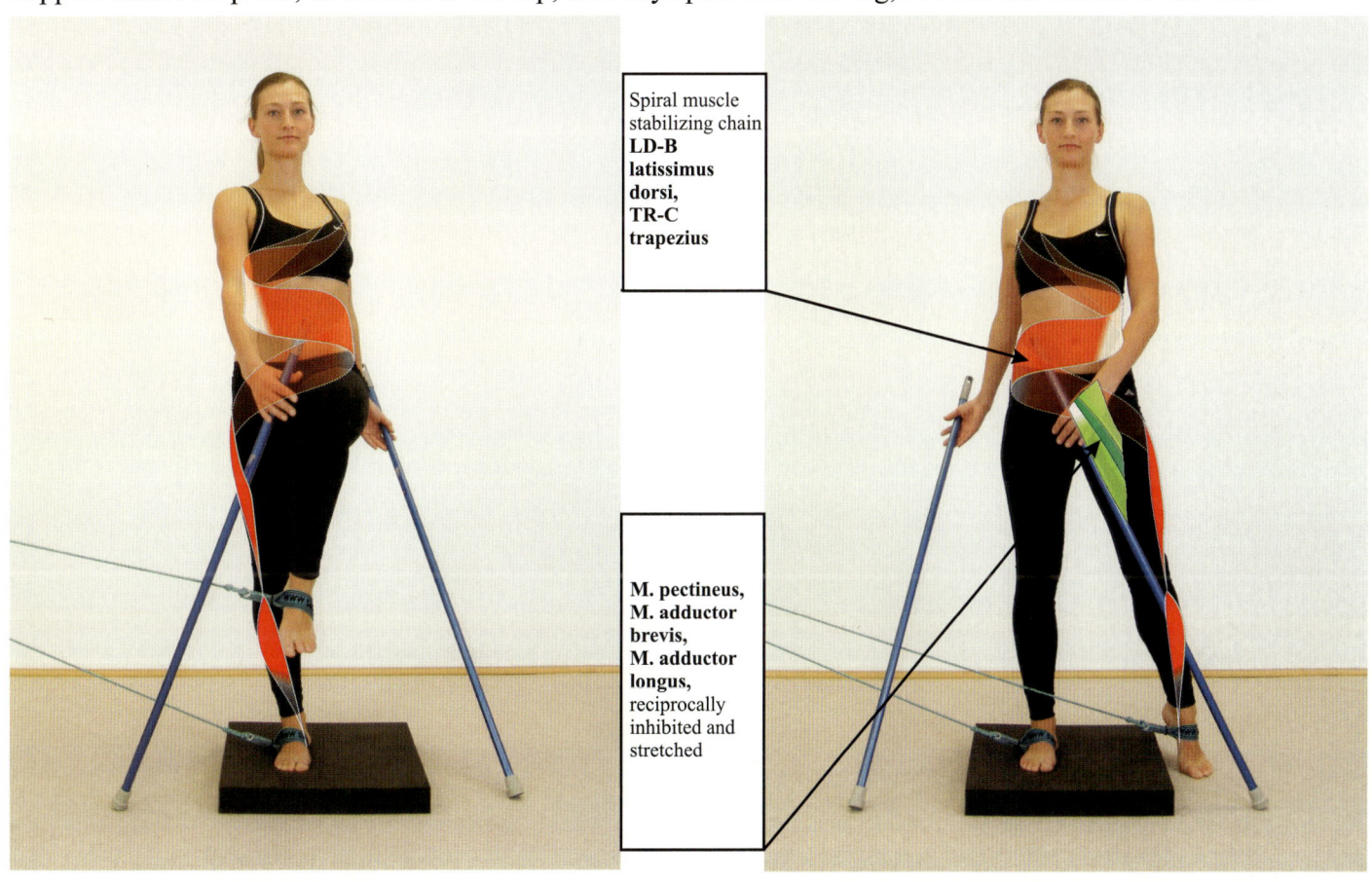

Spiral muscle stabilizing chain **LD-B** latissimus dorsi, **TR-C** trapezius

M. pectineus, M. adductor brevis, M. adductor longus, reciprocally inhibited and stretched

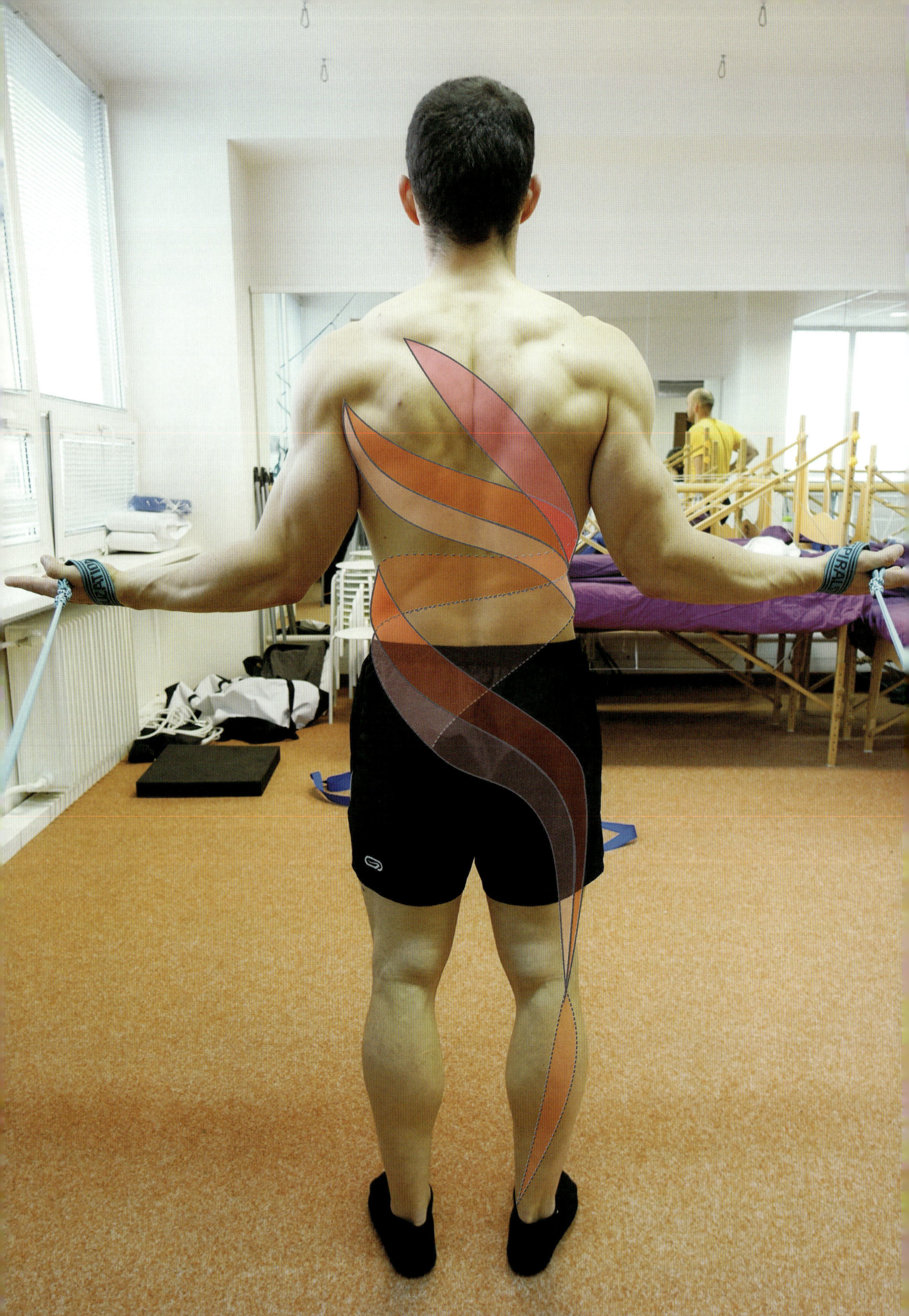

MANUAL TECHNIQUES AND EXERCISE ACCORDING TO MUSCLE ANALYSIS

Shoulder girdle
The posterior lower muscle group

Muscles with a tendency towards weakening:

M. trapezius
M. latissimus dorsi

Spine and chest autochthonous muscles and intercostal muscles

Muscles with a tendency towards weakening:

Mm. rotatores breves et longi
Mm. semispinales
Mm. multifidi
Mm. levatores costarum
Mm. intercostales externi

Anatomy
M. trapezius

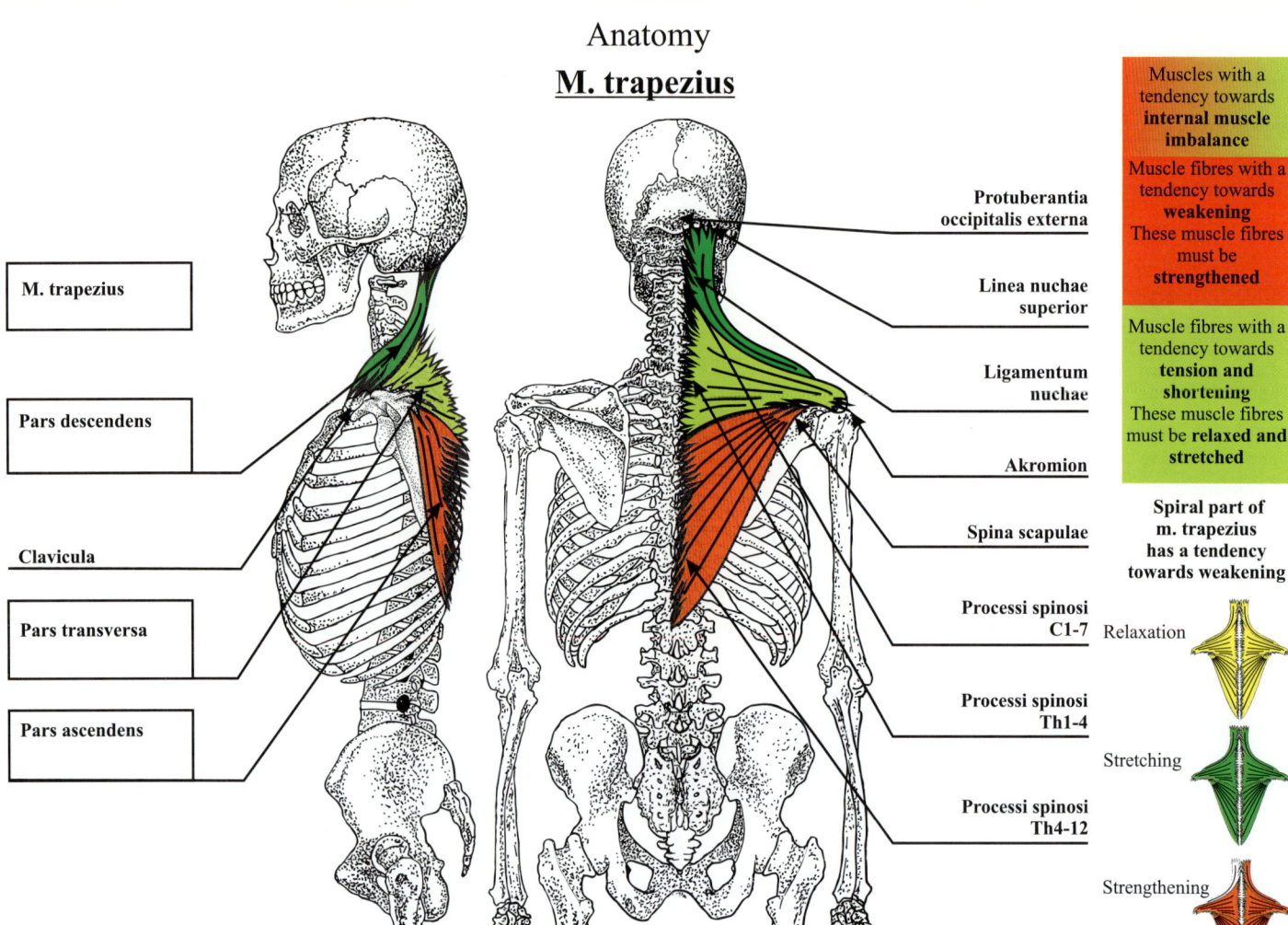

Labels (figure):
- M. trapezius
- Pars descendens
- Clavicula
- Pars transversa
- Pars ascendens
- Protuberantia occipitalis externa
- Linea nuchae superior
- Ligamentum nuchae
- Akromion
- Spina scapulae
- Processi spinosi C1-7
- Processi spinosi Th1-4
- Processi spinosi Th4-12

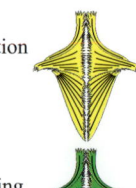

Legend:
- Muscles with a tendency towards **internal muscle imbalance**
- Muscle fibres with a tendency towards **weakening** — These muscle fibres must be **strengthened**
- Muscle fibres with a tendency towards **tension and shortening** — These muscle fibres must be **relaxed and stretched**
- Spiral part of m. trapezius has a tendency towards weakening
- Relaxation
- Stretching
- Strengthening
- Stabilization

M. trapezius
Origin: **- pars descendens** (descending - upper part)
- os occipitale (linea nuchalis superior, protuberantia occipitalis externa)
- ligamentum nuchae, processi spinosi C1-7
  - pars transversa (transverse - middle part)
- processi spinosi Th1-4
  - pars ascendens (ascending - lower part)
- processi spinosi Th5-12

Insertion: **- pars descendens**
- clavicula lateral third
  - pars transversa
- akromion
  - pars ascendens
- spina scapulae

Function: **- pars descendens**
- pulls the shoulder blade upwards
- turns the shoulder place outwards
  (synergically with the pars inferior m. serratus anterior)
- tilts the head towards the ipsilateral side
- turns the head towards the contralateral side
  (the punctum fixum is on the shoulder blade)
  - pars transversa
- pulls the shoulder blade medially
  - pars ascendens
- pulls the shoulder blade caudally and medially
- supports the rotational effect of the pars descendens
  - whole muscle
- fixes the shoulder blade to the chest

Innervation:
- n. accesorius XI, plexus cervicalis (C2-4)

M. trapezius
Muscle with internal muscle imbalance
- **pars descendens**
  has a tendency towards shortening
- **pars transversa**
  has a tendency towards weakening
- **pars ascendens**
  has a tendency towards weakening

Muscle chains
Spiral muscle chain TR - trapezius
The TR chain is activated by the backward movement of the shoulder blade - extension.

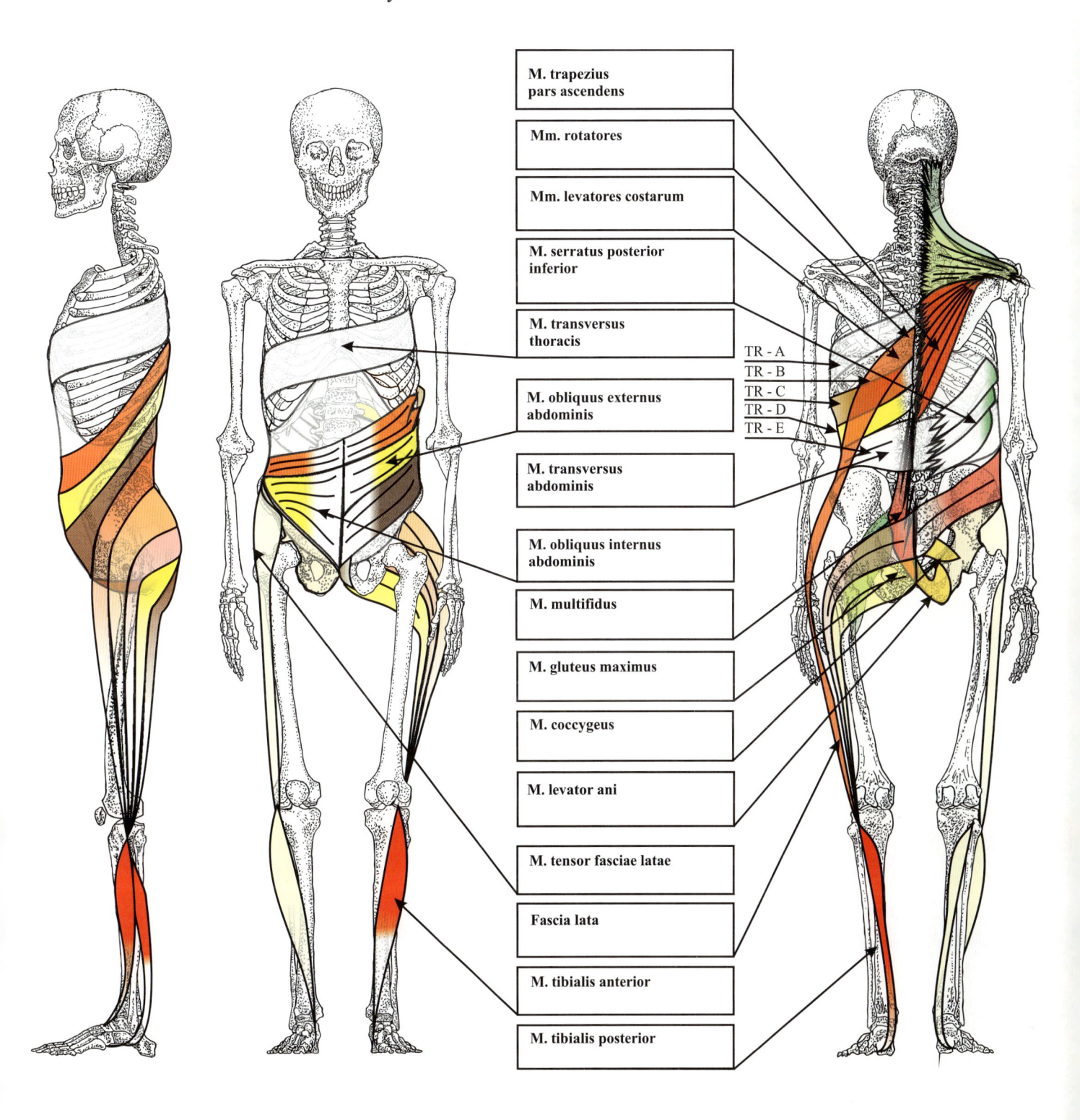

M. trapezius pars ascendens	
Mm. rotatores	
Mm. levatores costarum	
M. serratus posterior inferior	
M. transversus thoracis	TR - A
	TR - B
M. obliquus externus abdominis	TR - C
	TR - D
M. transversus abdominis	TR - E
M. obliquus internus abdominis	
M. multifidus	
M. gluteus maximus	
M. coccygeus	
M. levator ani	
M. tensor fasciae latae	
Fascia lata	
M. tibialis anterior	
M. tibialis posterior	

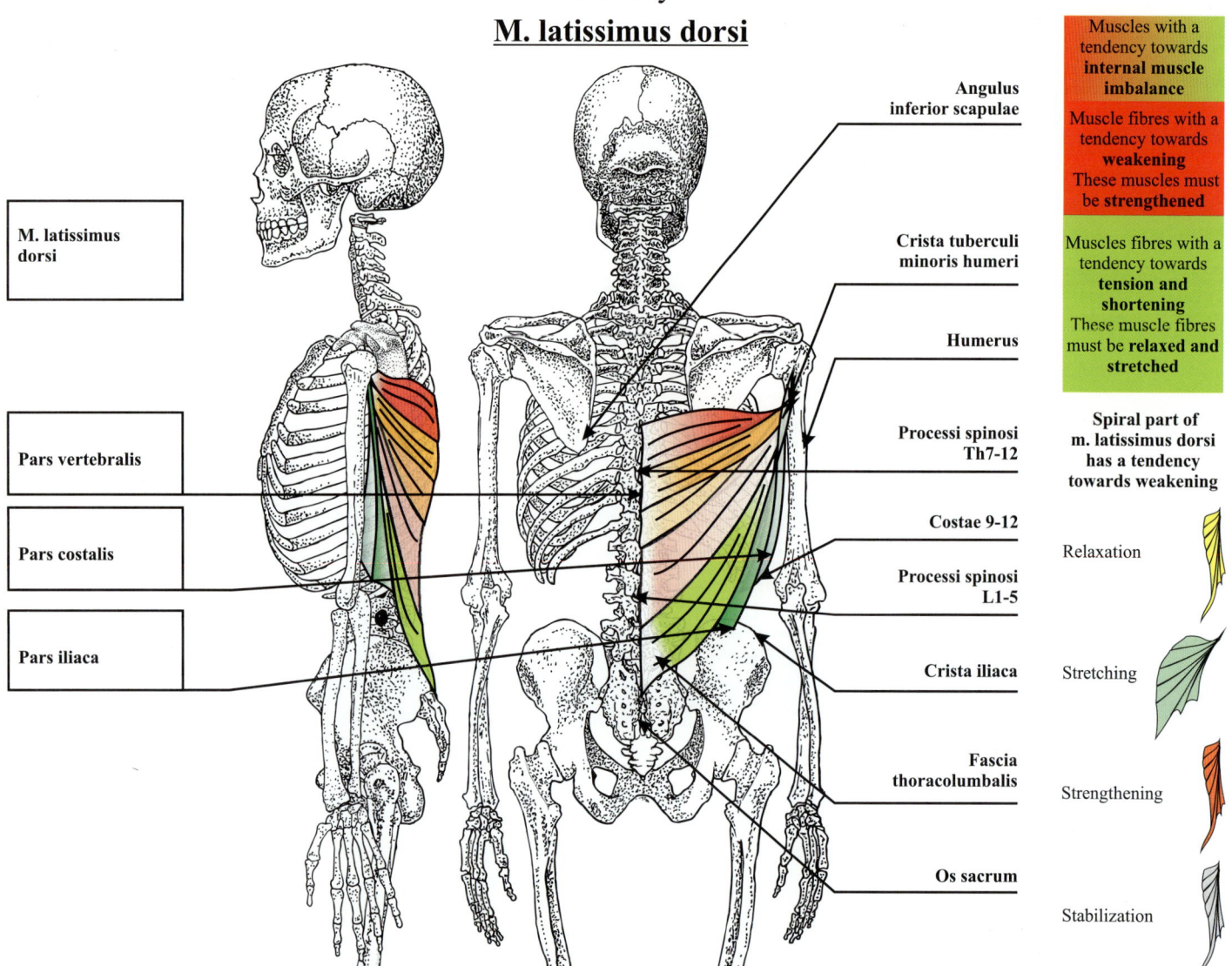

Anatomy
M. latissimus dorsi

M. latissimus dorsi	
Pars vertebralis	
Pars costalis	
Pars iliaca	

Labels (right side):
- Angulus inferior scapulae
- Crista tuberculi minoris humeri
- Humerus
- Processi spinosi Th7-12
- Costae 9-12
- Processi spinosi L1-5
- Crista iliaca
- Fascia thoracolumbalis
- Os sacrum

Muscles with a tendency towards internal muscle imbalance

Muscle fibres with a tendency towards **weakening**
These muscles must be **strengthened**

Muscles fibres with a tendency towards **tension and shortening**
These muscle fibres must be **relaxed and stretched**

Spiral part of m. latissimus dorsi has a tendency towards weakening

- Relaxation
- Stretching
- Strengthening
- Stabilization

M. latissimus dorsi
Origin: - **pars vertebralis:**
- processus spinosus Th7-12
- L1-5 through the fascia thoracolumbalis
- os sacrum
      - **pars iliaca:**
- posterior part of the crista iliaca
      - **pars costalis:**
- 9th-12th rib
Insertion:
- crista tuberculi minoris humeri
Function:
- internal rotation
- adduction (pulling in)
- retroversion (pulling the shoulder backwards and downwards)
- extension (stretching backwards)
- supports exhalation
- lifts the trunk from a hanging position
Innervation:
- n. thoracodorsalis (C6-C8)

M. latissimus dorsi
Muscles with internal muscle imbalance
- **pars vertebralis**
  has a tendency towards weakening
- **pars iliaca**
  has a tendency towards tension and shortening
- **pars costalis**
  has a tendency towards tension and shortening

Muscle chains
Spiral muscle chain LD - latissimus dorsi
The LD chain is activated by the backward movement of the arm - extension.

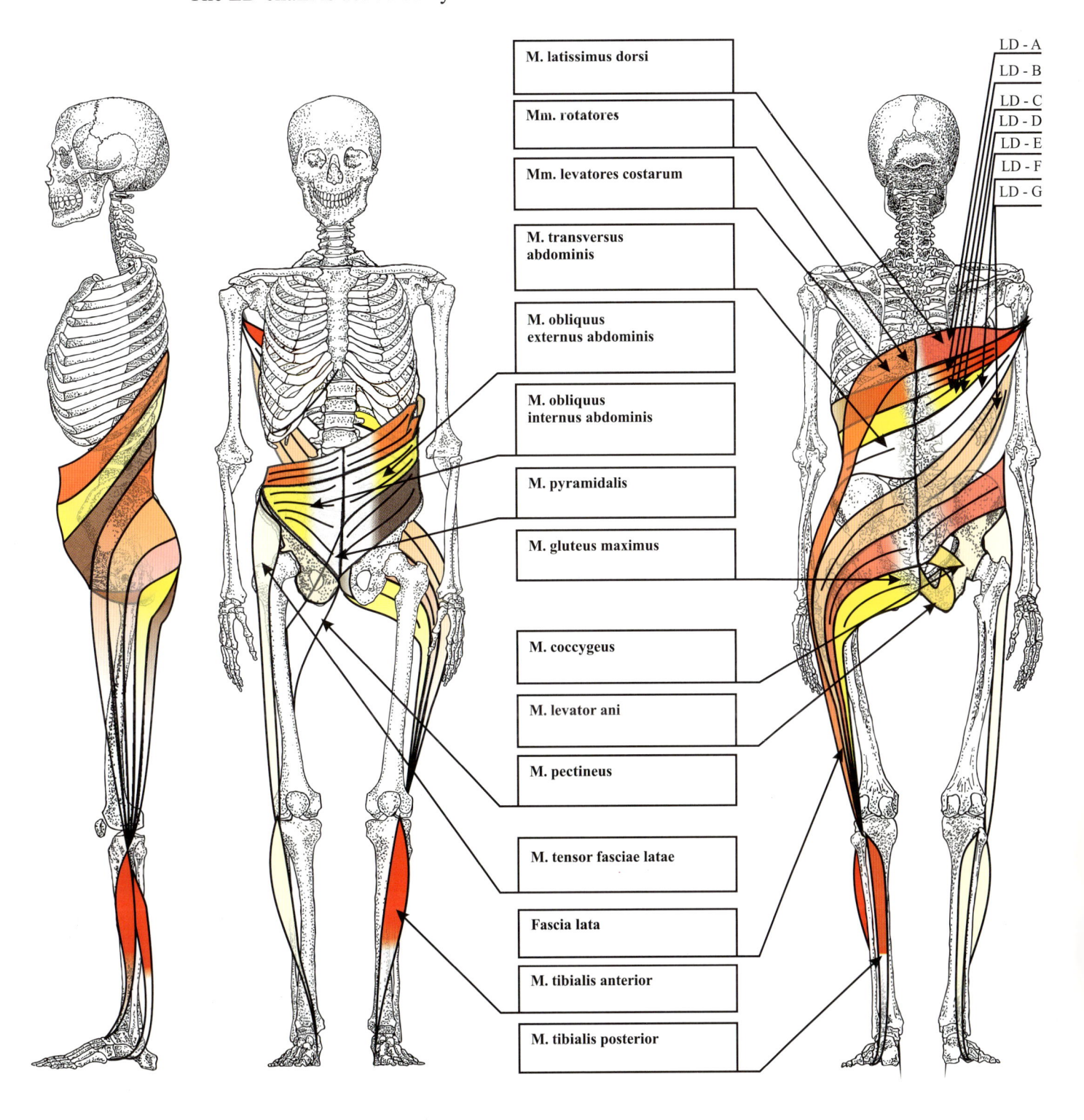

M. latissimus dorsi	LD - A
Mm. rotatores	LD - B
Mm. levatores costarum	LD - C
M. transversus abdominis	LD - D
M. obliquus externus abdominis	LD - E
M. obliquus internus abdominis	LD - F
M. pyramidalis	LD - G
M. gluteus maximus	
M. coccygeus	
M. levator ani	
M. pectineus	
M. tensor fasciae latae	
Fascia lata	
M. tibialis anterior	
M. tibialis posterior	

Anatomy
Mm. rotatores breves et longi, mm. semispinales, mm. multifidi

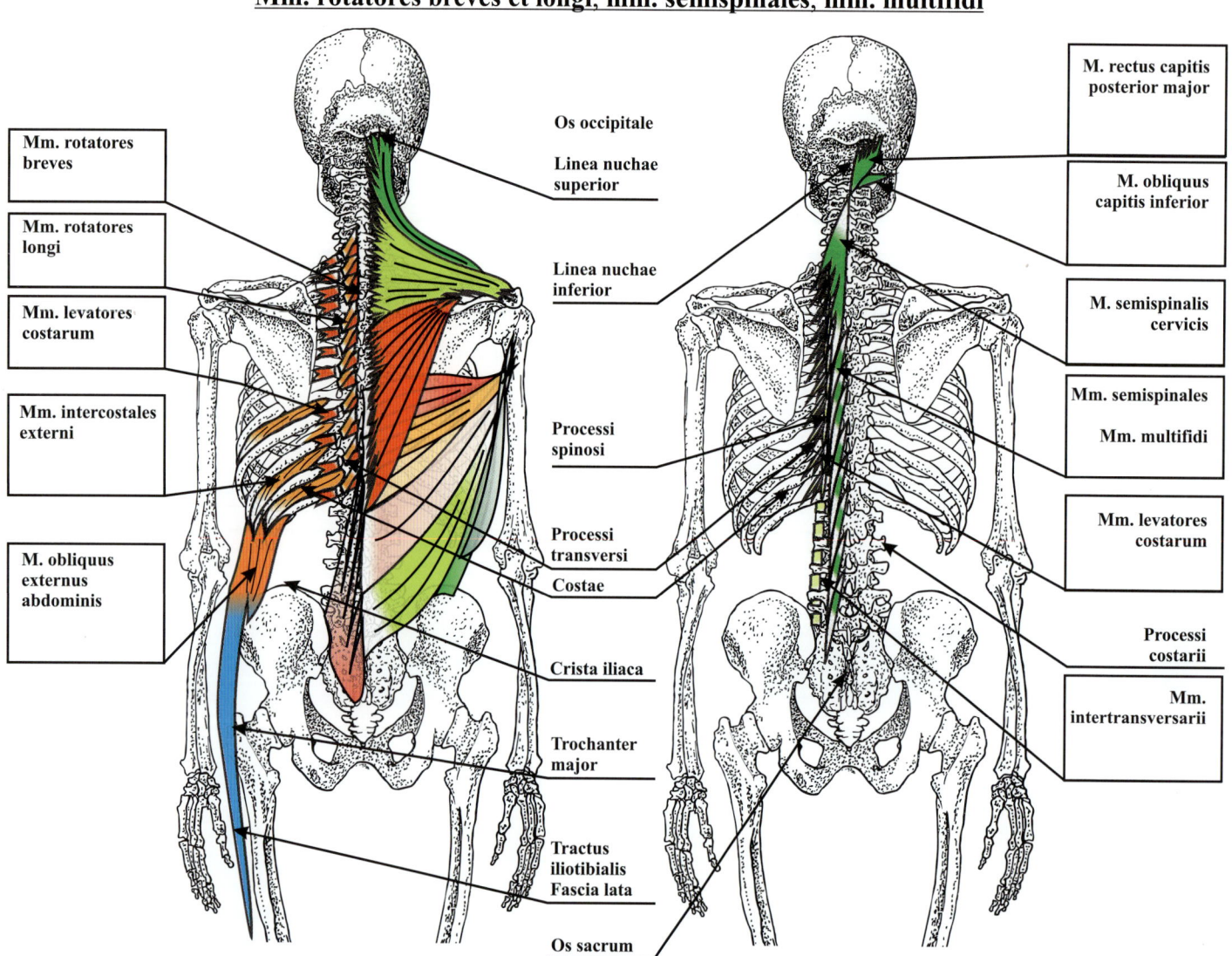

Labels (left figure):
- Mm. rotatores breves
- Mm. rotatores longi
- Mm. levatores costarum
- Mm. intercostales externi
- M. obliquus externus abdominis
- Os occipitale
- Linea nuchae superior
- Linea nuchae inferior
- Processi spinosi
- Processi transversi
- Costae
- Crista iliaca
- Trochanter major
- Tractus iliotibialis / Fascia lata
- Os sacrum

Labels (right figure):
- M. rectus capitis posterior major
- M. obliquus capitis inferior
- M. semispinalis cervicis
- Mm. semispinales
- Mm. multifidi
- Mm. levatores costarum
- Processi costarii
- Mm. intertransversarii

Mm. rotatores breves, longi
Origin:
- processi transversi Th1-12

Insertion:
- processi spinosi Th1-12
- breves - adjacent upper vertebra
- longi - second adjacent upper vertebra

Function:
- bilateral contraction - dorsal extension of the thoracic vertebrae
- unilateral contraction - rotation towards the contralateral side
- lateroflexion towards the ipsilateral side

Innervation:
- rr. dorsales of the spinal nerves Th

Mm. semispinales thoracis
Origin:
- processi transversi Th6-12

Insertion:
- processi spinosi C6-Th4
- intersects with 5 vertebrae

Function:
- bilateral contract - dorsal extension of the thoracic and cervical vertebrae
- unilateral contract - rotation towards the contralateral side
- lateroflexion towards the ipsilateral side

Innervation:
- rr. dorsales of the spinal nerves Th

Mm. levatores costarum breves, longi
Origin:
- processi transversi C7-Th1-11

Insertion:
- breves - angulus costae of the adjacent rib
- longi - angulus costae across two ribs

Function:
- bilateral contraction - dorsal extension of the thoracic vertebrae
- unilateral contraction - rotation towards the contralateral side
- lateroflexion towards the ipsilateral side

Innervation:
- rr. dorsales, rr. ventrales of the spinal nerves Th

Mm. intertransversarii
Origin and insertion:
- mm. intertransversarii mediales lumborum
- processi mamilares of the lumbar vertebrae
- mm. intertransversarii laterales lumborum
- processi costales of the lumbar vertebrae
- mm. intertransversarii posteriores cervicis
- tubercula posteriora of the 2nd-7th cervical vertebrae
- mm. intertransversarii anteriores cervicis
- tubercula anteriora of the 2nd-7th cervical vertebrae

Function:
- bilateral contraction - dorsal extension of the thoracic and cervical vertebrae
- unilateral contraction - rotation towards the contralateral side
- lateroflexion of the lumbar and cervical vertebrae towards the ipsilateral side

Innervation:
- rr. dorsales of the spinal nerves L, C:
- mm. intertransversarii mediales lumborum
- mm. intertransversarii posteriores lumborum
- mm. intertransversarii posteriores cervicis

- rr. ventrales of the spinal nerves L, C:
- mm. intertransversarii laterales lumborum
- mm. intertransversarii anteriores cervicis

Muscle chains
Latissimus dorsi, trapezius and erector spinae muscle chains - reciprocal relationships

Relationship between the agonist and antagonist
in the muscle chains, active relaxation, active stretching.
LD - latissimus dorsi and TR - trapezius spiral muscle chains (innervation n. acessorius, C1-S2)
inhibit the ES - erector spinae (innervation C1-L5)

Antagonist (opponent, inhibited muscle chain)	**Agonist** (player, activated muscle chain)
Vertical **ES - Erector spinae**	Spiral **LD - Latissimus dorsi**
	Spiral **TR - Trapezius**

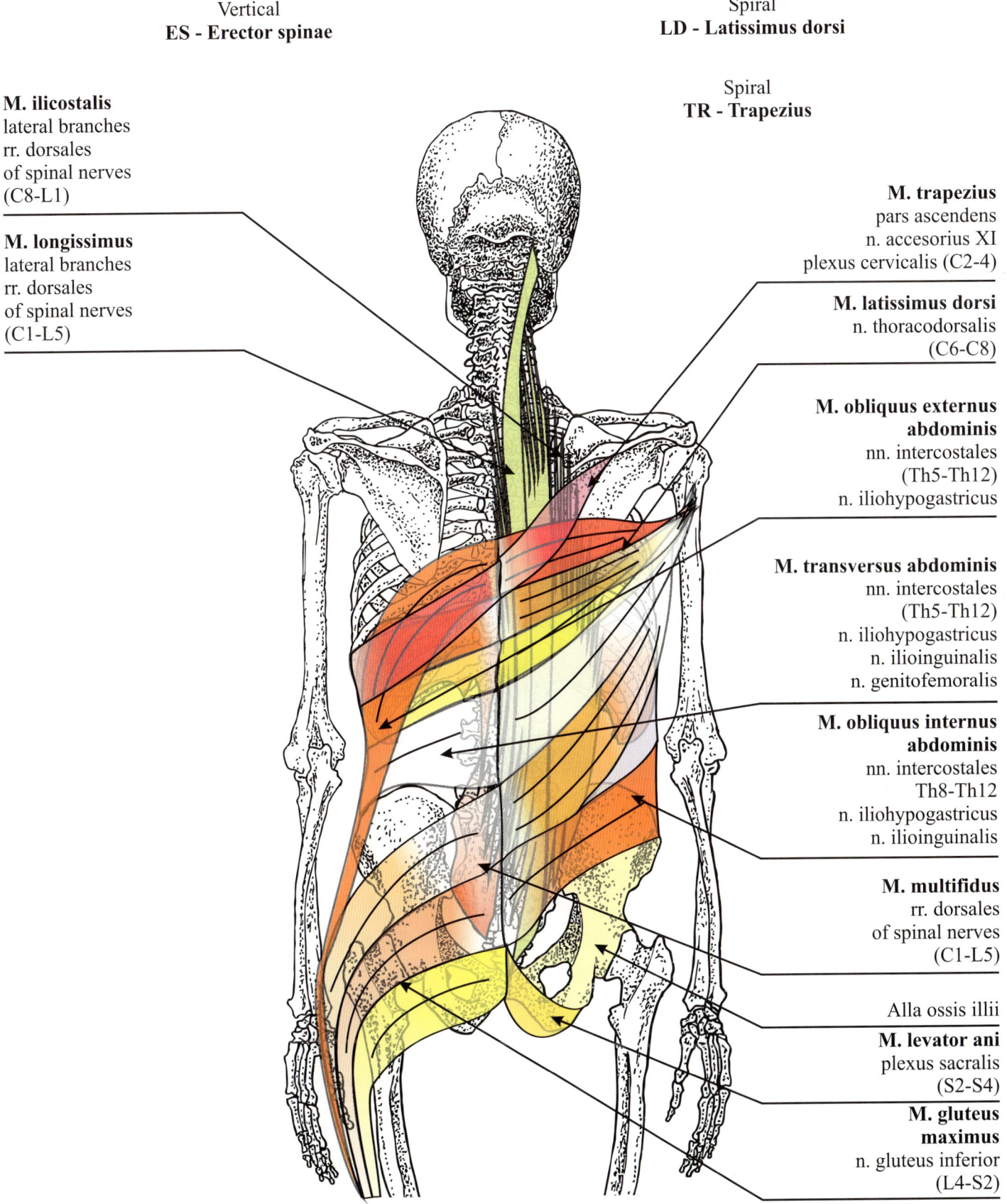

M. ilicostalis
lateral branches
rr. dorsales
of spinal nerves
(C8-L1)

M. longissimus
lateral branches
rr. dorsales
of spinal nerves
(C1-L5)

M. trapezius
pars ascendens
n. accesorius XI
plexus cervicalis (C2-4)

M. latissimus dorsi
n. thoracodorsalis
(C6-C8)

M. obliquus externus abdominis
nn. intercostales
(Th5-Th12)
n. iliohypogastricus

M. transversus abdominis
nn. intercostales
(Th5-Th12)
n. iliohypogastricus
n. ilioinguinalis
n. genitofemoralis

M. obliquus internus abdominis
nn. intercostales
Th8-Th12
n. iliohypogastricus
n. ilioinguinalis

M. multifidus
rr. dorsales
of spinal nerves
(C1-L5)

Alla ossis illii

M. levator ani
plexus sacralis
(S2-S4)

M. gluteus maximus
n. gluteus inferior
(L4-S2)

Muscle chains
Latissimus dorsi, trapezius and erector spinae muscle chains - reciprocal relationships

Relationship between the agonist and antagonist in the muscle chains
Spiral LD - latissimus dorsi, inhibits the vertical ES - erector spinae

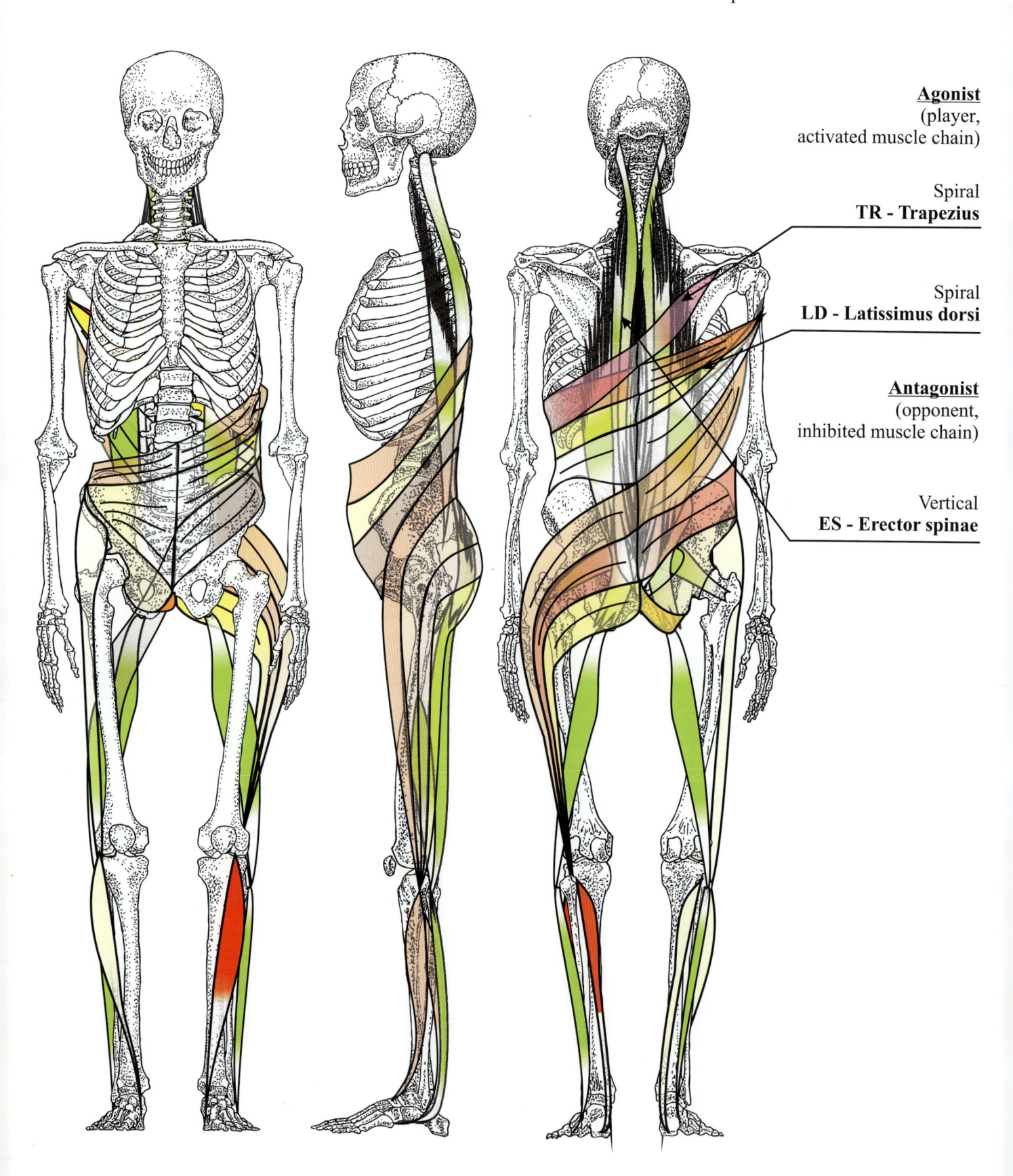

Agonist
(player,
activated muscle chain)

Spiral
TR - Trapezius

Spiral
LD - Latissimus dorsi

Antagonist
(opponent,
inhibited muscle chain)

Vertical
ES - Erector spinae

- 138 -

Manual techniques in a sitting position
M. latissimus dorsi, **m. trapezius** - passive stretching, strengthening

Exercise 1 - sitting facing the attachment of the elastic rope, backward pull with both arms

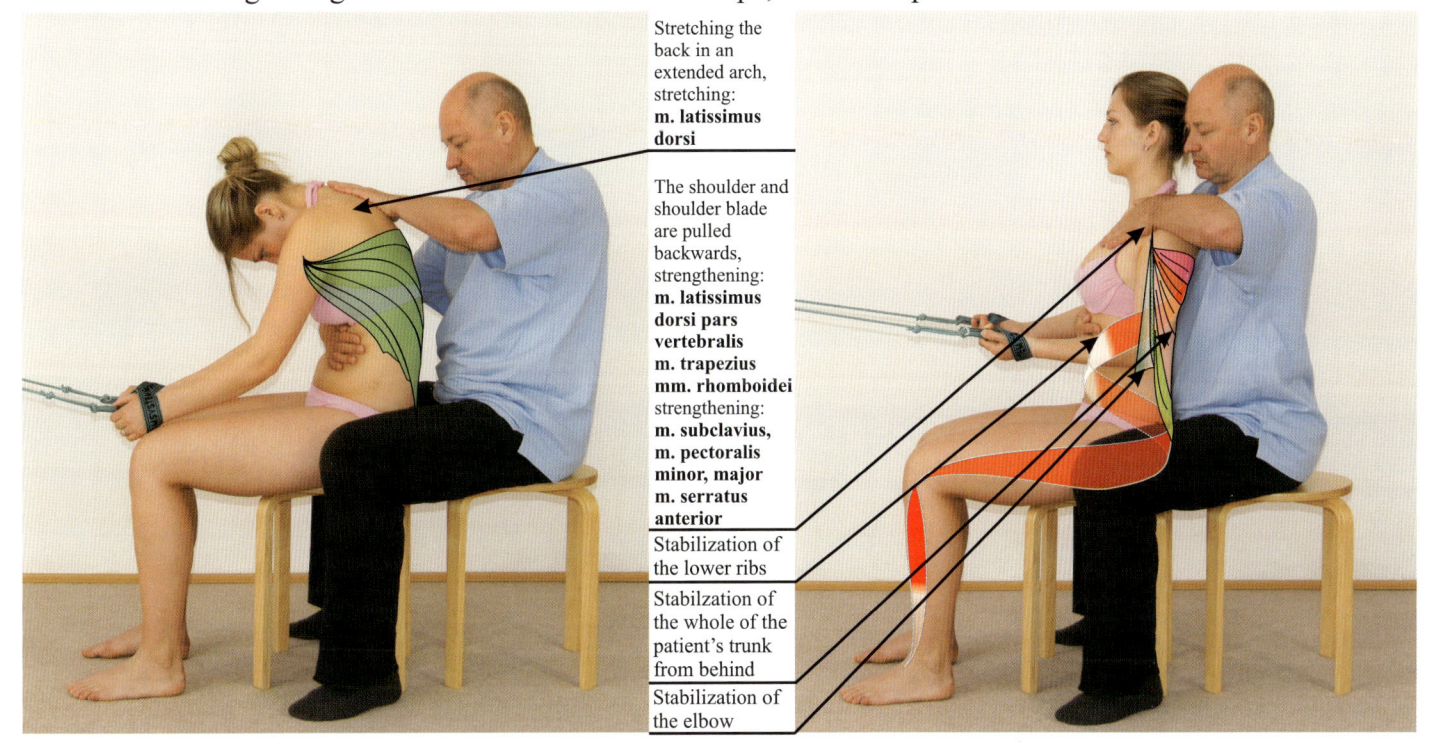

Stretching the back in an extended arch, stretching: **m. latissimus dorsi**

The shoulder and shoulder blade are pulled backwards, strengthening: **m. latissimus dorsi pars vertebralis m. trapezius mm. rhomboidei** strengthening: **m. subclavius, m. pectoralis minor, major m. serratus anterior**

Stabilization of the lower ribs

Stabilzation of the whole of the patient's trunk from behind

Stabilization of the elbow

M. latissimus dorsi - stretching the pars spinalis, strengthening the pars costalis

Exercise 6 - sitting with back to the attachment of the elastic rope, forward circles with both arms

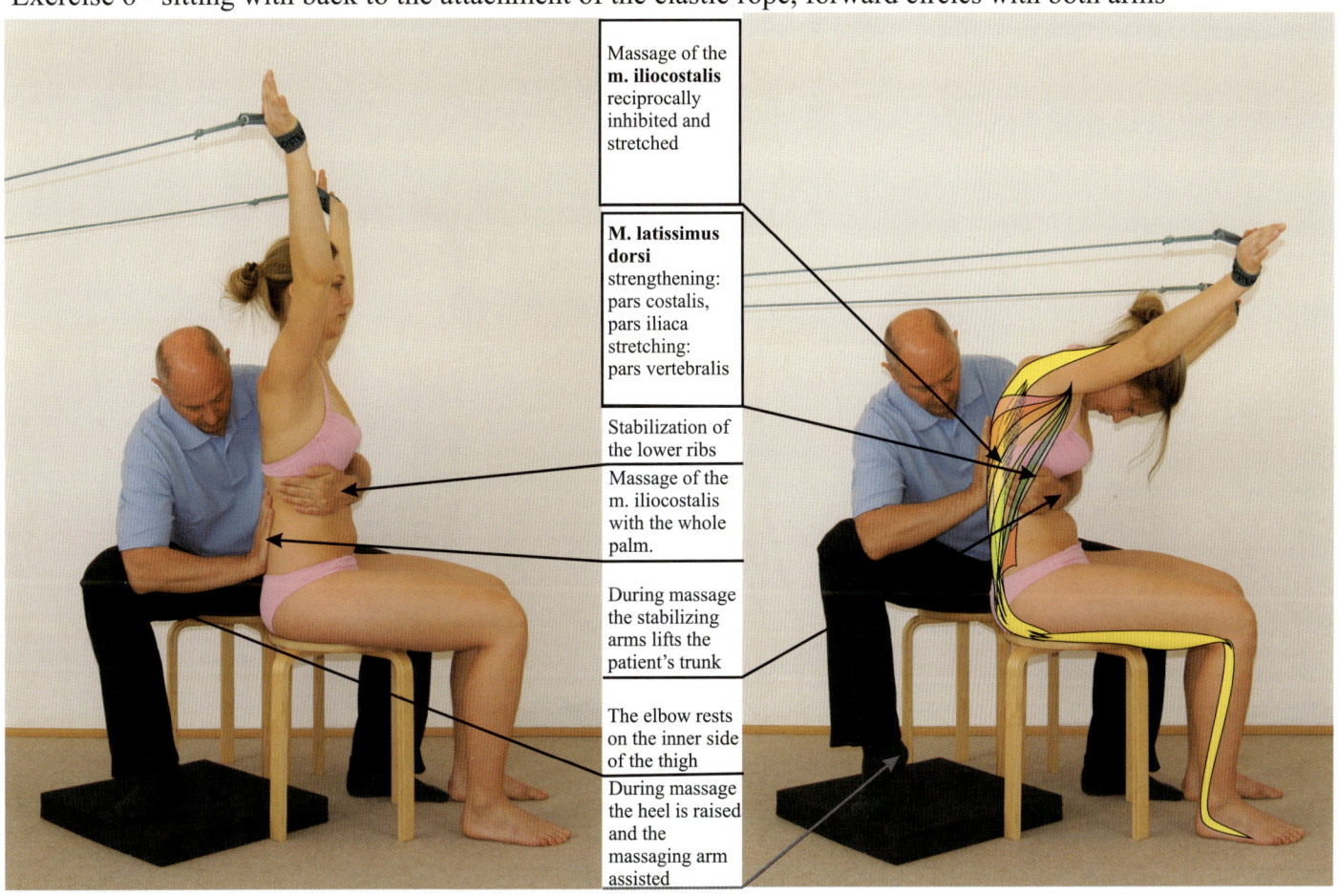

Massage of the **m. iliocostalis** reciprocally inhibited and stretched

M. latissimus dorsi strengthening: pars costalis, pars iliaca stretching: pars vertebralis

Stabilization of the lower ribs

Massage of the m. iliocostalis with the whole palm.

During massage the stabilizing arms lifts the patient's trunk

The elbow rests on the inner side of the thigh

During massage the heel is raised and the massaging arm assisted

Exercise - stabilization, stretching
M. trapezius, m. latissimus dorsi - strengthening, stretching
M. erector spinae - relaxation in reciprocal inhibition, stretching

The LD - latissimus dorsi and TR - trapezius chains are the agonists in the second part of the exercise.

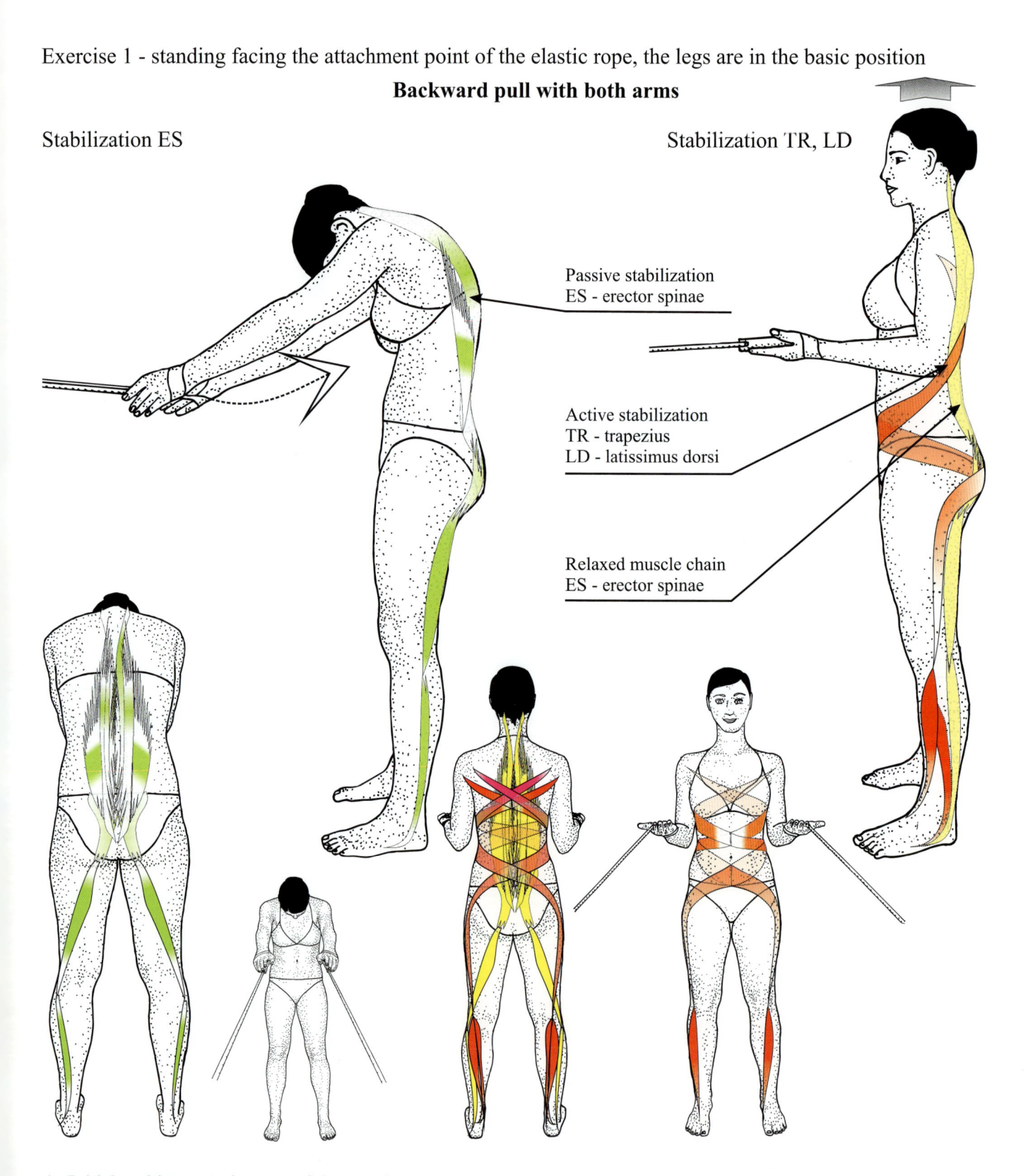

Exercise 1 - standing facing the attachment point of the elastic rope, the legs are in the basic position

Backward pull with both arms

Stabilization ES

Stabilization TR, LD

Passive stabilization
ES - erector spinae

Active stabilization
TR - trapezius
LD - latissimus dorsi

Relaxed muscle chain
ES - erector spinae

1 - Initial position - passive part of the exercise
The initial position is passively stabilized by the vertical chain ES - erector spinae, which is stretched at the same time.

2 - Performance - active part of the exercise
The active part of the exercise is stabilized by the spiral muscle chains
TR-C - trapezius, in this variant the trapezius predominates,
LD-B - latissimus dorsi.
The vertical muscle chain ES erector spinae relaxes in reciprocal inhibition.

- 140 -

Exercise - stabilization, stretching
M. trapezius, m. latissimus dorsi - strengthening, stretching
M. erector spinae - relaxation in reciprocal inhibition, stretching

The LD - latissimus dorsi and TR - trapezius chains are the agonists in the second part of the exercise.

Exercise 2 - standing sideways on to the attachment point of the elastic rope, the legs are in the basic position
Sideways pull with one arm

Stabilization ES   Stabilization TR, LD

Active muscle chain
LD - latissimus dorsi

Passive stabilization
ES - erector spinae

Relaxed muscle chain
ES - erector spinae

LD-A
latissimus dorsi

1 - Initial position
- passive part of the exercise
The initial position is passively
stabilized by the vertical chain
ES - erector spinae, which is
stretched at the same time.

2 - Performance - active part of the exercise
The active part of the exercise is stabilized by the spiral muscle chain
LD-B - latissimus dorsi and LD-A.
The vertical muscle chain ES - erector spinae relaxes.

Exercise
M. trapezius, m. latissimus dorsi - strengthening, stretching

Exercise 1 - standing facing the attachment point of the elastic rope, the legs are in the basic position

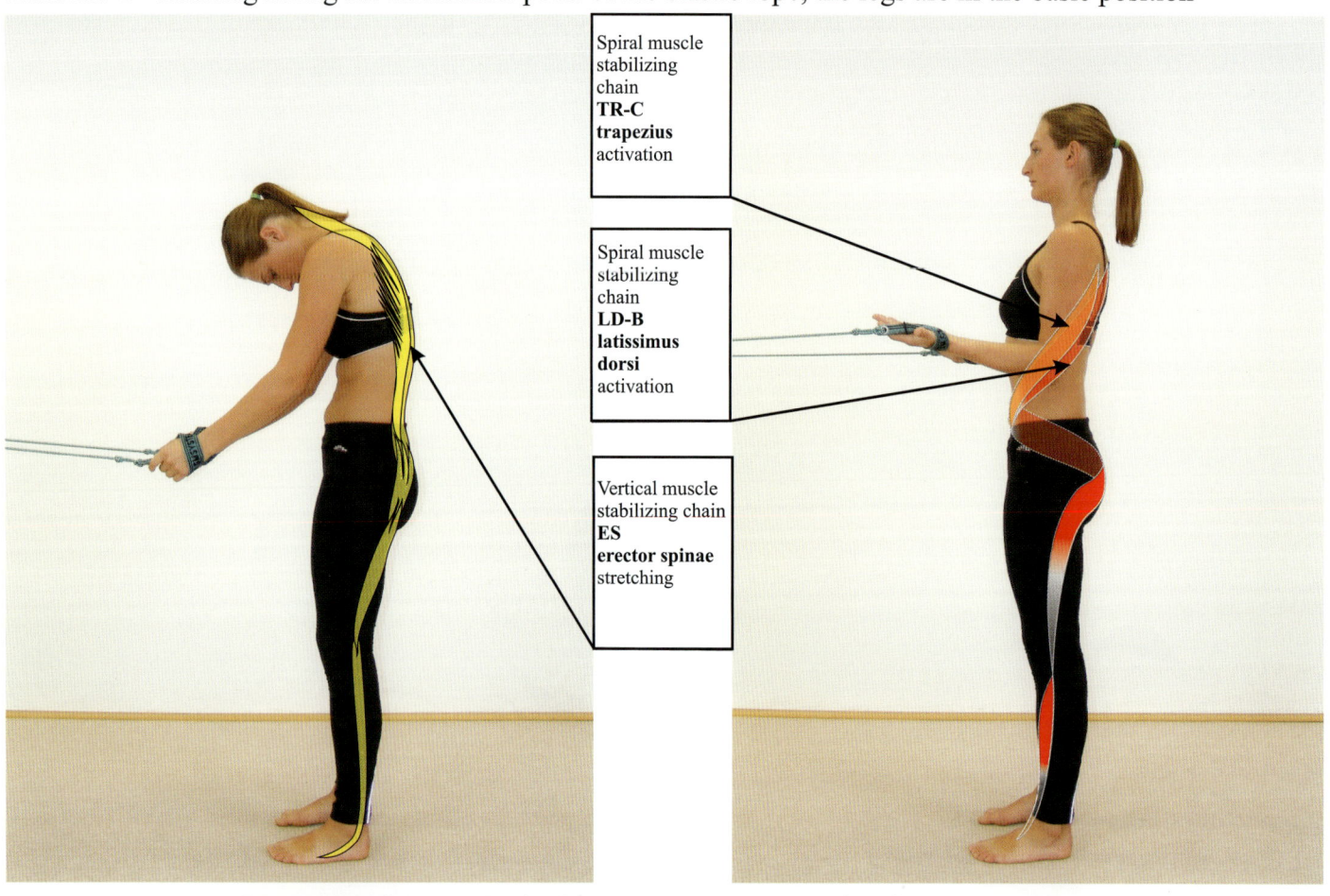

Spiral muscle stabilizing chain
TR-C trapezius activation

Spiral muscle stabilizing chain
LD-B latissimus dorsi activation

Vertical muscle stabilizing chain
ES erector spinae stretching

M. trapezius, m. latissimus dorsi - strengthening, stretching

Exercise 2 - standing sideways on the attachment of the elastic rope, the legs are in the basic position, sideways pull with one arm

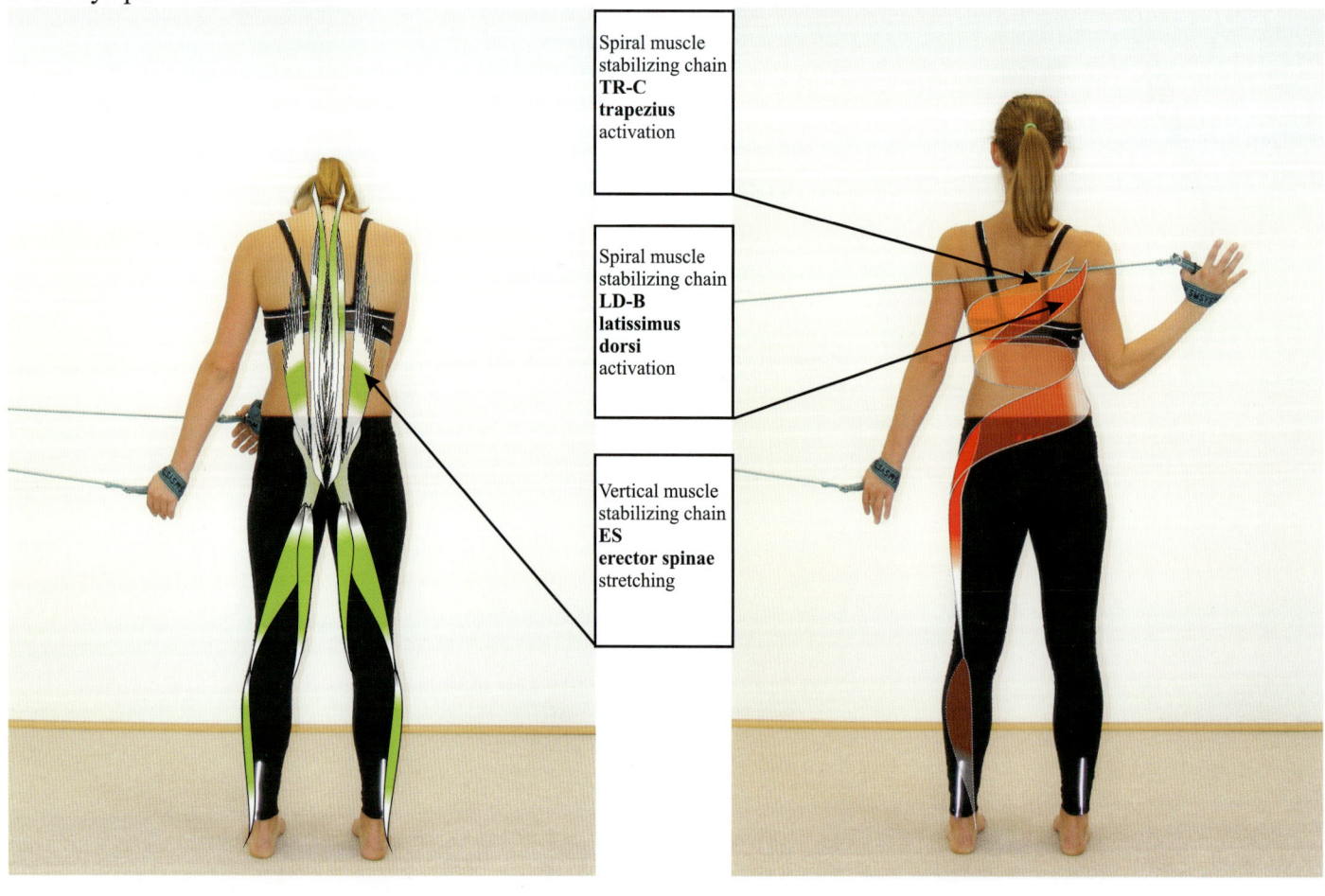

Spiral muscle stabilizing chain
TR-C trapezius activation

Spiral muscle stabilizing chain
LD-B latissimus dorsi activation

Vertical muscle stabilizing chain
ES erector spinae stretching

Exercise - stabilization, stretching
M. trapezius, m. latissimus dorsi - strengthening, stretching
M. erector spinae - relaxation in reciprocal inhibition, stretching

The PM - pectoralis major chain is agonist in the first part of the exercise,
the LD - latissimus dorsi and TR - trapezius chains are the agonists in the second part of the exercise.

Exercise 3 - standing with back to the attachment point of the elastic rope, the legs are in the basic position
Opening the arms backwards, pulling the shoulder blades towards each other

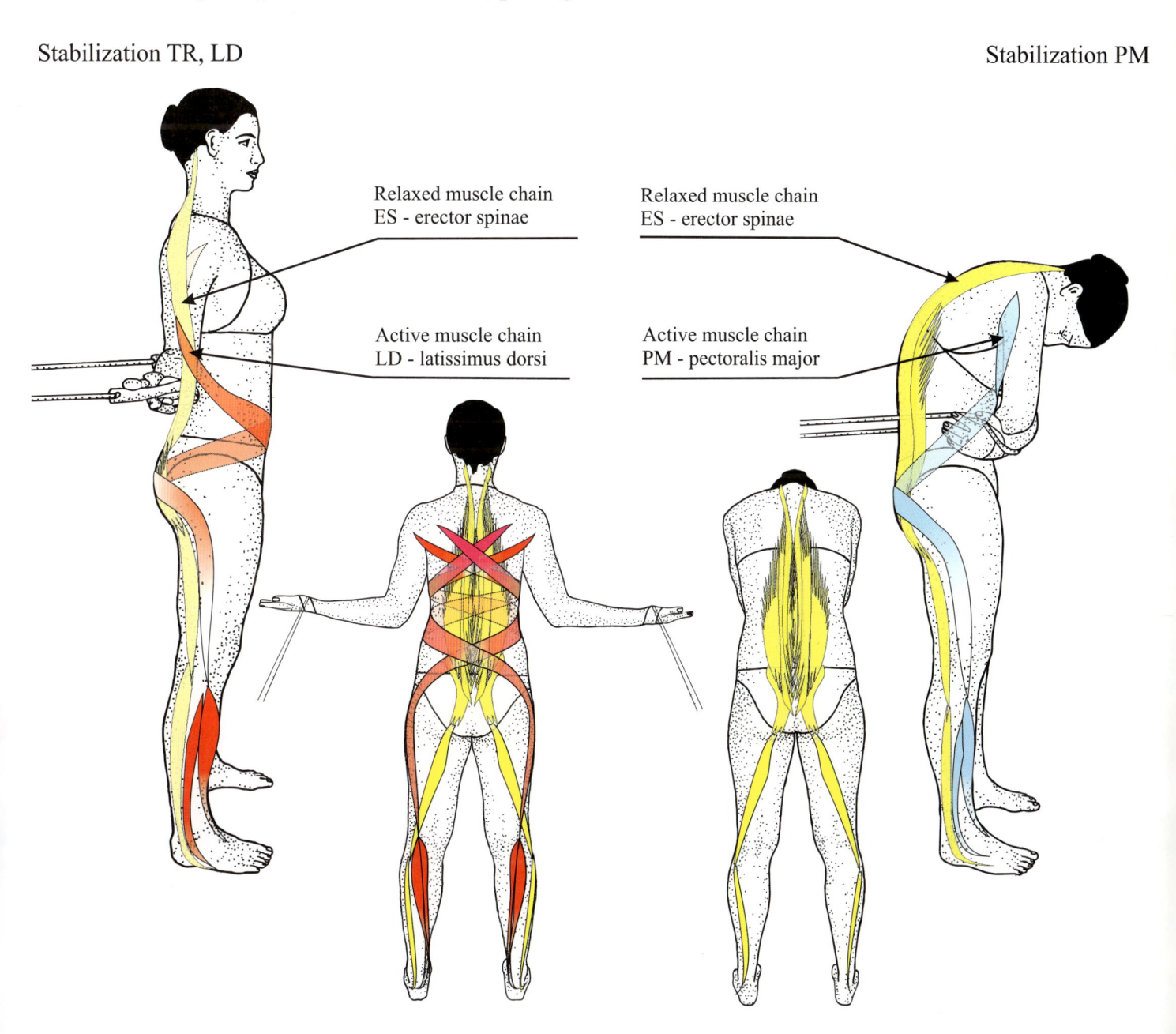

Stabilization TR, LD   Stabilization PM

Relaxed muscle chain ES - erector spinae

Relaxed muscle chain ES - erector spinae

Active muscle chain LD - latissimus dorsi

Active muscle chain PM - pectoralis major

2 - Performance - active part of the exercise
The active part of the exercise is stabilized by the spiral muscle chain
LD-B - latissimus dorsi
TR-C - trapezius.
The vertical muscle chain ES erector spinae relaxes.

1 - Initial position - active part of the exercise
The exercise is stabilized by the spiral chain
PM - pectoralis major.
It is active stabilization of the spine.
The vertical muscle chain ES - erector spinae relaxes.
In relaxation the ES is pulled across the active abdomen.

Exercise

M. trapezius, m. latissimus dorsi - strengthening, stretching

Exercise 3 - standing with back to the attachment of the elastic rope, the legs are in the basic position, opening the arms backward, pulling the shoulder blades toward each other

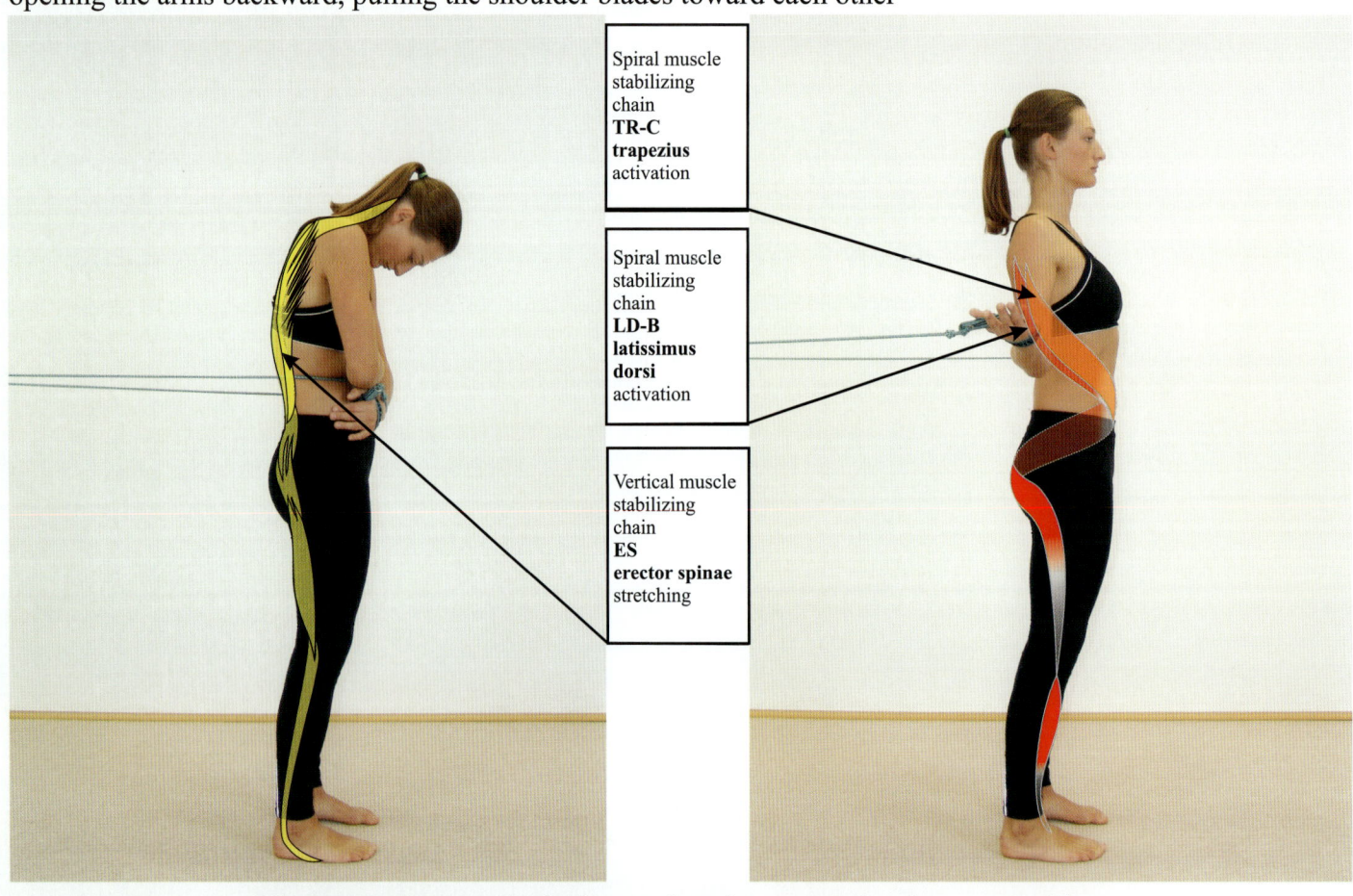

Spiral muscle stabilizing chain **TR-C trapezius** activation

Spiral muscle stabilizing chain **LD-B latissimus dorsi** activation

Vertical muscle stabilizing chain **ES erector spinae** stretching

M. trapezius, m. latissimus dorsi - strengthening, stretching

Exercise 11 - standing facing the attachment point of the elastic rope, crossed movement pattern, extension of the arm in the shoulder girdle and extension of the opposing leg in the pelvic girdle

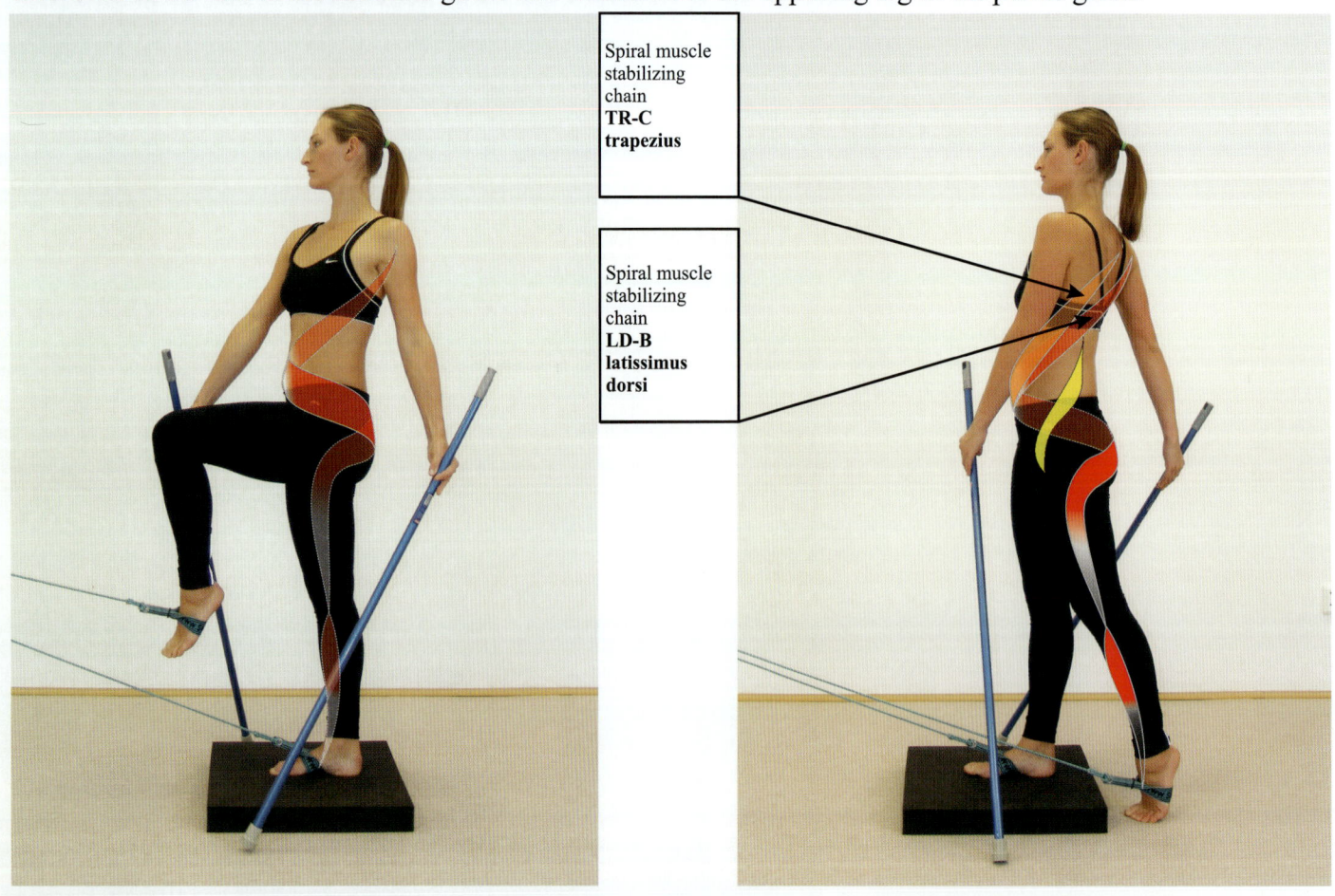

Spiral muscle stabilizing chain **TR-C trapezius**

Spiral muscle stabilizing chain **LD-B latissimus dorsi**

Exercise - stabilization, stretching

M. trapezius, m. latissimus dorsi - strengthening, stretching
M. erector spinae - relaxation in reciprocal inhibition, stretching

The LD - latissimus dorsi and TR - trapezius chains are the agonists in the second part of the exercise.

Exercise 7 - standing facing the attachment point of the elastic rope, one leg is placed forward on the mat

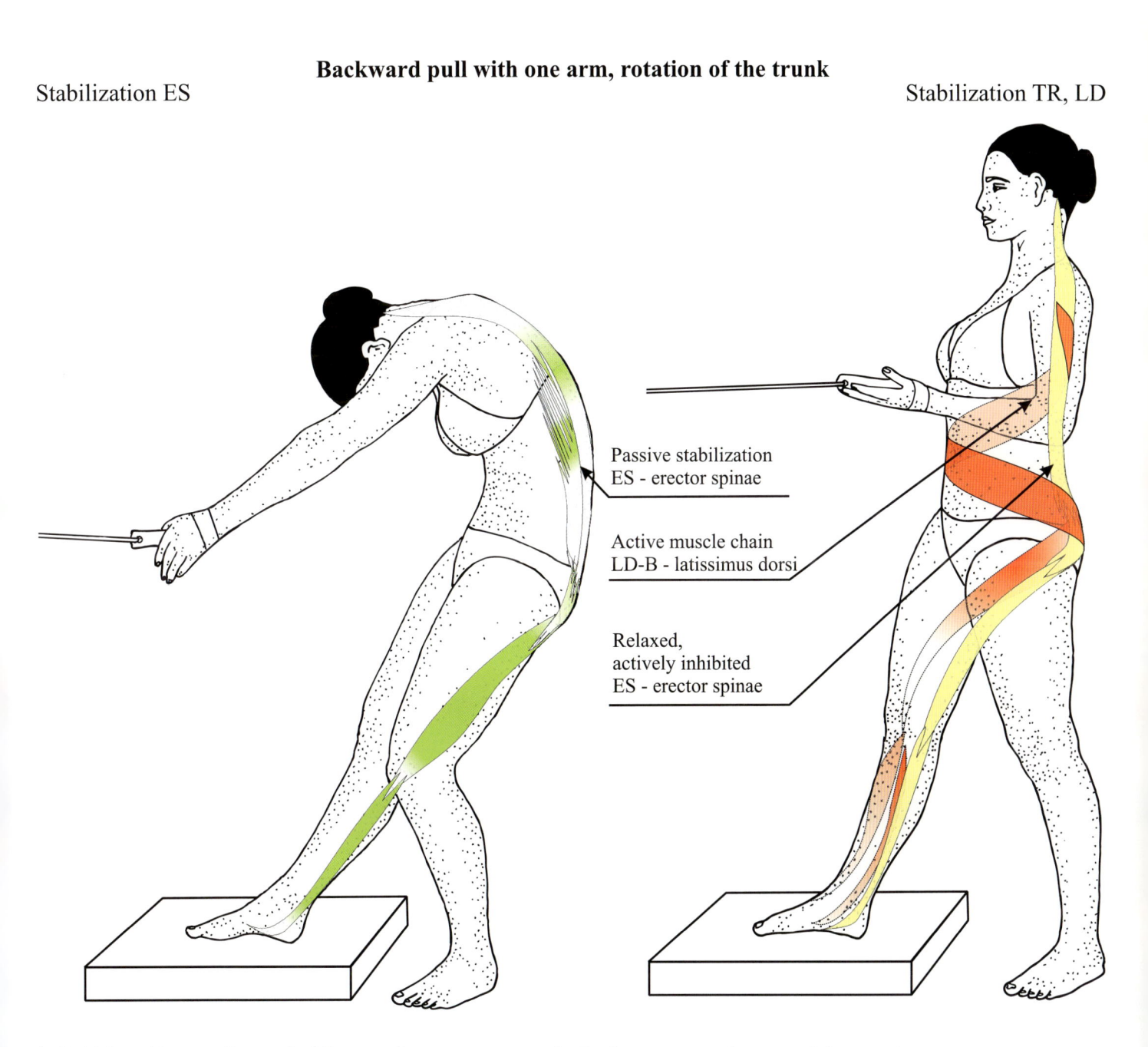

Backward pull with one arm, rotation of the trunk

Stabilization ES   Stabilization TR, LD

Passive stabilization
ES - erector spinae

Active muscle chain
LD-B - latissimus dorsi

Relaxed,
actively inhibited
ES - erector spinae

1 - Initial position - active part of the exercise
The initial position is actively stabilized by the vertical chain ES - erector spinae, which is stretched at the same time.

2 - Performance - active part of the exercise
The active part of the exercise is stabilized by the spiral muscle chain LD-B - latissimus dorsi.
The vertical muscle chain ES - erector spinae relaxes.

As the backward movement of the arm and shoulder blade come to an end, the trunk rotates backwards.
This vigorously engages the spinal rotators.
- Mm. rotatores breves, longi
- Mm. semispinales
- Mm. multifidi
- Mm. levatores costarum

Exercise - stabilization, stretching
M. trapezius, m. latissimus dorsi - strengthening, stretching
M. erector spinae - relaxation in reciprocal inhibition, stretching

The LD - latissimus dorsi and TR - trapezius chains are the agonists in the second part of the exercise.

Exercise 8 - standing sideways on to the attachment point of the elastic rope, one leg is placed forward on the mat

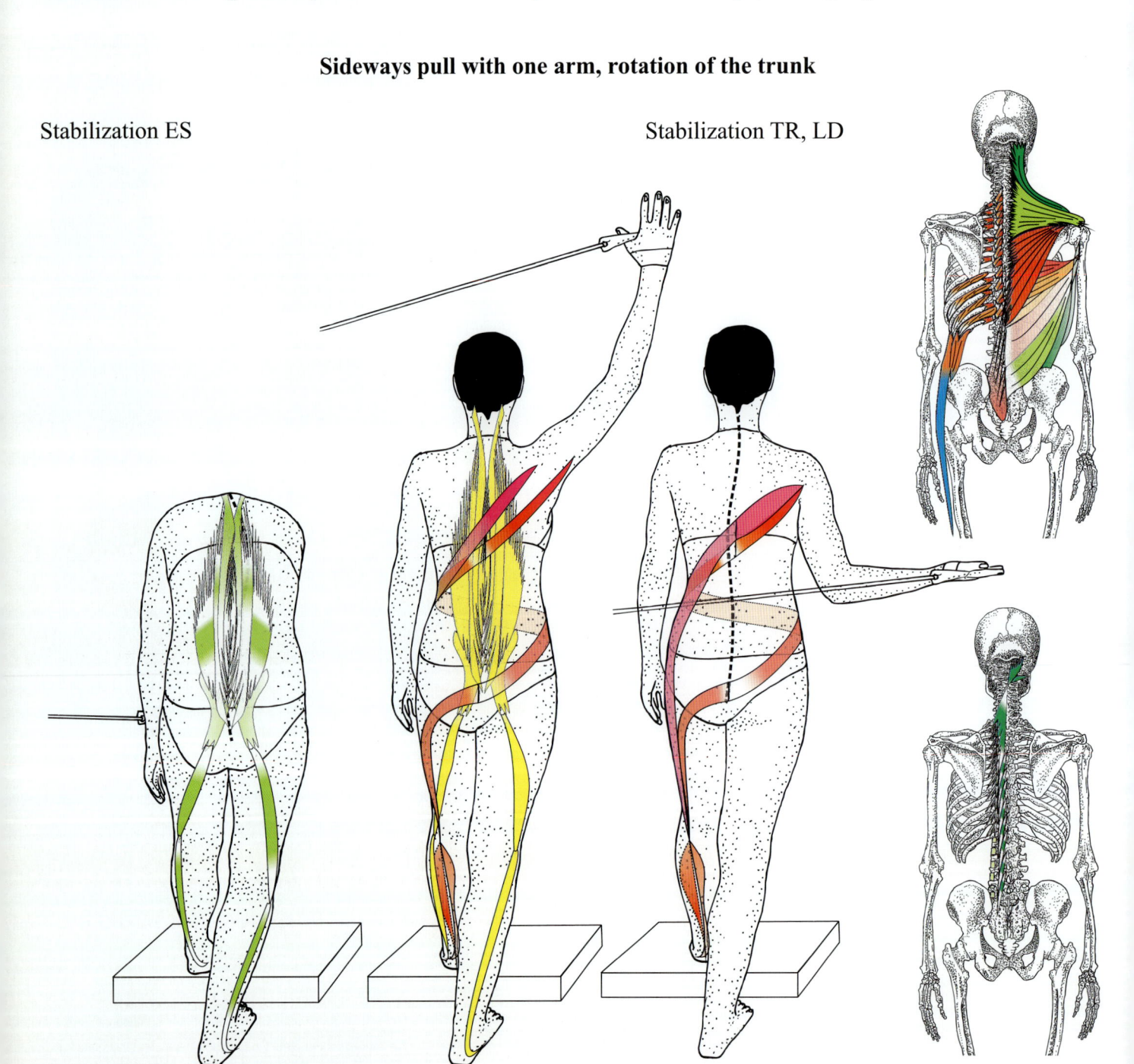

Sideways pull with one arm, rotation of the trunk

Stabilization ES   Stabilization TR, LD

1 - Initial position - active part of the exercise
The initial position is passively stabilized by the vertical chain ES - erector spinae, which is stretched at the same time.

2 - Performance - active part of the exercise
The active part of the exercise is stabilized by the spiral muscle chain LD-B - latissimus dorsi.
The vertical muscle chain ES - erector spinae relaxes.

As the backward movement of the arm and shoulder blade come to an end, the trunk rotates.
This vigorously engages the spinal rotators.
- Mm. rotatores breves, longi
- Mm. semispinales
- Mm. multifidi
- Mm. levatores costarum

Exercise

M. trapezius, m. latissimus dorsi - strengthening, stretching

Exercise 7 - standing facing the attachment point of the elastic rope, one leg is placed forward on the mat, backward pull with one arm, rotation of the trunk

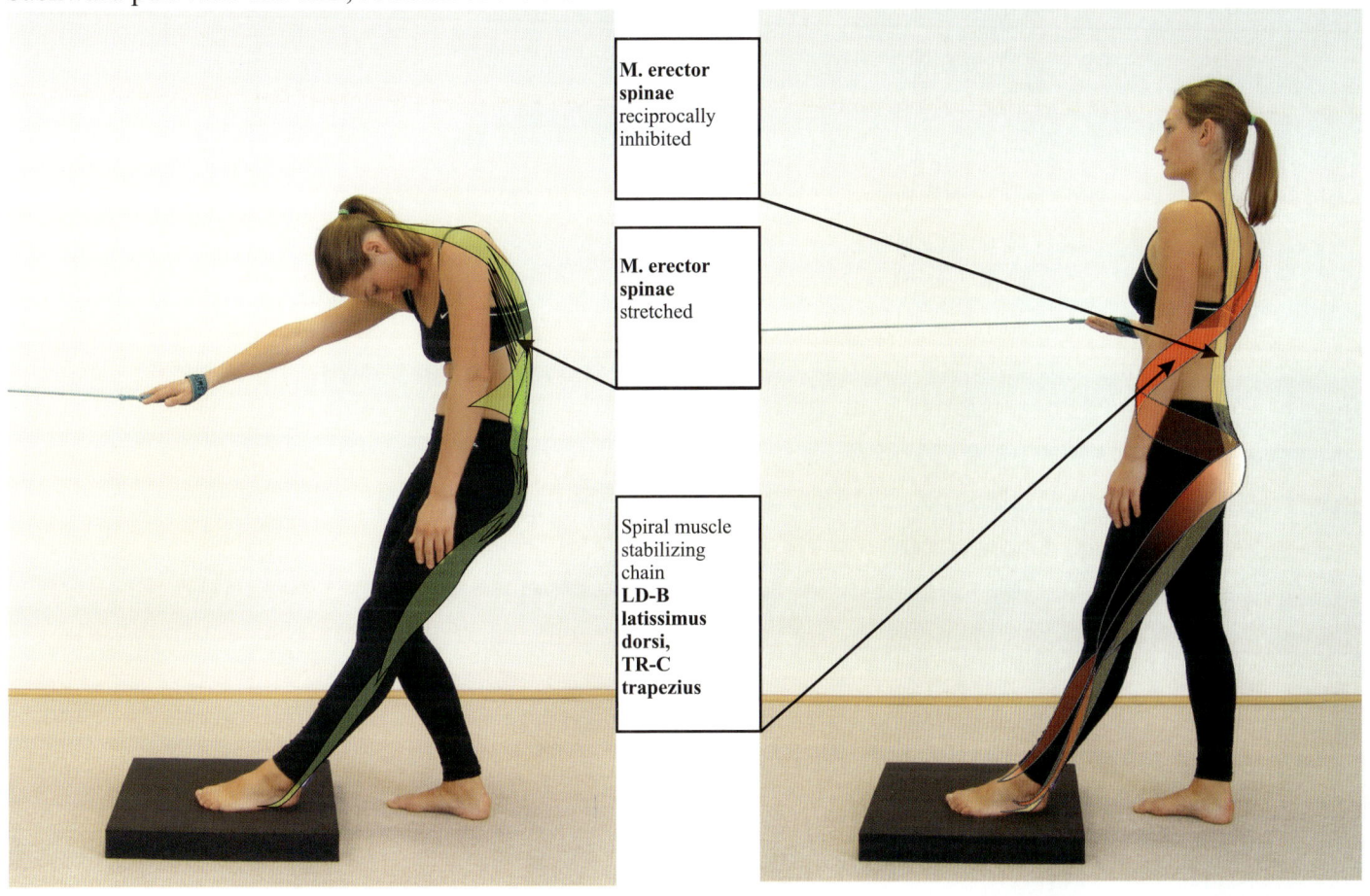

- M. erector spinae reciprocally inhibited
- M. erector spinae stretched
- Spiral muscle stabilizing chain **LD-B latissimus dorsi, TR-C trapezius**

M. trapezius, m. latissimus dorsi - strengthening, stretching

Exercise 8 - standing sideways on to the attachment of the elastic rope, one leg is placed forward on the mat, sideways pull with one arm, rotation of the trunk

- M. erector spinae reciprocally inhibited
- M. erector spinae stretched
- Spiral muscle stabilizing chain **LD-B latissimus dorsi, TR-C trapezius**

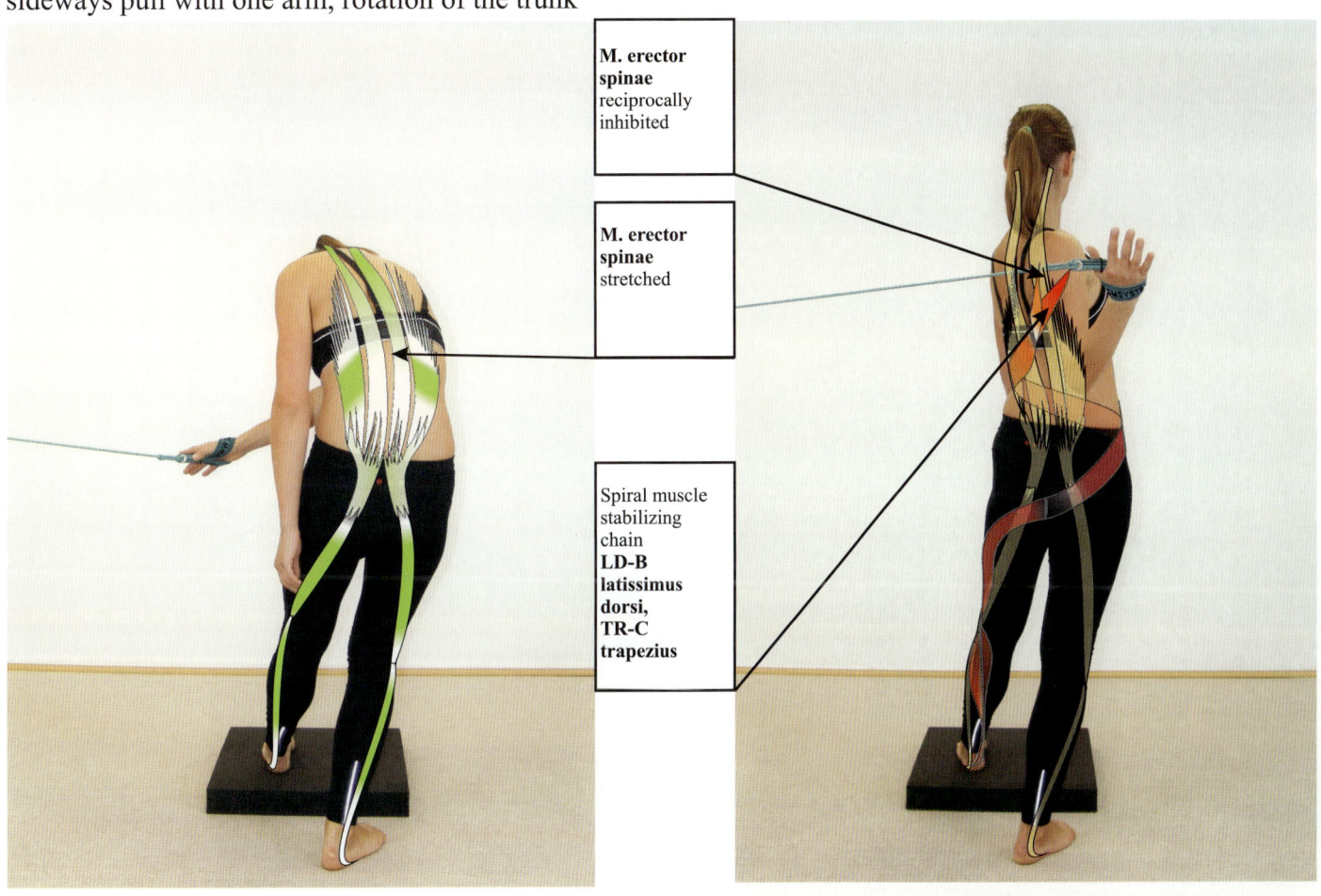

- 148 -

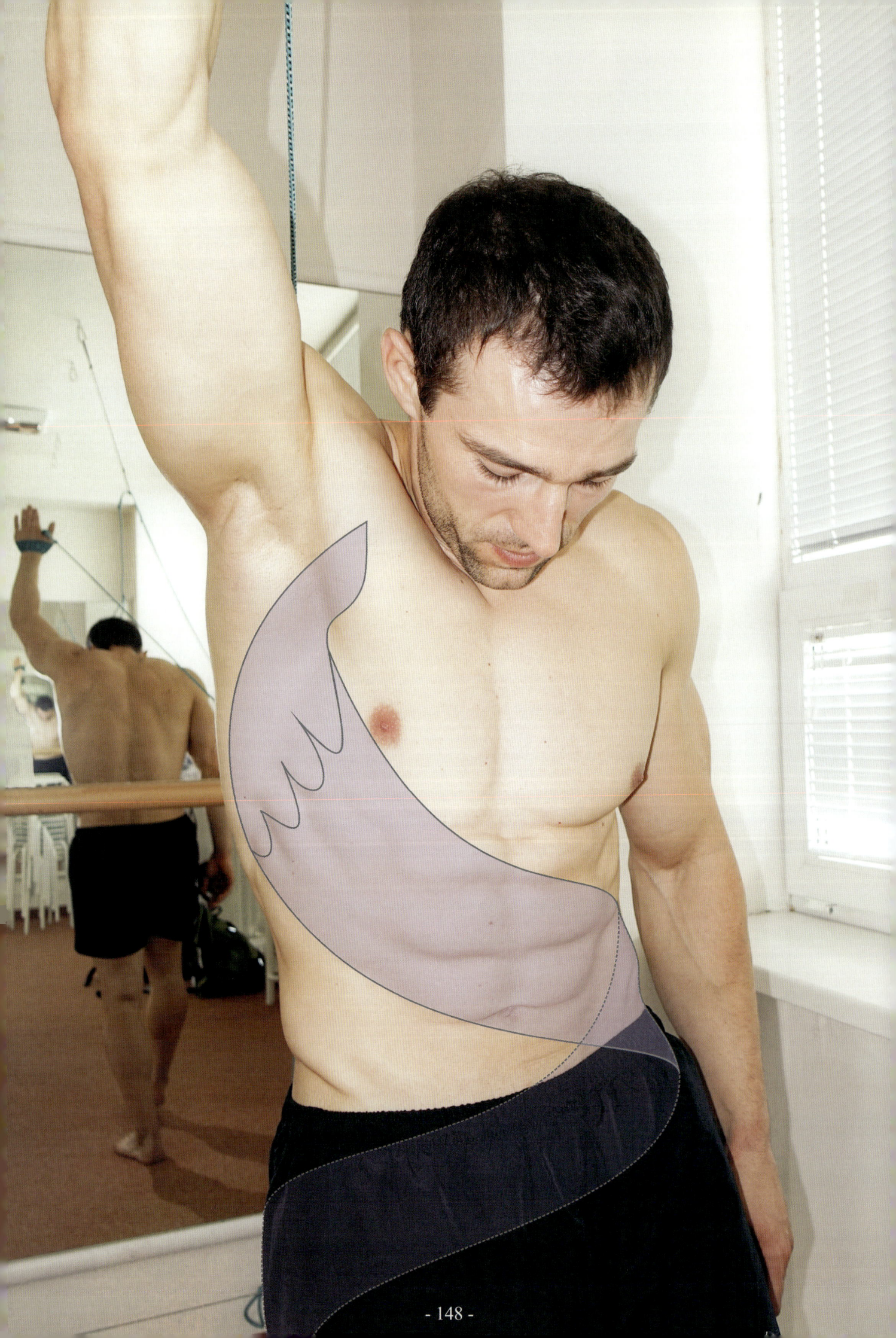

MANUAL TECHNIQUES AND EXERCISE ACCORDING TO MUSCLE ANALYSIS

Shoulder girdle
The lateral muscle group

Muscles with a tendency towards weakening:

M. serratus anterior
M. rhomboideus minor, major

Anatomy
M. serratus anterior

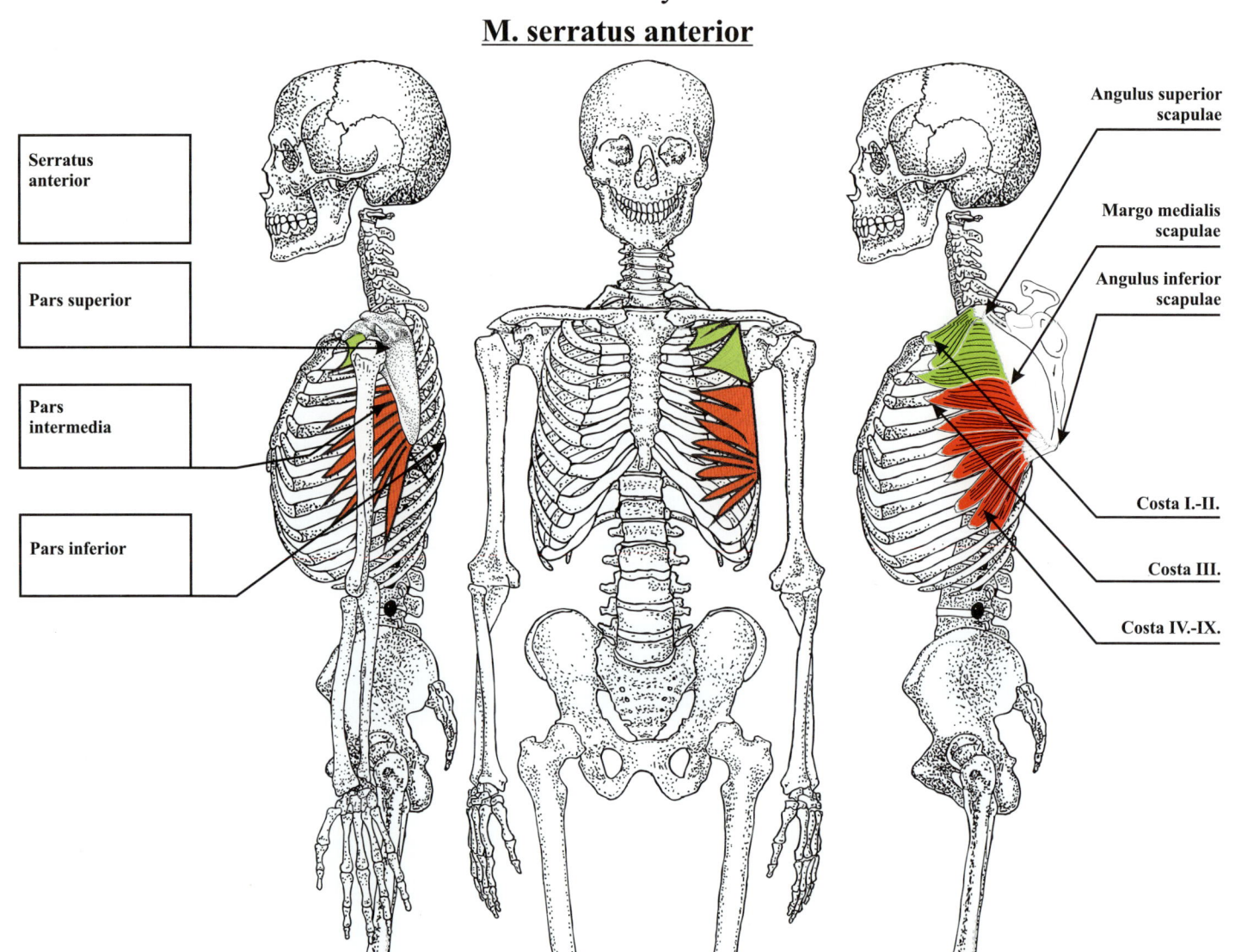

| Serratus anterior |
| Pars superior |
| Pars intermedia |
| Pars inferior |

Angulus superior scapulae
Margo medialis scapulae
Angulus inferior scapulae
Costa I.-II.
Costa III.
Costa IV.-IX.

M. serratus anterior
Origin: - **pars superior**
- 1st - 2nd rib
         - **pars intermedia**
- 3rd rib
         - **pars inferior**
- 4th - 9th rib
Insertion: scapula
         - **pars superior**
- angulus superior
         - **pars intermedia**
- margo medialis
         - **pars inferior**
- angulus inferior
Function:
- moves the shoulder blade laterally and ventrally (whole muscle)
- auxiliary respiratory muscle when the shoulder girdle is fixed
- pars inferior:
  - rotation of the shoulder blade, turning the angulus inferior laterally and ventrally
  (enables elevation of the arm above 90°)
- pars superior:
  - return of an elevated arm (works antagonistically against the pars inferior)
Innervation:
- n. thoracicus longus (C5-7)

Muscles with a tendency towards **internal muscle imbalance**

Muscle fibres with a tendency towards **weakening**
These muscles must be **strengthened**

Muscles with a tendency towards **tension and shortening**
These muscles must be **relaxed and stretched**

Relaxation
Stretching
Strengthening
Stabilization

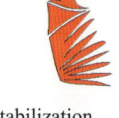

The spiral part of m. serratus anterior has a tendency towards weakening

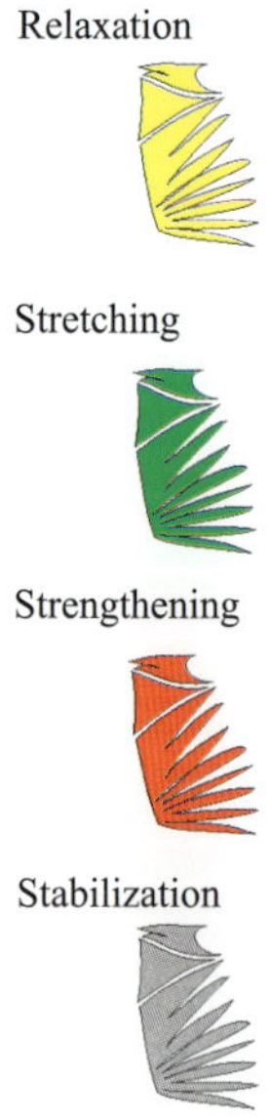

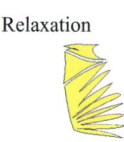

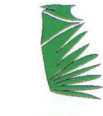

M. serratus anterior
A muscles with internal muscle imbalance
- **pars superior**
  has a tendency towards tension and shortening
- **pars intermedia**
  has a tendency towards weakening
- **pars inferior**
  has a tendency towards weakening

Muscle chains
Spiral muscle chain SA - serratus anterior
The SA chain is activated by forward movement of the shoulder blade - flexion.

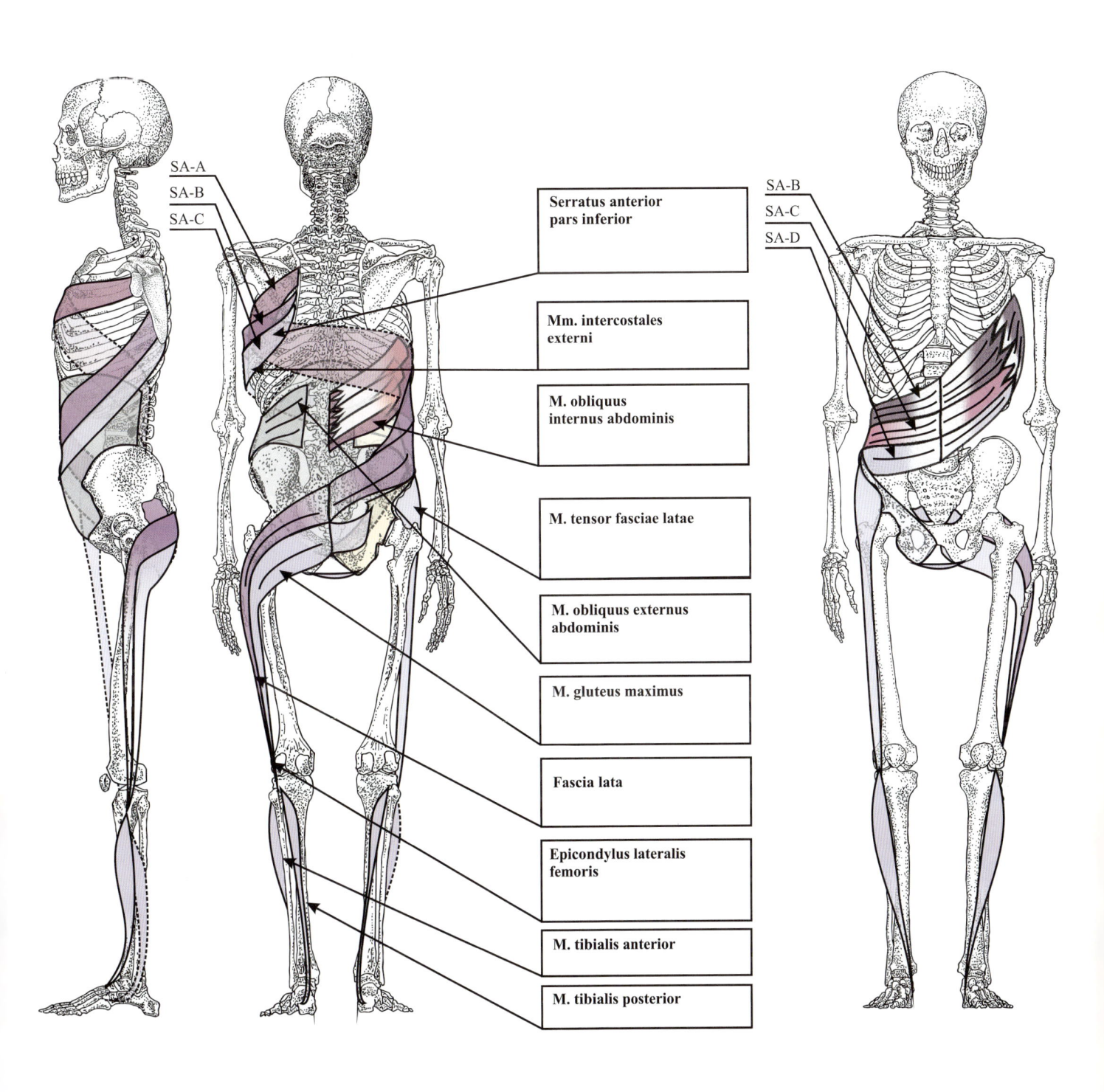

- Serratus anterior pars inferior
- Mm. intercostales externi
- M. obliquus internus abdominis
- M. tensor fasciae latae
- M. obliquus externus abdominis
- M. gluteus maximus
- Fascia lata
- Epicondylus lateralis femoris
- M. tibialis anterior
- M. tibialis posterior

- 151 -

Anatomy
M. rhomboideus minor, major

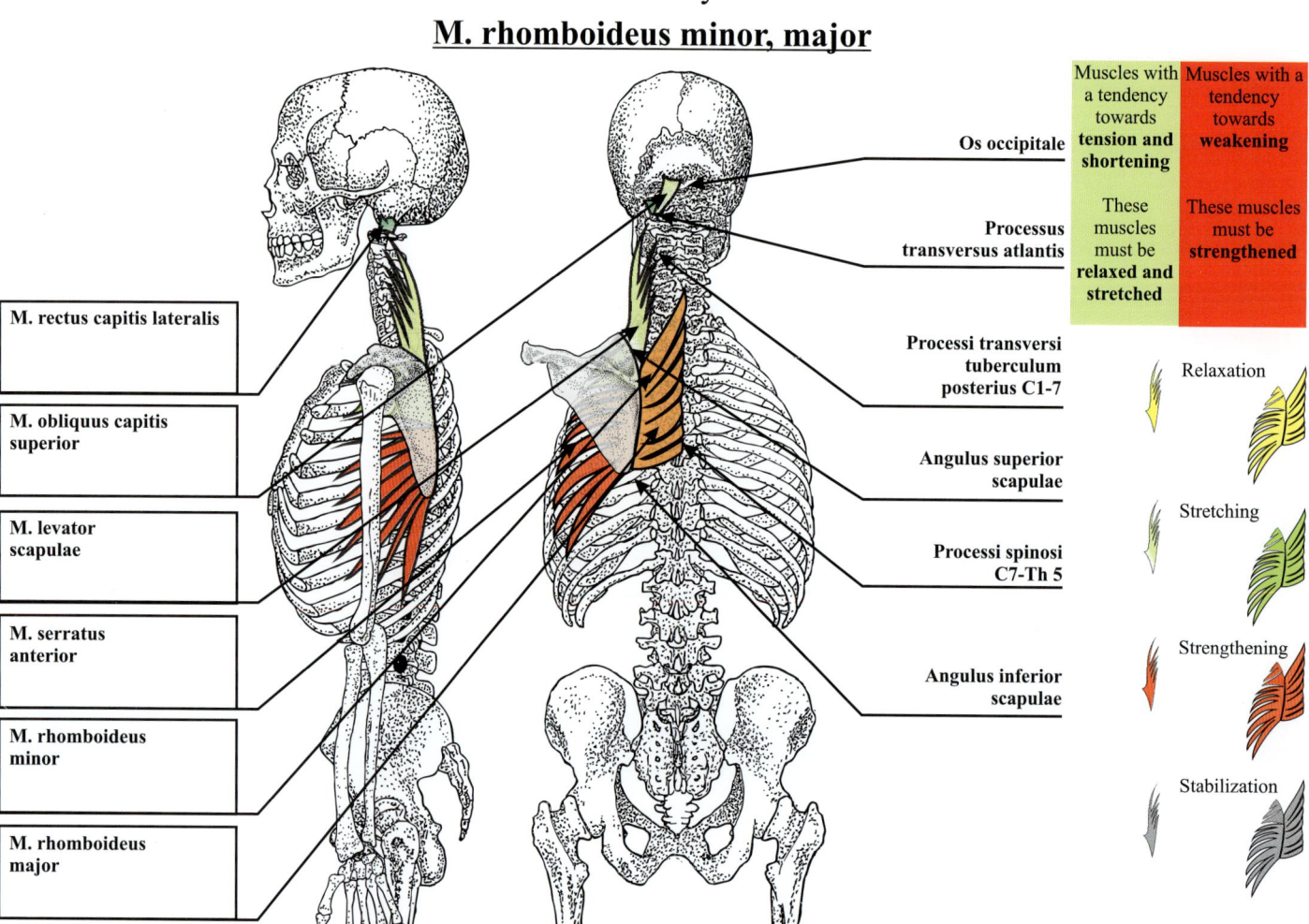

Muscles with a tendency towards **tension and shortening**	Muscles with a tendency towards **weakening**
These muscles must be **relaxed and stretched**	These muscles must be **strengthened**

Labels (figure):
- M. rectus capitis lateralis
- M. obliquus capitis superior
- M. levator scapulae
- M. serratus anterior
- M. rhomboideus minor
- M. rhomboideus major
- Os occipitale
- Processus transversus atlantis
- Processi transversi tuberculum posterius C1-7
- Angulus superior scapulae
- Processi spinosi C7-Th 5
- Angulus inferior scapulae

Legend:
- Relaxation
- Stretching
- Strengthening
- Stabilization

M. rhomboideus minor
Origin:
- processi spinosi C6-7

Insertion:
- margo medialis scapulae, above the spina scapulae

Function:
- lower fixation of the shoulder blade
- pulls the shoulder blade cranially and medially (upwards and towards the centre)

Innervation:
- n. dorsalis scapulae C4-5

M. rhomboideus major
Origin:
- processi spinosi Th1-4

Insertion:
- margo medialis scapulae, below the spina scapulae

Function:
- lower fixation of the shoulder blade
- pulls the shoulder blade cranially and medially (upwards and towards the centre)

Innervation:
- n. dorsalis scapulae C4-5

M. levator scapulae
Origin:
- processi transversi C1-4

Insertion:
- angulus superior scapulae

Function :
- pulls the shoulder blade cranially and medially (upwards and towards the centre)
- tilting side when the punctum fixum is on the shoulder blade

Innervation:
- n. dorsalis scapulae C4-5

M. rectus capitis lateralis
Origin:
- processus transversus atlantis

Insertion:
- os occipitale, pars basilaris, laterally from the condyli occipitales

Function:
- lateral flexion in the atlanto occipital joint - unilaterally
- ventral flexion in the atlanto occipital joint - bilaterally
- connects the pull of the m. levator scapulae, m. scalenus anterior to the head

Innervation:
- ramus ventralis C1

Manual techniques lying on one side
M. serratus anterior - massage, relaxation and passive stretching

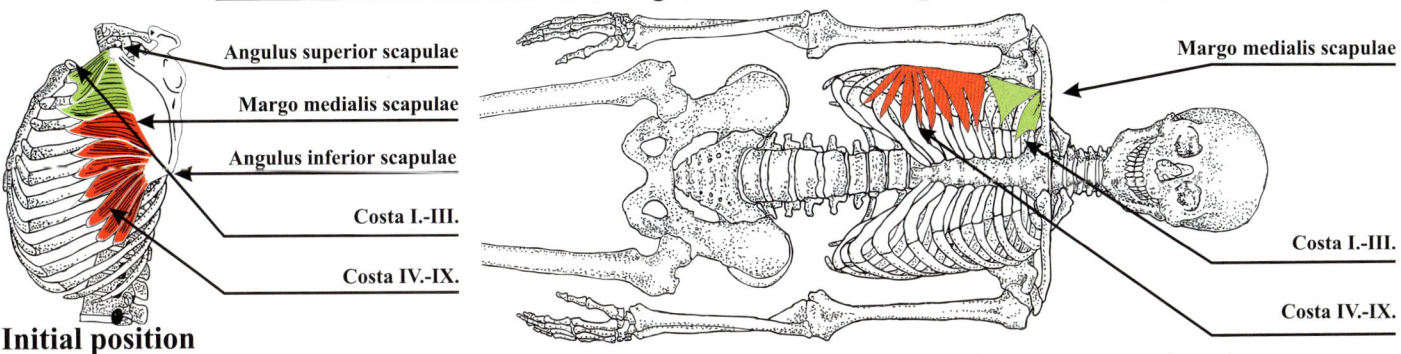

Angulus superior scapulae
Margo medialis scapulae
Angulus inferior scapulae
Costa I.-III.
Costa IV.-IX.

Margo medialis scapulae
Costa I.-III.
Costa IV.-IX.

Initial position

The therapist kneels behind the patient and stabilizes the patient's trunk with his right leg (punctum fixum).
The right palm is placed on the shoulder with the fingers pointing dorsally (backwards).
The palm and fingers of the left hand rest against the shoulder blade from behind. The patient breathes in.

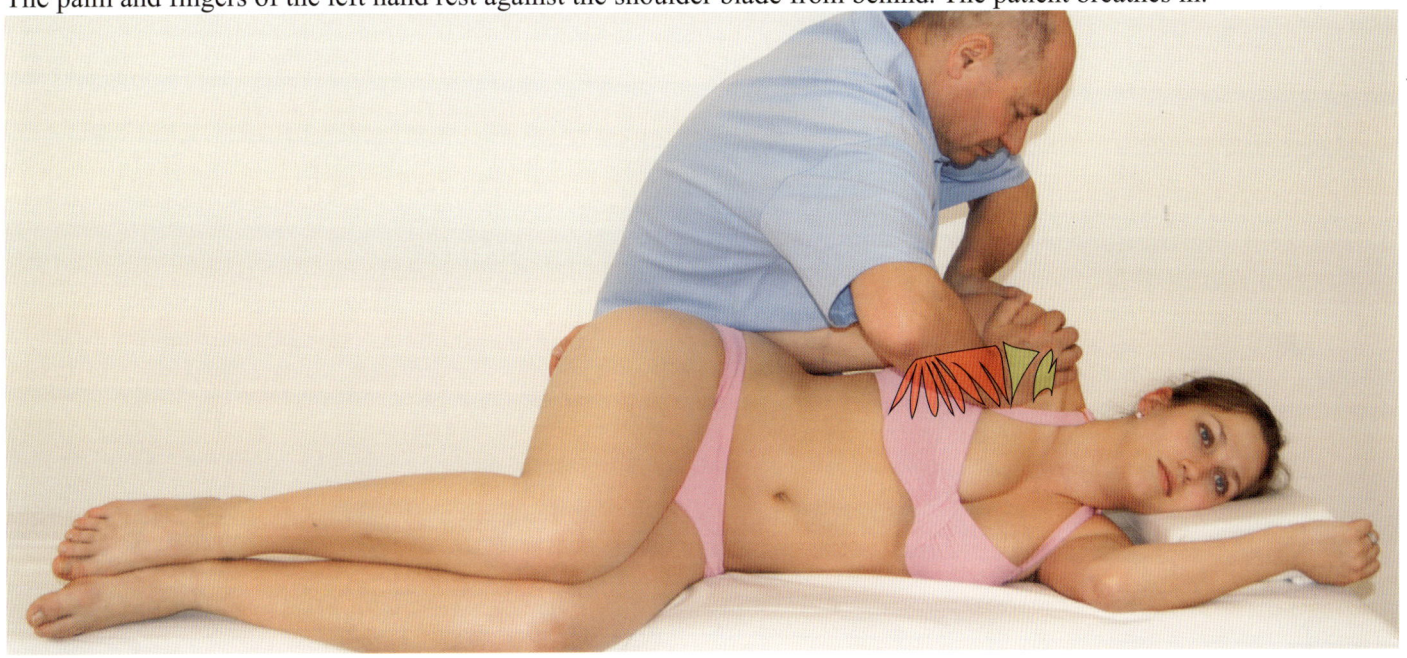

Performance

The therapist shifts the weight of the body to the right arm and shifts the shoulder blade dorsally (backwards), (punctum mobile). This stretches the m. serratus anterior to the full extent. This initiates the massage of the m. serratus anterior and m. subscapularis. The patient breathes out slowly. The pulling is slackened and the stretching is repeated 6 times. At the end of the technique the therapist pauses for about 3 seconds.

PIR. The extension is held and the patient breathes in. This causes a counter-pressure. When breathing out, the patient achieves further stretching. The process is repeated 3 times. In the same way, the technique is applied towards the 3rd, 4th and 5th ribs. This technique stretches the m. serratus anterior and other muscles of the anterior side of the shoulder girdle. This prepares the patient for the correct extent of backward movement of the shoulder blade during exercise.

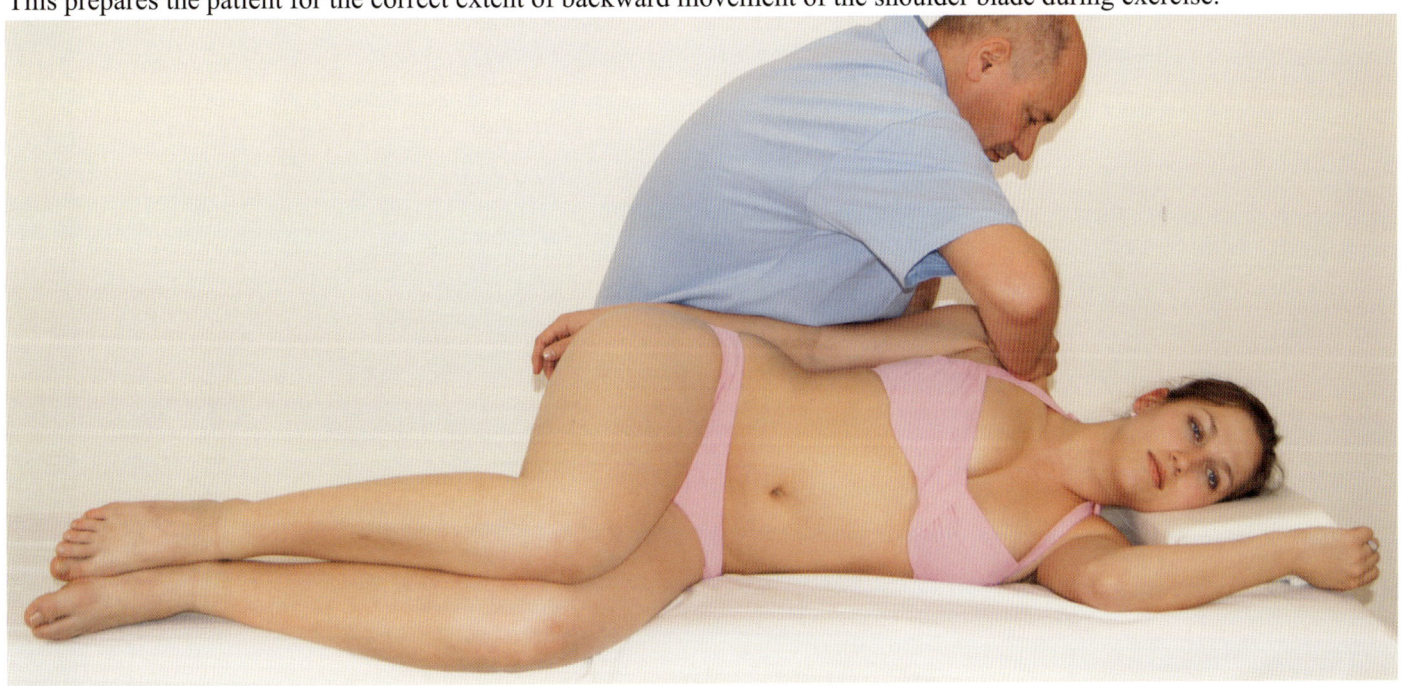

Manual techniques lying on one side
M. serratus anterior - massage, relaxation and passive stretching

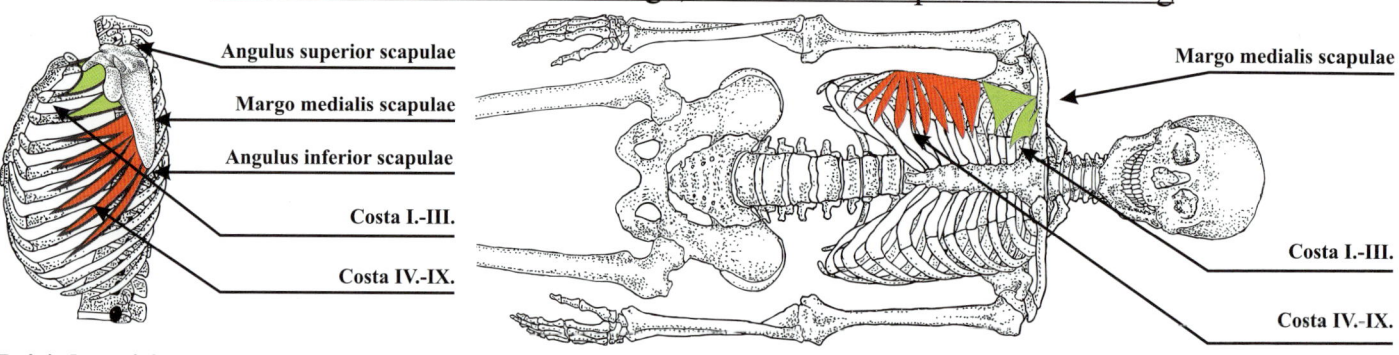

Angulus superior scapulae
Margo medialis scapulae
Angulus inferior scapulae
Costa I.-III.
Costa IV.-IX.

Margo medialis scapulae
Costa I.-III.
Costa IV.-IX.

Initial position

The therapist kneels behind the patient and stabilizes the patient's trunk with his right leg (punctum fixum). The right palm is placed on the shoulder from above, the fingers point downwards and the elbow is raised towards the head. The palm and fingers of the left hand rest against the shoulder blade from behind. The patient breathes in.

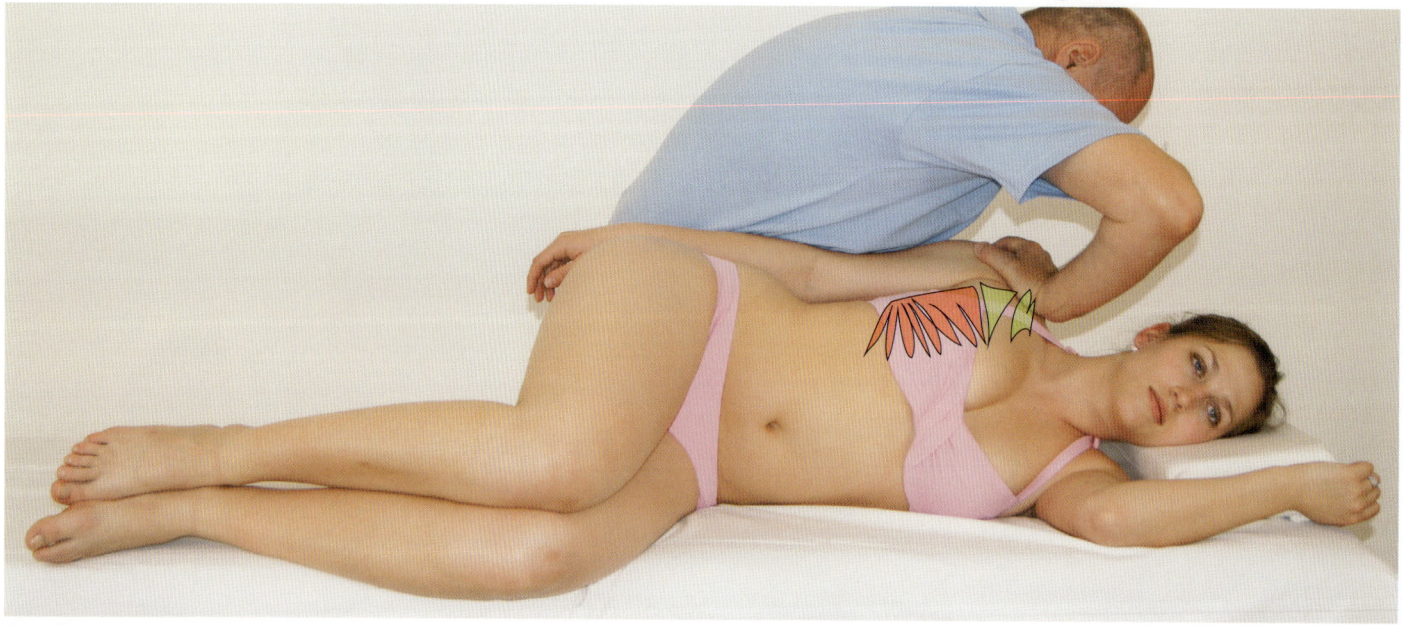

Performance

The therapist shifts the weight of the body to the right arm and shifts the shoulder blade caudally (downwards), (punctum mobile). The shoulder blade is constantly pressed against the trunk with the left arm. This stretches the upper part of the m. serratus anterior attached to the 1st to 3rd ribs. The upper part of the m. serratus anterior has a distinct tendency towards tension and shortening, and it is very important to stretch it. The patient breathes out slowly. The pulling is slackened and repeated 6 times. At the end of the technique the therapist pauses for about 3 seconds.

PIR. The extension is held and the patient breathes in. This causes a counter-pressure. When breathing out, the patient achieves further stretching. The process is repeated 3 times. In the same way the technique is applied towards the 3rd, 4th and 5th ribs. This technique stretches the m. serratus anterior and other muscles of the anterior side of the shoulder girdle. This prepares the patient for the correct extent of backward movement of the shoulder blade during exercise. The whole of this technique can be performed at once, beginning with the backward movement of the shoulder blade with the addition of the downward movement.

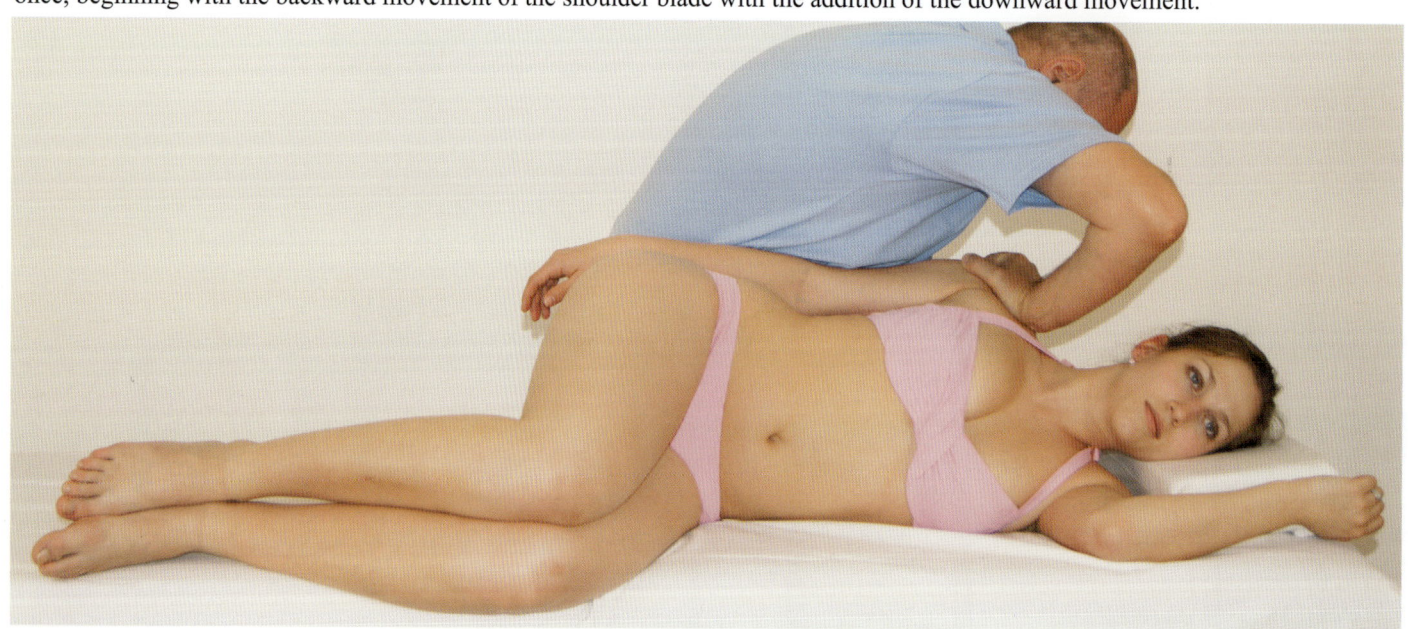

Manual techniques in a sitting position
M. serratus anterior - active relaxation, stretching

Exercise 3 - sitting with back to the attachment point of the elastic rope, opening the arms backwards, pulling the shoulder blades towards each other, performance with assistance, massage and correction

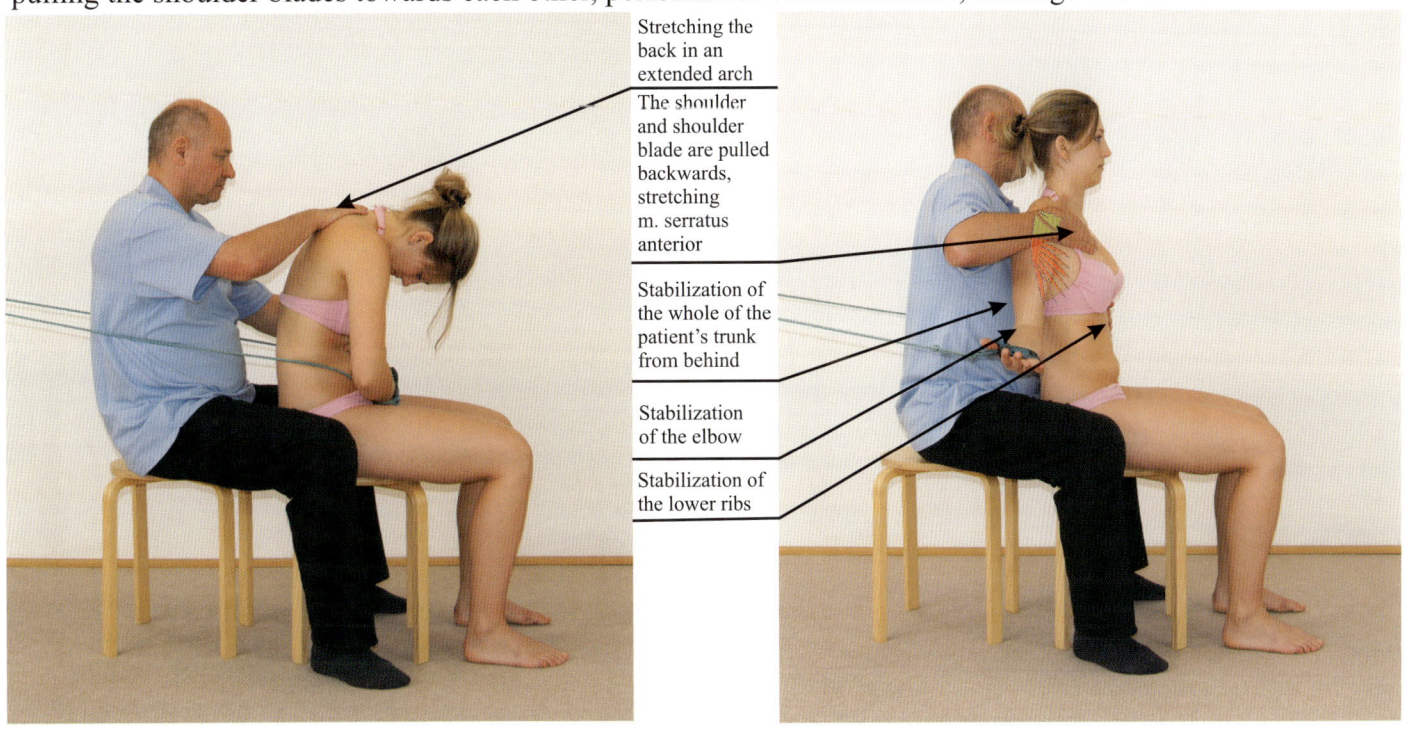

- Stretching the back in an extended arch
- The shoulder and shoulder blade are pulled backwards, stretching m. serratus anterior
- Stabilization of the whole of the patient's trunk from behind
- Stabilization of the elbow
- Stabilization of the lower ribs

M. serratus anterior - active relaxation, stretching

Exercise 3 - sitting with back to the attachment point of the elastic rope, opening the arms backwards, pulling the shoulder blades towards each other, performance with assistance, massage and correction

- **M. serratus anterior** reciprocally inhibited and stretched
- Spiral muscle stabilization chain **LD-B latissimus dorsi, TR-C trapezius**
- Spiral muscle stabilization chain **PM pectoralis major**
- **M. erector spinae** reciprocally inhibited and stretched

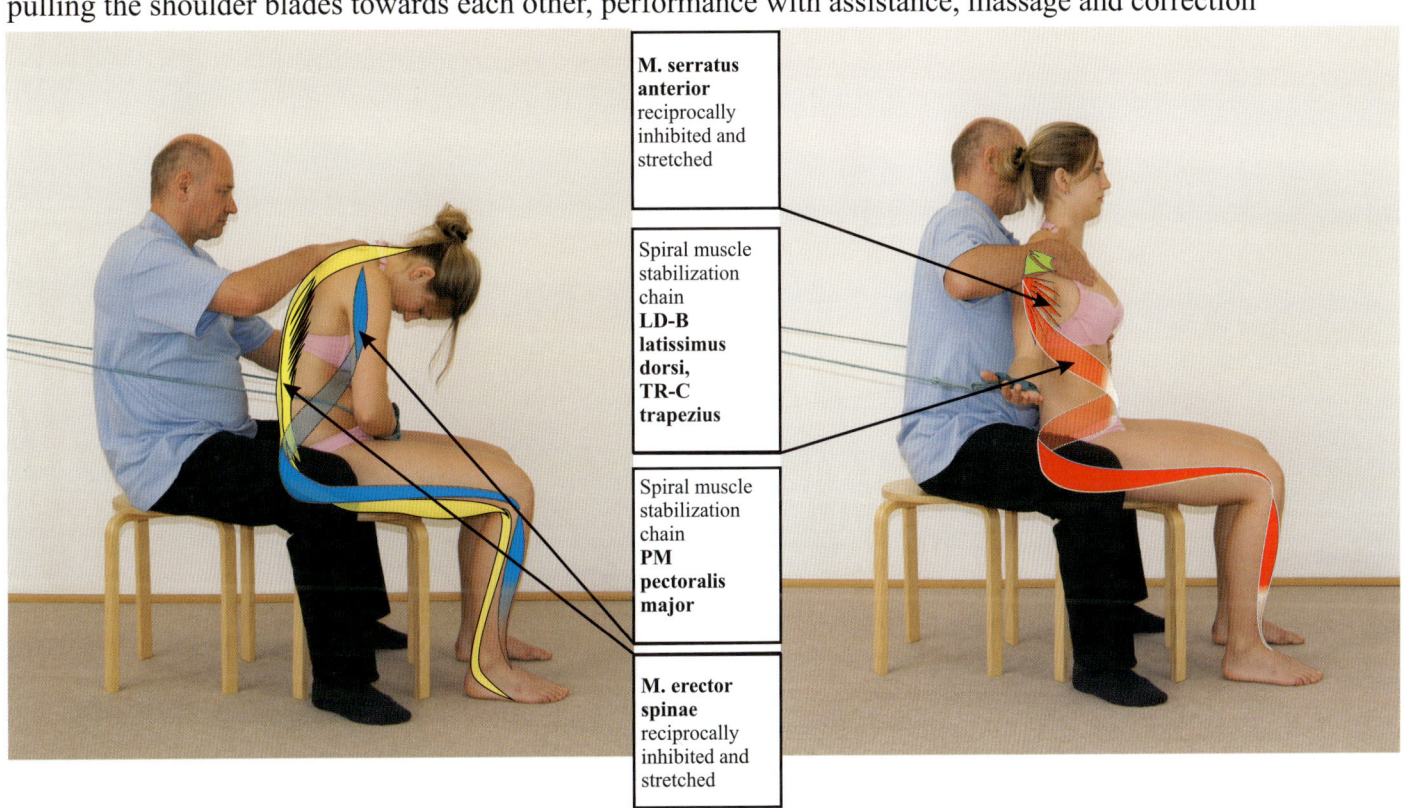

Stretching the m. serratus anterior inhibited in reciprocal inhibition.
The agonist is the spirals TR and LD, which stabilize the body.
The M. serratus anterior is reciprocally inhibited and stretched at the same time.

Exercise - stabilization, stretching
M. serratus anterior - relaxation, stretching, strengthening
M. erector spinae - relaxation in reciprocal inhibition, stretching

The LD - latissimus dorsi and TR - trapezius chains are the agonists in the first part of the exercise, the SA - serratus anterior chain is the agonist in the second part of the exercise.

Exercise 6 - standing with back to the attachment of the elastic rope, one leg is placed forward on the mat

Forward circles with both arms

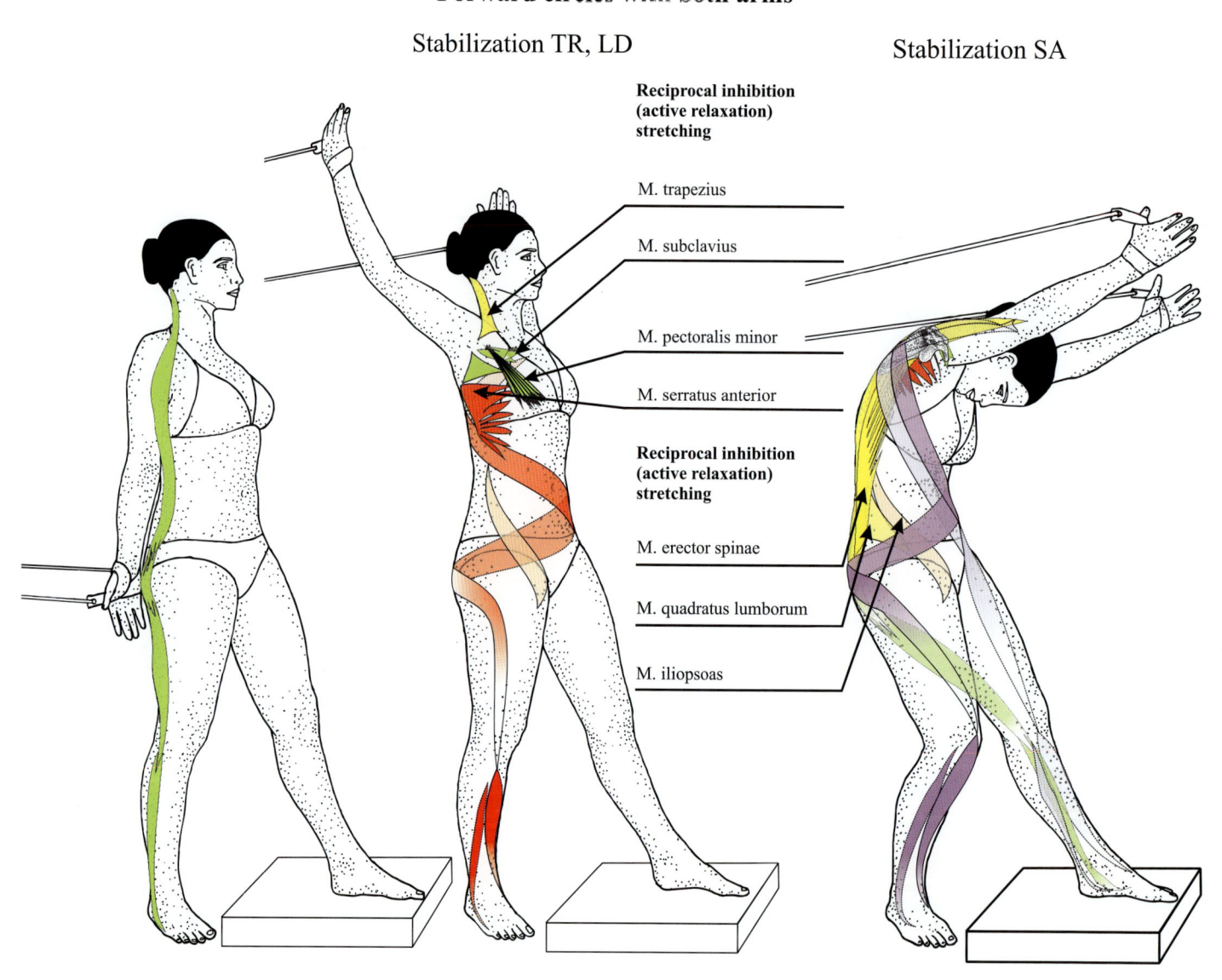

Stabilization TR, LD   Stabilization SA

Reciprocal inhibition (active relaxation) stretching
- M. trapezius
- M. subclavius
- M. pectoralis minor
- M. serratus anterior

Reciprocal inhibition (active relaxation) stretching
- M. erector spinae
- M. quadratus lumborum
- M. iliopsoas

1 - In the first part of performance - active part of the exercise
The muscles in the anterior side of the shoulder girdle are stretched:
- m. subclavius
- m. pectoralis minor
- m. pectoralis major
- m. serratus anterior

The muscles in the upper side of the shoulder girdles relax:
- m. trapezius pars descendens
- m. levator scapulae
- mm. scaleni
- m. semispinalis capitis, cervicis etc.

The first part of the exercise is stabilized by the chains LD and TR.

2 - In the second part of performance - active part of the exercise
The actively inhibited back muscles are stretched:
- m. erector spinae
- m. quadratus lumborum
- m. iliopsoas

The second part of the exercise is stabilized by the SA chain.

Exercise
M. serratus anterior - active relaxation, stretching, strengthening

Exercise 6 - sitting with back to the attachment point of the elastic rope, forward circles with both arms

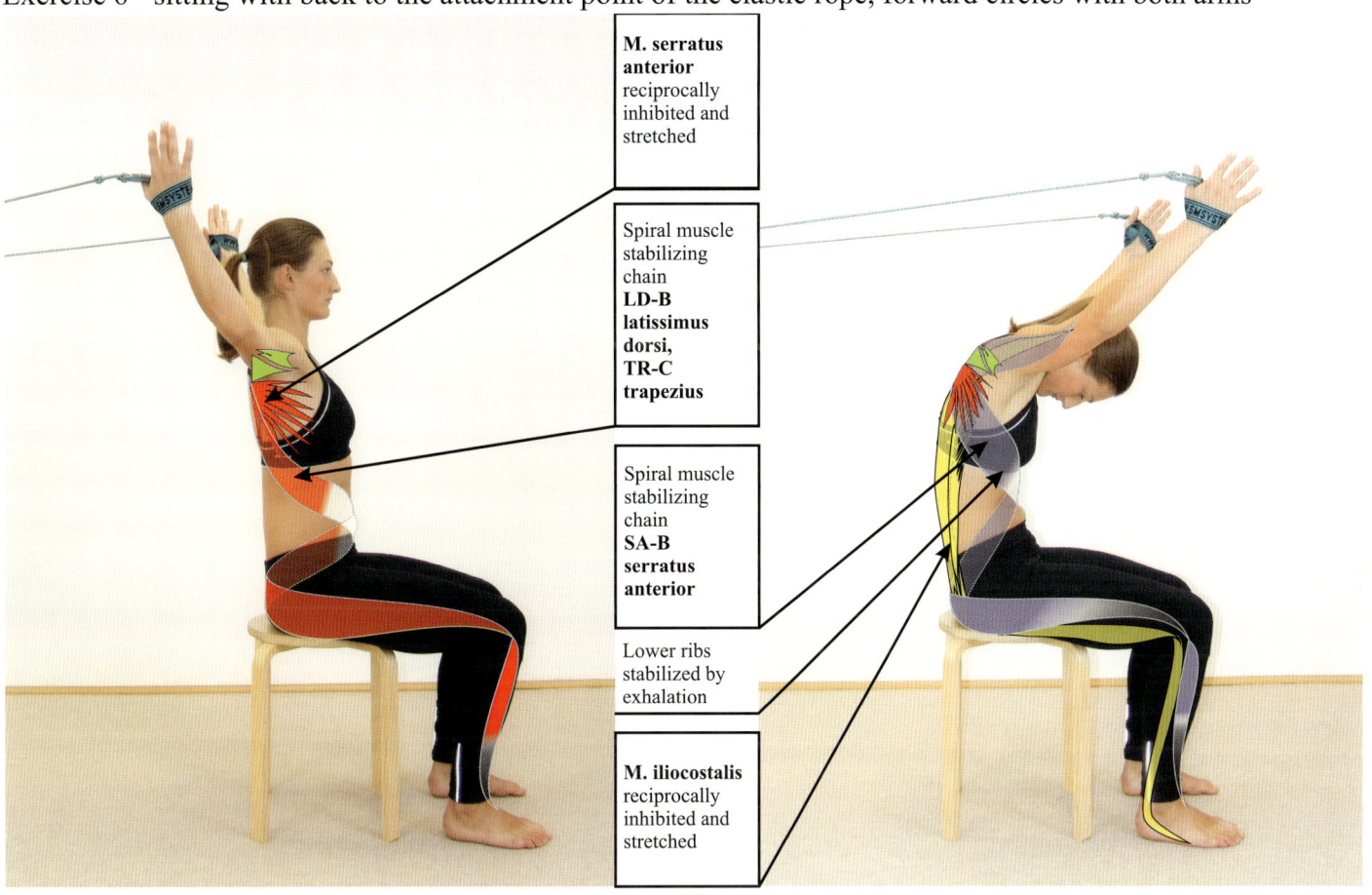

- **M. serratus anterior** reciprocally inhibited and stretched
- Spiral muscle stabilizing chain **LD-B latissimus dorsi, TR-C trapezius**
- Spiral muscle stabilizing chain **SA-B serratus anterior**
- Lower ribs stabilized by exhalation
- **M. iliocostalis** reciprocally inhibited and stretched

M. serratus anterior - active relaxation, stretching, strengthening

Exercise 6 - standing with back to the attachment point of the elastic rope, one leg placed forward on the mat, forward circles with both arms

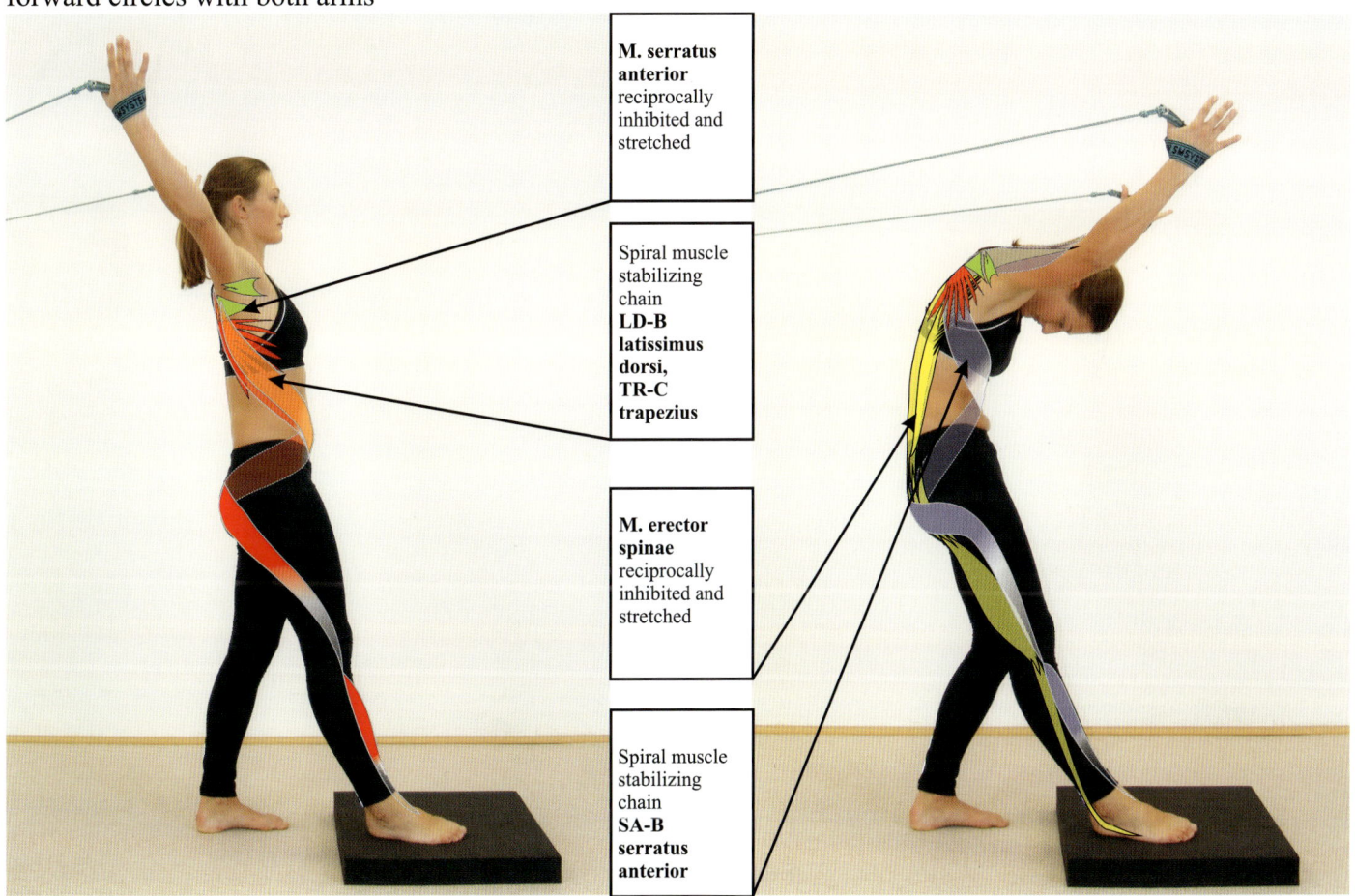

- **M. serratus anterior** reciprocally inhibited and stretched
- Spiral muscle stabilizing chain **LD-B latissimus dorsi, TR-C trapezius**
- **M. erector spinae** reciprocally inhibited and stretched
- Spiral muscle stabilizing chain **SA-B serratus anterior**

Exercise - stabilization, stretching
M. serratus anterior - relaxation, stretching
- relaxation in reciprocal inhibition, stretching

The PM - pectoralis major and SA - serratus anterior chains are agonists in the first part of the exercise, the LD - latissimus dorsi and TR - trapezius chains are the agonists in the second part of the exercise.

Exercise 3 - standing with back to the attachment point of the elastic rope, the legs are in the basic position

Opening the arms backwards, pulling the shoulder blades towards each other

Stabilization TR, LD   Stabilization SA, PM

- M. trapezius pars descendens
- M. subclavius
- M. pectoralis minor
- M. serratus anterior
- M. erector spinae

- M. erector spinae
- M. trapezius pars descendens

2 - Performance - active part of the exercise
In the active part of the exercise the muscles in the anterior side of the shoulder girdle are stretched:
- m. subclavius
- m. pectoralis minor
- m. pectoralis major
- m. serratus anterior

In the upper part of the shoulder girdle the neck muscles relax:
- m. trapezius pars descendens
- m. levator scapulae
- mm. scaleni
- m. semispinalis capitis, cervicis and other muscles.

The first part of the exercise is stabilized by the chains LD and TR.

1 - Initial position - active part of the exercise
In the initial position the
m. erector spinae, actively inhibited by the chain PM - pectoralis major, is stressed.
The movement is stopped by the tension in the ligamenta interspinalia.

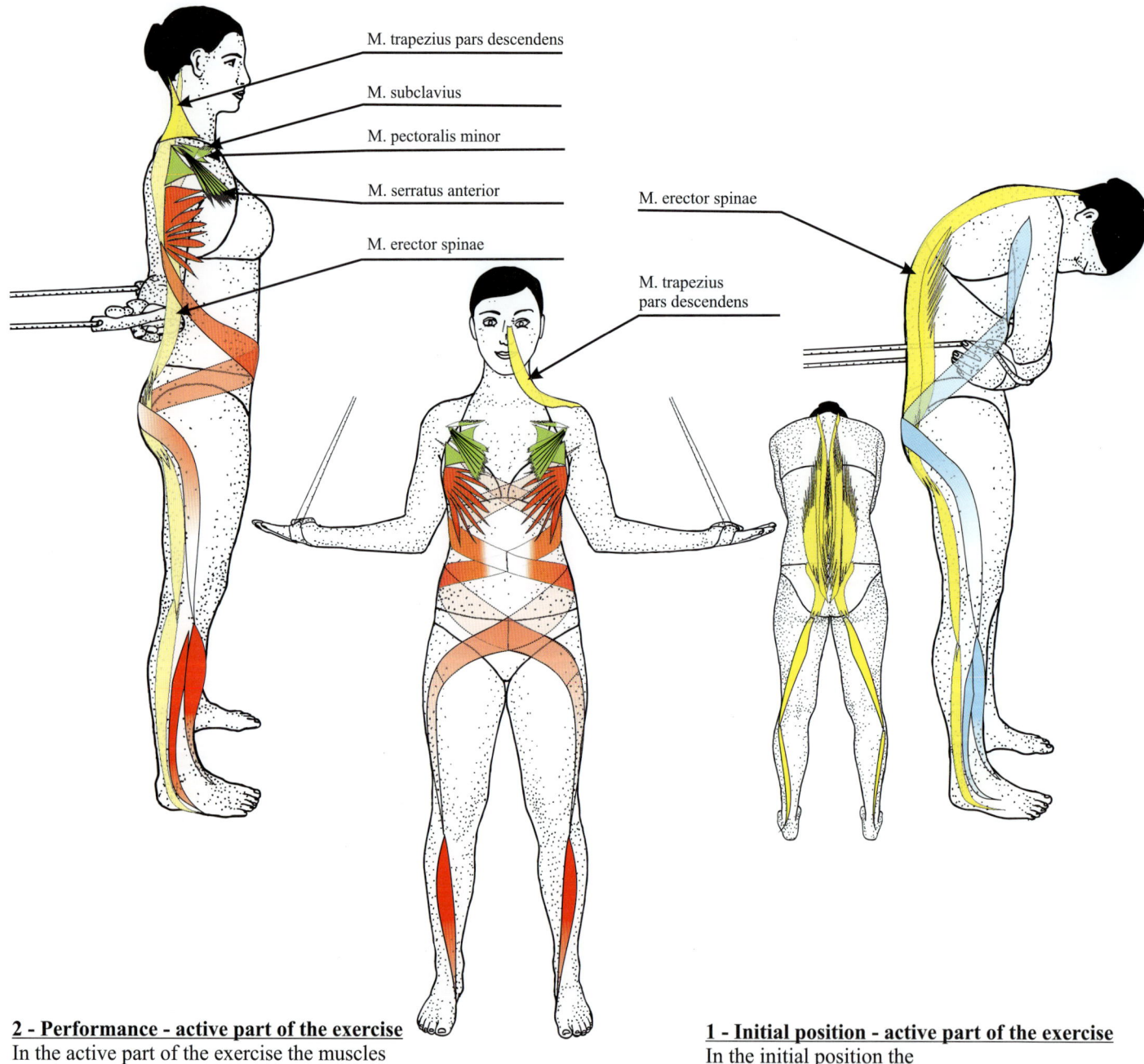

Exercise

M. serratus anterior - active relaxation and stretching

Exercise 3 - sitting with back to the attachment point of the elastic rope, the legs are in the basic position, opening the arms backwards, pulling the shoulder blades towards each other

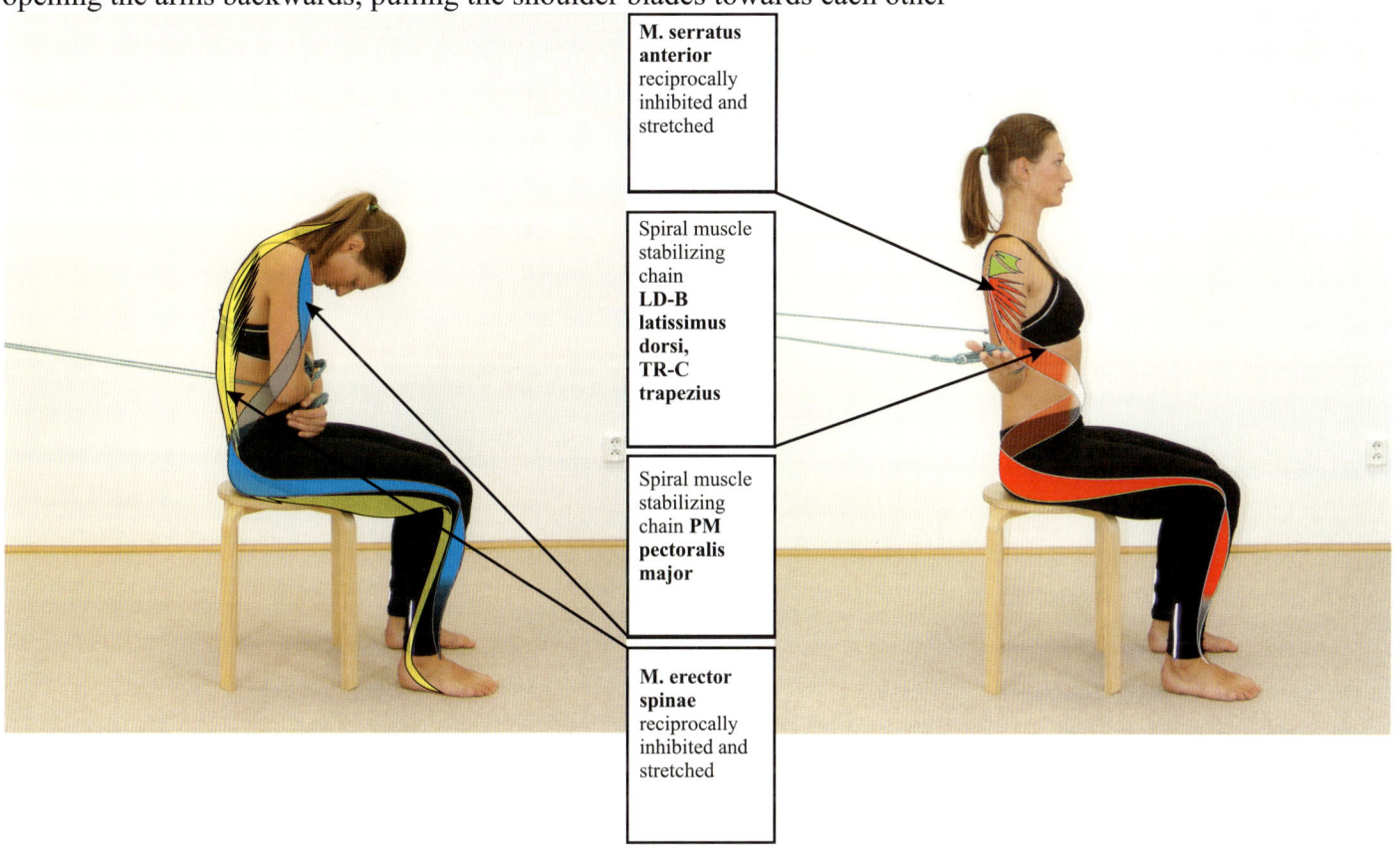

M. serratus anterior reciprocally inhibited and stretched

Spiral muscle stabilizing chain **LD-B** latissimus dorsi, **TR-C** trapezius

Spiral muscle stabilizing chain **PM** pectoralis major

M. erector spinae reciprocally inhibited and stretched

M. serratus anterior - active relaxation and stretching

Exercise 3 - standing with back to the attachment point of the elastic rope, the legs are in the basic position, opening the arms backwards, pulling shoulder blades towards each other

M. serratus anterior reciprocally inhibited and stretched

Spiral muscle stabilizing chain **PM** pectoralis major

Spiral muscle stabilizing chain **LD-B** latissimus dorsi, **TR-C** trapezius

M. erector spinae reciprocally inhibited and stretched

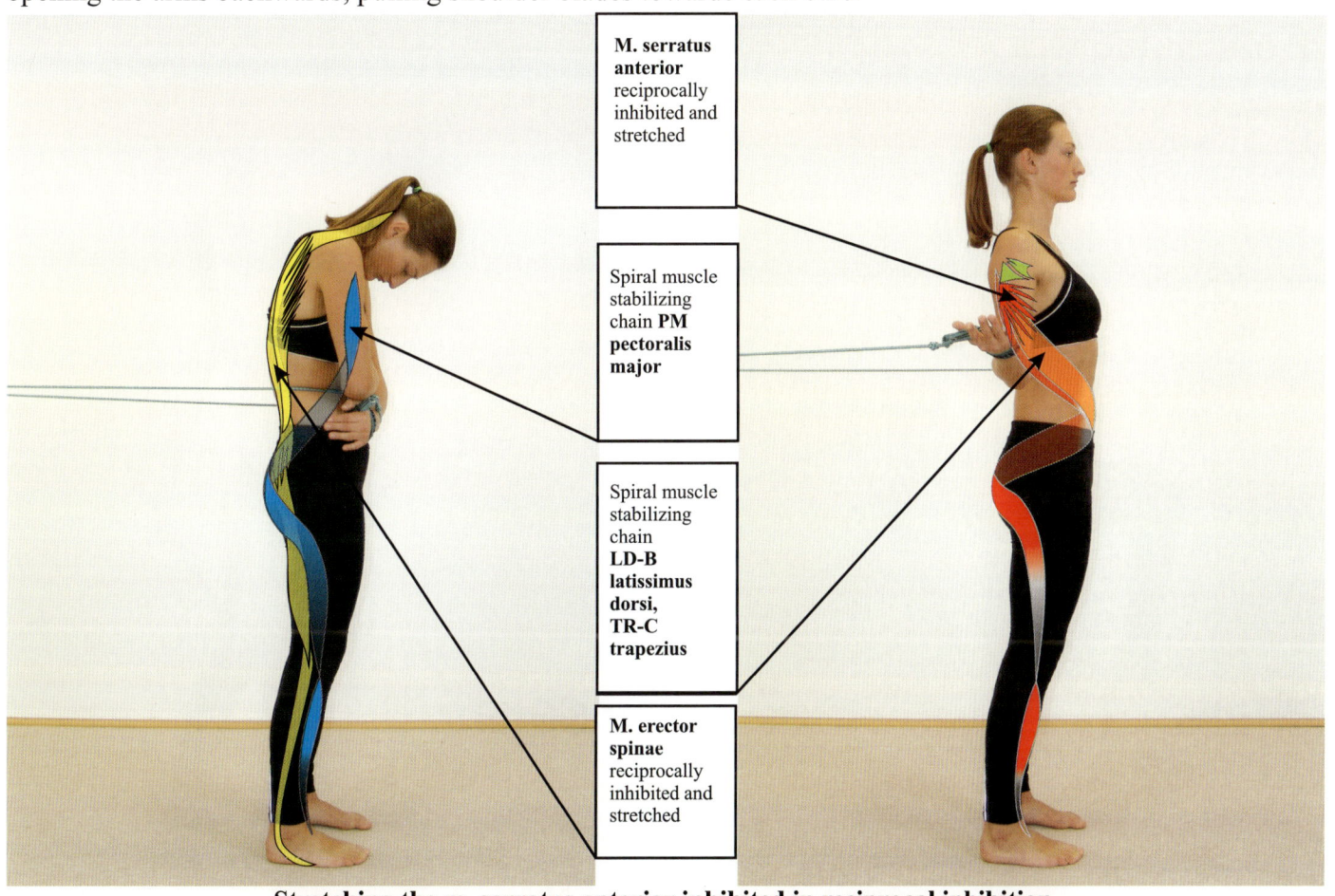

Stretching the m. serratus anterior inhibited in reciprocal inhibition.
The agonist is the spirals LD and TR, which stabilize the body. The m. serratus anterior is reciprocally inhibited and stretched.

Exercise
M. serratus anterior - relaxation, stretching, strengthening

Exercise 6 - standing with back to the attachment point of the elastic rope, one leg is placed forward on the mat, forward circles with one arm

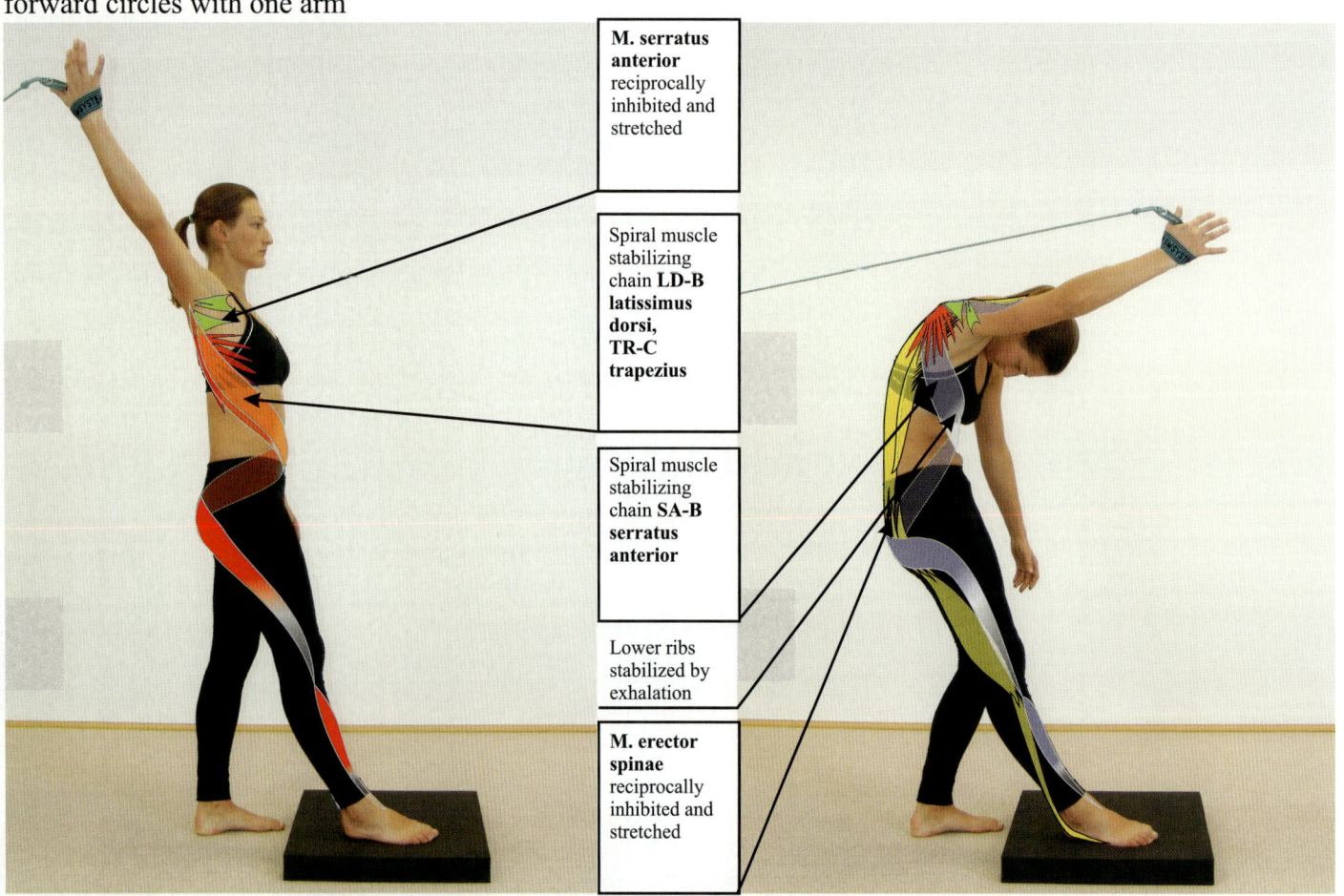

- **M. serratus anterior** reciprocally inhibited and stretched
- Spiral muscle stabilizing chain **LD-B** latissimus dorsi, **TR-C** trapezius
- Spiral muscle stabilizing chain **SA-B** serratus anterior
- Lower ribs stabilized by exhalation
- **M. erector spinae** reciprocally inhibited and stretched

M. serratus anterior - strengthening, stretching

Exercise 11 - standing facing the attachment point of the elastic rope, crossed movement pattern, extension of the arm in the shoulder girdle and extension of the opposing leg in the pelvic girdle. In both phases of the exercise, the TR, LD, SA and PM spirals are activated at the same time

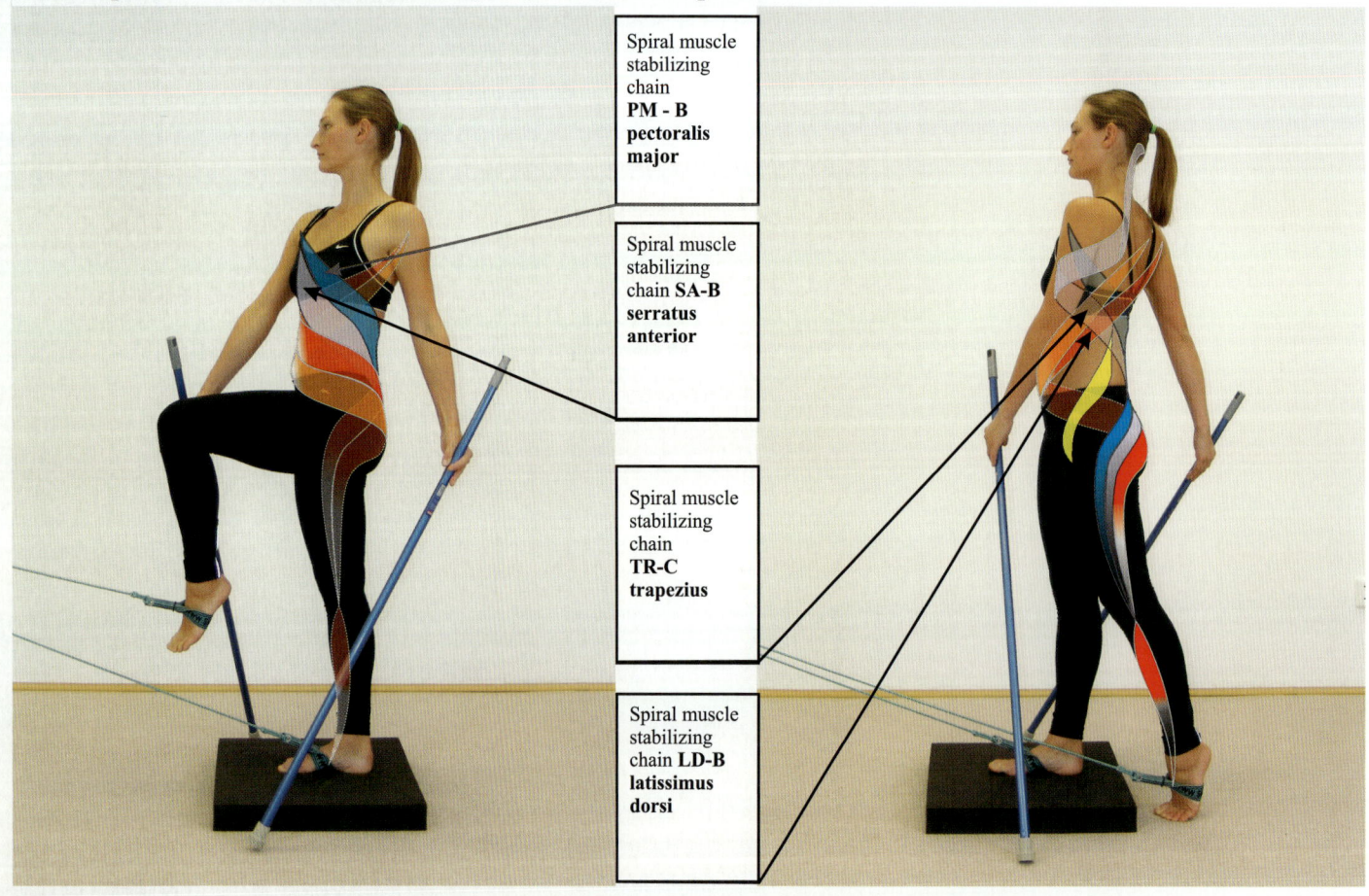

- Spiral muscle stabilizing chain **PM - B** pectoralis major
- Spiral muscle stabilizing chain **SA-B** serratus anterior
- Spiral muscle stabilizing chain **TR-C** trapezius
- Spiral muscle stabilizing chain **LD-B** latissimus dorsi

MANUAL TECHNIQUES AND EXERCISE ACCORDING TO MUSCLE ANALYSIS

Shoulder girdle
The anterior muscle group

Muscles with a tendency towards weakening:

M. pectoralis major

Anatomy
M. pectoralis major

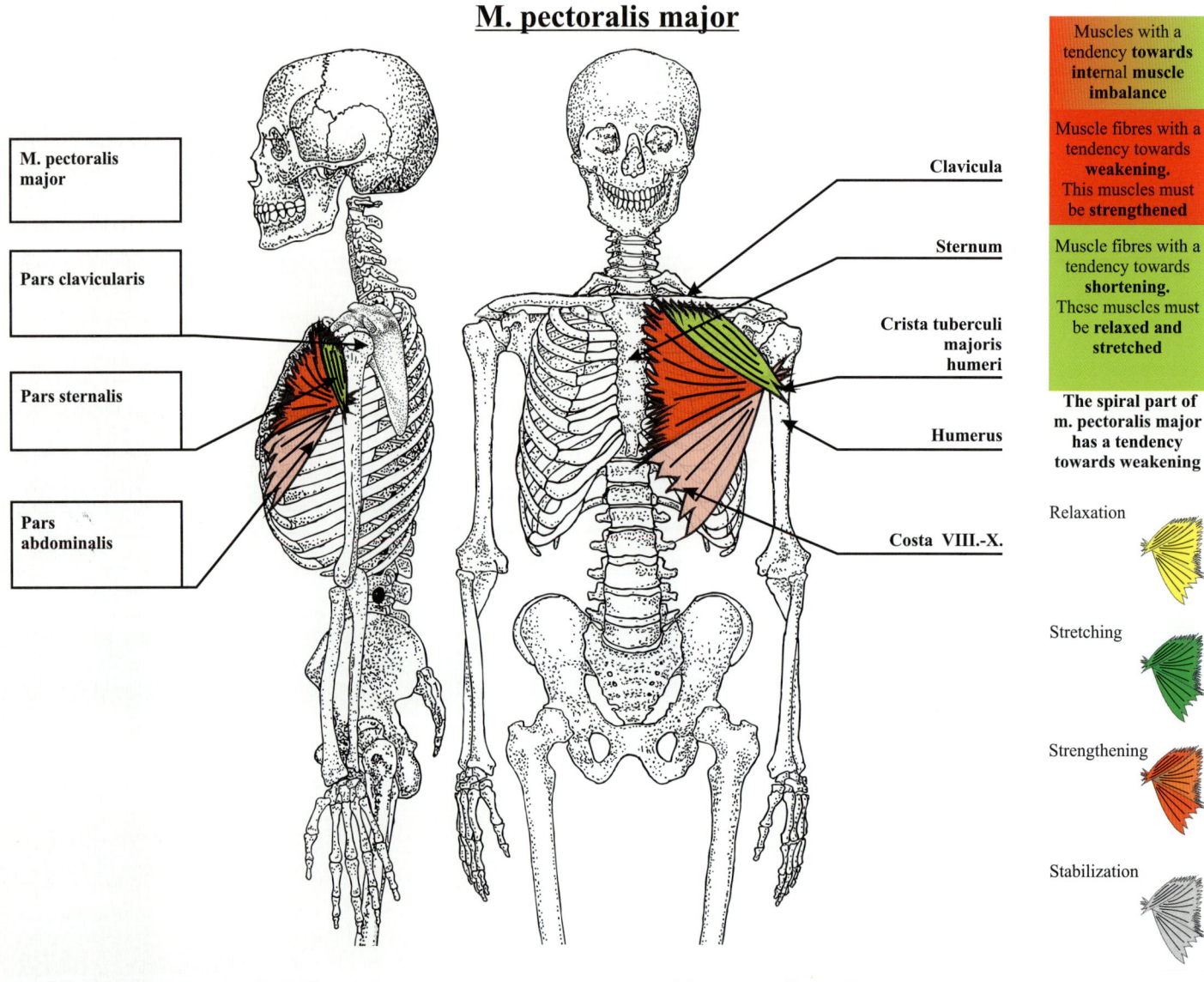

Labels (left figure): M. pectoralis major; Pars clavicularis; Pars sternalis; Pars abdominalis

Labels (right figure): Clavicula; Sternum; Crista tuberculi majoris humeri; Humerus; Costa VIII.-X.

Legend:
- Muscles with a tendency towards internal muscle imbalance
- Muscle fibres with a tendency towards **weakening**. This muscles must be **strengthened**
- Muscle fibres with a tendency towards **shortening**. These muscles must be **relaxed and stretched**

The spiral part of m. pectoralis major has a tendency towards weakening

- Relaxation
- Stretching
- Strengthening
- Stabilization

M. pectoralis major

Origin: - **pars clavicularis**
- medial half of the clavicle
         - **pars sternalis**
- sternum, cartilage 2nd-7th ribs
         - **pars abdominalis**
- cartilage 8th-10th ribs, lamina anterior m. recti abdominis

Insertion:
- crista tuberculi majoris humeri

Function:
- adduction, internal rotation (whole muscle)
- anteversion (pars clavicularis, sternalis)
- auxiliary respiratory muscle when the shoulder is fixed

Innervation:
- nn. pectorales mediales et laterales (C5-Th1)

M. pectoralis major
Muscle with internal muscle imbalance

- **pars clavicularis**
  has a tendency towards tension and shortening
- **pars sternalis**
  has a tendency towards weakening
- **pars abdominalis**
  has a tendency towards weakening

Muscle chains
Spiral muscle chains PM - pectoralis major
The PM chain is activated by the forward movement of the arm - flexion.

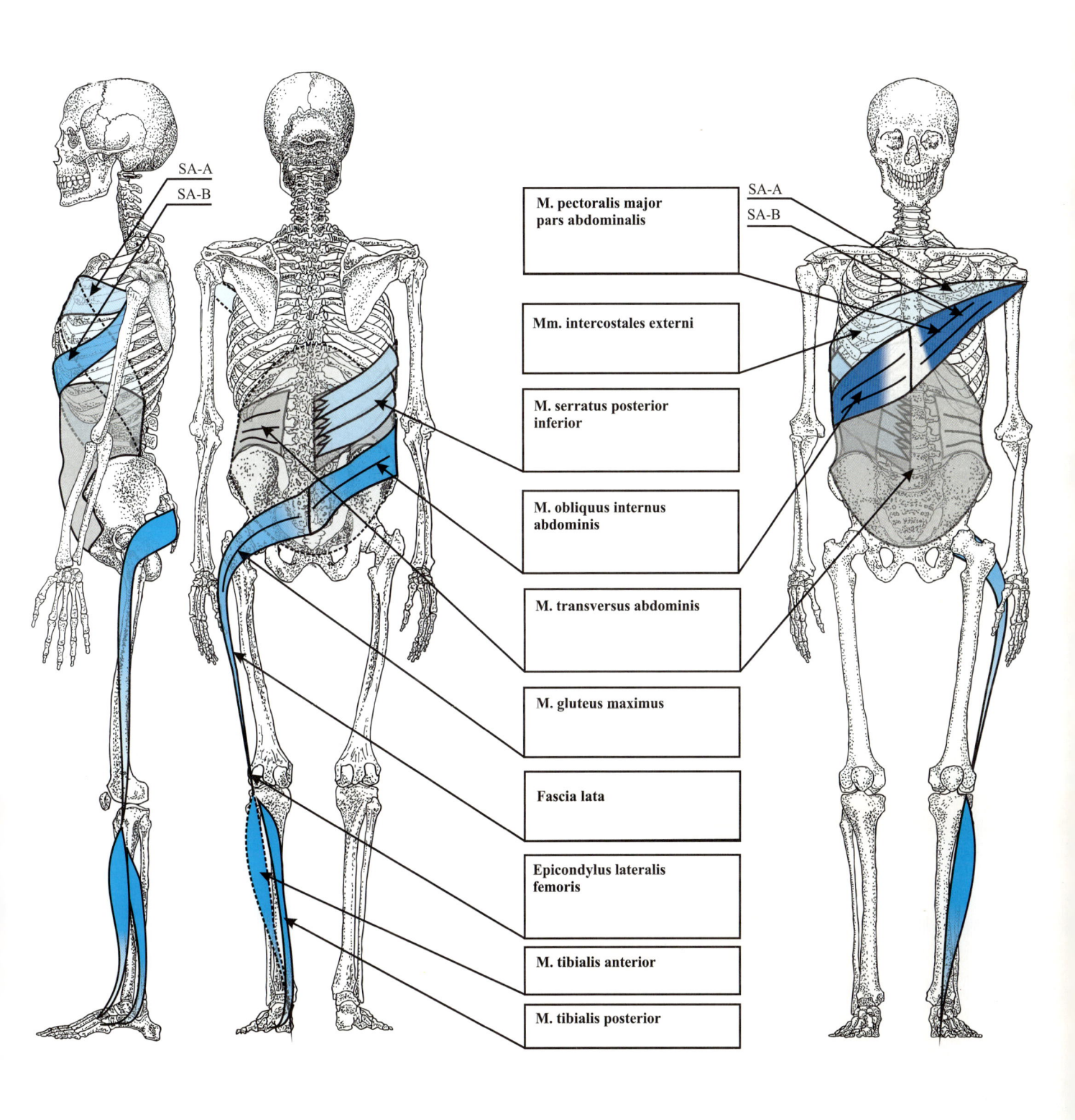

- M. pectoralis major pars abdominalis
- Mm. intercostales externi
- M. serratus posterior inferior
- M. obliquus internus abdominis
- M. transversus abdominis
- M. gluteus maximus
- Fascia lata
- Epicondylus lateralis femoris
- M. tibialis anterior
- M. tibialis posterior

- 163 -

Manual techniques in a sitting position
M. pectoralis major - stretching

Exercise 1 - sitting facing the attachment point of the elastic rope, backward pull with both arms

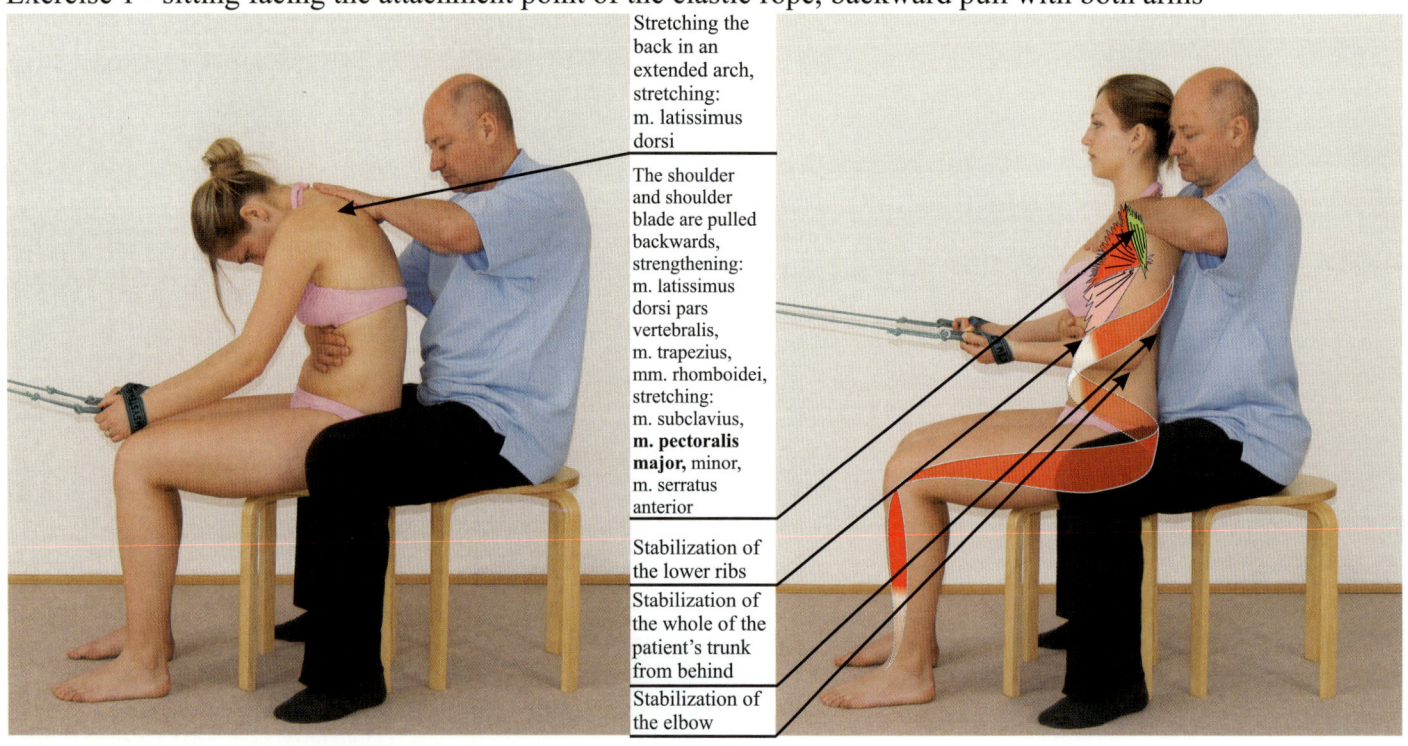

Stretching the back in an extended arch, stretching: m. latissimus dorsi

The shoulder and shoulder blade are pulled backwards, strengthening: m. latissimus dorsi pars vertebralis, m. trapezius, mm. rhomboidei, stretching: m. subclavius, **m. pectoralis major,** minor, m. serratus anterior

Stabilization of the lower ribs

Stabilization of the whole of the patient's trunk from behind

Stabilization of the elbow

M. pectoralis major - stretching

Exercise 2 - sitting sideways on to the attachment point of the elastic rope, sideways pull with one arm, the elastic rope is pulled over the head, performance with assistance, massage and correction

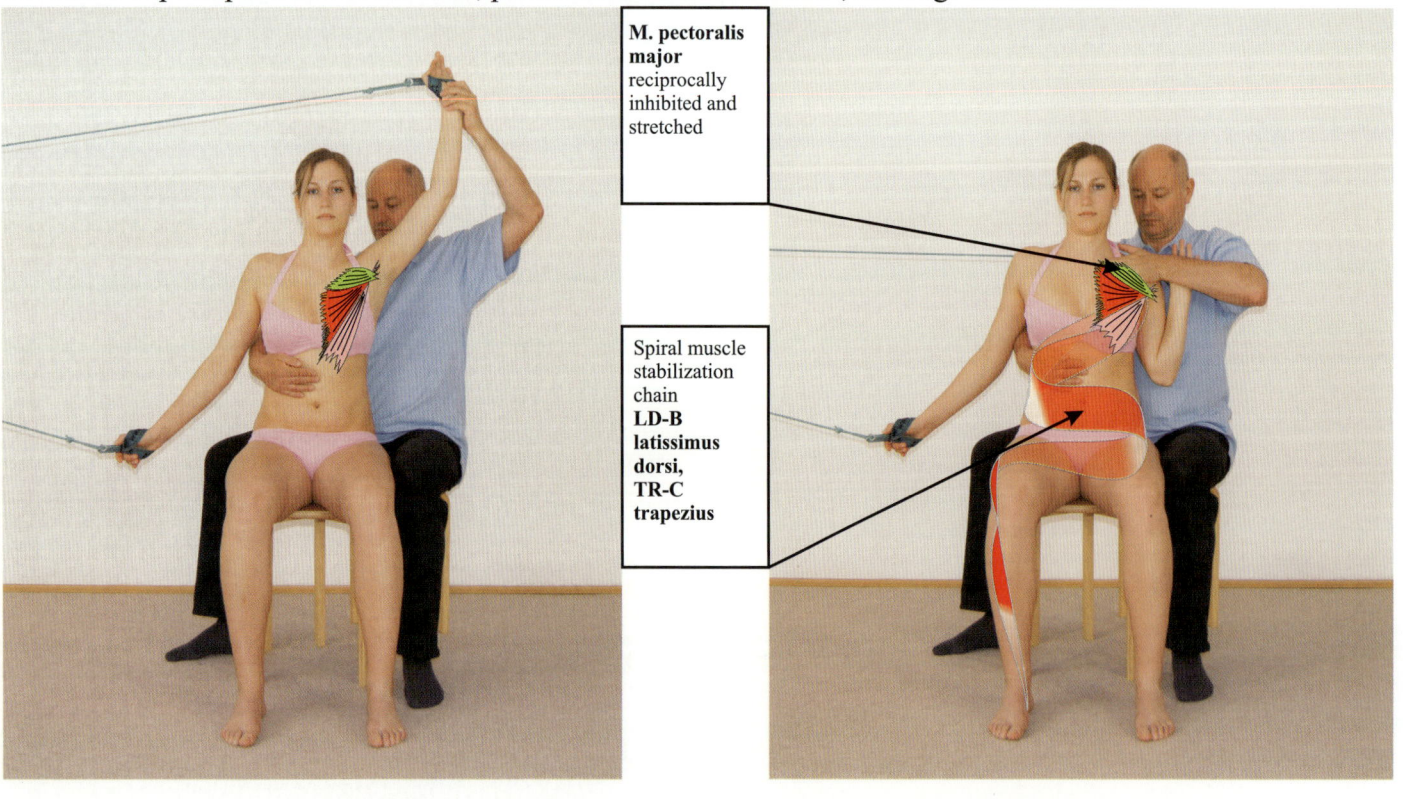

M. pectoralis major reciprocally inhibited and stretched

Spiral muscle stabilization chain **LD-B latissimus dorsi, TR-C trapezius**

Stretching the m. pectoralis major inhibited in reciprocal inhibition.
The agonist is the spirals TR and LD, which stabilize the body.
The m. pectoralis major is reciprocally inhibited and stretched at the same time.

Exercise - stabilization, stretching
M. pectoralis major - strengthening

The LD - latissimus dorsi and TR - trapezius chains are the agonists in the first part of the exercise, the SA - serratus anterior and PM - pectoralis major chains are the agonists in the second part of the exercise.

Exercise 10 - standing with the corresponding side of the body to the attachment point of the elastic rope, one leg is placed forward on the mat

Pulling in one arm in front of the centre of the abdomen, rotation of the trunk

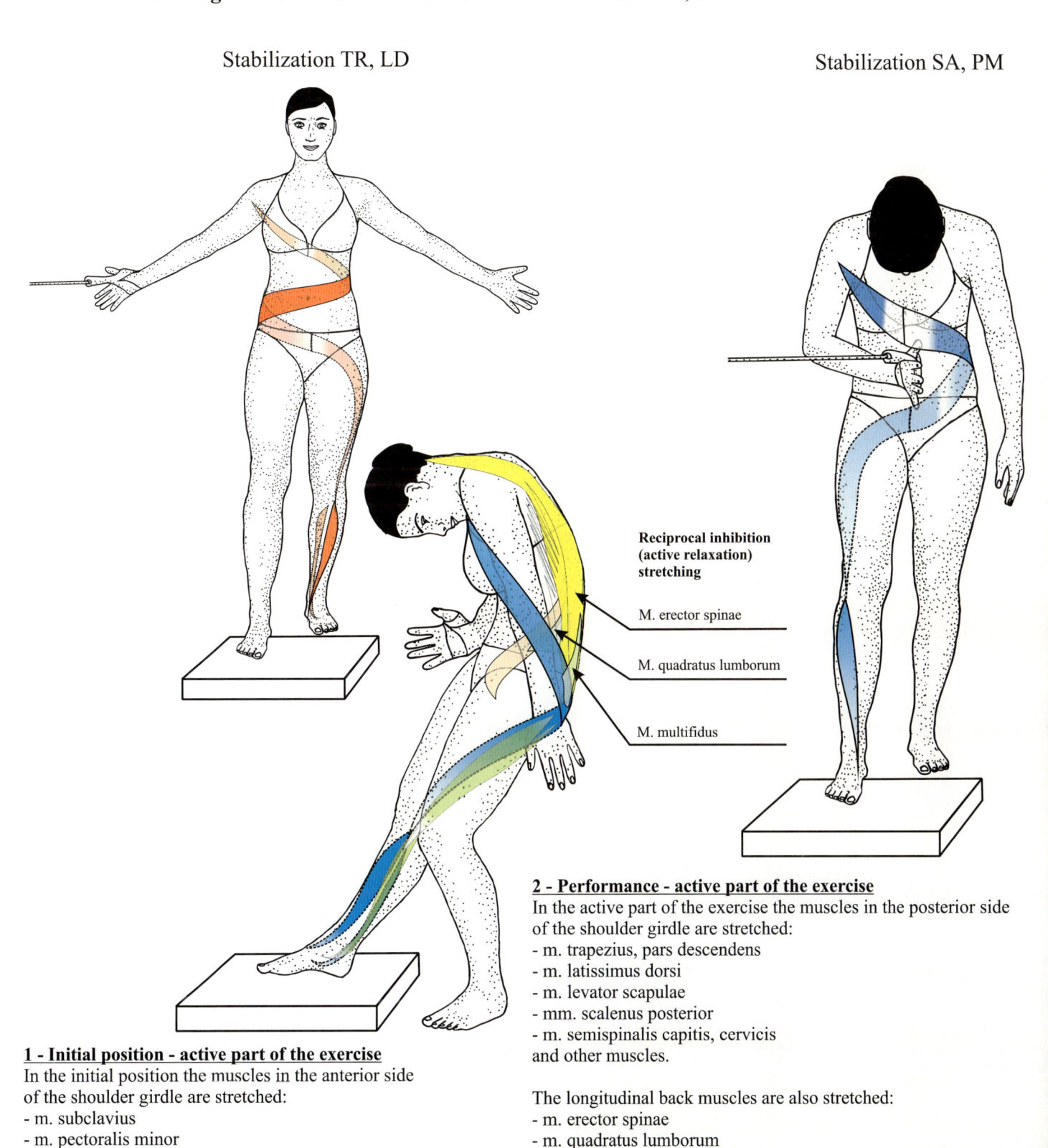

Stabilization TR, LD

Stabilization SA, PM

Reciprocal inhibition (active relaxation) stretching
- M. erector spinae
- M. quadratus lumborum
- M. multifidus

1 - Initial position - active part of the exercise
In the initial position the muscles in the anterior side of the shoulder girdle are stretched:
- m. subclavius
- m. pectoralis minor
- m. pectoralis major
- m. serratus anterior

2 - Performance - active part of the exercise
In the active part of the exercise the muscles in the posterior side of the shoulder girdle are stretched:
- m. trapezius, pars descendens
- m. latissimus dorsi
- m. levator scapulae
- mm. scalenus posterior
- m. semispinalis capitis, cervicis
and other muscles.

The longitudinal back muscles are also stretched:
- m. erector spinae
- m. quadratus lumborum
- m. multifidus

Exercise

M. pectoralis major - strengthening

Exercise 10 - standing with the corresponding side to the attachment point of the elastic rope, one leg is placed forward on the mat, pulling in one arm in front of the centre of the abdomen, rotation of the trunk

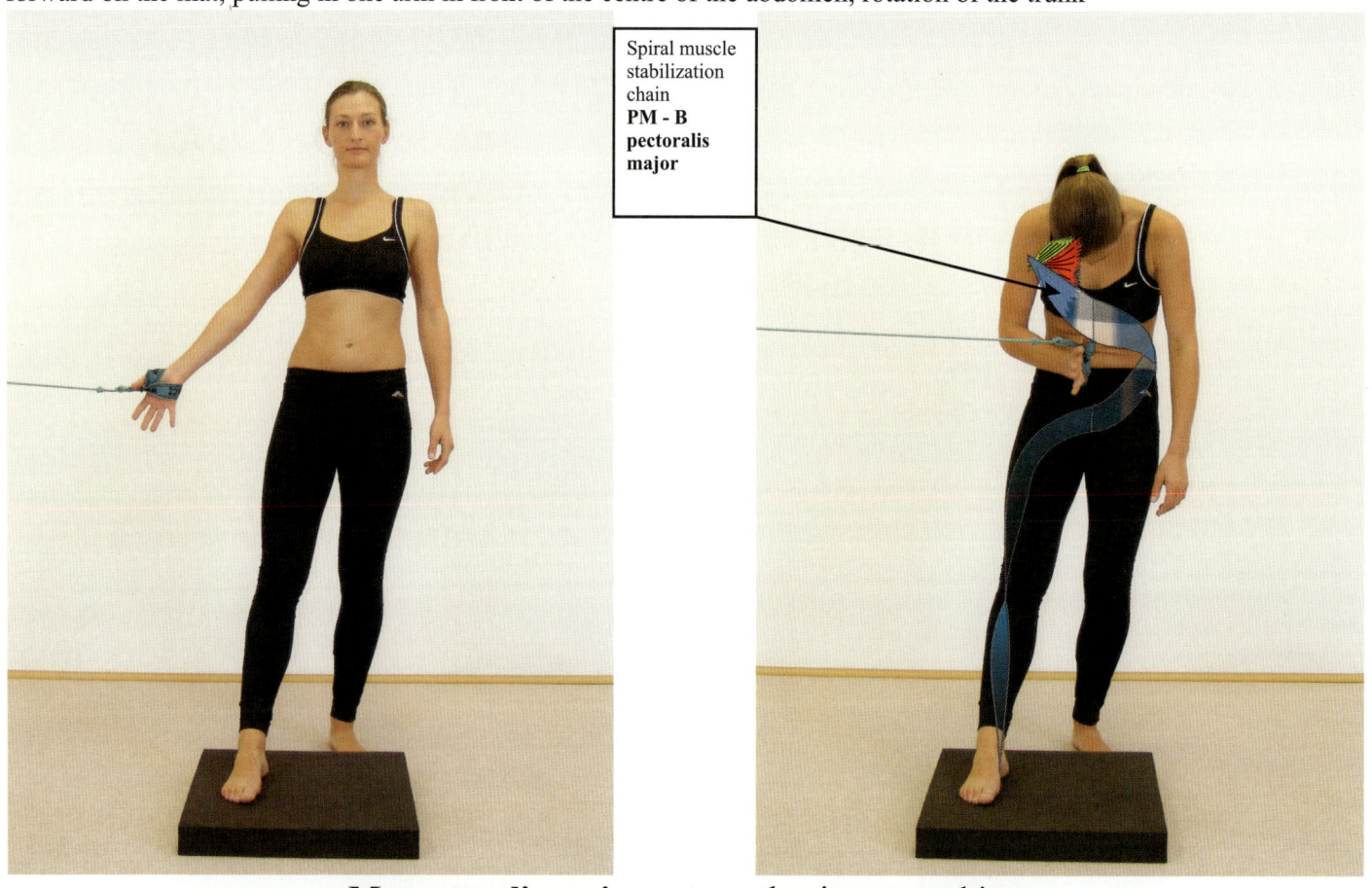

Spiral muscle stabilization chain
PM - B pectoralis major

M. pectoralis major - strengthening, stretching

Exercise 11 - standing facing the attachment point of the elastic rope, crossed movement pattern, extension of the arm in the shoulder girdle and extension of the opposing leg in the pelvic girdle. In both phases of the exercise, the TR, LD, SA and PM spirals are activated.

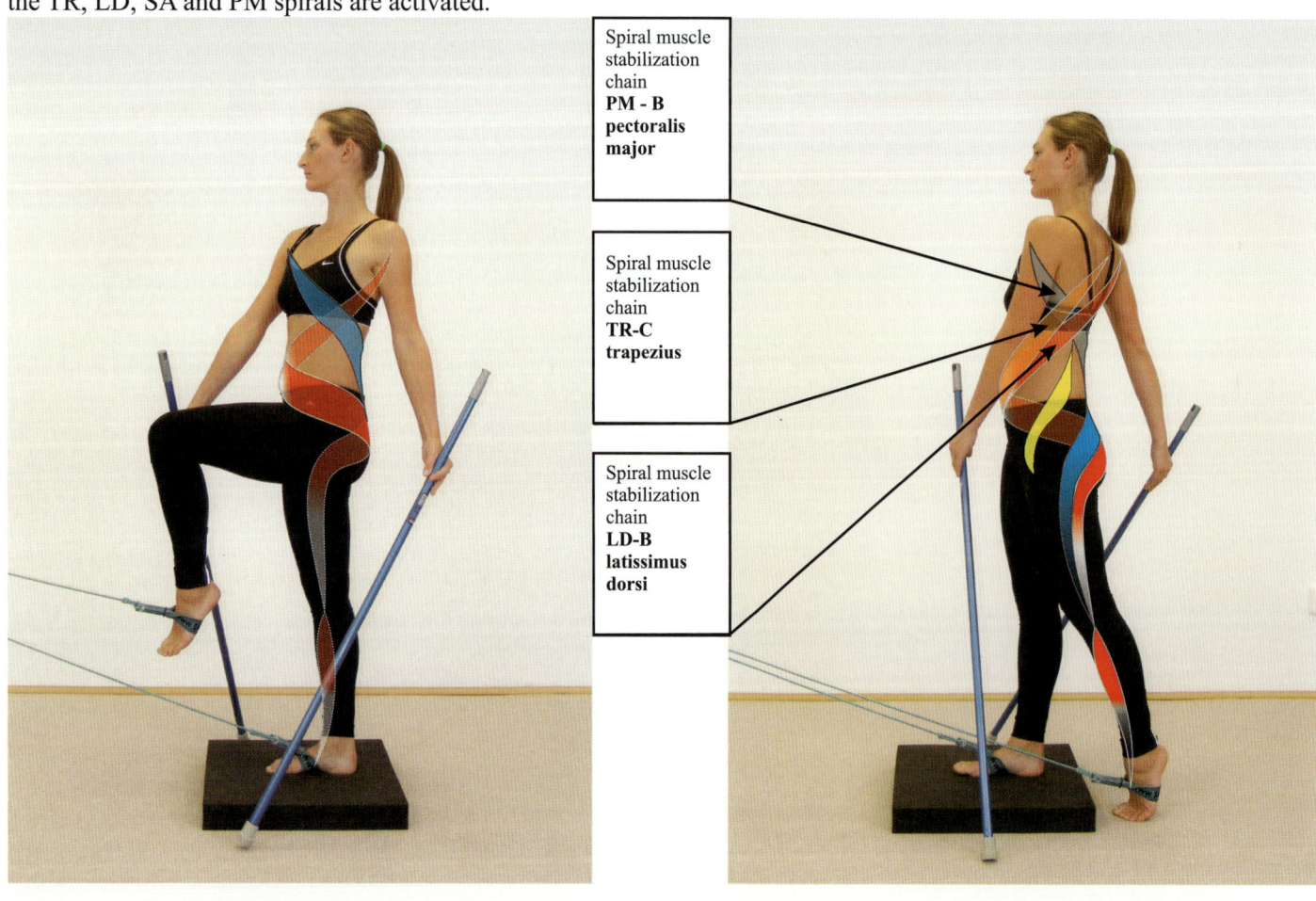

Spiral muscle stabilization chain
PM - B pectoralis major

Spiral muscle stabilization chain
TR-C trapezius

Spiral muscle stabilization chain
LD-B latissimus dorsi

Exercise
M. pectoralis major - strengthening, relaxation, stretching

Exercise 3 - standing with back to the attachment point of the elastic rope, the legs are in the basic position, opening the arms backwards, pulling the shoulder blades towards each others

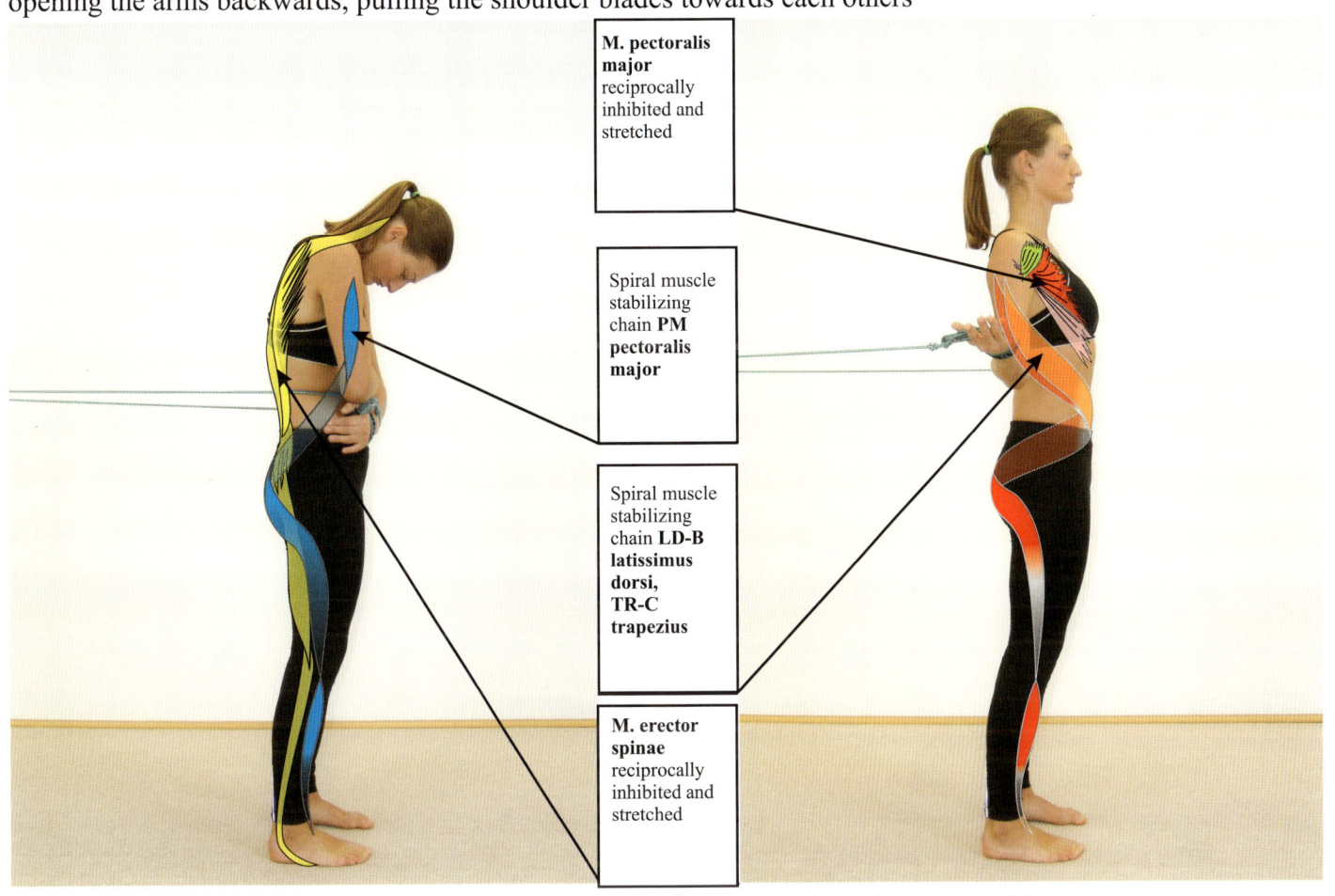

- **M. pectoralis major** reciprocally inhibited and stretched
- Spiral muscle stabilizing chain **PM pectoralis major**
- Spiral muscle stabilizing chain **LD-B latissimus dorsi, TR-C trapezius**
- **M. erector spinae** reciprocally inhibited and stretched

M. pectoralis major - strengthening, relaxation, stretching

Exercise 3 - standing with back to the attachment point of the elastic rope, one leg is placed forward on the mat, opening the arms backwards, pulling the shoulder blades towards each other

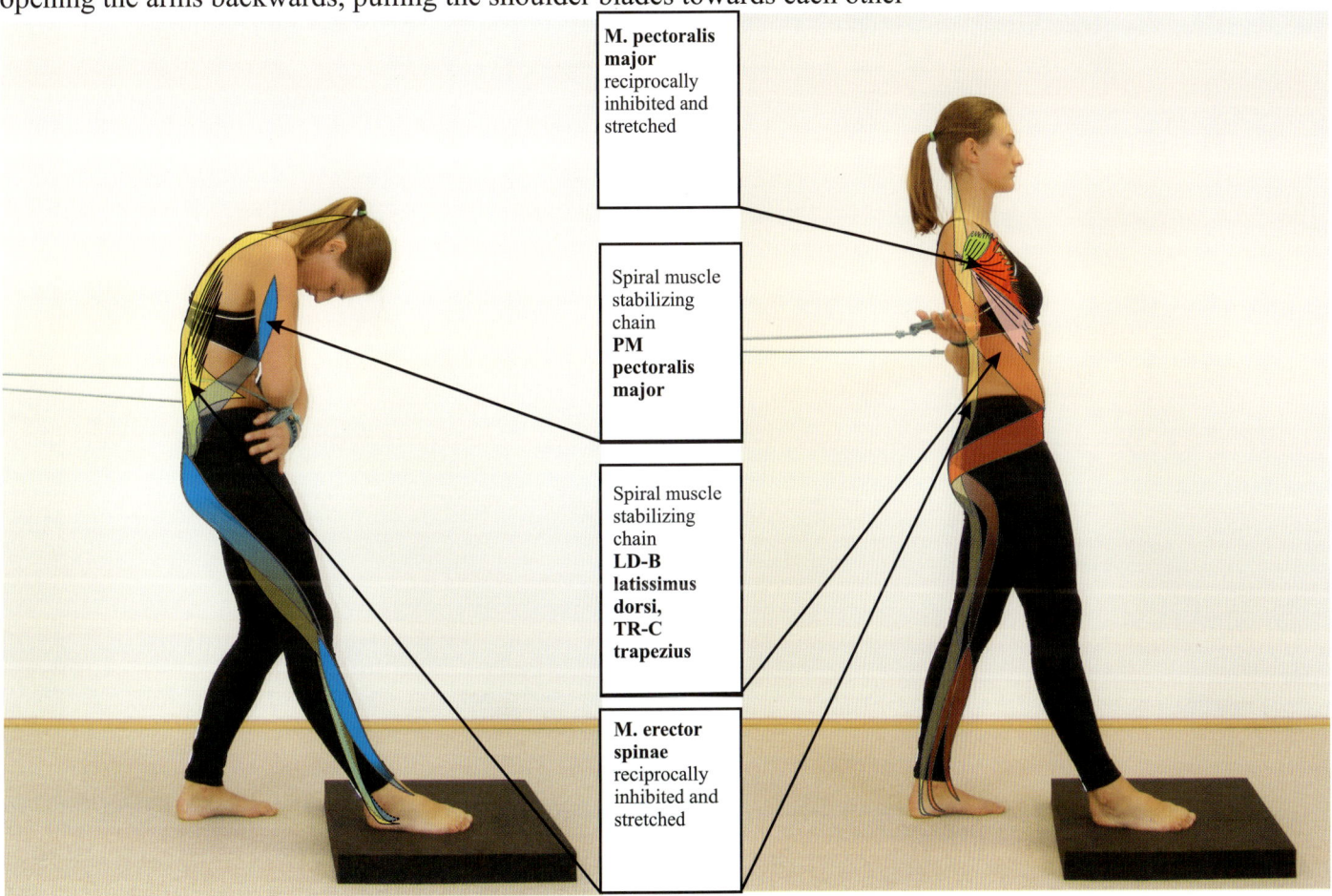

- **M. pectoralis major** reciprocally inhibited and stretched
- Spiral muscle stabilizing chain **PM pectoralis major**
- Spiral muscle stabilizing chain **LD-B latissimus dorsi, TR-C trapezius**
- **M. erector spinae** reciprocally inhibited and stretched

- 168 -

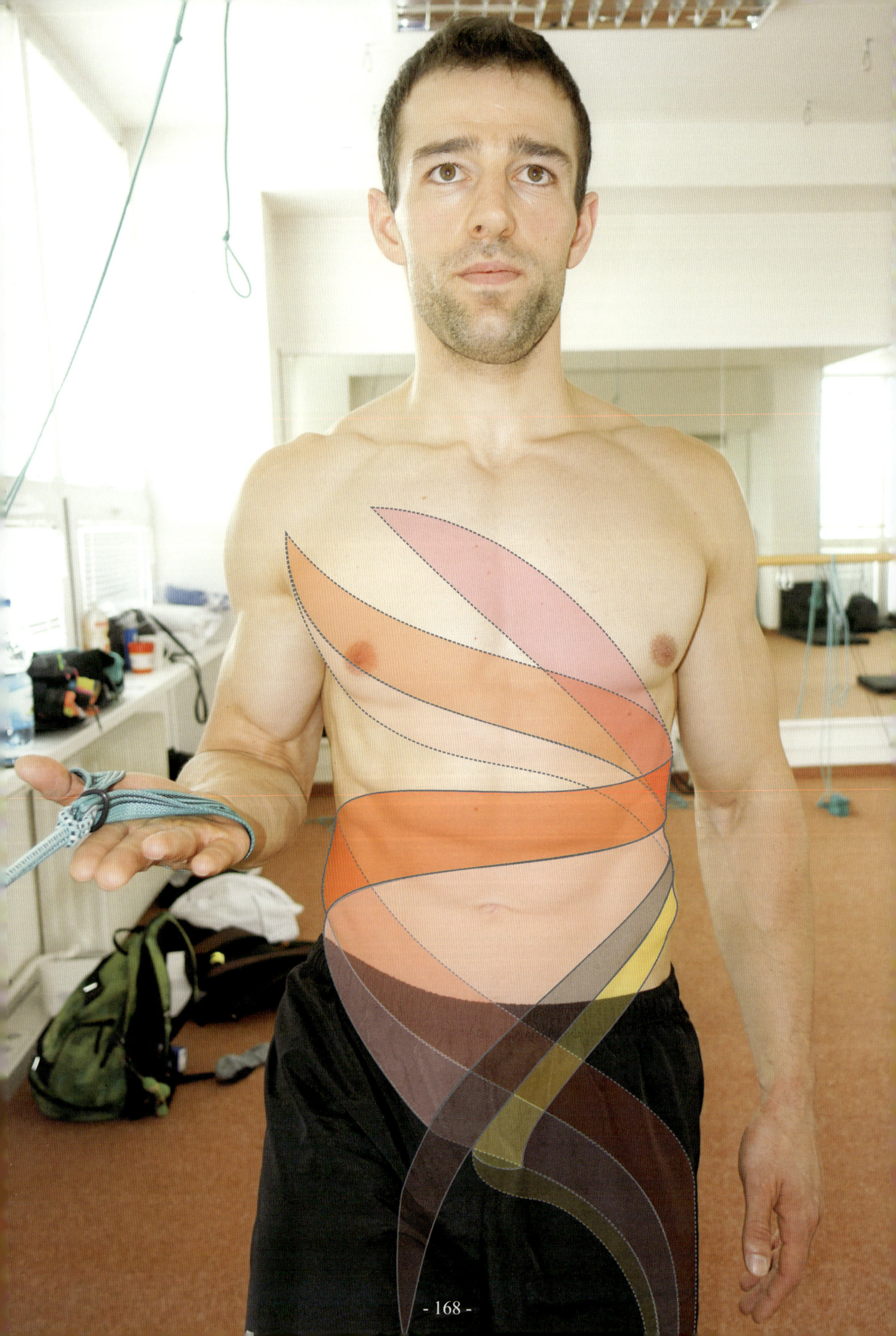

MANUAL TECHNIQUES AND EXERCISE ACCORDING TO MUSCLE ANALYSIS

Trunk
The anterior muscle group

Muscles with a tendency towards weakening:

M. obliquus externus abdominis
M. obliquus internus abdominis
M. transversus abdominis
M. rectus abdominis

Anatomy
M. obliquus externus abdominis

Costa 5.-12.
Processus xiphoideus
Linea alba
M. serratus anterior
M. latissimus dorsi
M. obliquus externus abdominis
Mm. intercostales externi
Costa X.-XII.
Labium externum cristae iliacae
Ligamentum inguinale
M. pyramidalis
Fascia lata
Symphysis

M. obliquus externus abdominis
Origin:
- outer surface of the ribs 5th-12th ribs
Insertion:
- crista iliaca, labium externum
- lamina anterior vaginae of the mm. recti abdominis
- linea alba
- os pubis
Function: - unilateral:
- lateral flexion (tilt) of the trunk towards the ipsilateral side
- rotation of the trunk towards the contralateral
    - bilaterally:
- ventral flexion of the trunk
- straightening the back
- abdominal press
- respiratory muscle - expiration
Innervation:
- nn. intercostales (Th5-Th12)
- n. iliohypogastricus

Anatomy
M. obliquus internus abdominis

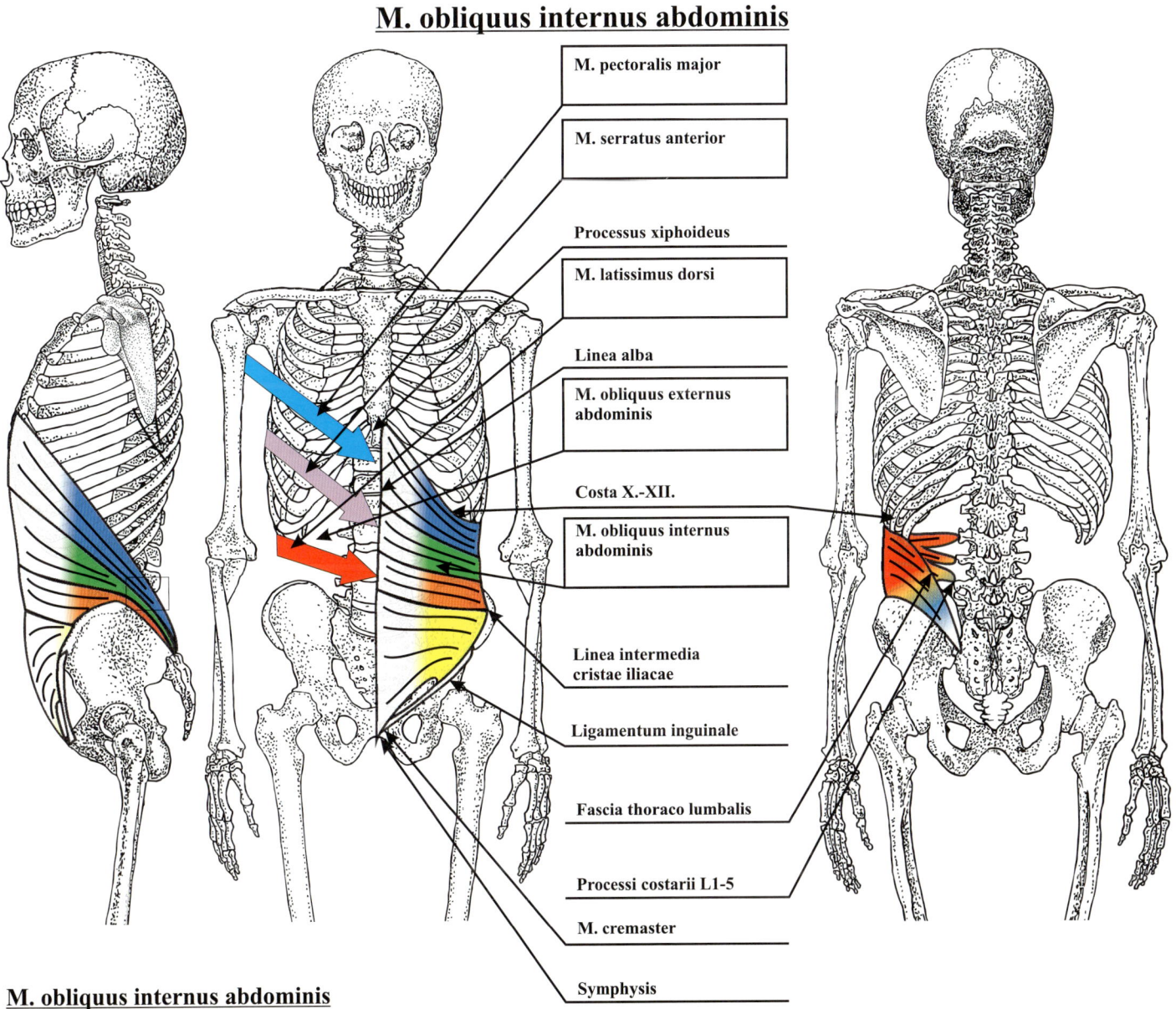

Labels:
- M. pectoralis major
- M. serratus anterior
- Processus xiphoideus
- M. latissimus dorsi
- Linea alba
- M. obliquus externus abdominis
- Costa X.-XII.
- M. obliquus internus abdominis
- Linea intermedia cristae iliacae
- Ligamentum inguinale
- Fascia thoraco lumbalis
- Processi costarii L1-5
- M. cremaster
- Symphysis

M. obliquus internus abdominis

Origin:
- deep lamina of the thoracolumbar fascia - processi costarii
- crista iliaca, linea intermedia
- spina iliaca anterior superior
- lateral half of the ligamentum inguinale

Insertion:
- lower edge 10th-12th ribs
- anterior and posterior lamina vaginae of the mm. recti abdominis
- linea alba
- transition to m. cremaster

Function: - unilateral:
- lateral flexion (tilt) of the trunk towards the ipsilateral
- rotation of the trunk towards the ipsilateral side
    - bilateral:
- ventral flexion of the trunk
- straightening the back
- abdominal press
- respiratory muscle - expiration

Innervation:
- nn. intercostales (Th8-Th12)
- n. iliohypogastricus
- n. ilioinguinalis
- m. cremaster: - ramus genitalis nervi genitofemoralis

Muscle chains
M. obliquus externus abdominis
M. obliquus internus abdominis

Activation of m. obliquus externus abdominis, m. obliquus internus abdominis, m. transversus abdominis through m. pectoralis major, m. serratus anterior, m. latissimus dorsi and m. trapezius.

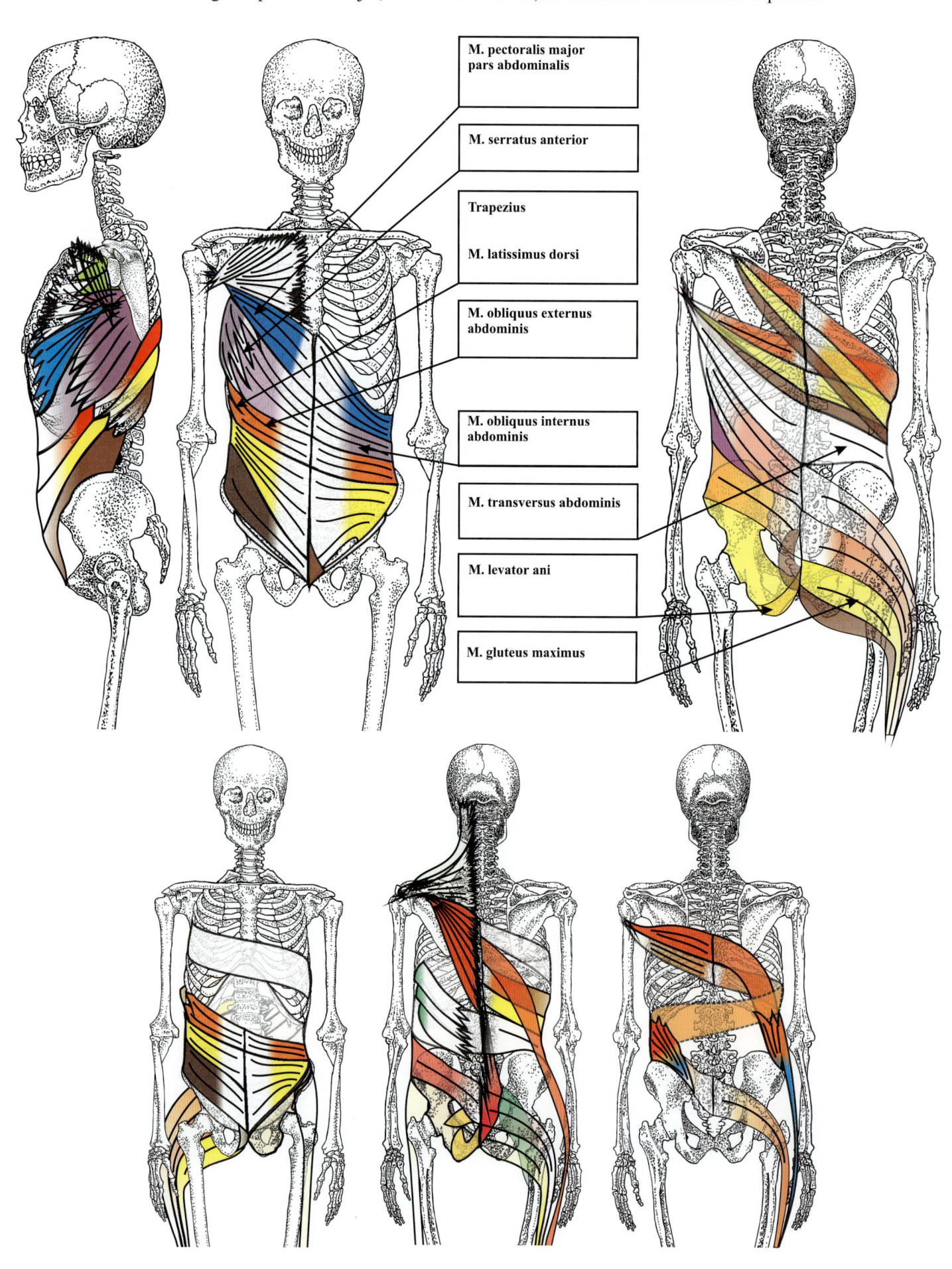

| M. pectoralis major pars abdominalis |
| M. serratus anterior |
| Trapezius |
| M. latissimus dorsi |
| M. obliquus externus abdominis |
| M. obliquus internus abdominis |
| M. transversus abdominis |
| M. levator ani |
| M. gluteus maximus |

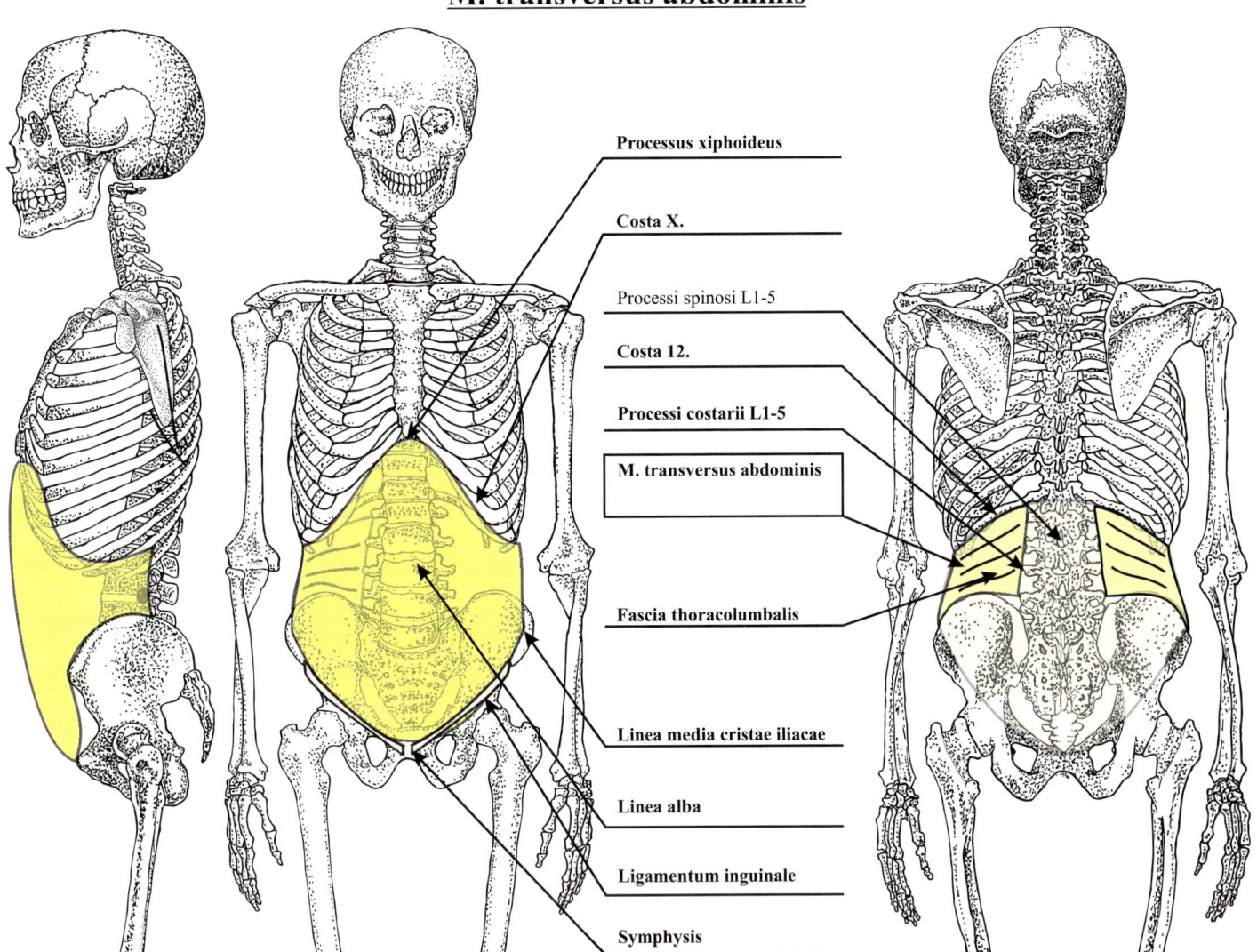

Anatomy
M. transversus abdominis

Processus xiphoideus
Costa X.
Processi spinosi L1-5
Costa 12.
Processi costarii L1-5
M. transversus abdominis
Fascia thoracolumbalis
Linea media cristae iliacae
Linea alba
Ligamentum inguinale
Symphysis

M. transversus abdominis
Origin:
- inner surface of the cartilage 7th-12th ribs
- deep lamina of the fascia thoracolumbalis
- processi costarii
- crista iliaca, labium internum
- spina iliaca anterior superior

Insertion:
- lamina interior vaginae of the mm. recti abdominis

Function: - unilateral:
- rotation of the trunk towards the ipsilateral side
  - bilateral:
- abdominal press
- respiratory muscle - expiration

Innervation:
- nn. intercostales (Th5-Th12)
- n. iliohypogastricus
- n. ilioinguinalis
- n. genitofemoralis

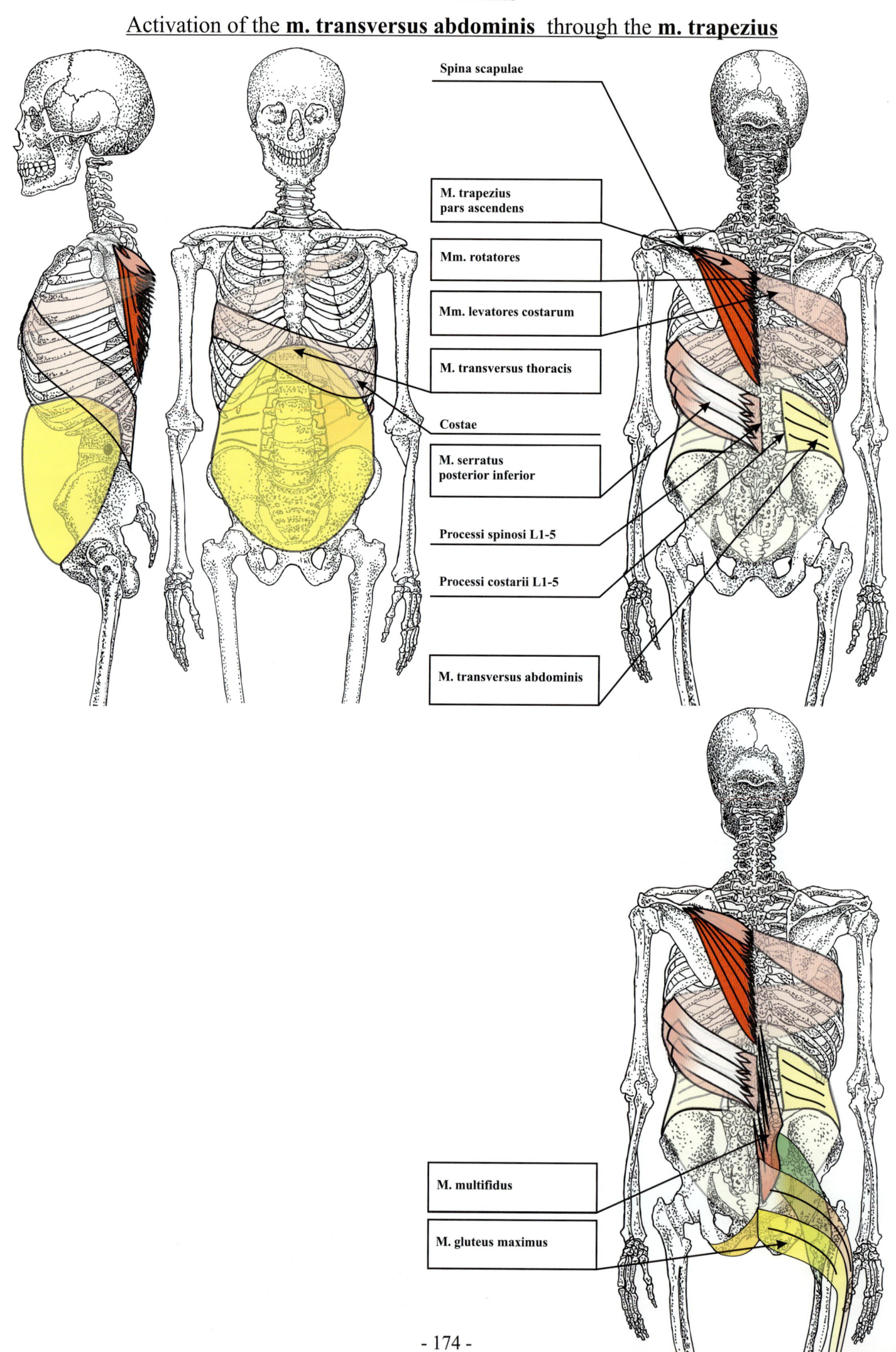

Muscle chains
Activation of the **m. transversus abdominis** through the **m. trapezius**

- Spina scapulae
- M. trapezius pars ascendens
- Mm. rotatores
- Mm. levatores costarum
- M. transversus thoracis
- Costae
- M. serratus posterior inferior
- Processi spinosi L1-5
- Processi costarii L1-5
- M. transversus abdominis
- M. multifidus
- M. gluteus maximus

- 174 -

Muscle chains
Activation of the m. transversus abdominis through the m. latissimus dorsi

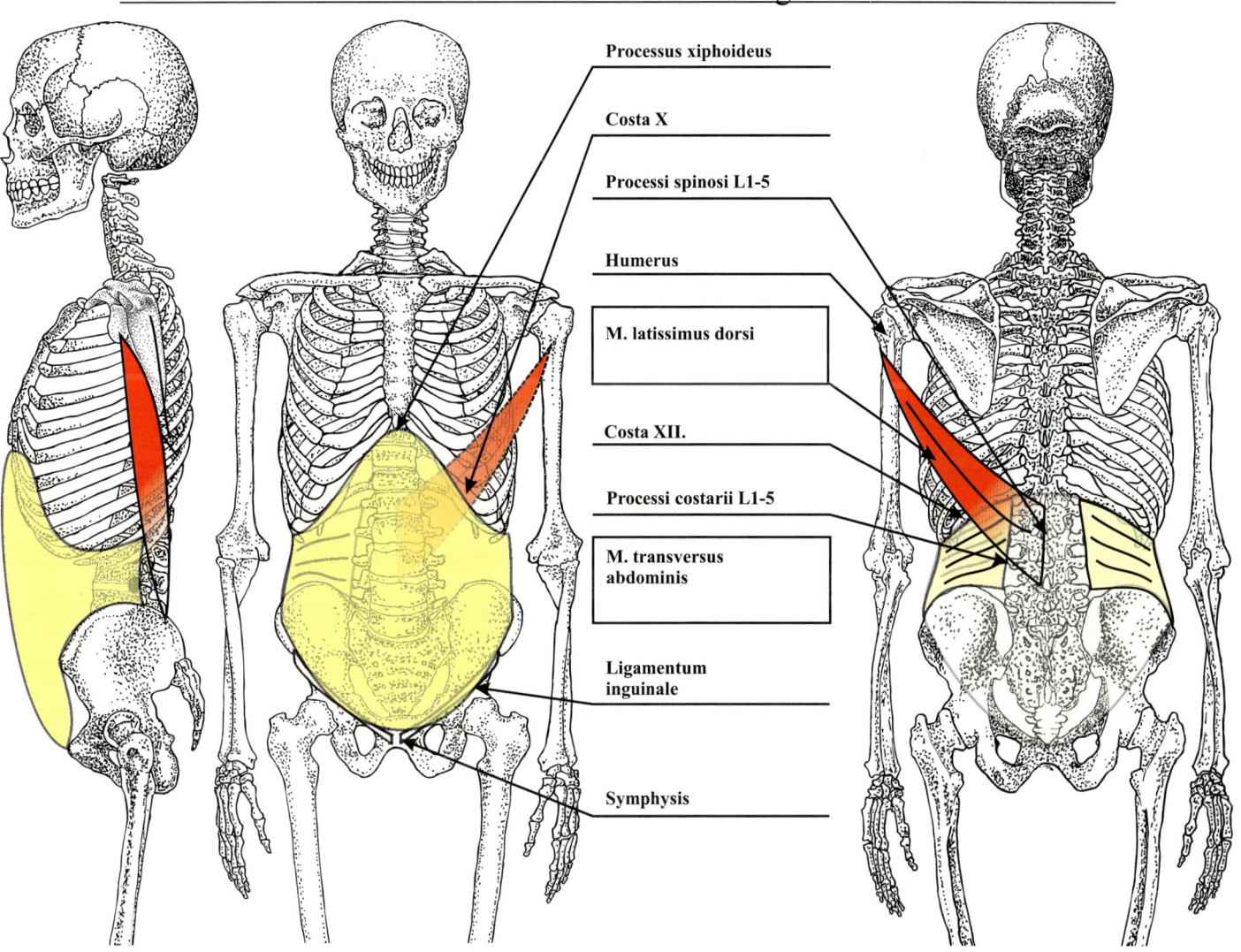

- Processus xiphoideus
- Costa X
- Processi spinosi L1-5
- Humerus
- M. latissimus dorsi
- Costa XII.
- Processi costarii L1-5
- M. transversus abdominis
- Ligamentum inguinale
- Symphysis

Muscle chains
Activation of the **m. transversus abdominis** through the **m. serratus anterior**

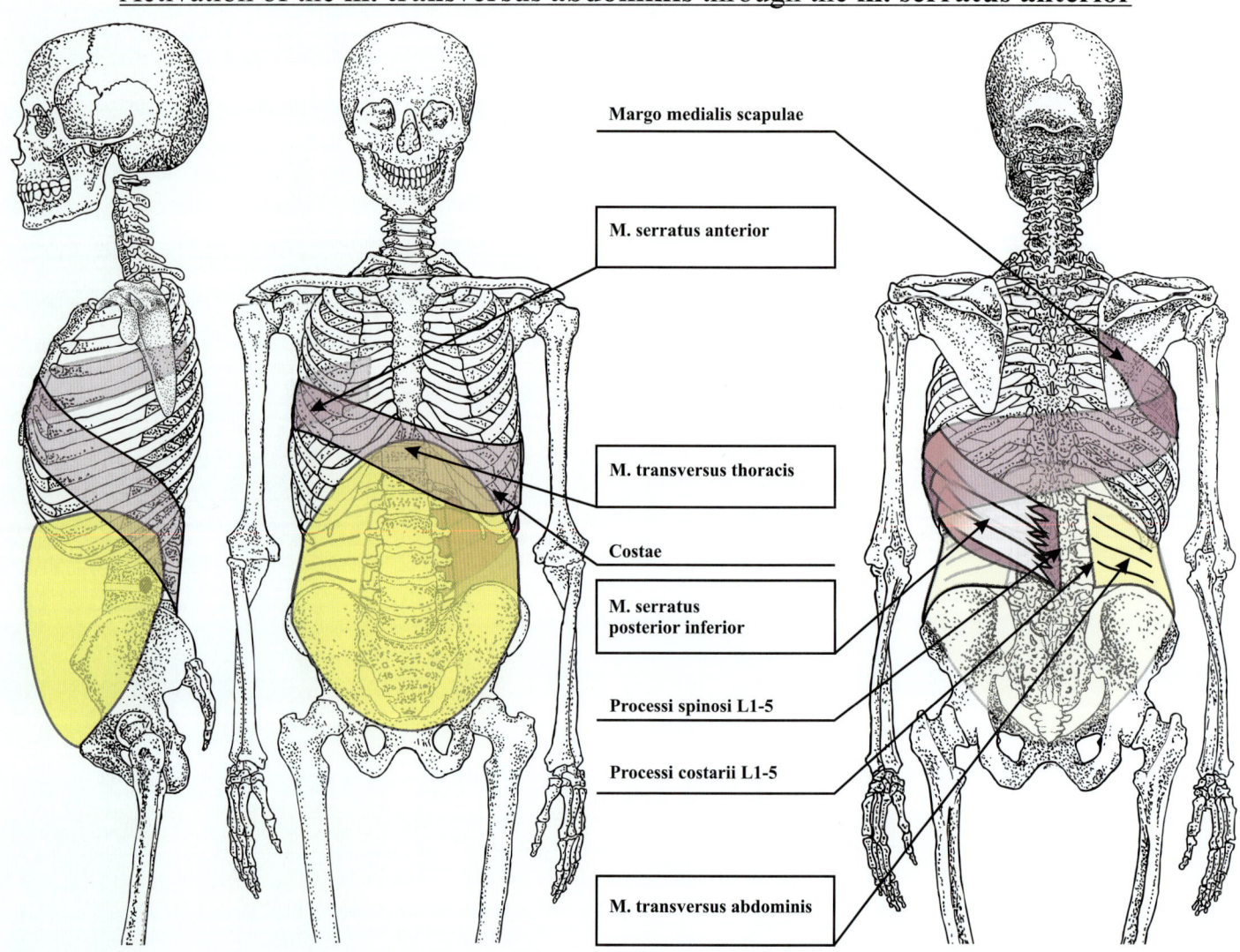

- Margo medialis scapulae
- M. serratus anterior
- M. transversus thoracis
- Costae
- M. serratus posterior inferior
- Processi spinosi L1-5
- Processi costarii L1-5
- M. transversus abdominis

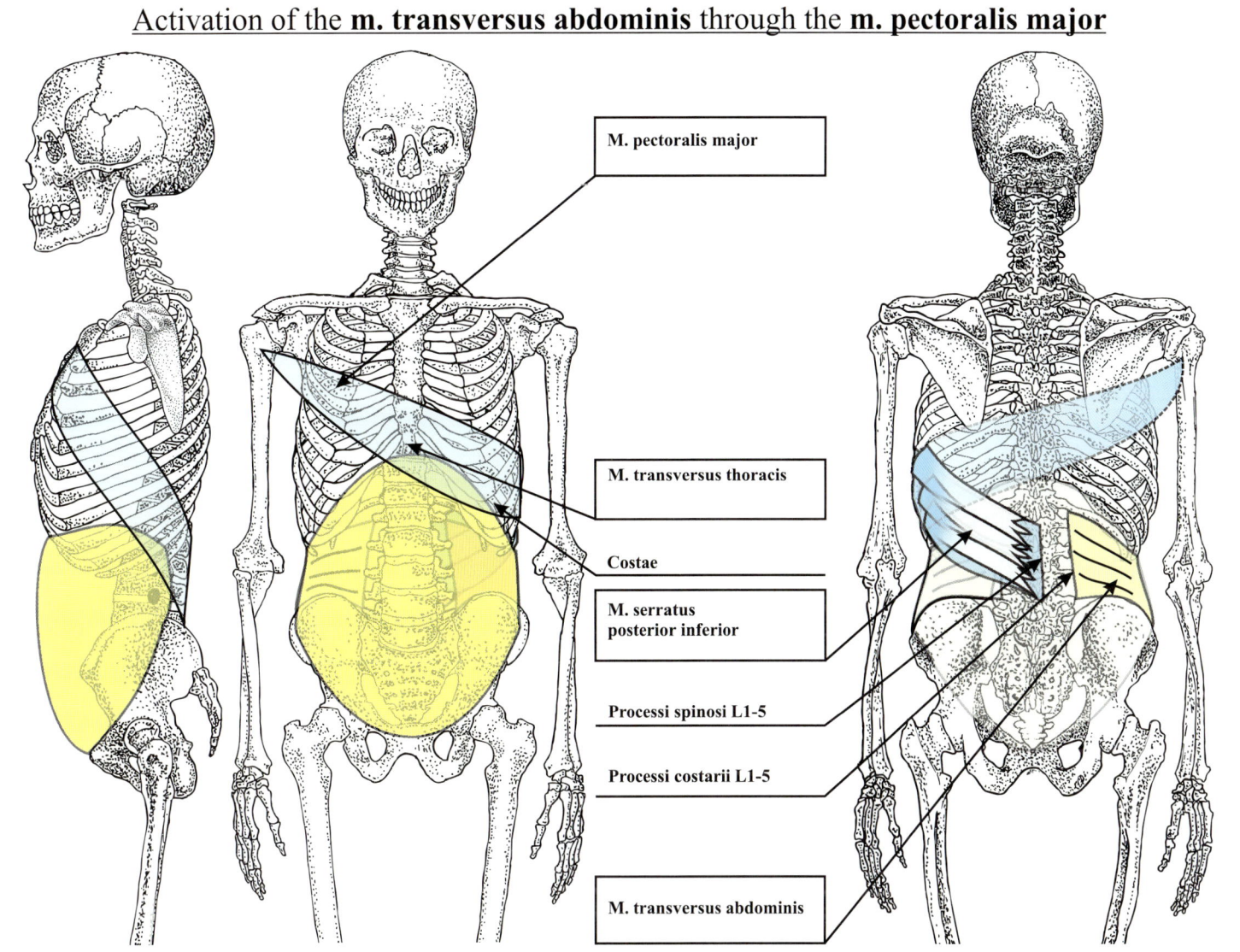

Muscle chains
Activation of the **m. transversus abdominis** through the **m. pectoralis major**

- M. pectoralis major
- M. transversus thoracis
- Costae
- M. serratus posterior inferior
- Processi spinosi L1-5
- Processi costarii L1-5
- M. transversus abdominis

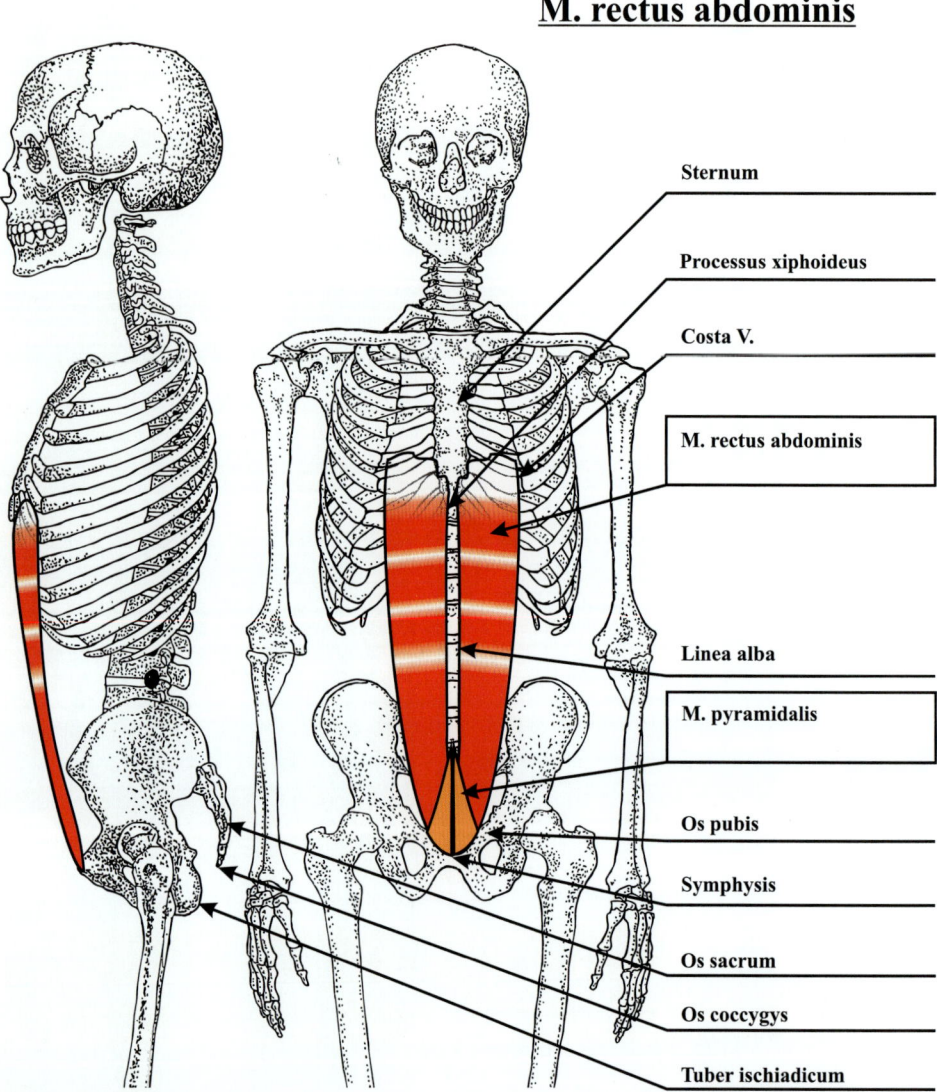

Anatomy
M. rectus abdominis

Sternum
Processus xiphoideus
Costa V.
M. rectus abdominis
Linea alba
M. pyramidalis
Os pubis
Symphysis
Os sacrum
Os coccygys
Tuber ischiadicum

M. rectus abdominis
Origin:
- cartilage 5th-7th ribs
- processus xiphoideus

Insertion:
- os pubis, between the tuberculum pubicum and the symphysis

Function:
- ventral flexion of the trunk
- stretching the back
- abdominal press
- respiratory muscle - expiration

Innervation:
- nn. intercostales (Th5-Th12)

M. pyramidalis
Origin:
- os pubis ventrally from the origin of the m. rectus abdominis

Insertion:
- linea alba

Function:
- tenses the linea alba

Innervation:
- n. subcostalis
  (n. intercostalis Th12)

Muscle chains
M. rectus abdominis - anatomical relationships

Clavicula
Processus coracoideus scapulae
Sternum
Processus xiphoideus
Costa III.-V.
M. rectus abdominis
M. iliocostalis
M. longissimus thoracis
Linea alba
M. pyramidalis
Os pubis
Symphysis
Os sacrum
Os coccygys
Tuber ischiadicum

Mutual balance of the anterior and posterior vertical muscle chains

The m. rectus abdominis in front, m. iliocostalis, and m. longus thoracis at the back mutually balance the posture of the chest and pelvis. This contributes significantly to the posture - the position of the body standing at rest.

Muscle chains
M. rectus abdominis

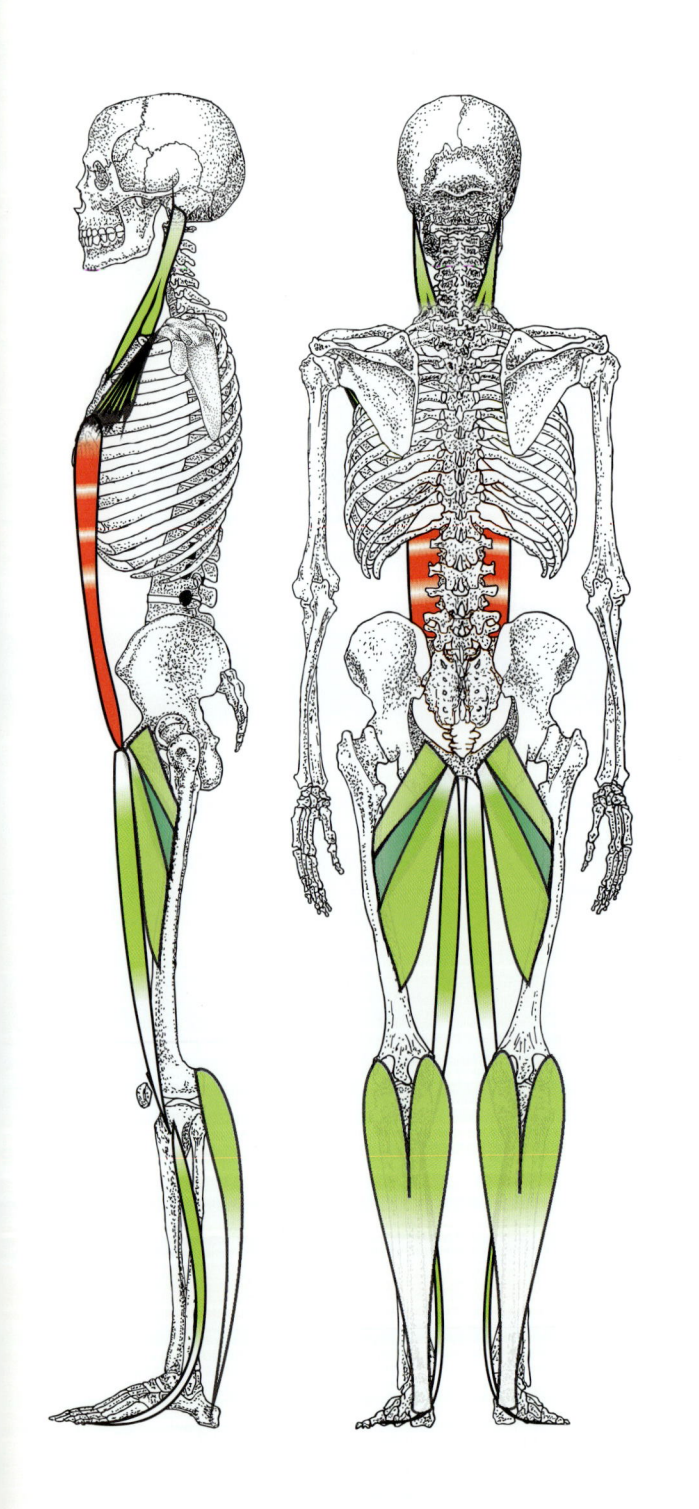

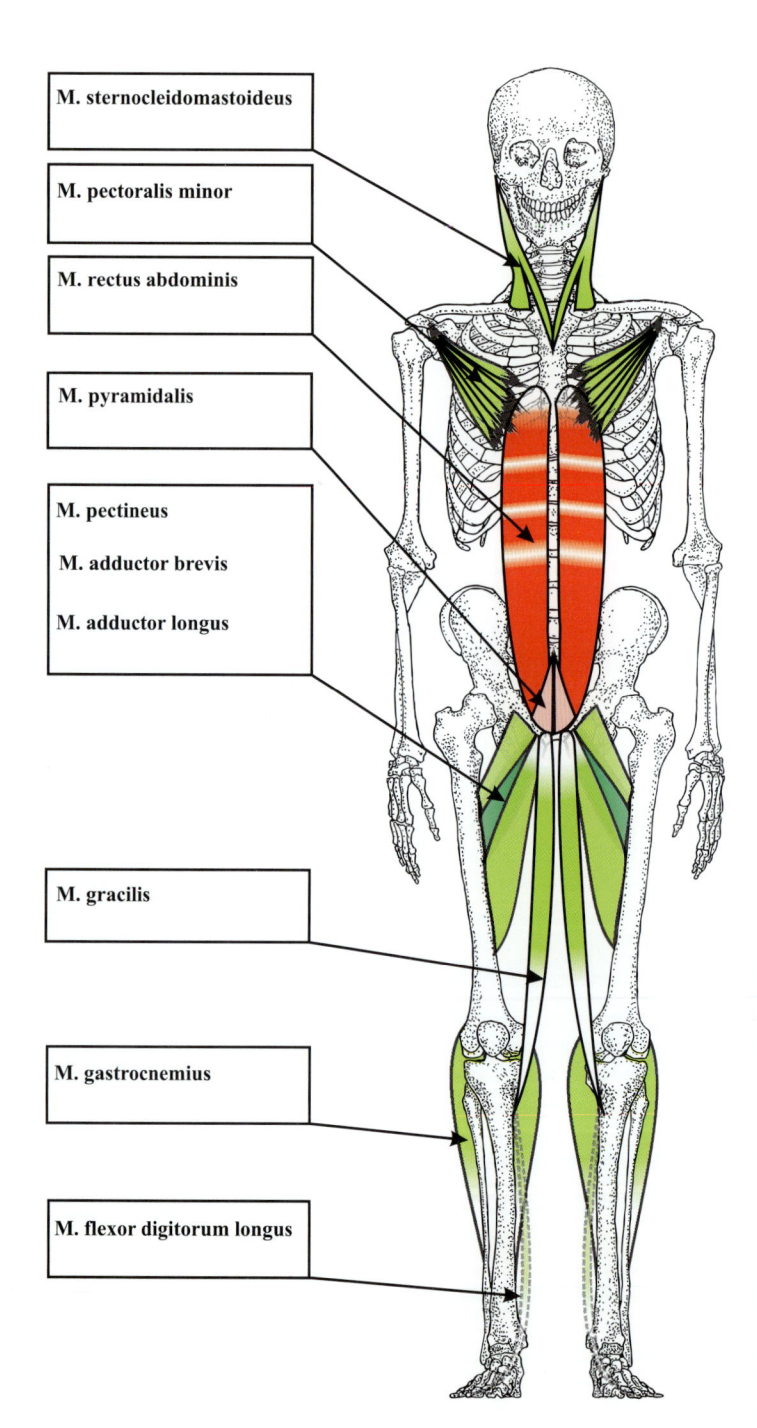

M. sternocleidomastoideus

M. pectoralis minor

M. rectus abdominis

M. pyramidalis

M. pectineus
M. adductor brevis
M. adductor longus

M. gracilis

M. gastrocnemius

M. flexor digitorum longus

MANUAL TECHNIQUES AND EXERCISE ACCORDING TO MUSCLE ANALYSIS

Pelvic girdle
The posterior lower muscle group

Muscles with a tendency towards weakening:

M. gluteus maximus

M. gluteus maximus

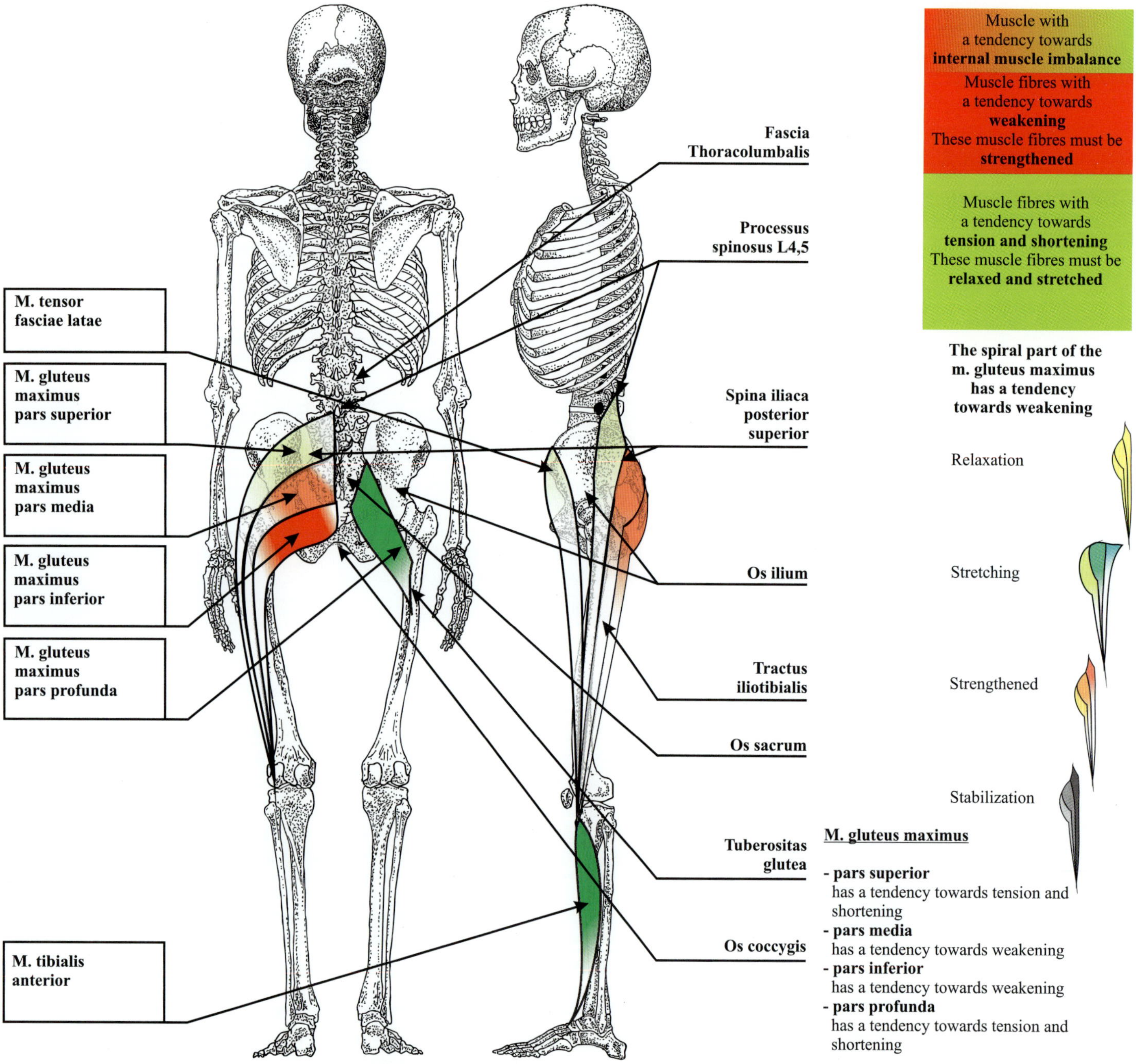

M. tensor fasciae latae
M. gluteus maximus pars superior
M. gluteus maximus pars media
M. gluteus maximus pars inferior
M. gluteus maximus pars profunda
M. tibialis anterior
Fascia Thoracolumbalis
Processus spinosus L4,5
Spina iliaca posterior superior
Os ilium
Tractus iliotibialis
Os sacrum
Tuberositas glutea
Os coccygis
Muscle with a tendency towards internal muscle imbalance
Muscle fibres with a tendency towards weakening These muscle fibres must be strengthened
Muscle fibres with a tendency towards tension and shortening These muscle fibres must be relaxed and stretched
The spiral part of the m. gluteus maximus has a tendency towards weakening
Relaxation
Stretching
Strengthened
Stabilization

M. gluteus maximus

- **pars superior** has a tendency towards tension and shortening
- **pars media** has a tendency towards weakening
- **pars inferior** has a tendency towards weakening
- **pars profunda** has a tendency towards tension and shortening

M. gluteus maximus

- pars superior

origin:
- fascia thoracolumbalis
- processi spinosi L4,5
- os ilium facies glutea

insertion:
- tractus iliotibialis - pars media,
- fascia lata

function: - hip:
- extension of the hip joint
- abduction (pulling away) of the thigh
- outward rotation of the thigh
- stabilization of the hip

- pelvis:
- straightens the pelvis from anteversion (tilting forward and downward)

- knee:
- extension
- outward rotation
- lateral stabilization

Innervation - all parts:
- n. gluteus inferior (L4-S2)

- pars media

origin:
- os sacrum (connects with the m. obliquus internus abdominis)
- ligamentum sacrotuberale

Insertion:
- tractus iliotibialis - pars media
- fascia lata

function: - hip:
- extension of the hip joint
- abduction (pulling away) of the thigh
- outward rotation of the thigh
- stabilization of the hip

- pelvis:
- straightens the pelvis from anteversion (tilting forward and downward)

- knee:
- extension
- outward rotation
- lateral stabilization

- pars inferior

origin:
- os coccygis (connects with the m. levator ani - pelvic floor)

insertion:
- tractus iliotibialis - pars posterior
- fascia lata

function: - hip:
- hyperextension (extending the hip joint from the vertical to full extension - sprint)
- adduction (pulling in) of the thigh
- outward rotation of the thigh
- stabilization of the hip

- pelvic:
- straightens the pelvis from anteversion (tilting forward and downward)

- knee:
- extension
- outward rotation
- lateral stabilization

- pars profunda

origin:
- os sacrum (connects to the m. iliocostalis)

insertion:
- tuberositas glutea

function: - hip:
- extension of the hip joint
- abduction (pulling away) of the thigh
- outward rotation of the thigh
- stabilization of the hip

- pelvis:
- straightens the pelvis from anteversion (tilting forward and downward)

Muscle chains
Spiral muscle chain **TR - trapezius**
The TR chain activates the m. gluteus maximus by a backward movement of the shoulder blade - extension.

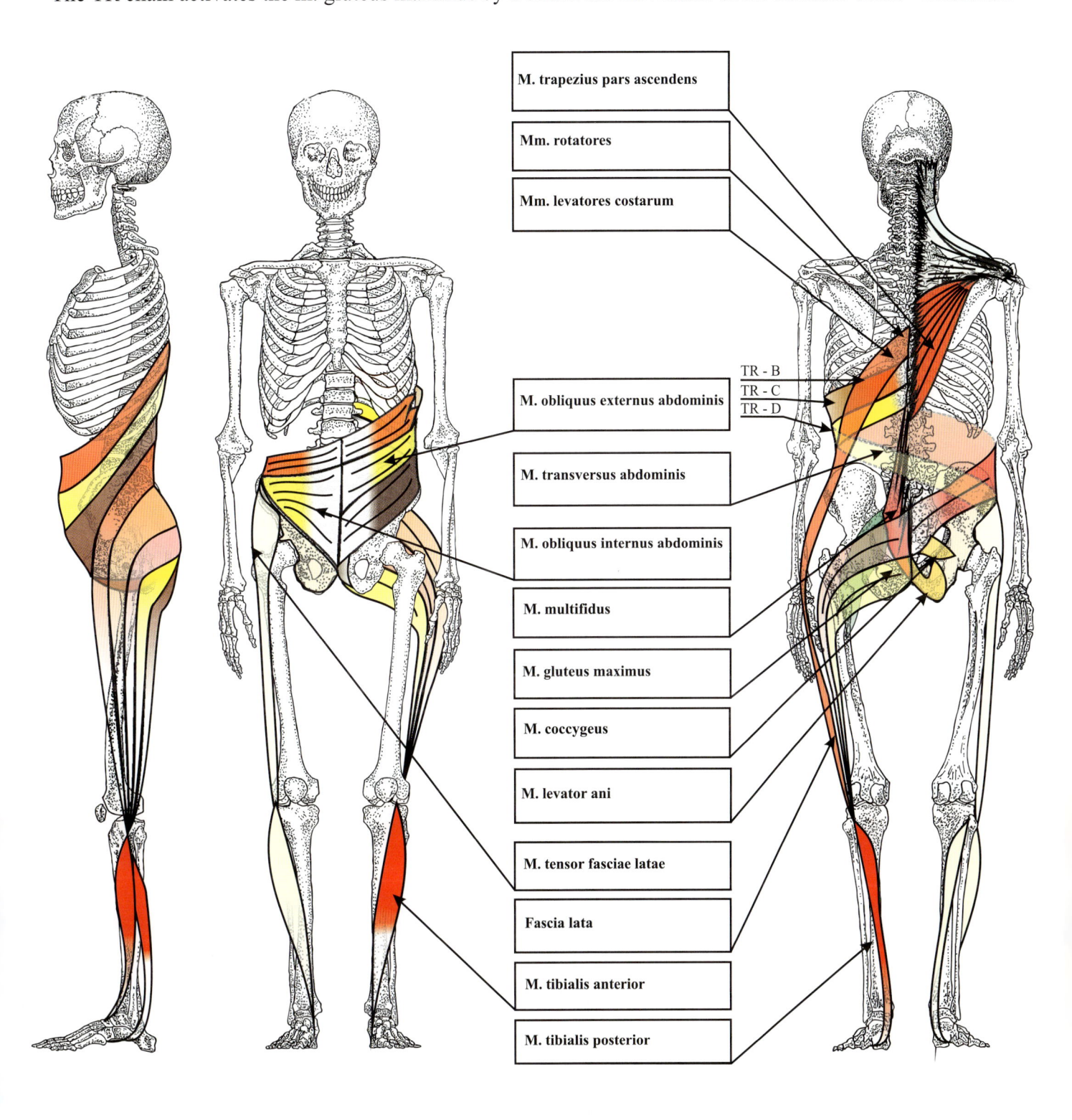

- M. trapezius pars ascendens
- Mm. rotatores
- Mm. levatores costarum
- M. obliquus externus abdominis
- M. transversus abdominis
- M. obliquus internus abdominis
- M. multifidus
- M. gluteus maximus
- M. coccygeus
- M. levator ani
- M. tensor fasciae latae
- Fascia lata
- M. tibialis anterior
- M. tibialis posterior

TR - B
TR - C
TR - D

- 183 -

Muscle chains
Spiral muscle chain LD - latissimus dorsi
The LD chain activates the m. gluteus maximus by a backward movement of the arm - extension.

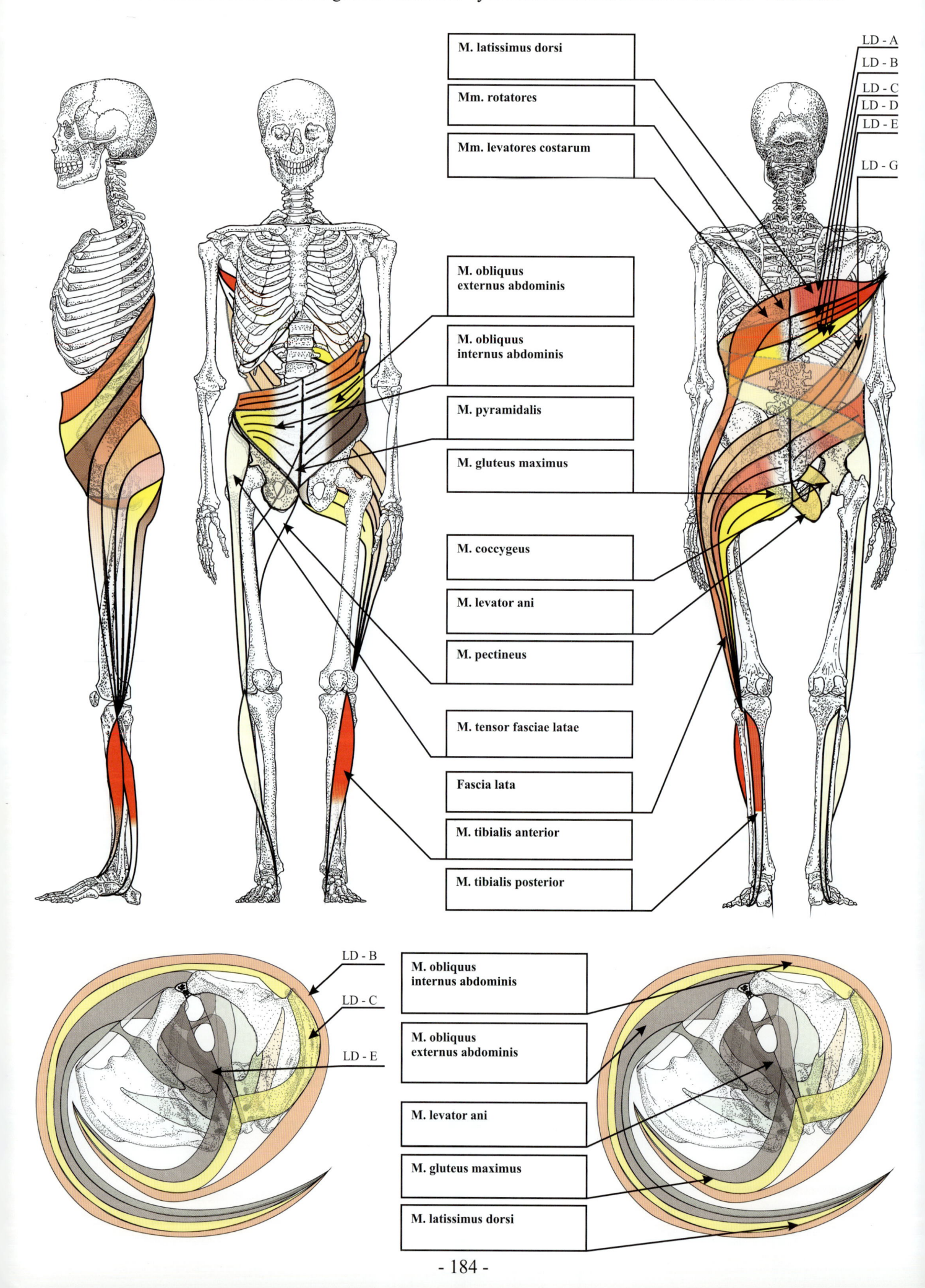

- M. latissimus dorsi
- Mm. rotatores
- Mm. levatores costarum
- M. obliquus externus abdominis
- M. obliquus internus abdominis
- M. pyramidalis
- M. gluteus maximus
- M. coccygeus
- M. levator ani
- M. pectineus
- M. tensor fasciae latae
- Fascia lata
- M. tibialis anterior
- M. tibialis posterior

LD - A
LD - B
LD - C
LD - D
LD - E
LD - G

- M. obliquus internus abdominis
- M. obliquus externus abdominis
- M. levator ani
- M. gluteus maximus
- M. latissimus dorsi

LD - B
LD - C
LD - E

Muscle chains
Spiral muscle chain LD-E - latissimus dorsi
Muscle chain LD activates the m. gluteus maximus by a backward movement of the arm - extension.

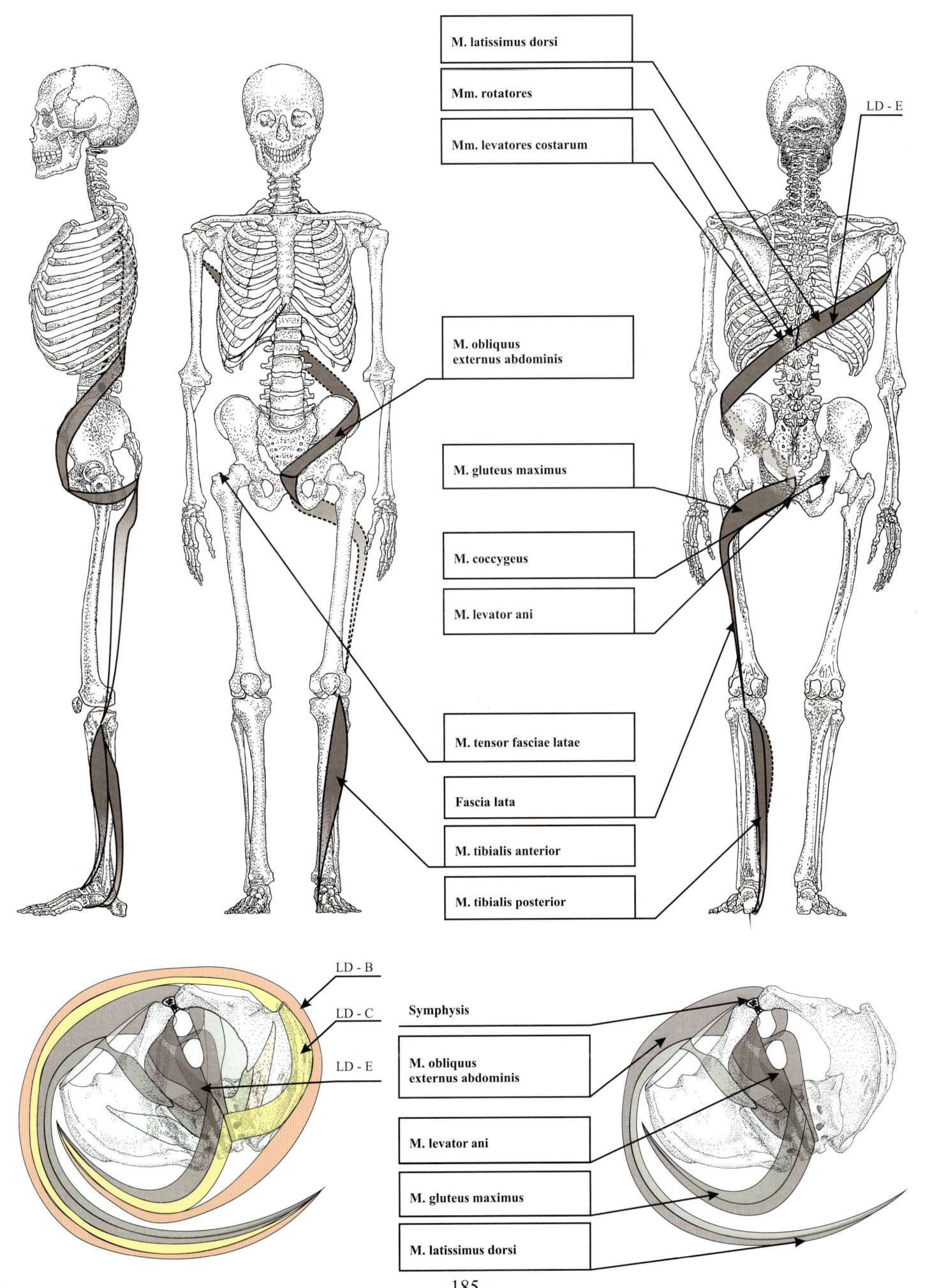

- M. latissimus dorsi
- Mm. rotatores
- Mm. levatores costarum
- M. obliquus externus abdominis
- M. gluteus maximus
- M. coccygeus
- M. levator ani
- M. tensor fasciae latae
- Fascia lata
- M. tibialis anterior
- M. tibialis posterior

LD - E

LD - B
LD - C
LD - E

Symphysis

- M. obliquus externus abdominis
- M. levator ani
- M. gluteus maximus
- M. latissimus dorsi

Muscle chain
Spiral muscle chain SA - serratus anterior

The SA chain activates the m. gluteus maximus by a forward movement of the shoulder blade - flexion.
A precondition of activation is to start from previous extension.

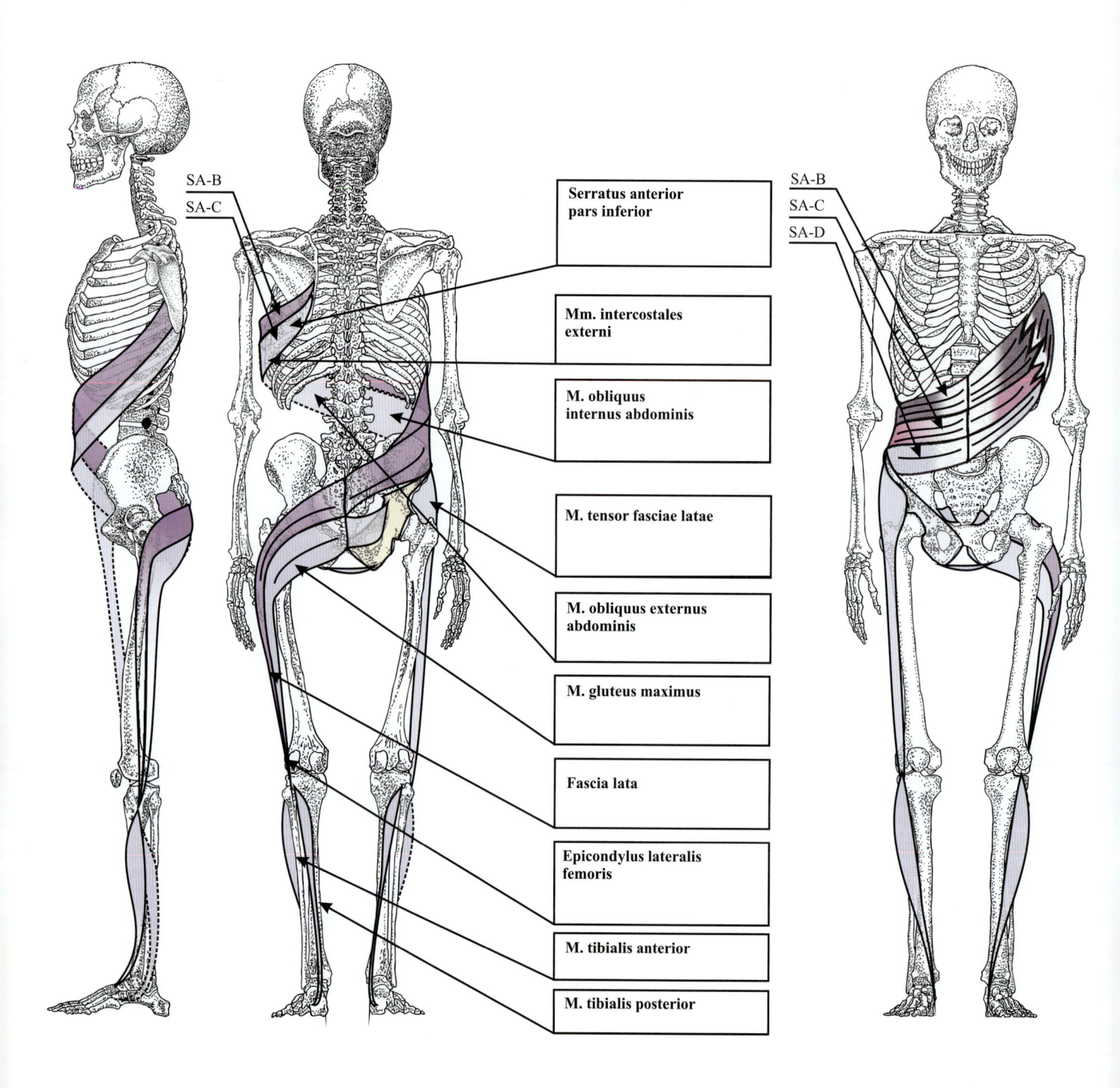

- Serratus anterior pars inferior
- Mm. intercostales externi
- M. obliquus internus abdominis
- M. tensor fasciae latae
- M. obliquus externus abdominis
- M. gluteus maximus
- Fascia lata
- Epicondylus lateralis femoris
- M. tibialis anterior
- M. tibialis posterior

Muscle chains
Spiral muscle chain **PM - pectoralis major**

The PM chain activates the m. gluteus maximus by a forward movement of the arm - flexion.
A precondition of activation is to start from previous extension.

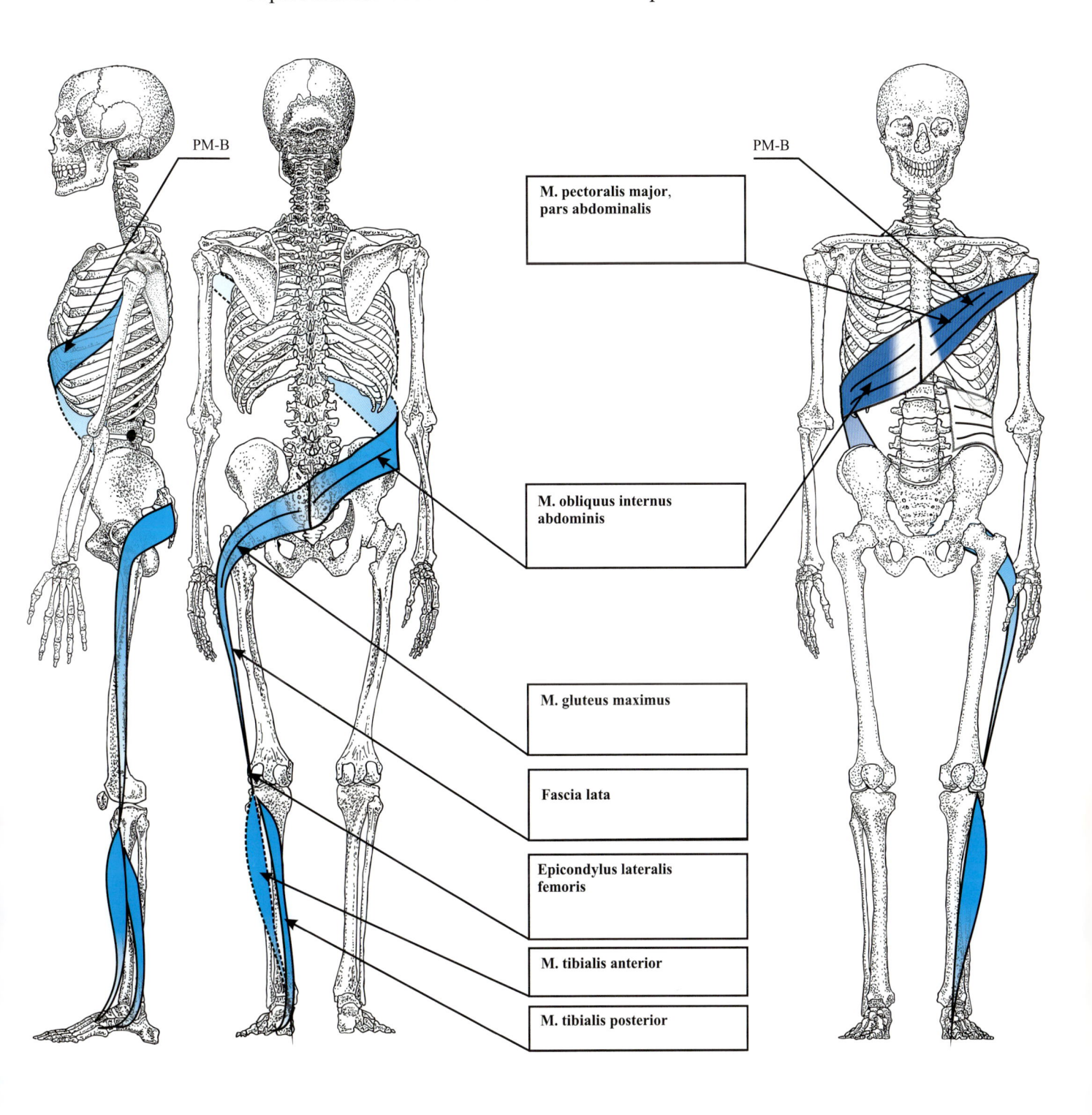

PM-B

M. pectoralis major, pars abdominalis

M. obliquus internus abdominis

M. gluteus maximus

Fascia lata

Epicondylus lateralis femoris

M. tibialis anterior

M. tibialis posterior

Exercise
M. gluteus maximus - strengthening, stretching

Exercise 11 - standing facing the attachment point of the elastic rope, crossed movement pattern, extension of the arm in the shoulder girdle and extension of the opposing leg in the pelvic girdle. In both phases of the exercise the TR, LD, SA and PM spirals are activated at the same time.

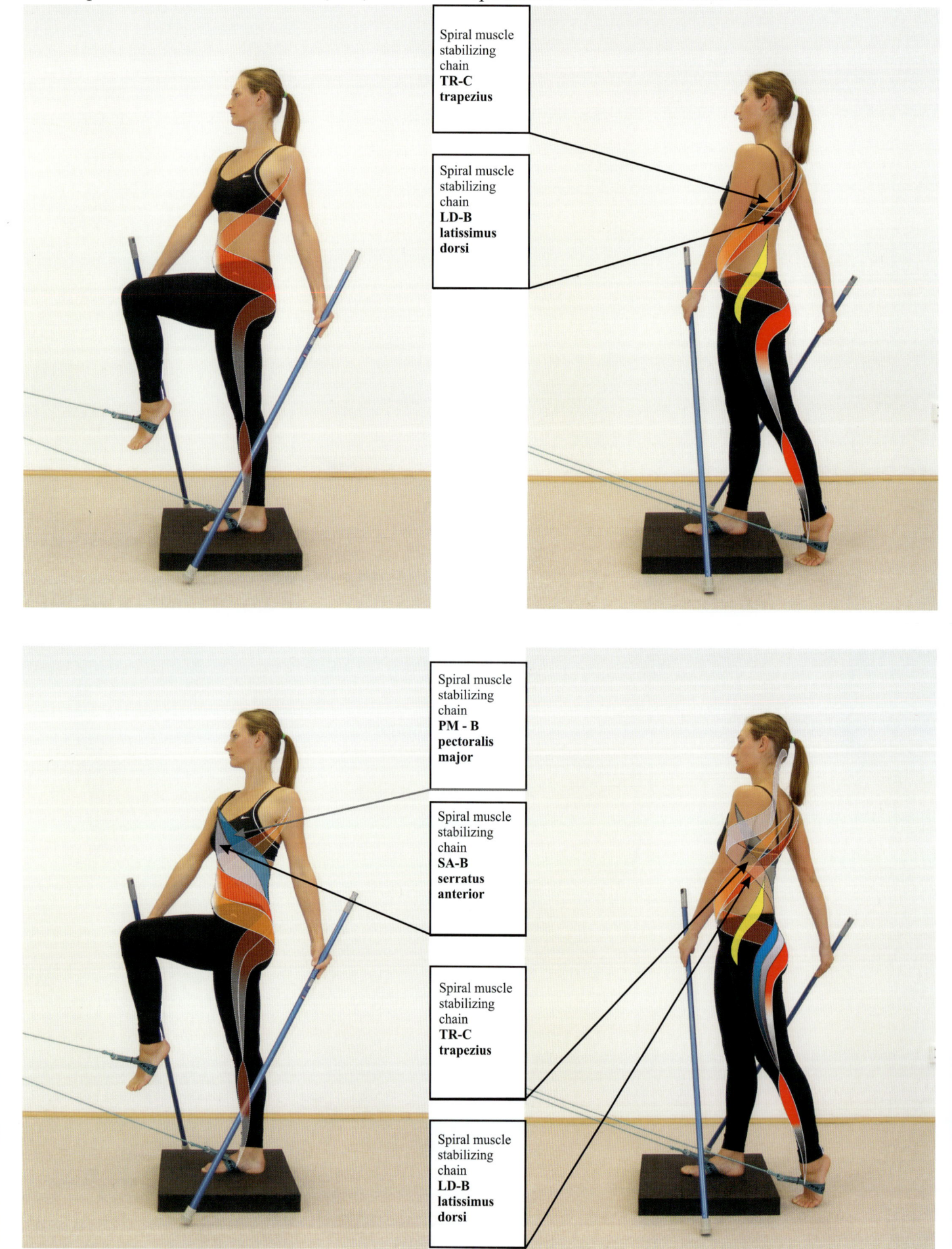

Spiral muscle stabilizing chain **TR-C trapezius**

Spiral muscle stabilizing chain **LD-B latissimus dorsi**

Spiral muscle stabilizing chain **PM - B pectoralis major**

Spiral muscle stabilizing chain **SA-B serratus anterior**

Spiral muscle stabilizing chain **TR-C trapezius**

Spiral muscle stabilizing chain **LD-B latissimus dorsi**

DISORDER OF MUSCLE RELAXATION
TP - trigger points
Fibromyalgia

Eliminating pathological muscle tension
Eliminating TP - trigger points

Muscle contraction and relaxation

Muscle, muscle cell, sarcomere

Skeletal transversely striated muscle
The muscle is located in a ligament sheet - muscle fascia.
The muscle is divided into muscle cords, which are separated by ligament.
The muscle contains a large number of muscle cells between which run arteries, veins and nerves.

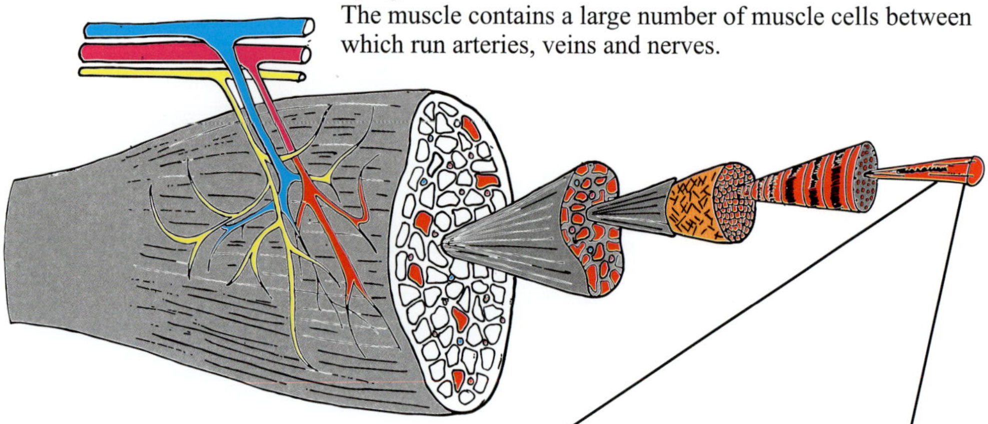

Muscle cell (myocytes)
The muscle cell contains a large number of sarcomeres - units which are able to contract and relax.

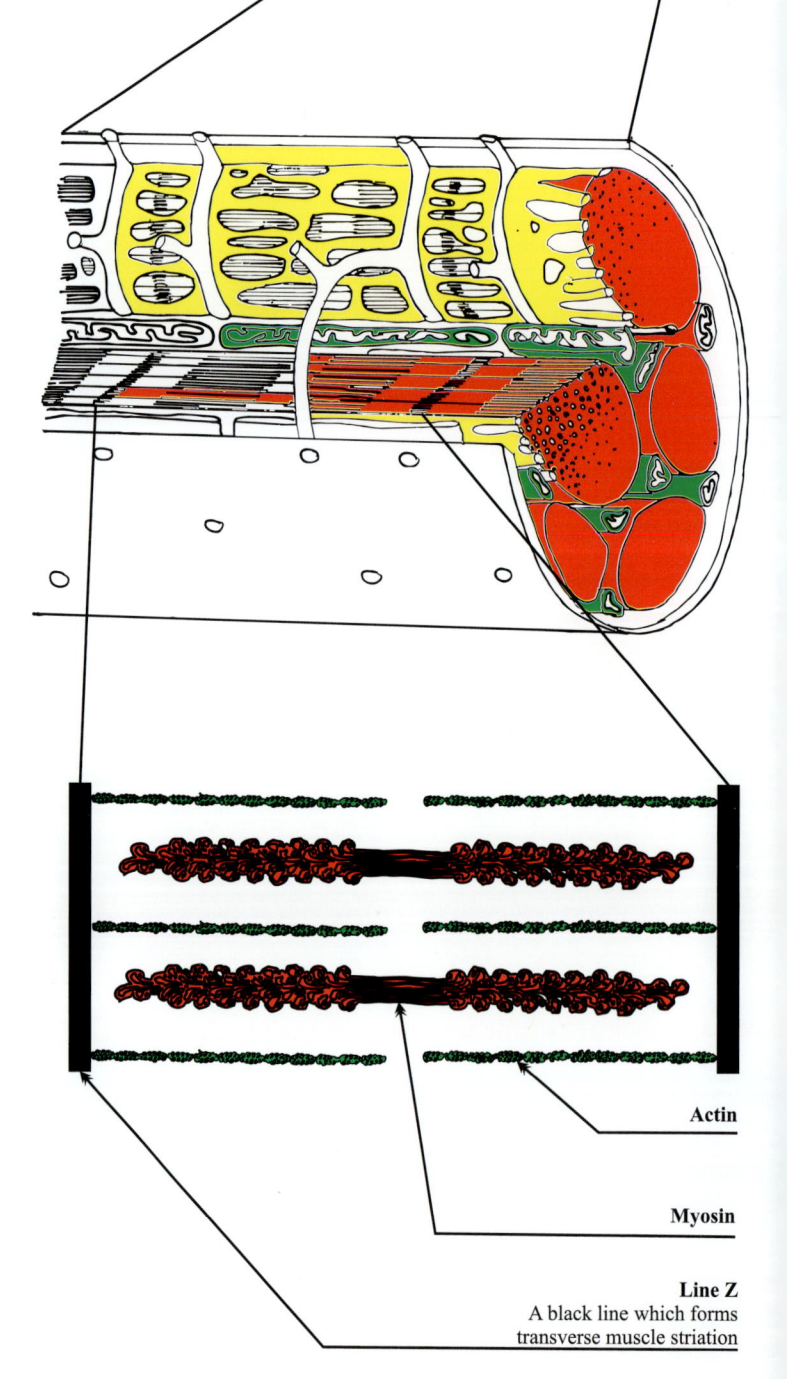

Sarcomere
A sacromere is a unit in which muscle contraction takes place. During contraction, the proteins actin and myosin bind.

Actin

Myosin

Line Z
A black line which forms transverse muscle striation

Muscle contraction and relaxation

Blood supply during muscle contraction and relaxation, muscle pump

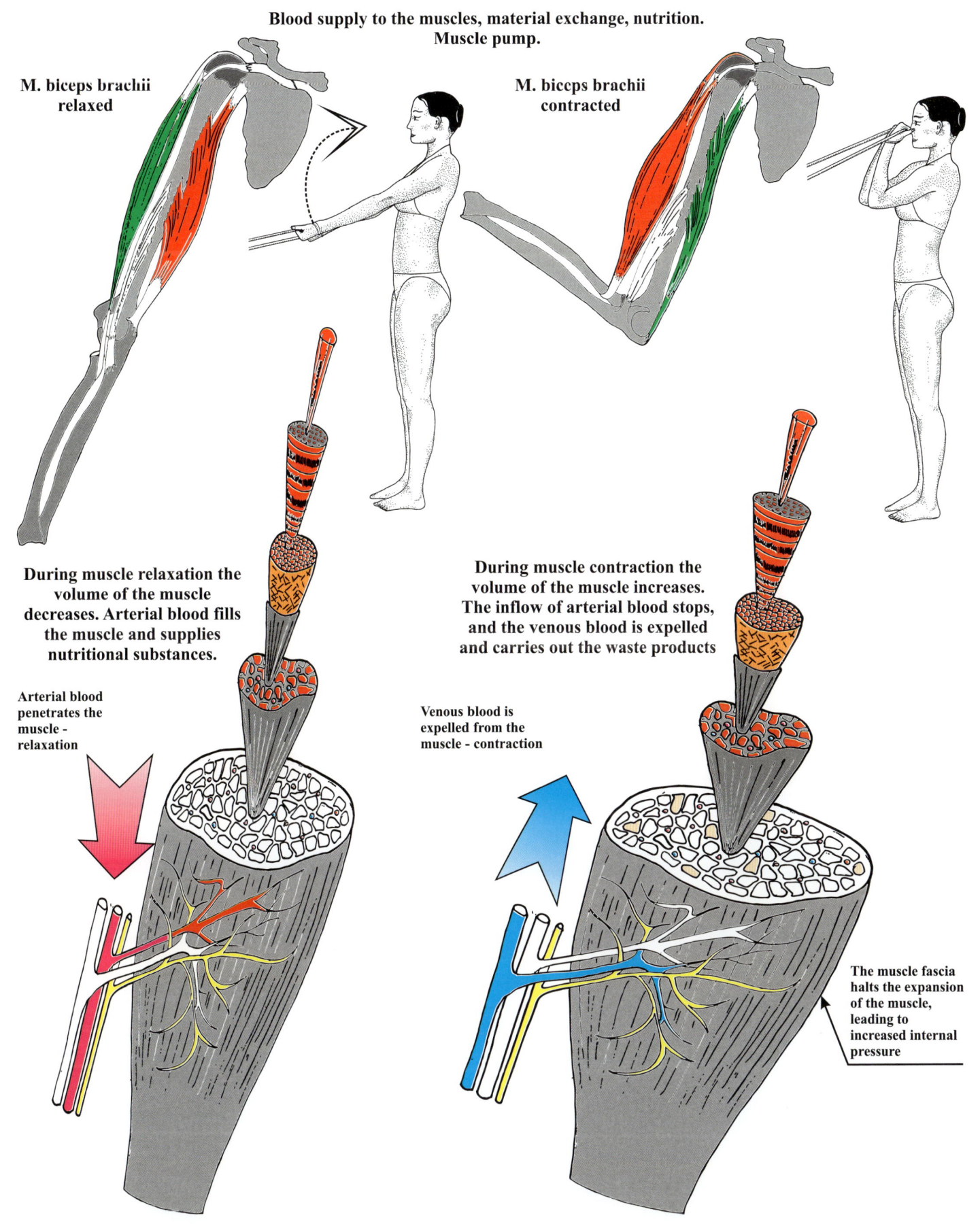

**Blood supply to the muscles, material exchange, nutrition.
Muscle pump.**

M. biceps brachii relaxed

M. biceps brachii contracted

During muscle relaxation the volume of the muscle decreases. Arterial blood fills the muscle and supplies nutritional substances.

Arterial blood penetrates the muscle - relaxation

During muscle contraction the volume of the muscle increases. The inflow of arterial blood stops, and the venous blood is expelled and carries out the waste products

Venous blood is expelled from the muscle - contraction

The muscle fascia halts the expansion of the muscle, leading to increased internal pressure

The transversely striated muscles need alternating contraction and relaxation.
The alternation of tension and relaxation of a muscle ensures a good blood supply and sufficient material exchange.
  When a muscle is tensed for a long time, the material exchange is disrupted and the muscle suffers an energy crisis.
The mitochondria located in the muscle do not have a sufficient supply of material for the metabolism and cannot create ATP (adenosine triphosphate) energy, which is necessary for muscle relaxation.
The muscle then remains permanently tense and prevents itself from having a good blood supply.
This leads to muscle degeneration.

Muscle contraction and relaxation

**Muscle contraction originates in the sarcomeres when the Z lines come closer together.
A sarcomere is a functional unit consisting of actin and myosin.
The edge of a sarcomere is delineated by black lines - striations.
The striations give skeletal muscle its appearance - transversely striated muscle.**

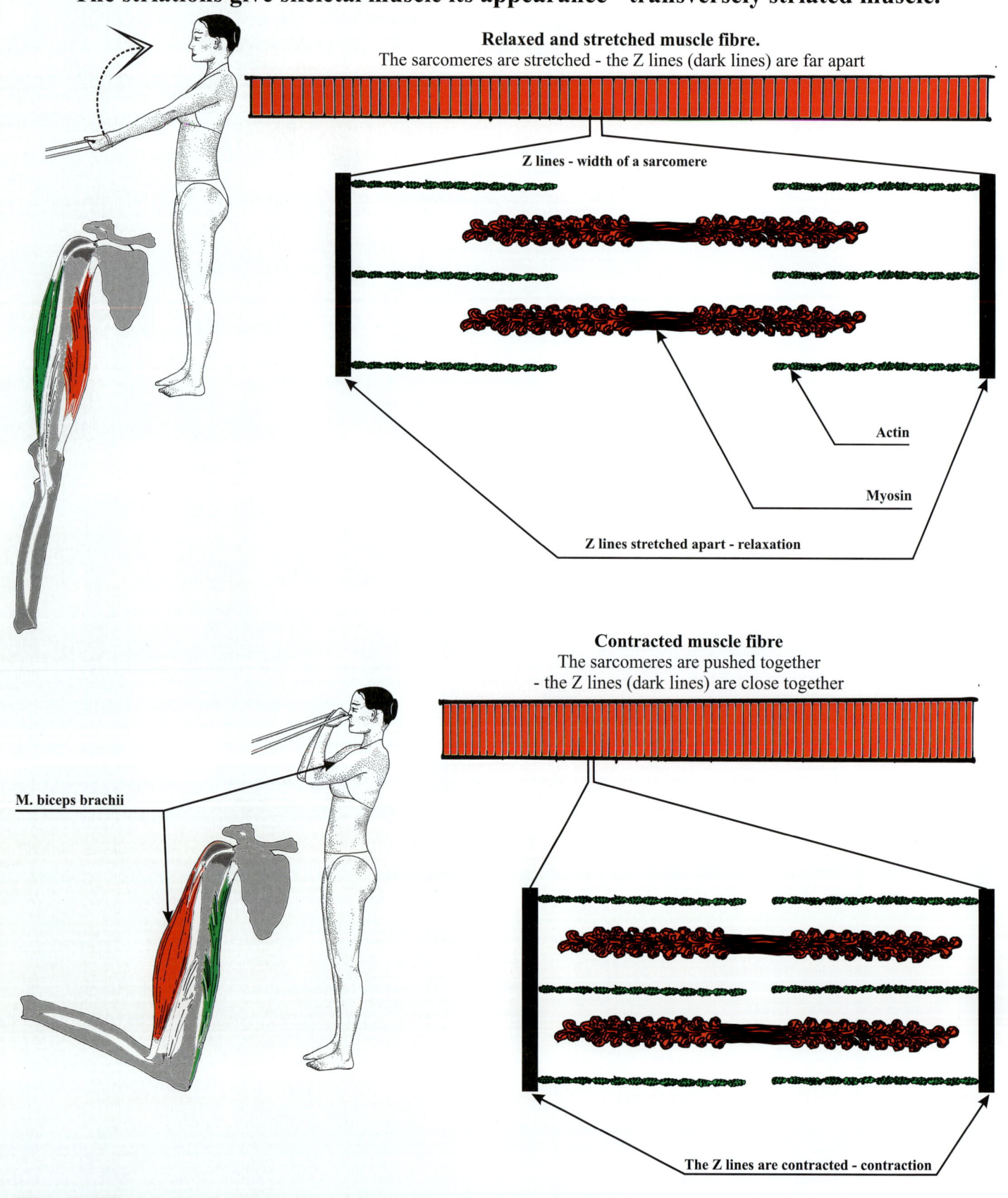

Relaxed and stretched muscle fibre.
The sarcomeres are stretched - the Z lines (dark lines) are far apart

Z lines - width of a sarcomere

Actin

Myosin

Z lines stretched apart - relaxation

Contracted muscle fibre
The sarcomeres are pushed together
- the Z lines (dark lines) are close together

M. biceps brachii

The Z lines are contracted - contraction

When the Z lines in the sarcomeres come closer together, the muscle contracts.
When the Z lines move apart, the muscle relaxes.

Muscle contraction and relaxation

Muscle contraction occurs when the black Z lines come closer together in the sarcomeres. The Z lines approach through the outflow of the Ca++ calcium ions from the endoplasmic reticulum between the actin and myosin, which bind chemically.
Muscle relaxation arises when the Z lines move apart.
Relaxation occurs after the expulsion of the Ca++ ions from the region of the sarcomeres to the endoplasmic reticulum.

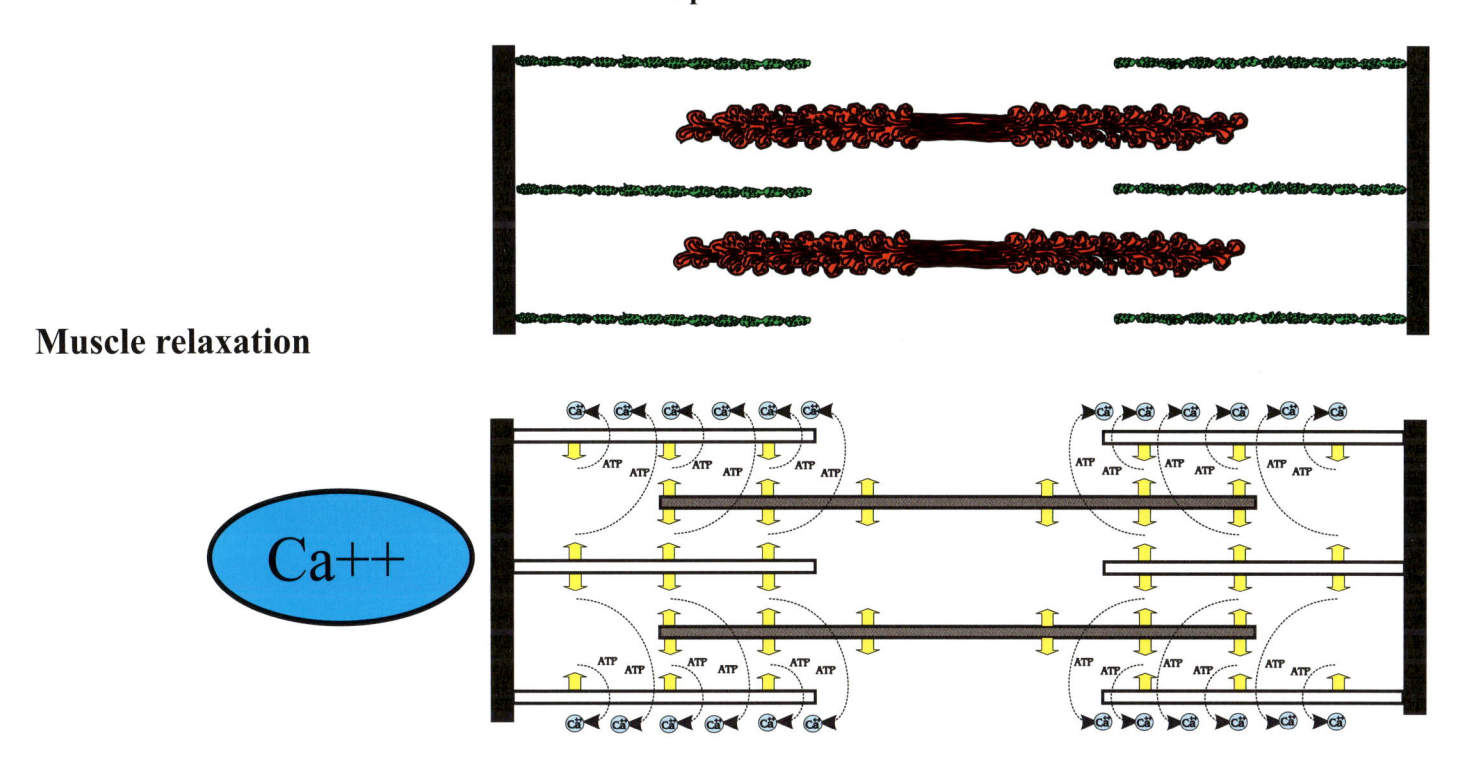

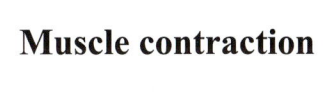

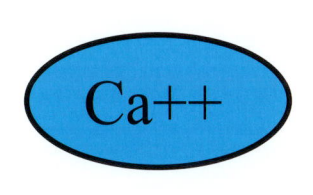

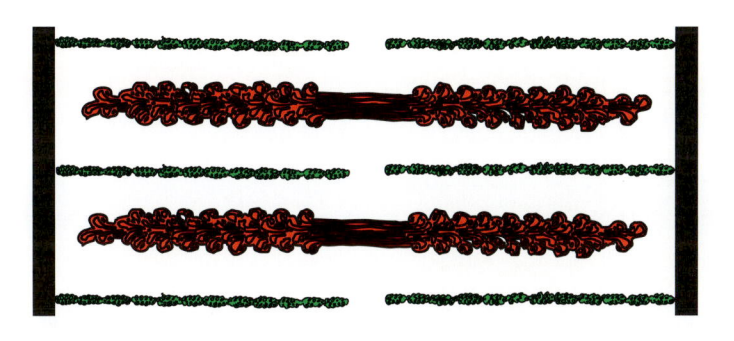

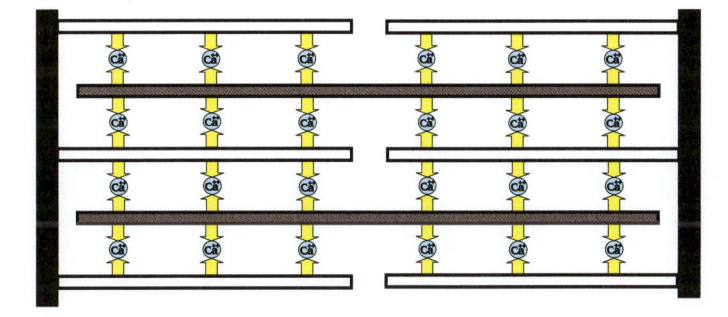

Muscle relaxation

Muscle contraction

Muscle contraction is caused by the outflow of Ca++ ions from the endoplasmic reticulum to the area between the actin and myosin. Muscle contraction is a not an energy-intensive process.
Muscle relaxation is caused by the pumping out of Ca++ions from the area between the actin and myosin into the endoplasmic reticulum. This is an active process known as the calcium pump. Pumping out the Ca++ ions requires a large amount of energy.
   An example of this is an exhausted sportsman who, after a long run, has no energy for relaxation and has, therefore, tense muscles and muscle cramp.

Muscle contraction and relaxation

Muscle contraction occurs when the Z lines come closer together in the sarcomeres. The Z lines approach through the outflow of the Ca++ calcium ions from the endoplasmic reticulum between the actin and myosin, which bind chemically.

Relaxed and stretched muscle fibres
The sarcomeres are stretched apart - the Z lines (dark lines) move far apart.
The calcium ions are pumped out into the endoplasmic reticulum.

Z lines - width of a sarcomere

Actin

Myosin

The Z lines are stretched - relaxation

Ca++ ions are pumped out into the endoplasmic reticulum. The proteins actin and myosin are free and can unbind and move apart.

The mitochondrion creates ATP energy in the Krebs cycle

The endoplasmic reticulum is the supplying, exporting and resorption organ for Ca++ ions.

M. triceps brachii

M. biceps brachii

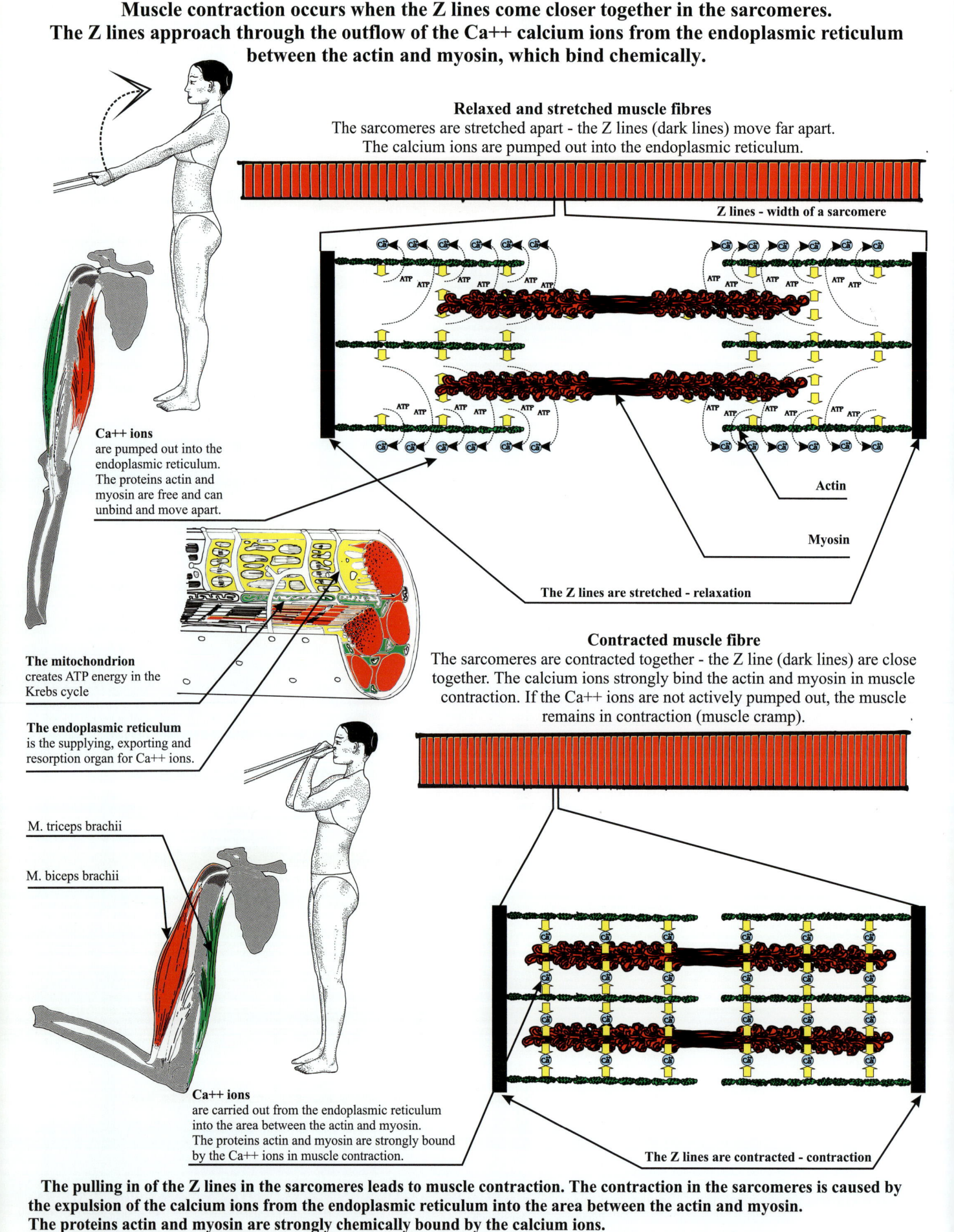

Contracted muscle fibre
The sarcomeres are contracted together - the Z line (dark lines) are close together. The calcium ions strongly bind the actin and myosin in muscle contraction. If the Ca++ ions are not actively pumped out, the muscle remains in contraction (muscle cramp).

Ca++ ions are carried out from the endoplasmic reticulum into the area between the actin and myosin. The proteins actin and myosin are strongly bound by the Ca++ ions in muscle contraction.

The Z lines are contracted - contraction

The pulling in of the Z lines in the sarcomeres leads to muscle contraction. The contraction in the sarcomeres is caused by the expulsion of the calcium ions from the endoplasmic reticulum into the area between the actin and myosin. The proteins actin and myosin are strongly chemically bound by the calcium ions.
The stretching apart of the Z lines leads to muscle relaxation. The calcium pump expels calcium ions from the area between the actin and myosin into the endoplasmic reticulum. The pumping of the calcium ions is an energy-intensive process which requires ATP (adenosine triphosphate) energy, which is produced in the neighbouring mitochondrion.
The mitochondrion requires a good blood supply to the muscle to have a sufficient supply of substances (glucose, lipids and oxygen) to create ATP.

Muscle contraction and relaxation

Muscle cells, organelles - mitochondrion, endoplasmic reticulum, muscle fibres

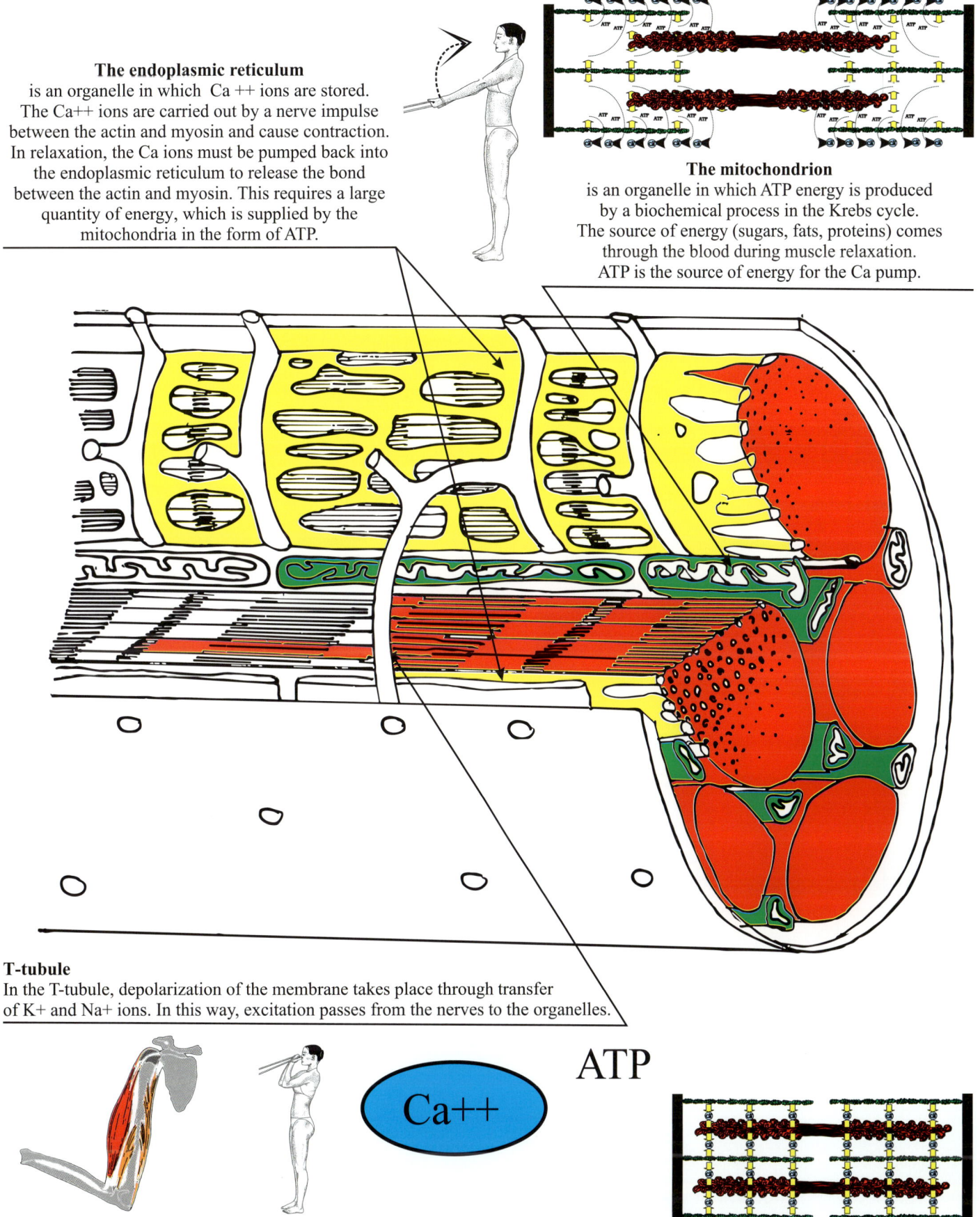

The endoplasmic reticulum
is an organelle in which Ca ++ ions are stored. The Ca++ ions are carried out by a nerve impulse between the actin and myosin and cause contraction. In relaxation, the Ca ions must be pumped back into the endoplasmic reticulum to release the bond between the actin and myosin. This requires a large quantity of energy, which is supplied by the mitochondria in the form of ATP.

The mitochondrion
is an organelle in which ATP energy is produced by a biochemical process in the Krebs cycle. The source of energy (sugars, fats, proteins) comes through the blood during muscle relaxation. ATP is the source of energy for the Ca pump.

T-tubule
In the T-tubule, depolarization of the membrane takes place through transfer of K+ and Na+ ions. In this way, excitation passes from the nerves to the organelles.

Ca++   ATP

The pulling in of the Z lines in the sarcomeres leads to muscle contraction. The contraction in the sarcomeres is caused by the expulsion of the calcium ions from the endoplasmic reticulum into the area between the actin and myosin. The proteins actin and myosin are strongly chemically bound by the calcium ions.

The stretching apart of the Z lines leads to muscle relaxation. The calcium pump expels calcium ions from the area between the acin and myosin into the endoplasmic reticulum. The pumping of the calcium ions is an energy-intensive process that requires ATP energy (adenosine triphosphate), which is produced in the neighbouring mitochondrion. The mitochondrion requires a good blood supply to the muscle to have a sufficient supply of substances (glucose, lipids and oxygen) to create ATP.

Muscle contraction and relaxation

TP - Trigger point

TP arises when there is a poor supply of blood to the muscle and an insufficient transfer of nutrients to the muscle cell. Because of a disorder of the vascular supply, the exchange of materials is disrupted, as is the nutrition of the muscle. The mitochondria do not have enough energy resources to create ATP , and the muscle suffers an energy crisis. The muscle does not have enough energy to relax. The calcium ions remain between the actin and myosin and the muscle is blocked in contraction (tension). The muscle tension prevents the supply of blood to the muscles. Over vigorous stretching of the muscle can damage it. Stretching exercises are, therefore, completely inappropriate in this situation.

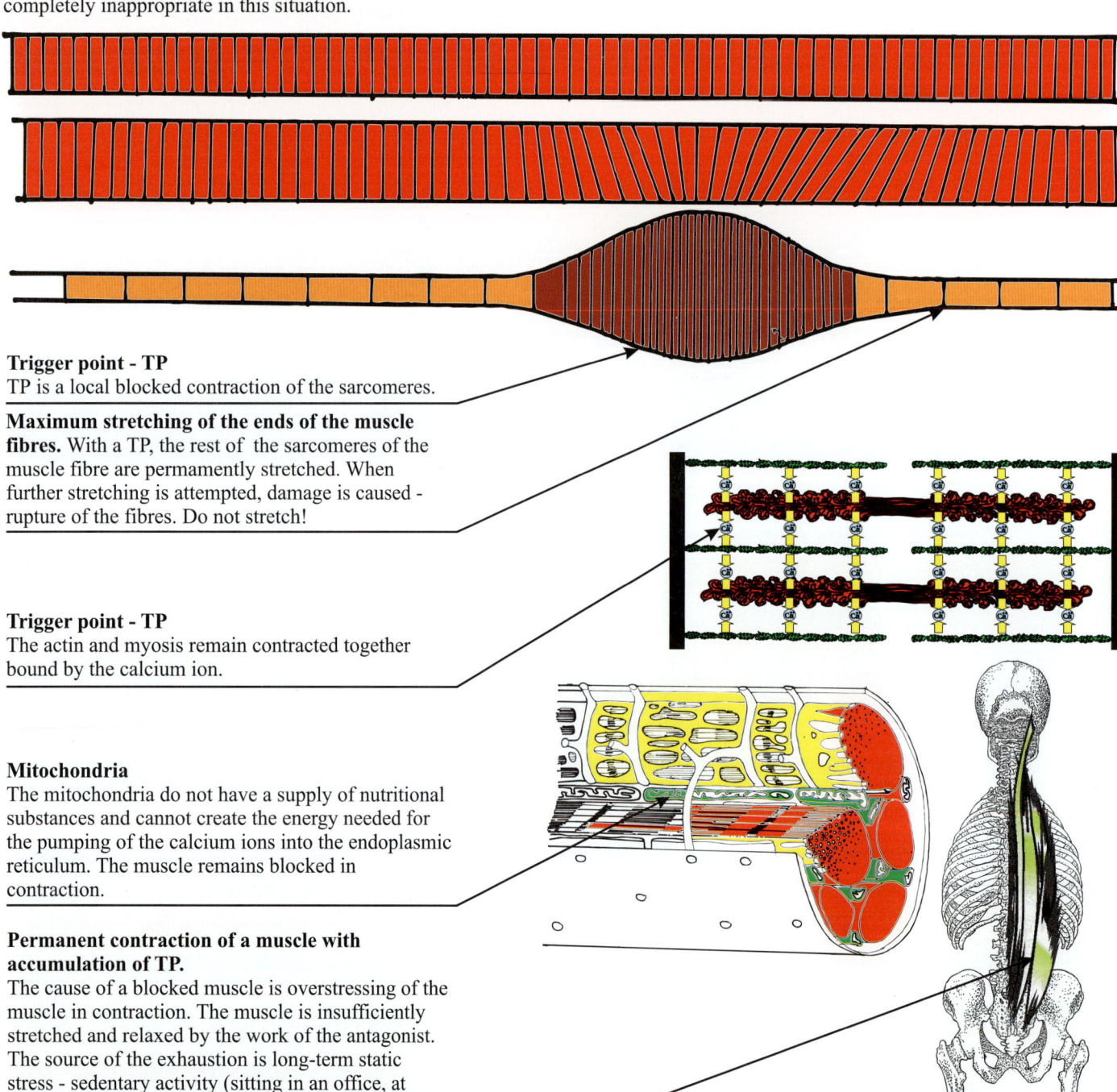

Trigger point - TP
TP is a local blocked contraction of the sarcomeres.

Maximum stretching of the ends of the muscle fibres. With a TP, the rest of the sarcomeres of the muscle fibre are permanently stretched. When further stretching is attempted, damage is caused - rupture of the fibres. Do not stretch!

Trigger point - TP
The actin and myosis remain contracted together bound by the calcium ion.

Mitochondria
The mitochondria do not have a supply of nutritional substances and cannot create the energy needed for the pumping of the calcium ions into the endoplasmic reticulum. The muscle remains blocked in contraction.

Permanent contraction of a muscle with accumulation of TP.
The cause of a blocked muscle is overstressing of the muscle in contraction. The muscle is insufficiently stretched and relaxed by the work of the antagonist. The source of the exhaustion is long-term static stress - sedentary activity (sitting in an office, at school, in a car), bodybuilding without sufficient regeneration, sports with one-sided stress (hockey, floorball, tennis, golf).

An accumulation of TPs causes a stiff, painful point in the muscle. The muscle loses its ability to stretch and also to contract. The sufferer loses mobility, and his work and sports performance declines. The tense points are painful. When 18 painful points in different quadrants are identified, the situation is called fibromyalgia syndrome. The patient feels pain, but according to laboratory tests, X-rays and MRI there are no signs of pathology. He is often considered to be a malingerer. After a long period of muscle tension and poor nutrition, the muscle atrophies, the TP s become necrotized (myogelosis), and the muscle is transformed into inactive and stiff ligament. The ligament tissue over-stresses the spine and joints, which are contracted together. In the region of the spine, herniations of the intervertebral discs occur, as well as deformity of the vertebral units (spondylosis) and intervertebral joints (spondylarthrosis). In the region of the large joints, this leads to disruption of the cartilage and arthrosis. The stiff, tense muscles do not have a sufficient blood supply, and the mitochondria do not consume the sugars and fats. These fats and sugars therefore accumulate in the blood vessels. The levels of sugars and fats can be measured in a laboratory. Increased levels are diagnosed as type 2 diabetes and dyslipidemia. The correct way to solve this situation is a very gentle movement programme to activate the agonists, relax the antagonists and ensure their blood supply. Only after several days of relaxation exercises can we begin to stretch the muscles slightly. The movement therapy must be regular (daily) and long-term (life-long). Relaxation and improved blood supply to the muscles are assisted by relaxation massage.

Muscle contraction and relaxation
Accumulation of TP trigger points - fibromyalgia

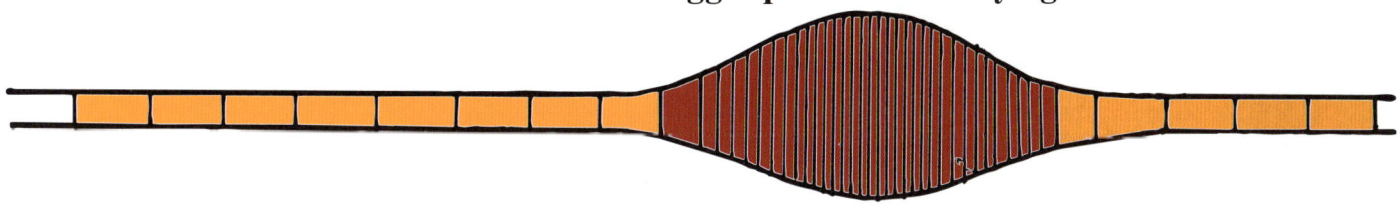

Locomotor apparatus - muscles, joint, spine
Trigger point - TP
Impact of TPs on the muscle cells:
Long-term persistent contraction and stretching cause damage to the sarcomeres.
There is damage to the affected muscle fibres.
The TPs prevent the healthy muscle fibres located in the region from functioning. This reduces the performance of the muscles.
Pain develops.
Increased stretching of fibres and permanent contraction is registered by the proprioceptors, while constant information from the muscles with TPs is registered by the CNS and leads to greater pain.
Muscles with permanent contraction have a poor blood supply. The metabolism in the cells is predominantly anaerobic, and acidic metabolic products are created. The acidic environment irritates the nerve endings and also leads to pain.
Impact of the TPs on the joints:
TPs damage the joints. Increased muscle tension compresses the joints. This restricts mobility. Increased muscle tension at the end of a movement halts the movement and intensively contracts the joint. The joint is mechanically damaged and ischemia occurs. Ischemia accelerates degeneration of the joint. This is first manifested in damage to the soft tissue (meniscus, cartilage of the joint), and later in deformity of the bones and the growth of osteophytes. Asymmetric muscle tension in the region of a joint disrupts the optimal position of the joint - decentration of the joint. An asymmetrically positioned joint degenerates more on the compressed side. A disorder of one joint causes the decentration of other joints.
Impact of TPs on the spine:
TPs damage the intervertebral discs. Compression of the intervertebral discs by the muscles located in front of, behind and along the spine (paravertebral muscles) leads to disruption of the nutrition of the discs through diffusion.
The discs degenerate and rupture - disc herniation. Later, the intervertebral joints become deformed - spondylarthrosis - as do the vertebral units - spondylosis.
Impact of the TPs on muscle performance:
Because of the blockage of a muscle in contraction, the number of muscle fibres which can contract is reduced and sports performance is reduced.
The TPs prevent the effective functioning of the muscle, causing rapid muscle fatigue.
Impact of TPs on the control of movement:
The TPs, which continually inform the CNS about the contraction of the muscles, cause disruption to the prioprioceptor information for the brain's control centre. On the basis of faulty information, the brain changes the stereotypical movement patterns. After some time, pathological movement patterns become fixed. The TPs make the muscle very irritable, and provoke the muscle spindle defensive reflex prematurely, thus continuing to prevent the relaxation and stretching of the muscle as well as its blood supply and nutrition. A vicious circle thus gradually develops.
Impact of the TPs on the whole metabolism:
TPs disrupt the nutrition of the whole muscle. The muscle, which is in contraction, is compressed in its ligament sheath.
Muscle ischemia occurs. Waste products accumulate in the muscle. The acidic products make the muscle more irritable and increase muscle tension. Because of the restricted ability to supply blood to the muscle, an accumulation of energy resources occurs in the blood outside the muscle - hyperglycemia and hyperlipoproteinemia. This is the basis for the development of type 2 diabetes and disruption of the metabolism of fats. These are the factors for the development of ischemic heart disease.
Impact on the cardiovascular system:
Increased muscle resistance leads to increased filling pressure and causes hypertension.
The blood filling pressure is greater for tense muscles and the vegetative system activates the sympathicus - sympathicotonia - and increases the strength of heart contraction. This is manifested in hypertension.
One organ which is very sensitive to a lack of nutrition and oxygen is the brain. Tension in the neck muscles and a projecting head posture inhibit the blood supply to the brain in the region of the arteria vertebralis and arteria carotis. The brain must be more strongly supplied with blood, with greater blood pressure, which comes from greater contraction of the heart.
This is a further reason for the development of hypertension.
Impact on the pulmonary system:
The lungs are squeezed by muscle tension in an immobile chest. The loss of mobility of the chest is caused by tension in the m. iliocostalis, m. semispinalis capitis and m. pectoralis minor. TPs worsen the vital capacity of the lungs, and the blood is insufficiently oxygenated. The compression of the lungs forces the right-hand part of the heart to work harder and causes its over-stressing.
Impact on the CNS - central nervous system:
An insufficient blood supply to the CNS leads to a feeling of fatigue, depression, burn-out syndrome and headaches.
The brain is constantly overloaded by an increased flow of information from tense muscles all over the body - information stress.
Processing this information requires increased brain activity, which needs a good supply of blood to the brain.

General over-stressing of the organism occurs.

Conclusion:
   The occurrence of TPs is the main cause of type 2 diabetes mellitus, hypertension, arteriosclerosis, ischemic heart disease, obesity, and metabolic syndrome. The correct solution is a long-term movement programme to activate muscle activity in the whole body.

Muscle contraction and relaxation

TP trigger points - fibromyalgia - causal treatment
Trigger point - TP

Disruption of the blood supply to a muscle, disruption of material exchange, disruption of nutrition. The muscle does not have energy for relaxation.

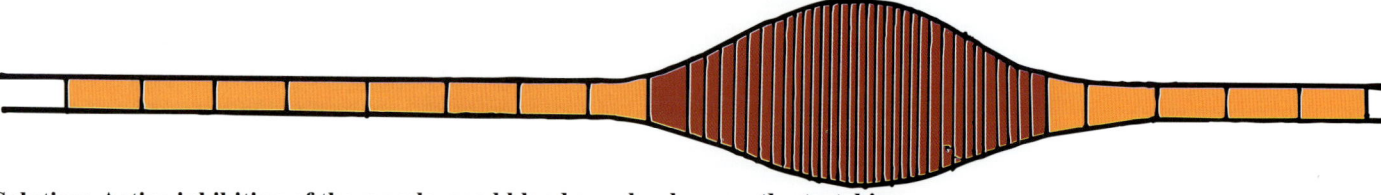

Solution: Active inhibition of the muscle, good blood supply, slow, gentle stretching.
- **reciprocal inhibition** in the region of:
  - a joint
  - a muscle girdle
  - the whole body - the muscle chains - exercise in a standing position is necessary
- **ensuring the blood supply:**
  - alternating moderate contraction with relaxation and appropriate stretching
  - engaging the muscle using little strength to avoid energy exhaustion
- **stretching:**
  - slow completion of the exercises in extreme positions to avoid the muscle spindle reflex
  - thorough stretching of the muscles, at first just slightly, then, after a warm-up, stretching to the extreme positions which are possible at that moment
  - extensive movement
  - fluent movement backwards and forwards. In the exercises there are no held positions which do not support the blood supply, and which are held with too much force when there are muscle imbalances.

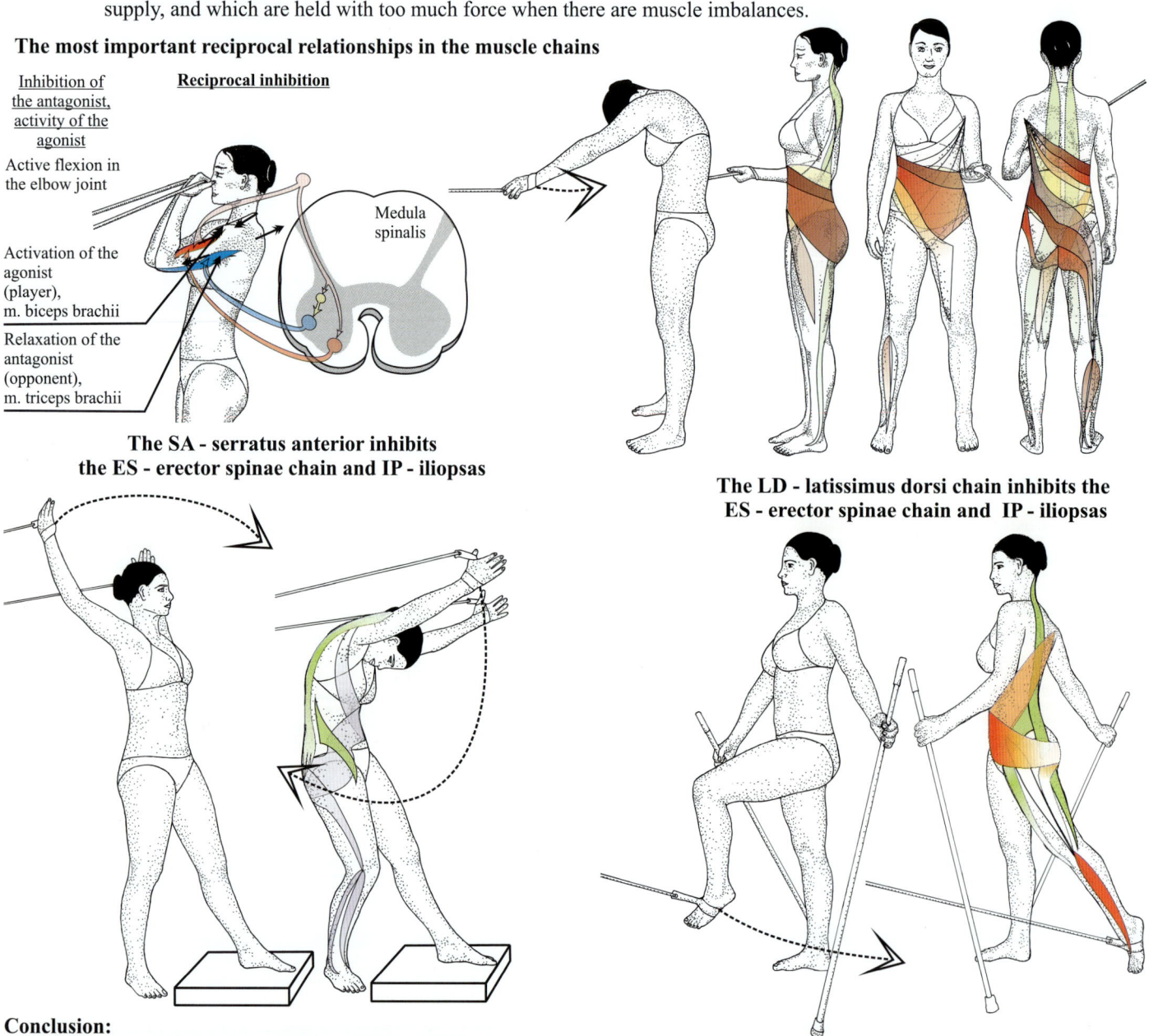

The most important reciprocal relationships in the muscle chains

Inhibition of the antagonist, activity of the agonist
Active flexion in the elbow joint
Activation of the agonist (player), m. biceps brachii
Relaxation of the antagonist (opponent), m. triceps brachii

Reciprocal inhibition
Medula spinalis

The SA - serratus anterior inhibits the ES - erector spinae chain and IP - iliopsas

The LD - latissimus dorsi chain inhibits the ES - erector spinae chain and IP - iliopsas

Conclusion:
It is the optimal form of condition training which regenerates the muscle tissue and eliminates TPs and is the primary form of treatment and prevention of type 2 diabetes, arteriosclerosis, ischemic heart disease, obesity and metabolic syndrome. In Germany, this movement programme is used preventively (the back school) and therapeutically (rehabilitative sport) for patients with fibromyalgia or cardiovascular disease.

DISORDER OF SPIRAL STABILIZATION
FBS - failed back surgery syndrome
Complications following an operation on an intervertebral disc

Treatment of FBS
Eliminating the negative factors
which lead to FBS

FB syndrome - failed back surgery syndrome
Aggravated back pain after an operation on the spine

A failing abdomen in front, a failing spine at the back - that is a clinical picture of back pain after an operation on the spine. The abdominal muscles are not strengthened by an operation, but through exercise. The choice of treatment of the causes of back failure is therefore clear. The abdominal muscles must be strengthened in cooperation with the other muscles which form the spiral stabilizing muscle corset - spiral stabilization of the spine. Tension in the back muscles must be relieved. The transverse muscle and the oblique abdominal muscles must be strengthened, not the straight muscles. This can be achieved only in a standing position by connecting the activity of the arm and leg with the abdominal muscles. We call the connection of muscle activity on the surface of the body "spiral stabilization", because the muscle chains are in the form of a descending spiral which constricts the girth and creates an upward force which increases the space between the vertebrae and regenerates the intervertebral discs and joint.

Because this principle is unknown to therapists and not used, problems develop after operations on the spine.

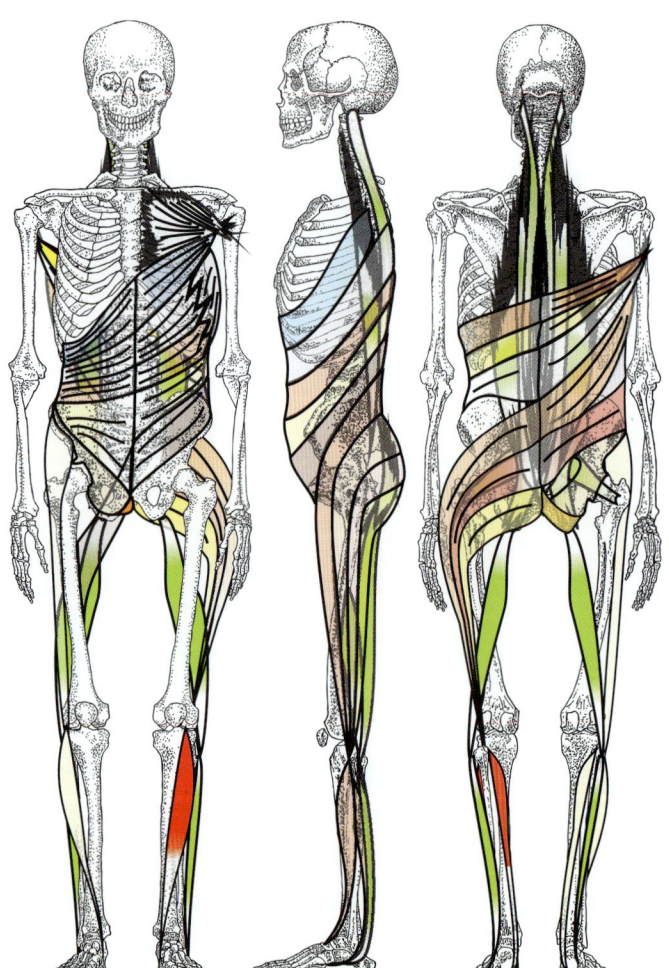

A failing abdomen in front, a failing spine at the back

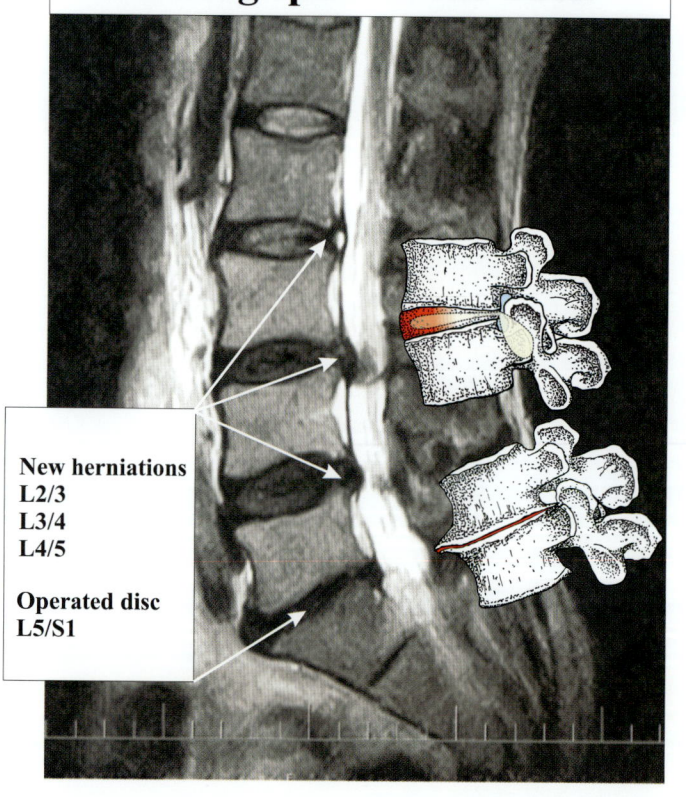

New herniations
L2/3
L3/4
L4/5

Operated disc
L5/S1

FB syndrome is a set of problems following a spinal operation which do not have a single cause. As the number of spinal operations increases, so does the number of failures. The current therapeutic approaches do not know how to deal with this disorder, so there are repeated operations. The patient's state of health usually worsens after further operations because the level of disability increases, while the cause of the problem is not eliminated. In affected patients we see a range of negative factors which lead to over-stressing of the spine after an operation. If we manage to eliminate these negative factors, it is usually possible to improve significantly or completely cure the patient's clinical state.

X-rays and MRI reveal a relapse of herniation in the same segment, over-stressing of that segment's intervertebral joints, closure of the foramina by a projection of the joint often enlarged by arthrosis, over-stressing of a vertebral unit and its productive change - spondylosis, folding in the ligamentum flavum, which closes the foramen, contraction of the nerve root by a scar, and touching vertebral processes.

An operation disrupts the structure of the muscles and the resulting scar disrupts their functioning.

In the neighbouring segments, because of the blockade in the operated segment, there is an increased demand on their functioning, causing over-stressing and accelerated degeneration. The neighbouring segments are mostly already affected by partial degeneration and so rapidly succumb to decay.

We nearly always find a disorder of the spiral stabilization of the spine caused by the muscle chain TR - trapezius, LD - latissimus dorsi A, B, C and a disorder of the reciprocal inhibition of the vertical chains ES - erector spinae, QL - quadratus lumborum and IP - iliopsoas.

Spiral stabilization of the spine enables therapeutic exercise at all stages of the body at the same time and can therefore eliminate many negative factors at the same time. That is why spiral stabilization is the method of choice for this multi-factor disease.

In our article we shall try to show the various negative factors which over-stress the spine and lead to FB syndrome. At the same time, we shall show the way to eliminate them in our pre-operation rehabilitation plan and the following rehabilitation plan.

1st negative factor
- shortened muscles in the anterior part of the shoulder girdle

Shortened muscles in the anterior part of the shoulder girdle:

M. subclavius
M. pectoralis minor
M. serratus anterior

Disrupted activation of the abdominal muscles by the LD latissimus dorsi chain

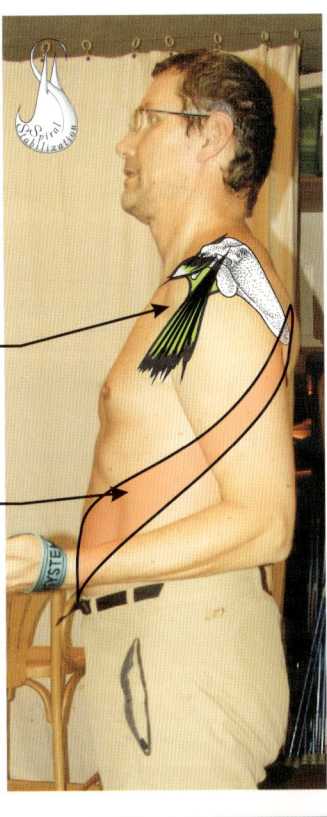

Shortened muscles:
- M. subclavius
- M. serratus anterior
- M. pectoralis minor

Weakened muscles:
- M. serratus anterior
- M. trapezius
- M. latissimus dorsi

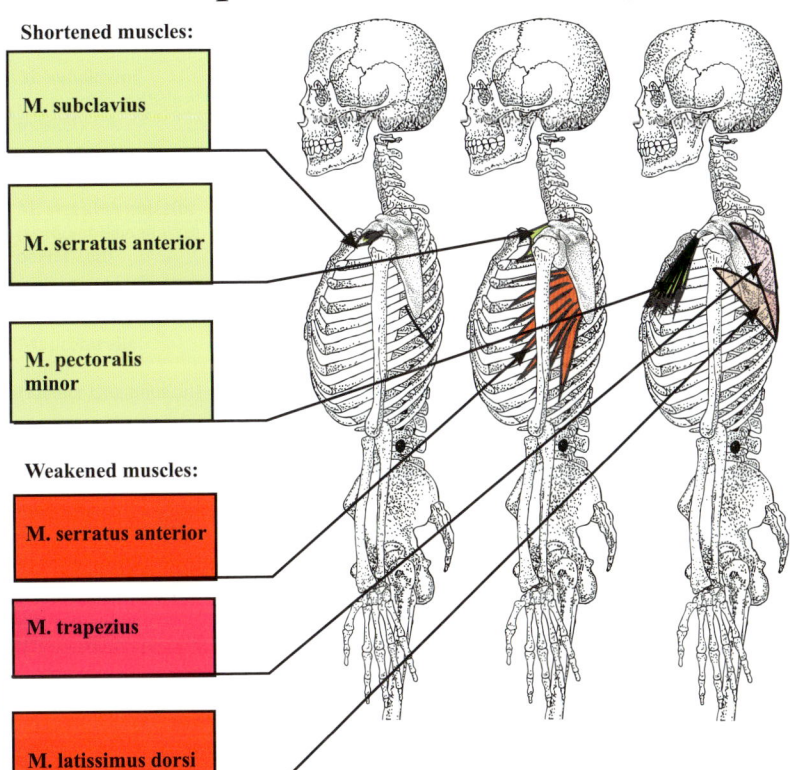

Incorrect performance of the exercise at the beginning:
The shoulder blade stays in front - protraction and up - elevation. This prevents activation of the abdomen by the TR and LD chains. Here it is necessary to halt the movement to avoid over-stressing of the back in the lumbar and cervical regions.

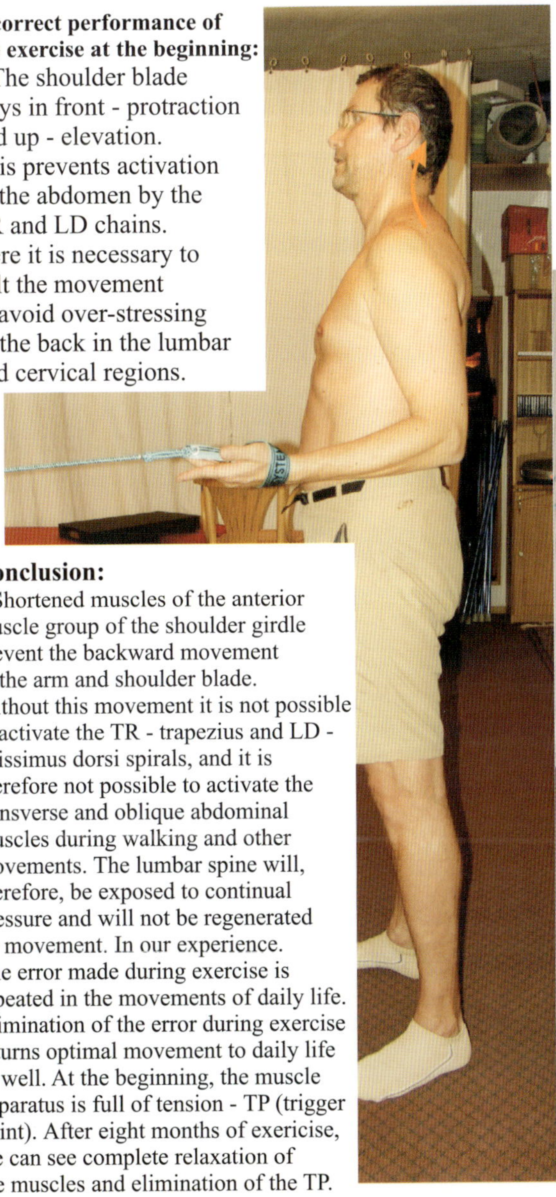

Optimal performance of the exercise:
This exercise relaxes and stretches the muscles in the anterior part of the shoulder girdle and activates the oblique abdominal muscles through the TR and LD chains.

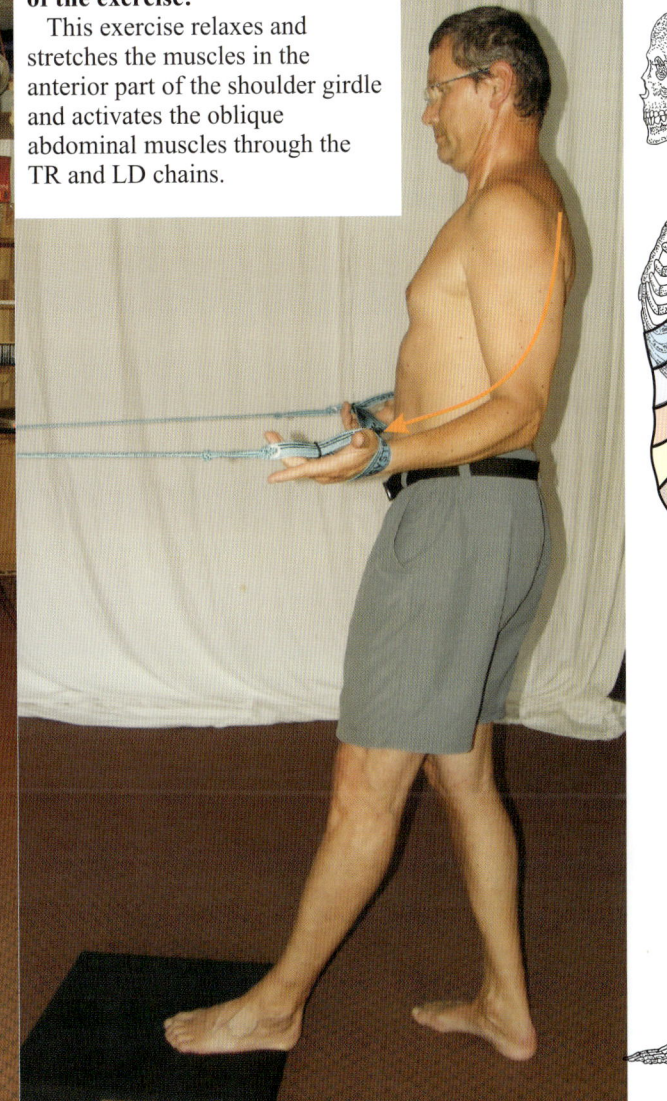

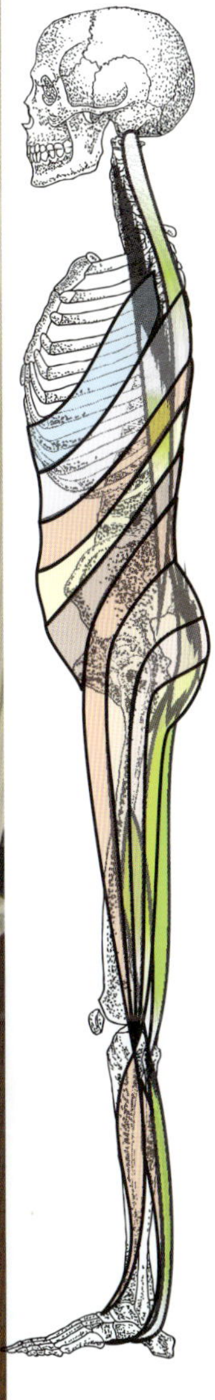

Conclusion:
Shortened muscles of the anterior muscle group of the shoulder girdle prevent the backward movement of the arm and shoulder blade. Without this movement it is not possible to activate the TR - trapezius and LD - latissimus dorsi spirals, and it is therefore not possible to activate the transverse and oblique abdominal muscles during walking and other movements. The lumbar spine will, therefore, be exposed to continual pressure and will not be regenerated by movement. In our experience. The error made during exercise is repeated in the movements of daily life. Elimination of the error during exercise returns optimal movement to daily life as well. At the beginning, the muscle apparatus is full of tension - TP (trigger point). After eight months of exercise, we can see complete relaxation of the muscles and elimination of the TP.

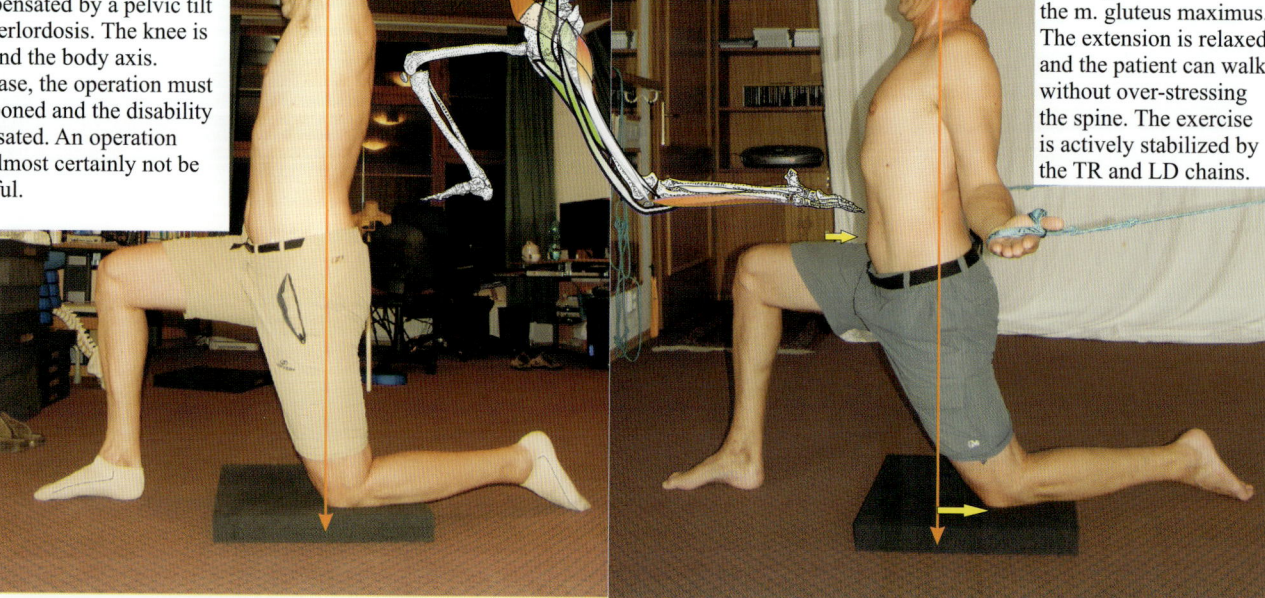

2nd negative factor
- shortened muscles in the anterior part of the pelvic girdle

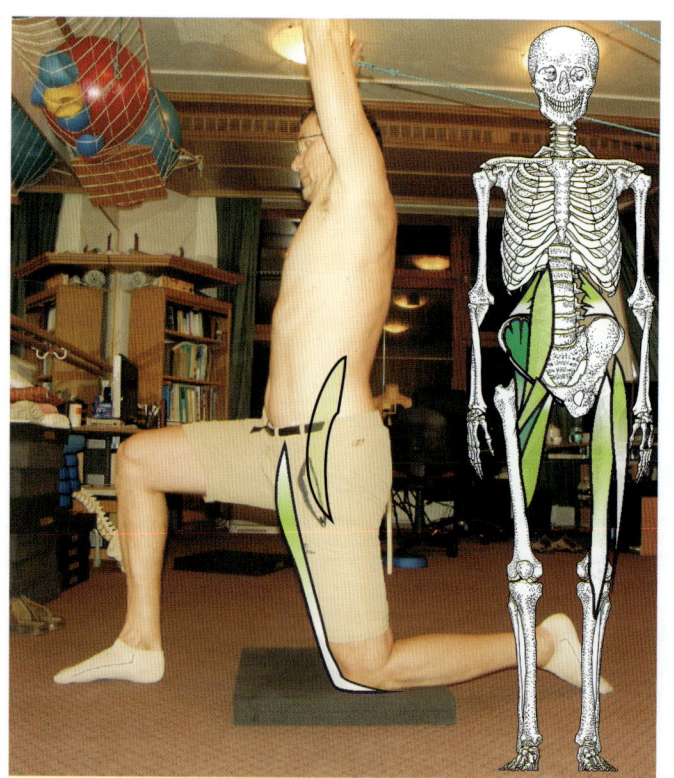

Shortened muscles:

- M. psoas major
- M. iliacus
- M. quadratus lumborum
- M. tensor fasciae latae
- M. rectus femoris
- M. pectineus
- M. adductor brevis
- M. adductor longus

Conclusion:

Tension in the hip flexors is caused by a sedentary life-style or inappropriate sport. The flexors restrict extension in the hip joint. During walking, the backward movement of the leg at the hip is halted by tension in the flexors and is compensated by the bending of the lumbar spine into hyperlordosis. This compresses the spine and causes damage. At the same time, the hip joint is over-stressed. The shortening of the flexors is then a joint cause of discopathy and arthrosis of the hip joint.

The muscles of the pelvic girdle and leg are the largest muscle mass in the human body. An accumulation of trigger points and blocking of the muscles in tension disrupt the metabolism of the whole of the human organism.

Incorrect performance of the exercise at the beginning:

The extent of movement does not enable extension in the hip joint. Further movement would be compensated by a pelvic tilt and hyperlordosis. The knee is not behind the body axis.
In this case, the operation must be postponed and the disability compensated. An operation would almost certainly not be successful.

Optimal performance of the exercise:

This exercise relaxes and stretches the muscles of the anterior part of the pelvic girdle and activates the m. gluteus maximus. The extension is relaxed and the patient can walk without over-stressing the spine. The exercise is actively stabilized by the TR and LD chains.

- 202 -

3rd negative factor
- shortened vertical back muscles

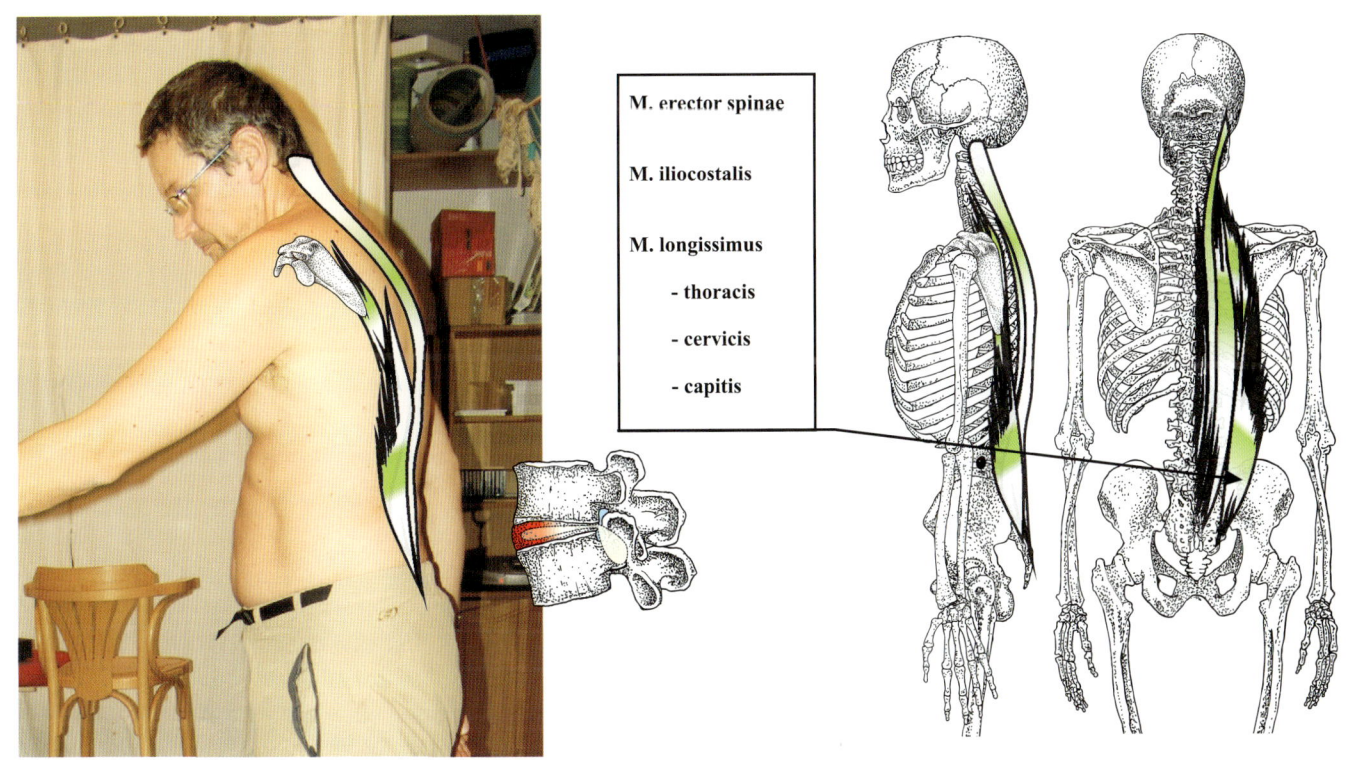

M. erector spinae

M. iliocostalis

M. longissimus
- thoracis
- cervicis
- capitis

Conclusion:

Increased tension in the m. erector spinae compresses the spine and prevents its regeneration. It is the main muscle which causes back pain. This muscle needs consistent relaxation and stretching. Some therapists, wrongly, strengthen it, thus worsening the patient's state of health. It should be noted that sit-ups strengthen and shorten this muscle, thus damaging the spine.

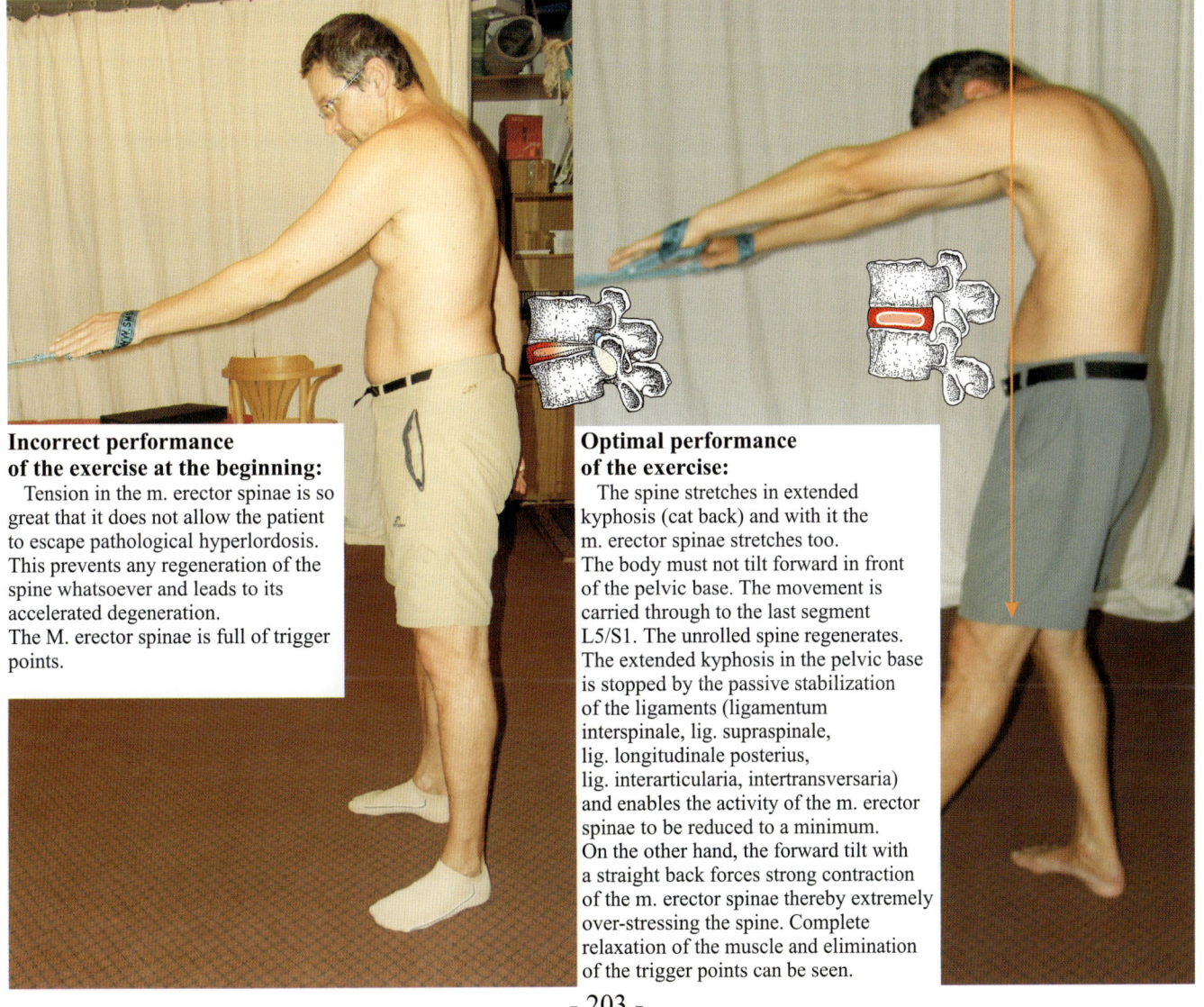

Incorrect performance of the exercise at the beginning:

Tension in the m. erector spinae is so great that it does not allow the patient to escape pathological hyperlordosis. This prevents any regeneration of the spine whatsoever and leads to its accelerated degeneration.
The M. erector spinae is full of trigger points.

Optimal performance of the exercise:

The spine stretches in extended kyphosis (cat back) and with it the m. erector spinae stretches too. The body must not tilt forward in front of the pelvic base. The movement is carried through to the last segment L5/S1. The unrolled spine regenerates. The extended kyphosis in the pelvic base is stopped by the passive stabilization of the ligaments (ligamentum interspinale, lig. supraspinale, lig. longitudinale posterius, lig. interarticularia, intertransversaria) and enables the activity of the m. erector spinae to be reduced to a minimum. On the other hand, the forward tilt with a straight back forces strong contraction of the m. erector spinae thereby extremely over-stressing the spine. Complete relaxation of the muscle and elimination of the trigger points can be seen.

4th negative factor
- shortened muscles in the posterior part of the pelvic girdle

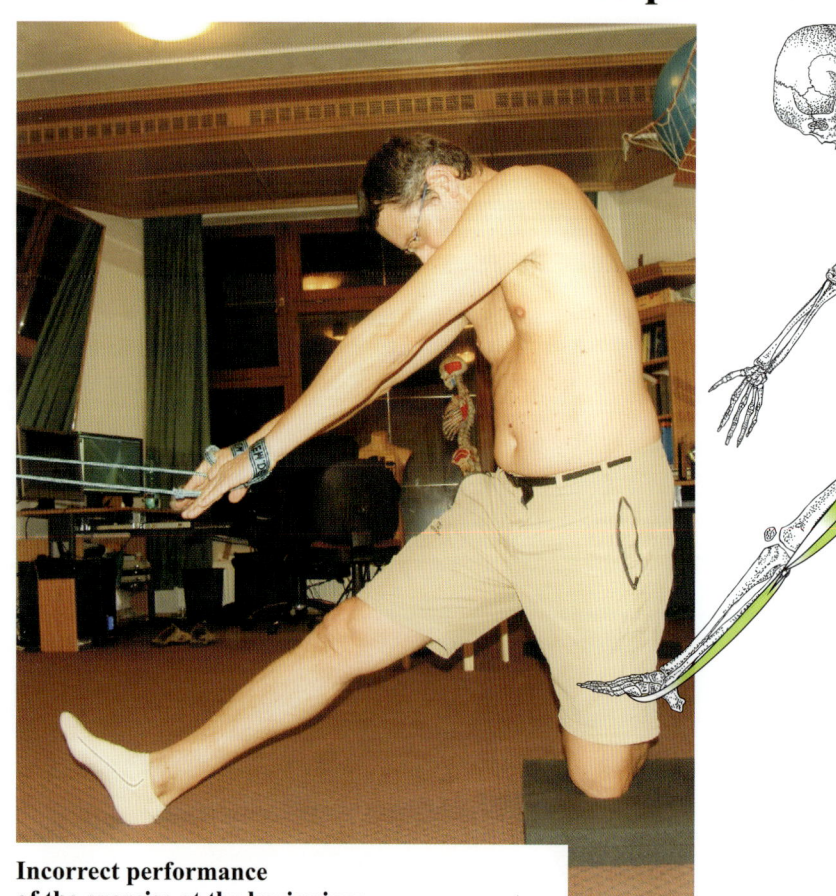

M. erector spinae

M. iliocostalis

M. longissimus
- thoracis
- cervicis
- capitis

M. spinalis

Stretching of the ischiocrural muscles:

M. adductor magnus

M. semimembranosus

M. semitendinosus

M. biceps femoris

Incorrect performance of the exercise at the beginning:
Tension in the ischiocrural muscles together with tension in the m. erector spinae - posterior vertical - stresses the spine in a forward tilt and during the forward movement of the leg. This prevents regeneration of the spine and leads to its accelerated degeneration. Stretching exercises must be very gentle and progress slowly. The muscle is full of trigger points.

Conclusion:
Increased tension in the posterior vertical is caused, for example, by sedentary work. Relaxing the muscle tension in the posterior vertical through exercise enables regeneration during walking and running.

Optimal performance of the exercise:
The ischiocrural muscles are stretched at the same time as the paravertebral muscles. In the active phase of the exercise, which is spirally stabilized, there is reciprocal inhibition of the paravertebral muscles and a good blood supply, which enables further stretching. The exercise also relaxes the pull of the whole posterior vertical. The elimination of the trigger points can be seen.

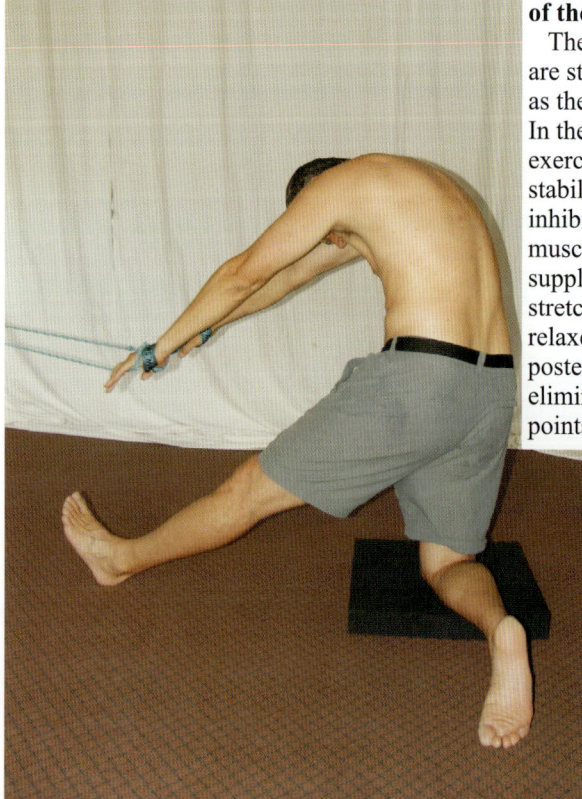

5th negative factor - shortened muscles in the anterior group of the neck and in the shoulder girdle

Anterior group of the neck:

- M. sternocleido-mastoideus
- Mm. suprahyoidei
- Mm. infrahyoidei
- M. scalenus anterior
- M. omohyoideus venter superior venter inferior
- M. trapezius pars descendens
- M. levator scapulae

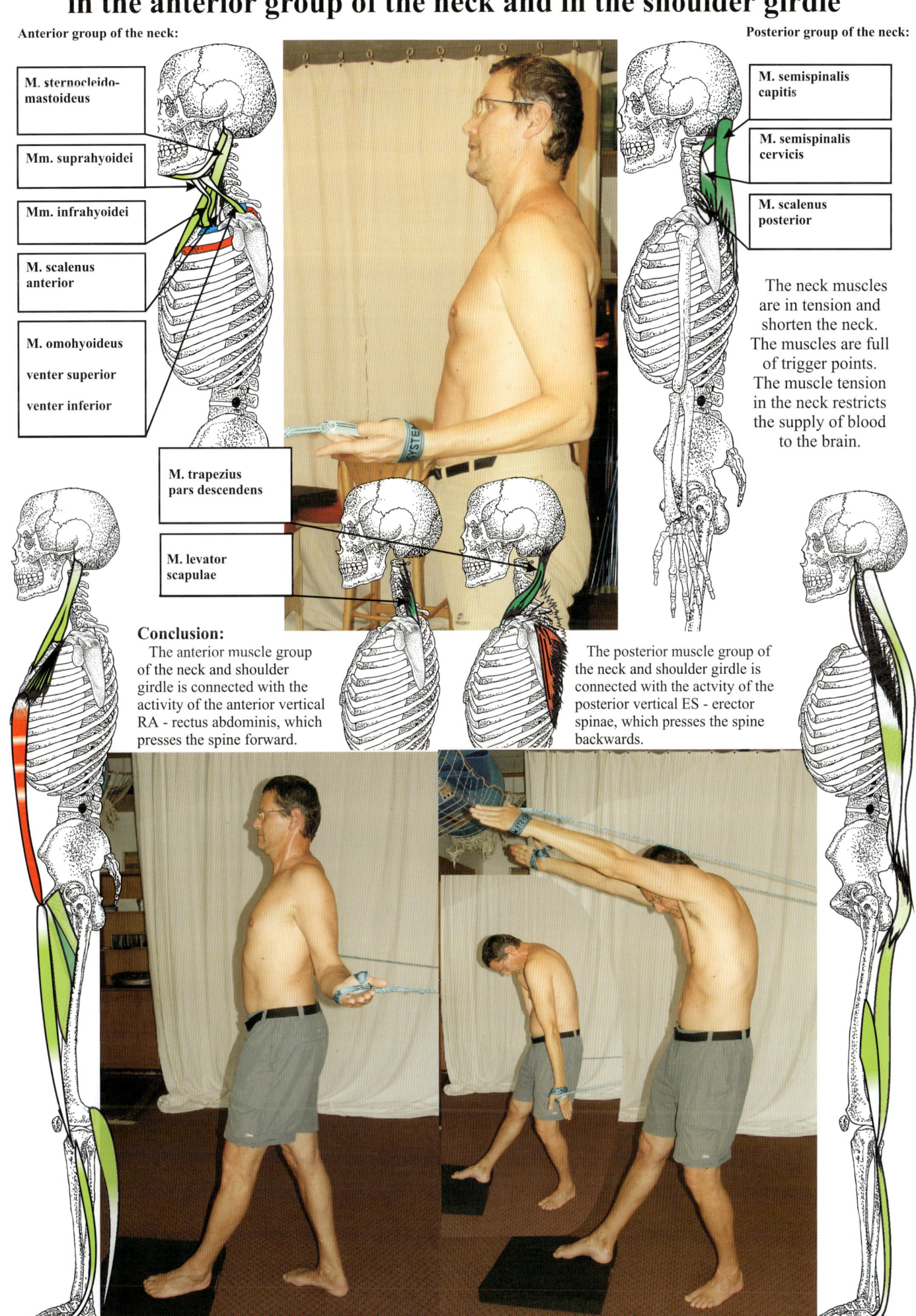

Posterior group of the neck:

- M. semispinalis capitis
- M. semispinalis cervicis
- M. scalenus posterior

The neck muscles are in tension and shorten the neck. The muscles are full of trigger points. The muscle tension in the neck restricts the supply of blood to the brain.

Conclusion:

The anterior muscle group of the neck and shoulder girdle is connected with the activity of the anterior vertical RA - rectus abdominis, which presses the spine forward.

The posterior muscle group of the neck and shoulder girdle is connected with the actvity of the posterior vertical ES - erector spinae, which presses the spine backwards.

6th negative factor
- disorder of reciprocal inhibition between the LD and ES chains

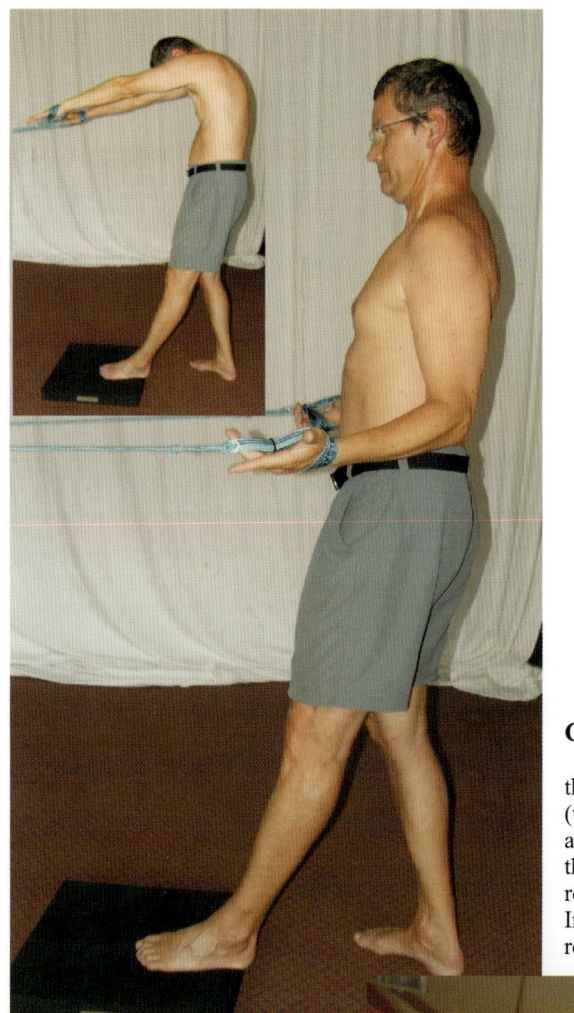

Initial state
Shortened back muscles prevent bending forward

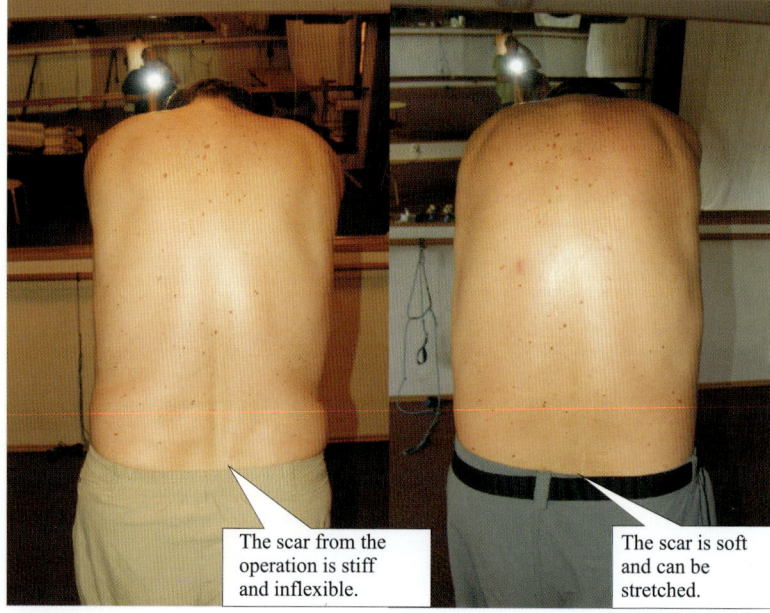

State after treatment
Back muscles are completely relaxed and stretched.

The scar from the operation is stiff and inflexible.

The scar is soft and can be stretched.

Conclusion:
A very important part of treatment is inducing reciprocal inhibition between the LD - latissimus dorsi chain (the agonist) and the ES erector spinae chain (the antagonist). The active LD spiral inhibits the ES vertical. The LD then has a clear path to pull the whole body up and to regenerate the whole of the spine through traction. Traction then enables the mobilization of all the sections in rotation - movement spread across the segments. This is then applied in walking. In the lower picture we can see the complete elimination of the TPs and complex relaxation of the ES inhibited in reciprocal inhibition by the LD spiral.

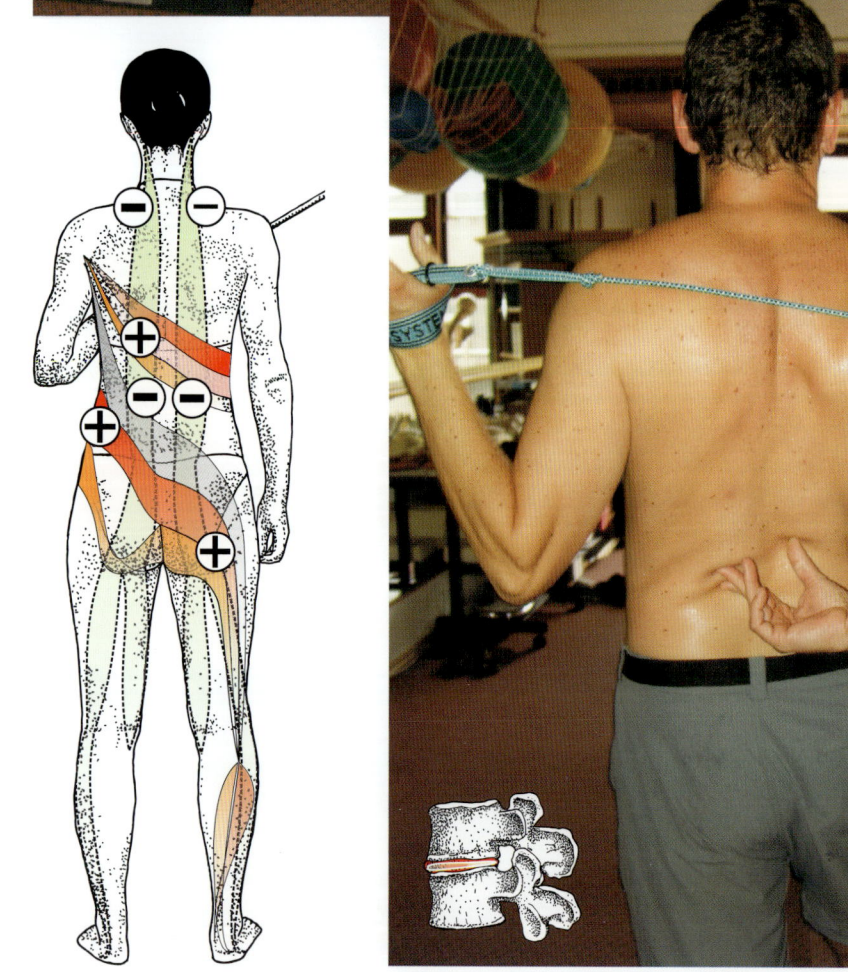

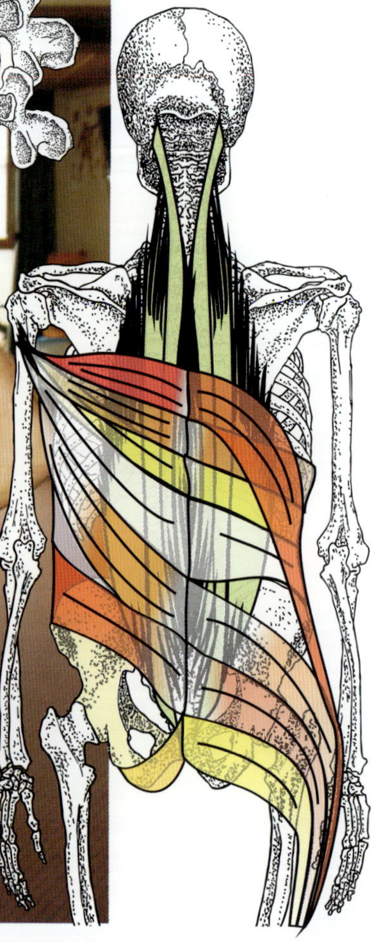

7th negative factor
- disorder of the coordination and stabilization of the gait

Mm. rotatores breves, longi , mm. semispinales, mm. multifidi

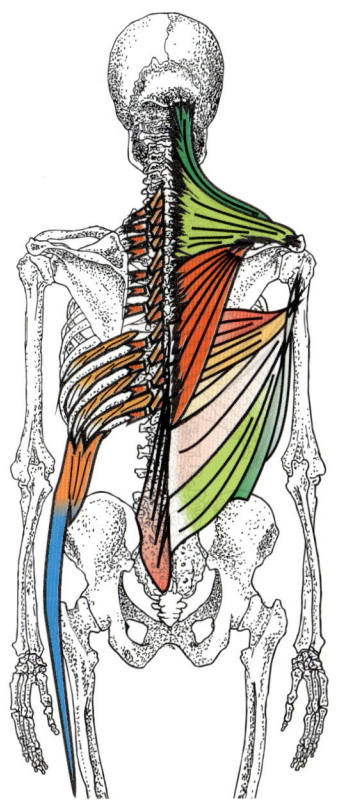

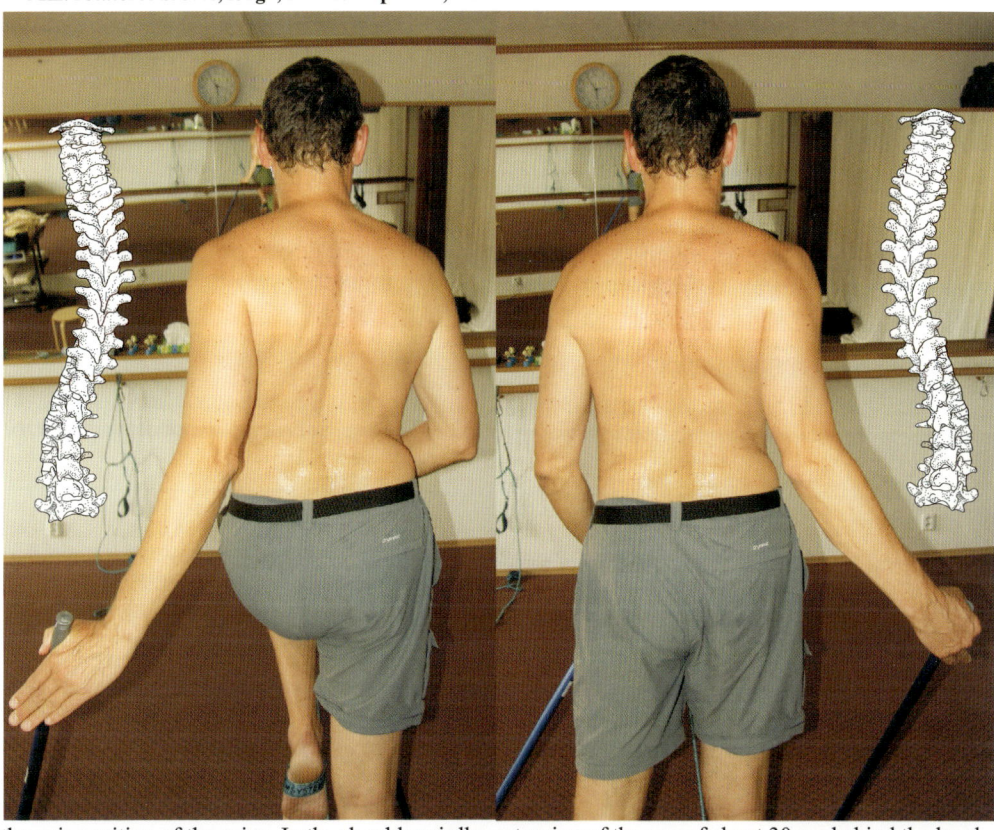

Conclusion:

Optimal gait coordination is achieved in the axis position of the spine. In the shoulder girdle, extension of the arm of about 30 cm behind the level of the body is combined with a backward and downward movement of the shoulder blade and a movement of the spine, which follows the movement of the shoulder blade. In the pelvic girdle, extension in the hip joint is combined with a movement of the SI joint
and a movement of the spine, which follows a movement of the leg and pelvis. The spine thus creates two "S" curves, which alternate during traction of the spine, which is performed by the spiral stabilizing chains TR, LD, SA, PM. The "S" curves spread the movement evenly to all segments. This is done through the short autochthonous muscles. At the same time, the ribs and chest are mobilized.

Optimal stabilization of the spine is ensured by the backward movement of the arm. This arm activates the LD - latissimus dorsi spiral chain. The backward movement of the shoulder blade activates the TR - trapezius chain. The forward movement of the arm activates the PM - pectoralis major chain. The forward movement of the shoulder blade activates the SA - serratus anterior chain. During walking, all the spiral chains are activated at the same time.

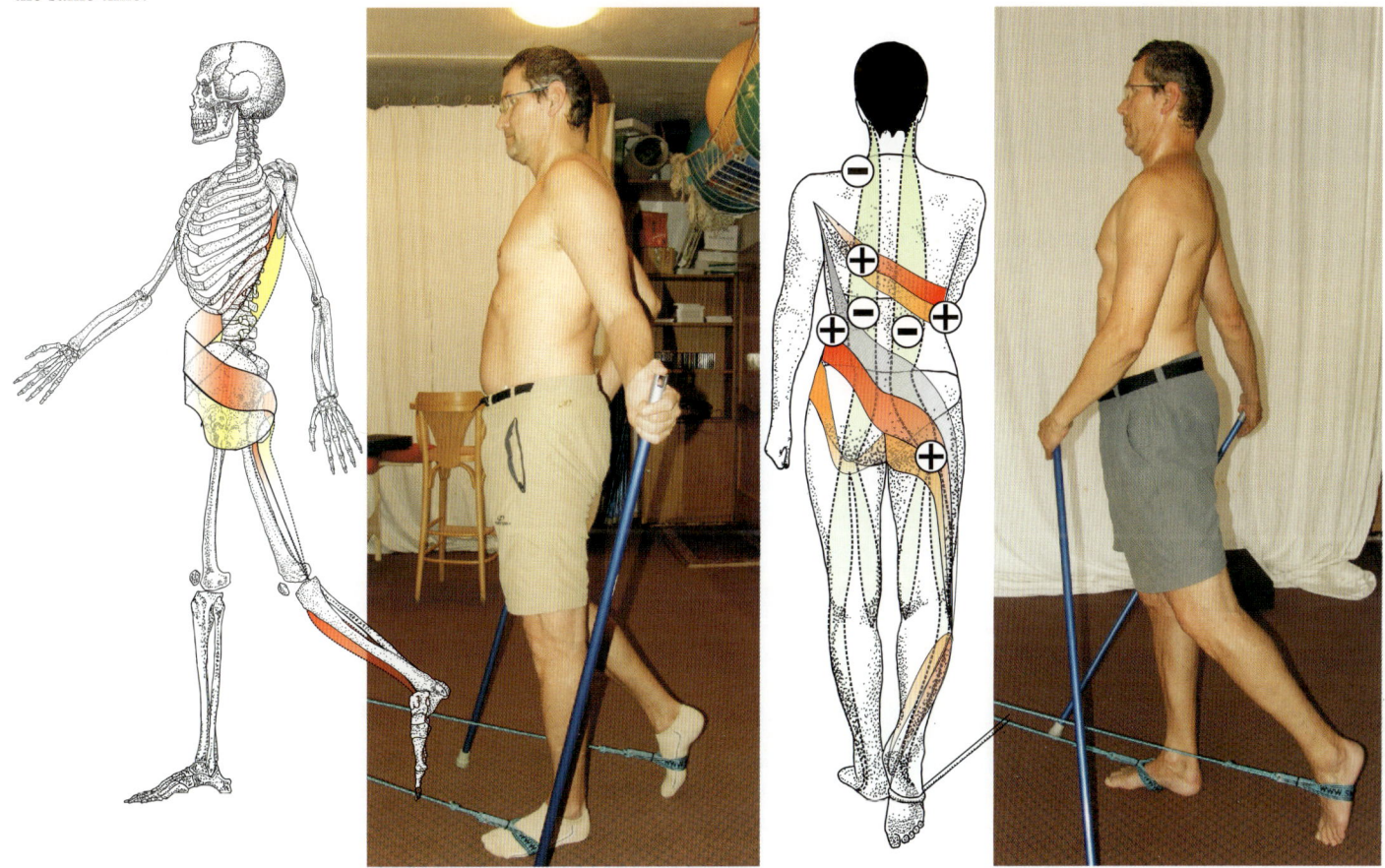

The clinical picture of our patient

Medical history:
I was suffering from back pain which extended down into my leg. The diagnosis was herniation of intervertebral disc L5/S1.
After the operation I had no pain for a year, but then the pains returned and gradually got stronger. The pain extends into my leg,
as before, but I also have a new pain, which is in my thigh at the back and front. They don't recommend another operation.
The rehabilitation isn't helping. I can't sit or stand. With every step I take, I get a sharp pain in my leg. I am unable to work.

Investigation - finding:
Tension in the anterior muscle group of the shoulder girdle prevents the backward movement of the shoulder blade.
The shoulder blade, blocked in a forward position, cannot activate the abdomen through the LD- latissimus dorsi muscle chain.
The passive abdomen does not relax the vertical back muscles. Tension in the vertical back muscles compresses the intervertebral discs of the lumbar spine towards each other. The pressure on the discs causes their degeneration and herniation.
An operation on a herniated disc lowers the height of intervertebral disc L5/S1, blocking the segment's movement.
That movement is compensated in the other segments, where degeneration has already occurred. They cannot withstand the strain,
and new herniations occur. Neither the doctors nor the physiotherapists know what to do about the problem.
A further operation would make the situation even worse, while classic physiotherapy fails, or even causes pain.
The patient is unable to work. The main principle of spiral stabilization - traction (stretching) of the spine - is disrupted in the patient.
Traction of the spine takes place through extension movements of the arm (backward movements), which activate the oblique abdominal muscles via the active LD - latissimus dorsi muscle chain, but they are restricted by muscle tension and the accumulation of trigger points.

A new treatment which eliminates the cause and leads to full health - spiral stabilization:
The situation can be resolved, if we treat the cause of the illness - the disruption of the spiral stabilization of movement.
Through exercise and massage we relieve the tension in the anterior muscle group of the shoulder girdle, practise the movement
of the shoulder blade backwards and downwards and activate the abdominal muscles through the LD- latissimus dorsi spiral chain. The abdominal muscles also engage the m. gluteus maximus, which stabilizes the pelvis and straightens the spine.
The LD spiral stabilizing chain contracts the girth, thereby lifting the intervertebral discs. The spine is regenerated and intensively treated.
Our patient improved after just one week of intensive therapy through exercise and manual traction techniques.
After 3 months of regular exercise he was completely free from pain. After 6 to 8 months he regained full performance and can even do sports (he plays golf). We have had a similar success with our other patients, who appreciated the active approach to treatment.

Conclusion:
From our example, it is clear that by gradually eliminating the negative factors which contribute to FB syndrome,
the body reaches a situation in which the spine is stretched upwards and sufficiently regenerated.
The patient feels no pain and is able to live, work and do sport happily.
Let us recall the negative factors which lead to the development of FB syndrome.

Social factors:
- neglecting the correct development of the muscle apparatus and the coordination and stabilization of movement during the growth period.
  Those responsible for this are parents, the staff of nursery schools, schools and sports clubs, and trainers.
- neglecting the regeneration of the locomotor apparatus during work and sport - conditioning, regeneration, and compensation of one-sided stress.

Main negative factors:
- muscle imbalance in the shoulder girdle
- muscle imbalance in the pelvic girdle
- muscle imbalance in the trunk
- muscle imbalance in the neck and head region
- muscle imbalance in the legs and feet
- muscle imbalance in the arms
- disorder of the posture at rest arising from those imbalances

- disorder of the function of the spiral stabilizing chains - TR - trapezius, LD - latissimus dorsi, SA - serratus anterior, PM - pectoralis major
- increased activity of the vertical stabilizing chains - ES - erector spinae, QL - quadratus lumborum, IP - iliopsoas, RA - rectus abdominis

- disorder of reciprocal inhibition in the joints, girdles, trunk and muscle chains
- disorder of the postural reaction and sensorimotor response

- disorder of the coordination and stabilization of the walking and running gait
  - disorder of the axis
  - disorder of the coordination in the shoulder girdle and chest
  - disorder of the coordination in the pelvic girdle and lumbar spine

- incorrect coordination and stabilization during exercise and sport

From the above information we may conclude that the accumulation of negative factors disrupts the functioning of the spiral stabilization
of the spine and the traction force which comes from it, and the spine therefore stops being regenerated.
This regenerating effect must be restored before an operation and continued afterwards. Of course, the most effective prevention
of FB syndrome is active, conservative treatment of the intervertebral disc without an operation. In our centre we have treated 4000 patients
for herniation of an intervertebral disc over 32 years, of whom we have sent only four for an operation.

Recommended therapeutic procedure
activate the oblique abdominal muscles and the longitudinal back muscles
1. Creating a muscle corset TR, LD

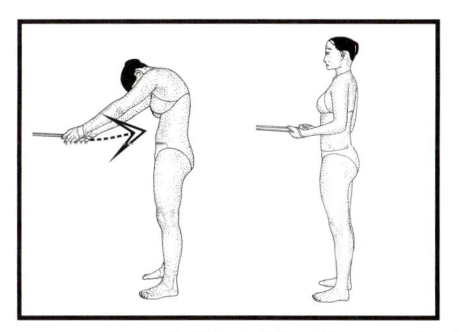

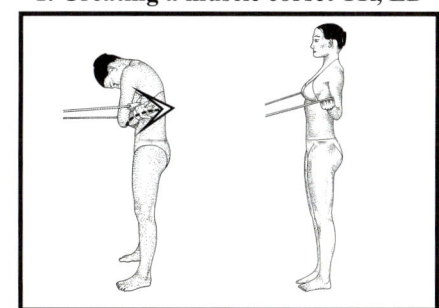

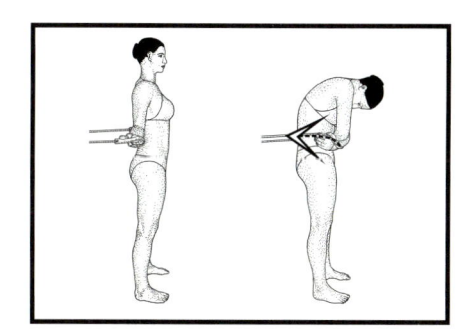

2. Stretching the muscles in the shoulder and pelvic girdles and trunk with stabilization by TR, LD

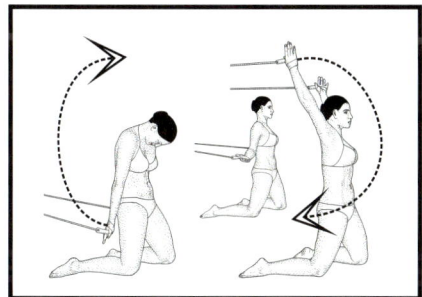

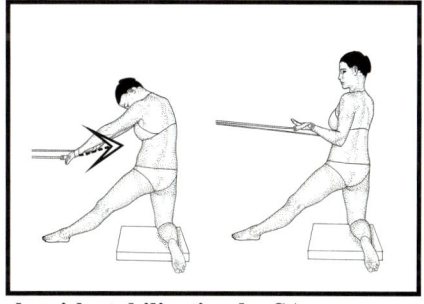

3. Stretching the paravertebral muscle with stabilization by SA

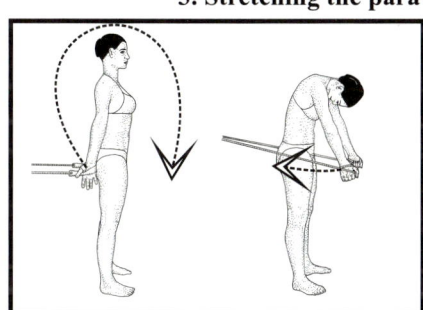

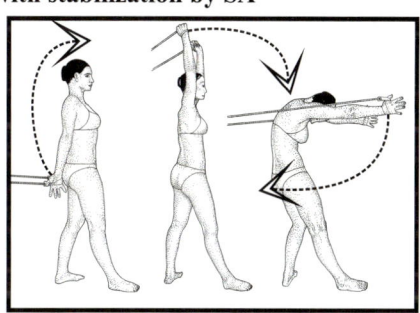

4. Mobilization of the spine and activation of the rotary autochthonous muscles with stabilization by TR, LD

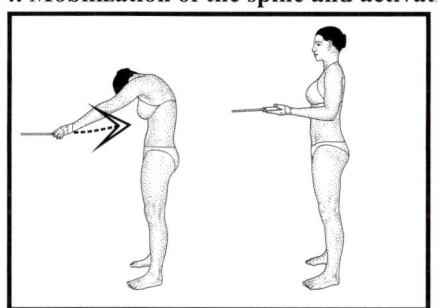

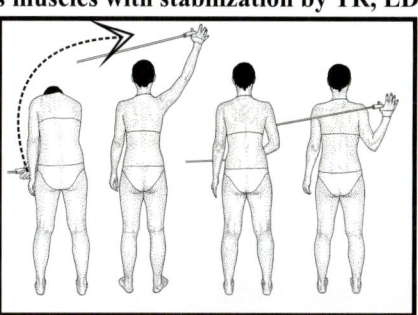

5. Strengthening the m. gluteus maximus and restoring gait coordination and stabilization with stabilization by TR, LD, SA, PM

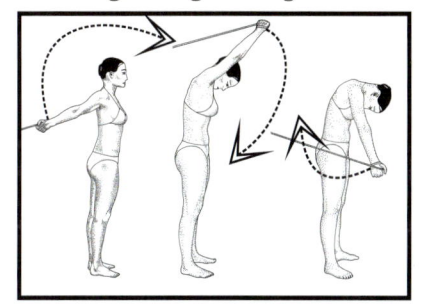

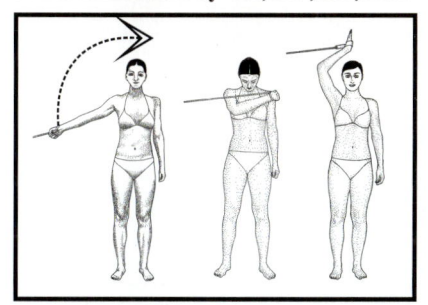

6. Gait stabilized by TR, LD, SA, PM

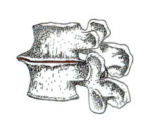

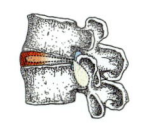

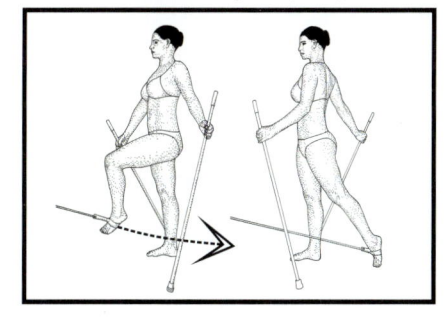

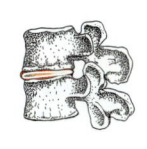

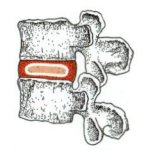

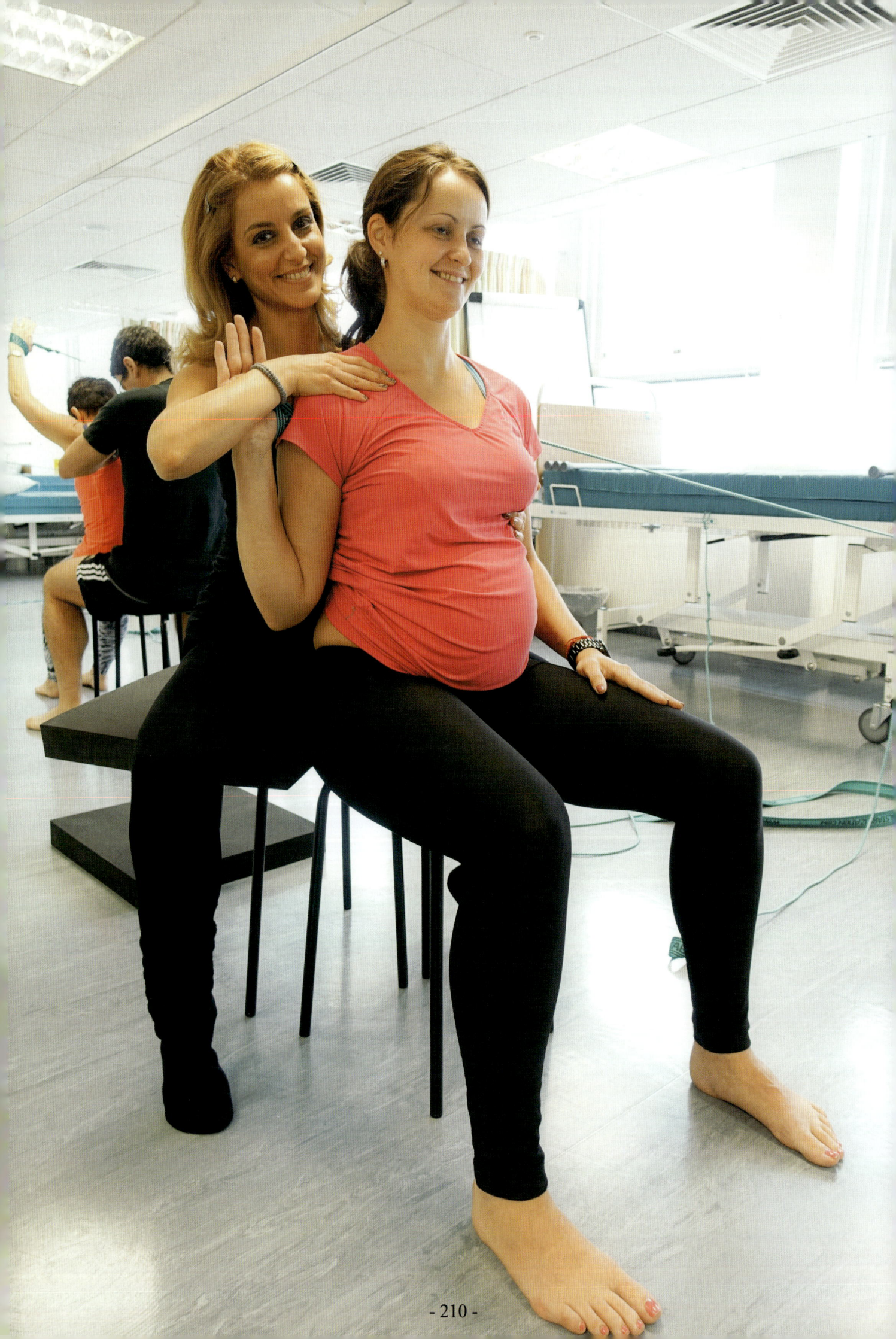

DISORDER OF SPIRAL STABILIZATION

Eliminating a disorder of spiral stabilization

Eliminating muscle imbalances

Eliminating pathological muscle tension
Eliminating TP - trigger points

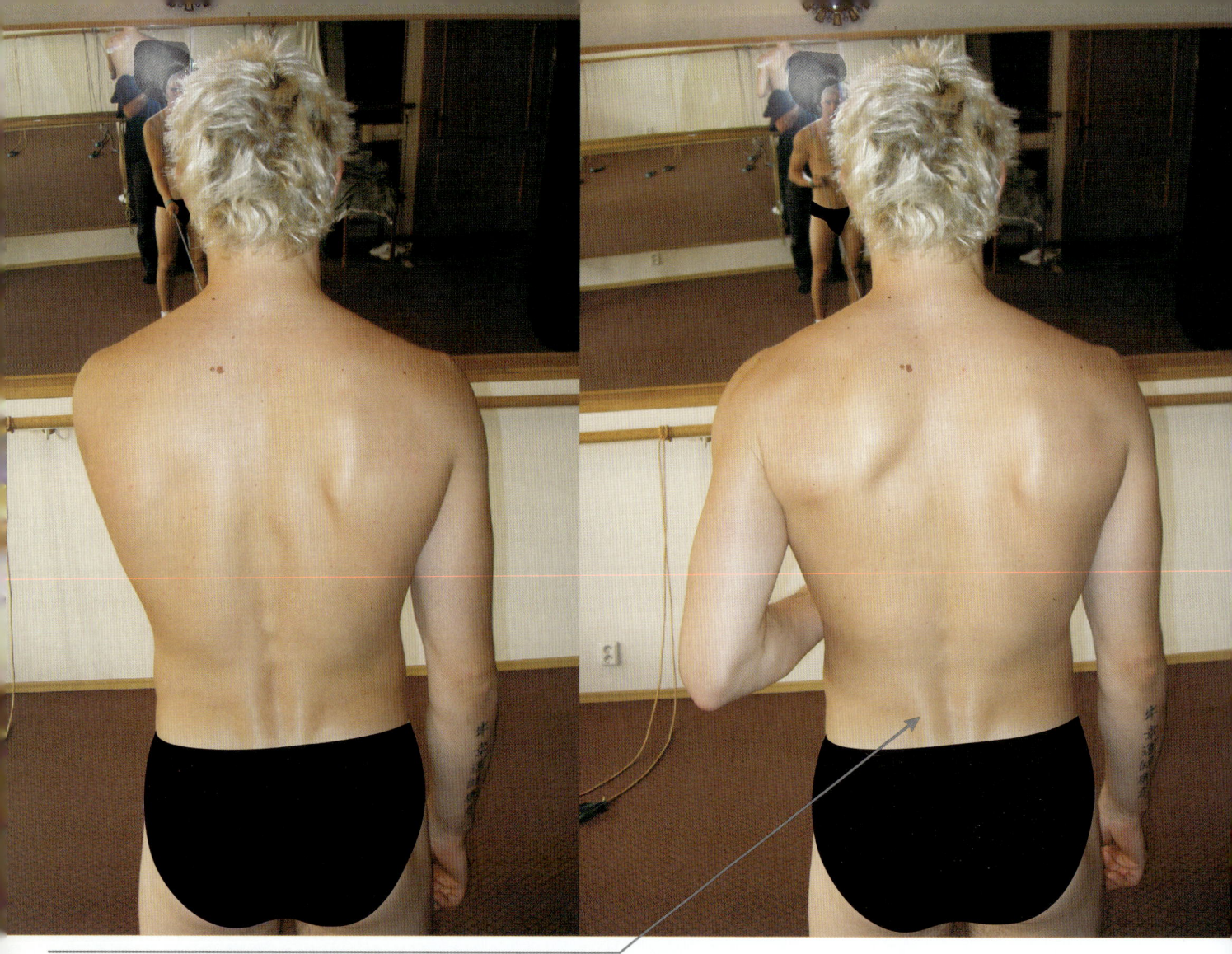

Disorder of spiral stabilization, the TR and LD chain is not activated, tension persists in the m. erector spinae (vertical stabilization ES)

After three months of exercise, the TR and LD chains are activated and the m. erector spinae is compeletely relaxed.

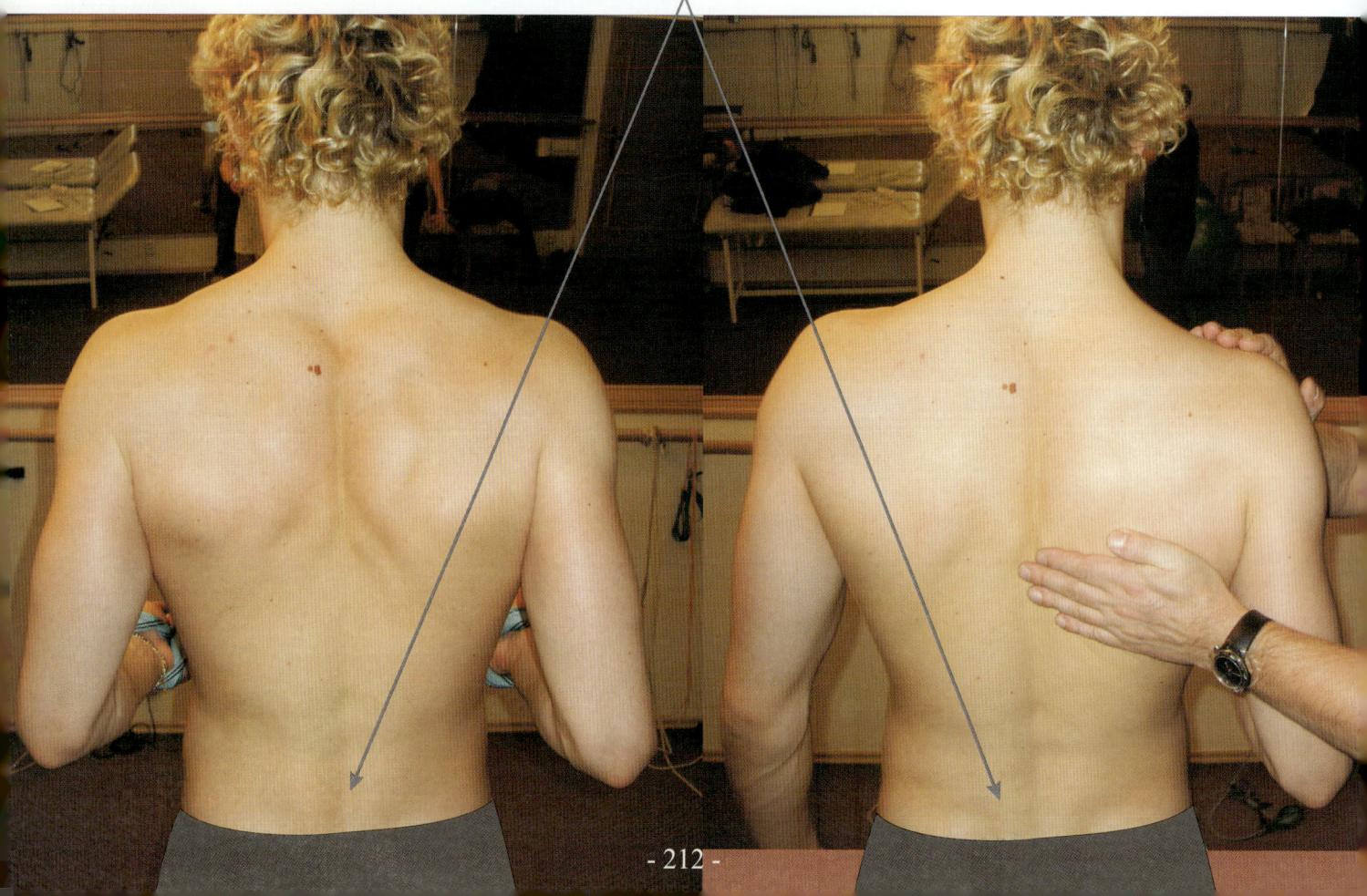

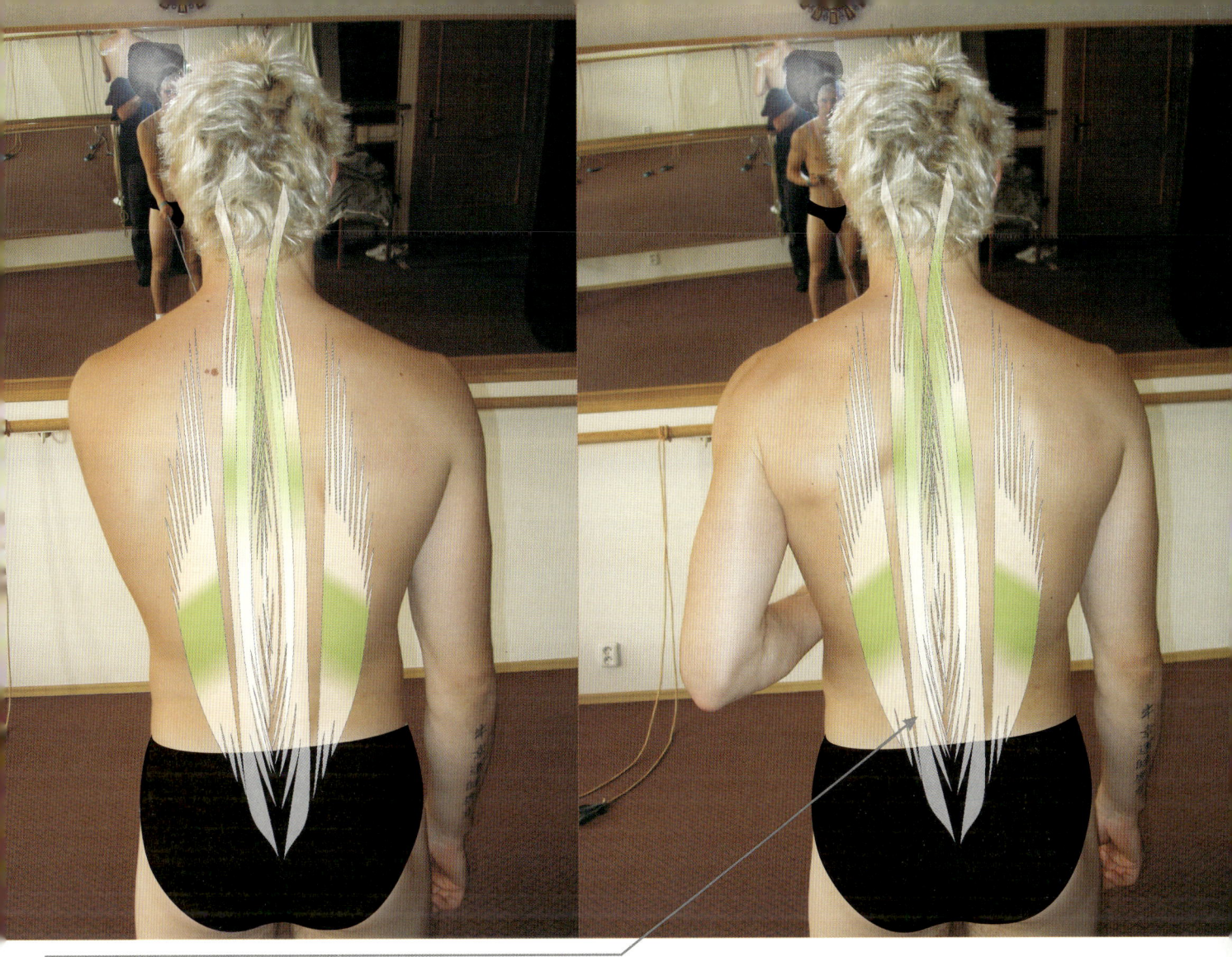

Disorder of spiral stabilization, the TR and LD chain is not activated, tension persists in the m. erector spinae (vertical stabilization ES)

After three months of exercise, the TR and LD chains are activated and the m. erector spinae is compeletely relaxed.

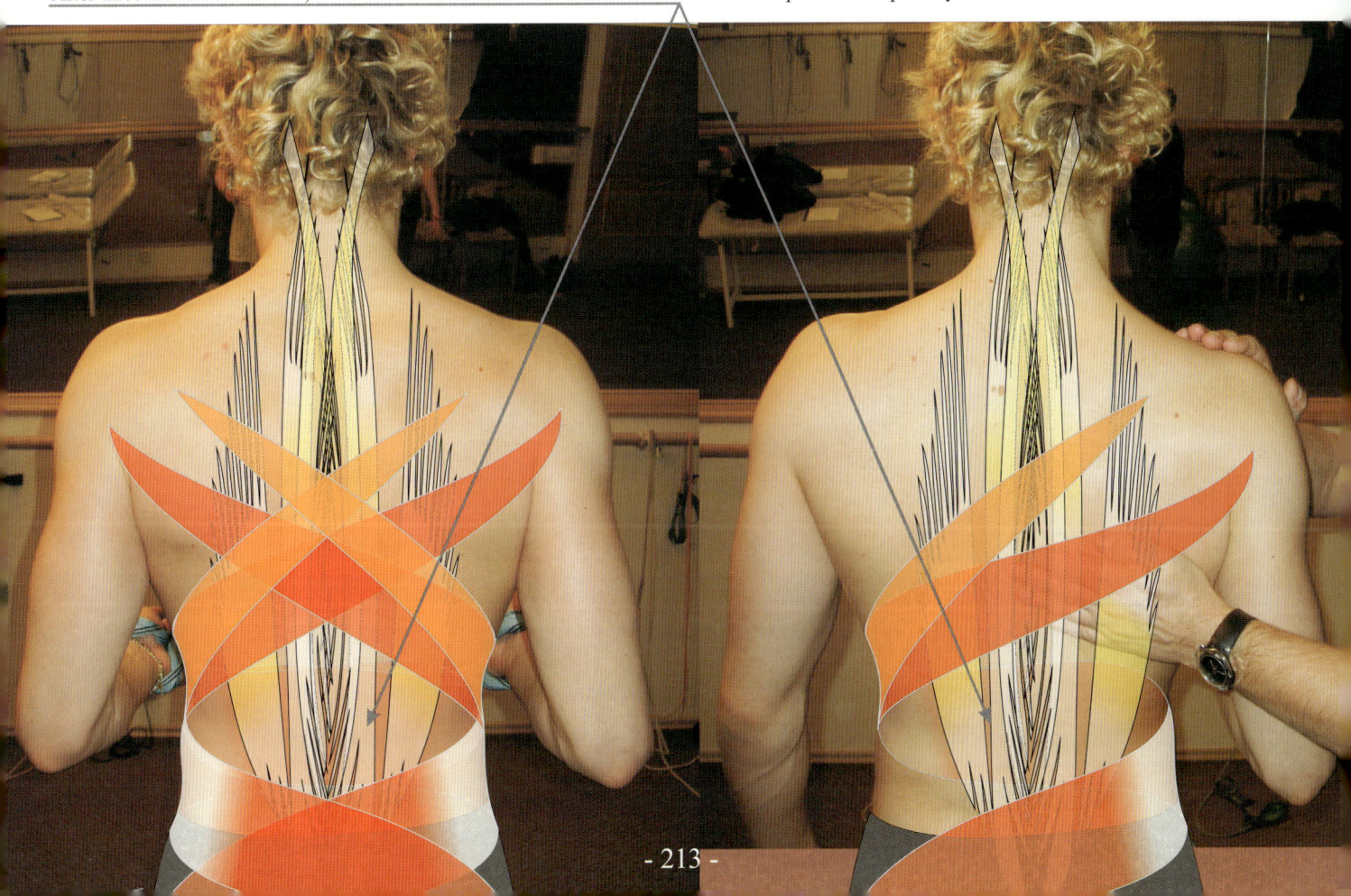

At the beginning
weak posture, severe muscle imbalance

After 3 months' exercise
balanced posture, muscle balance achieved

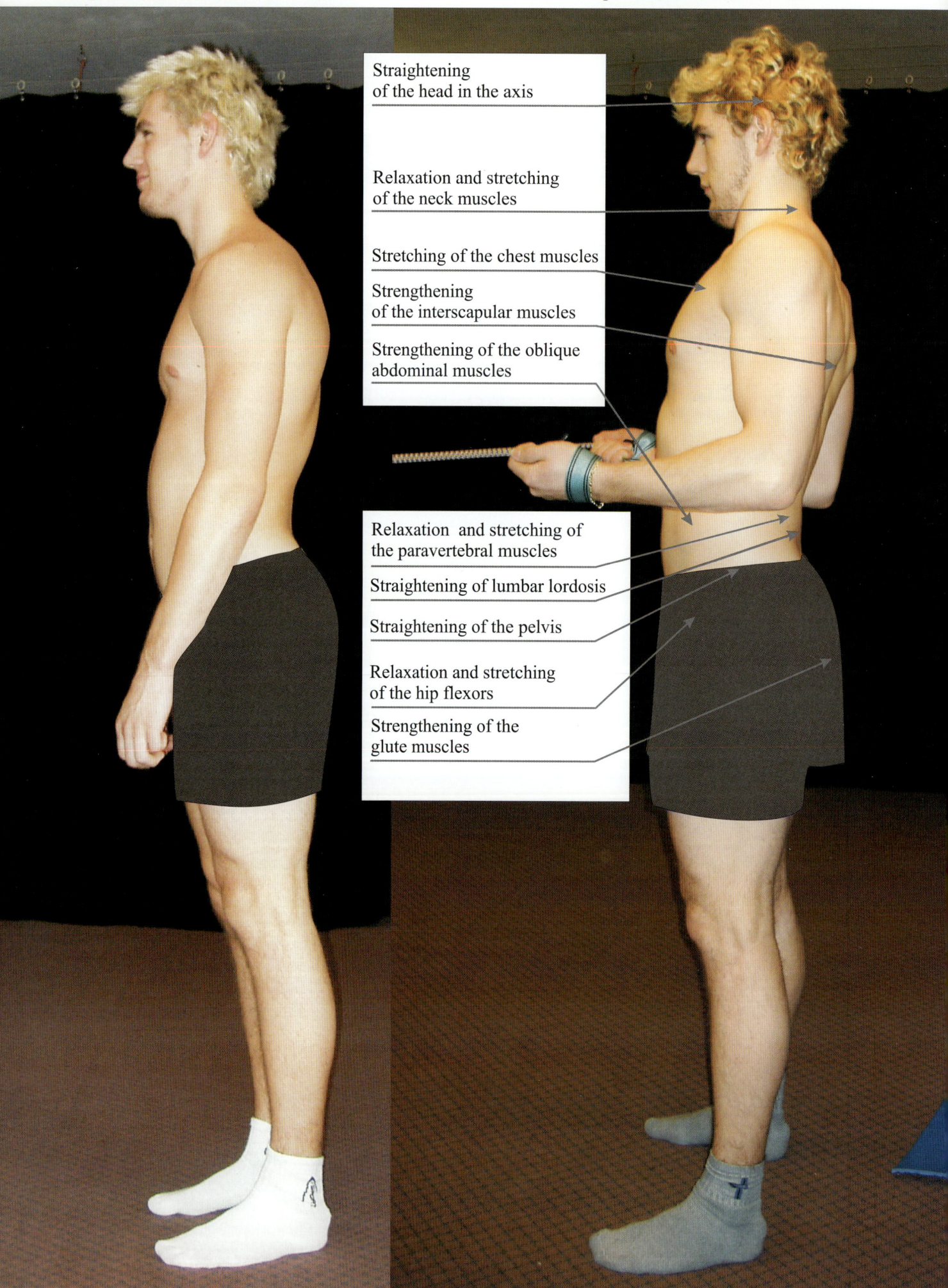

Straightening of the head in the axis

Relaxation and stretching of the neck muscles

Stretching of the chest muscles

Strengthening of the interscapular muscles

Strengthening of the oblique abdominal muscles

Relaxation and stretching of the paravertebral muscles

Straightening of lumbar lordosis

Straightening of the pelvis

Relaxation and stretching of the hip flexors

Strengthening of the glute muscles

At the beginning
vertical stabilization

After 3 months' exercise
spiral stabilization of movement, active relaxation of the vertical chains

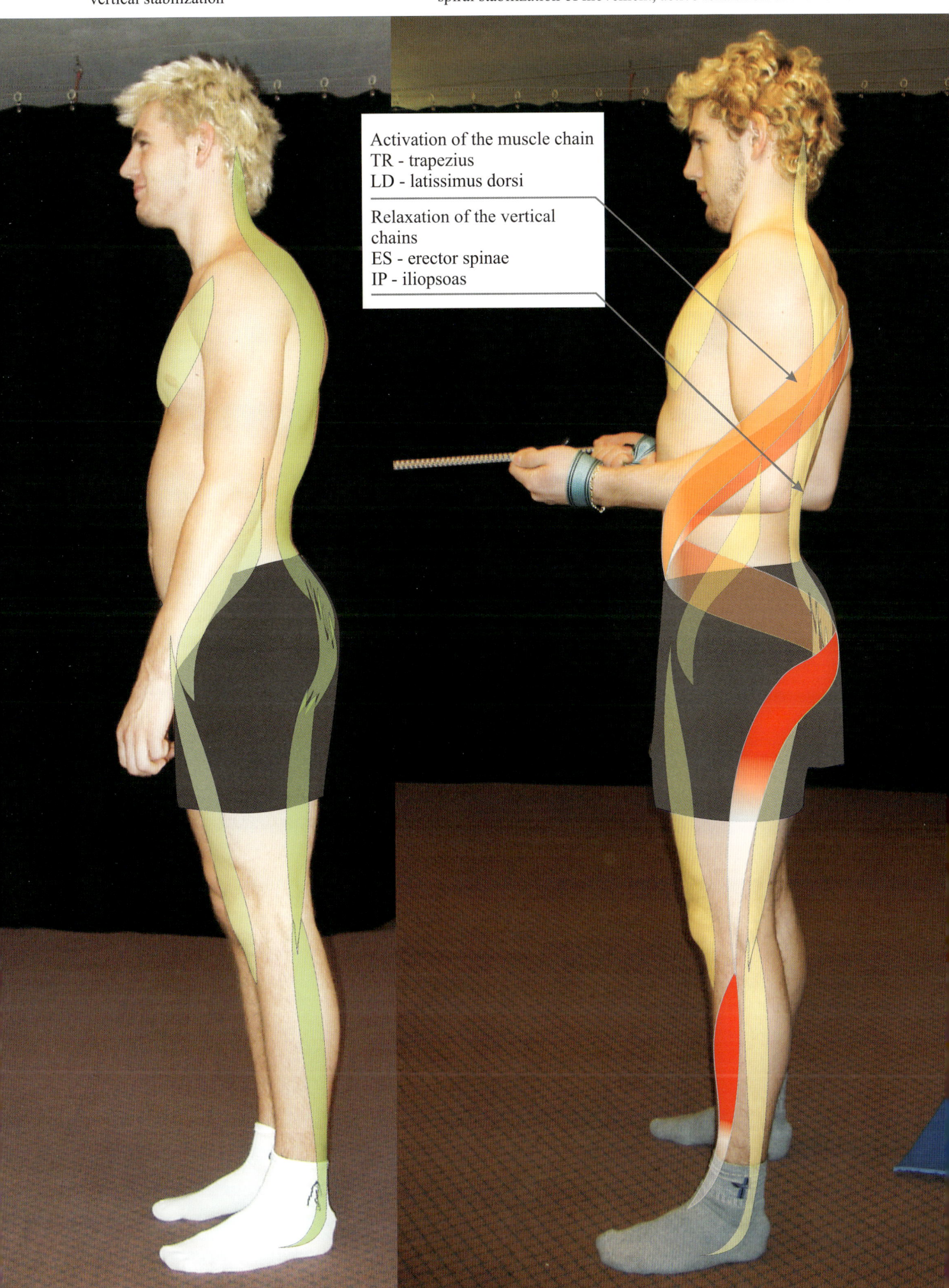

Activation of the muscle chain
TR - trapezius
LD - latissimus dorsi

Relaxation of the vertical chains
ES - erector spinae
IP - iliopsoas

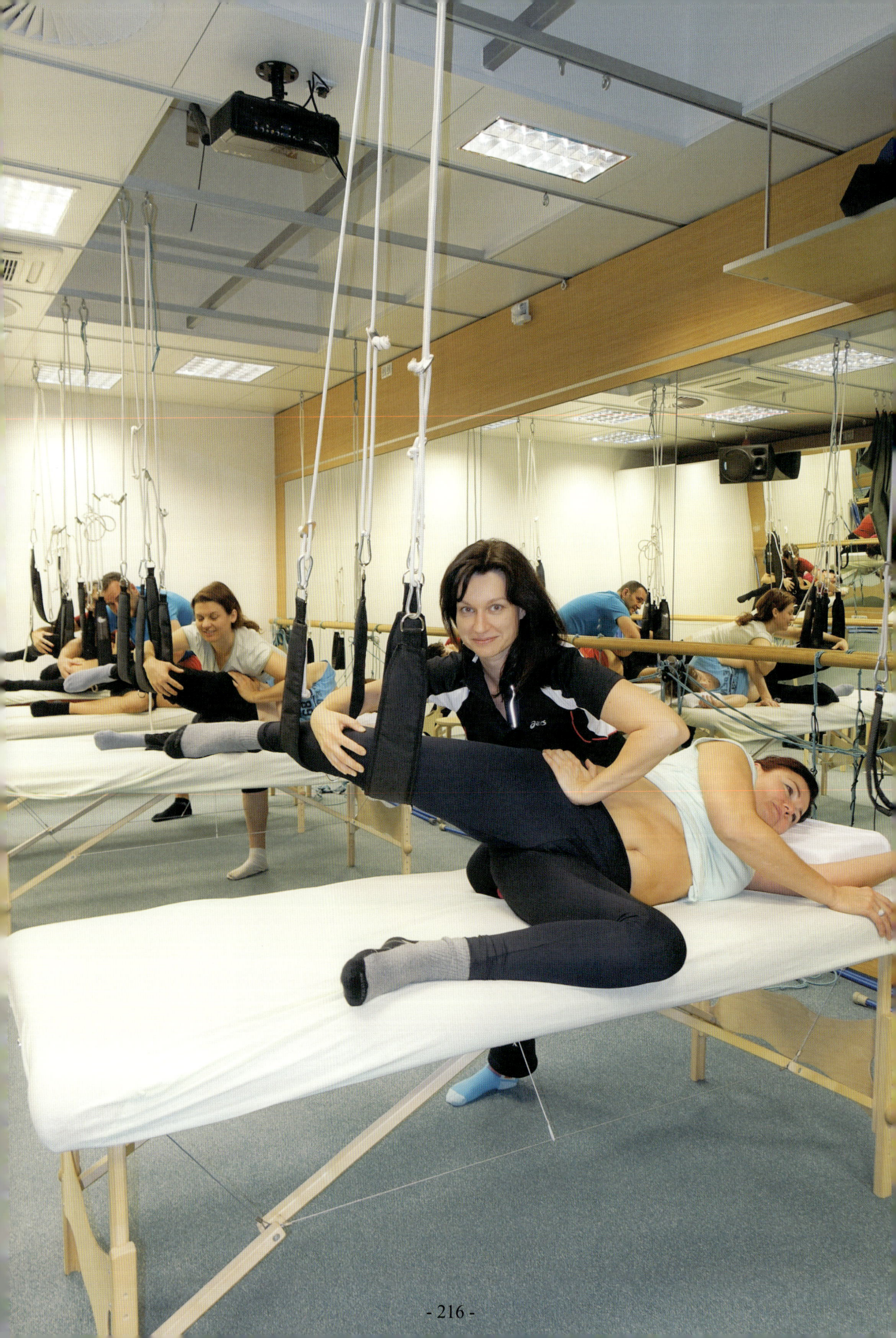

Parameters for measuring the extent and coordination of movement

Optimally coordinated movement engages the muscle spirals and inhibits the muscle verticals

The activity of the muscle spirals regenerates the spine and large joints

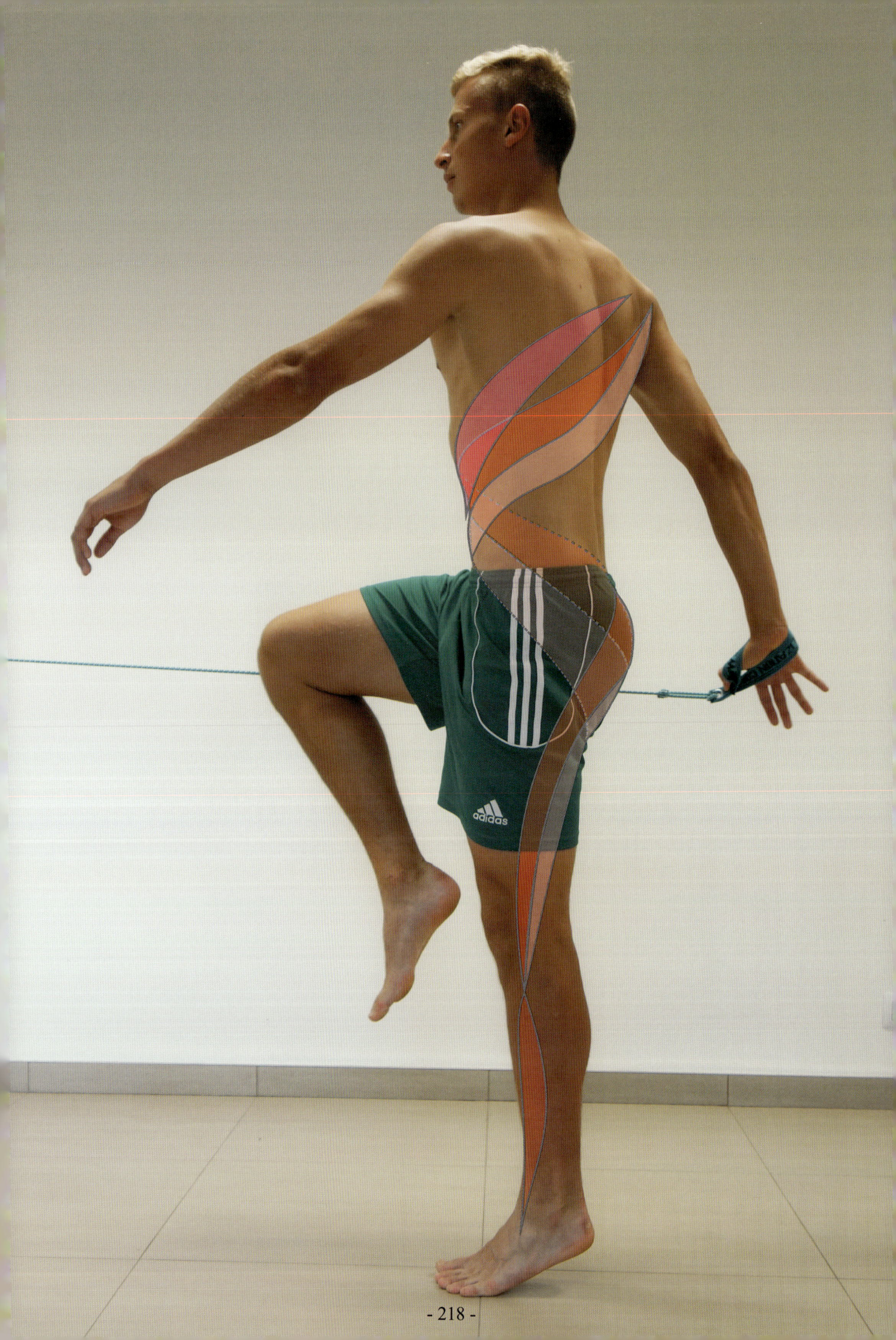

The most important parameter

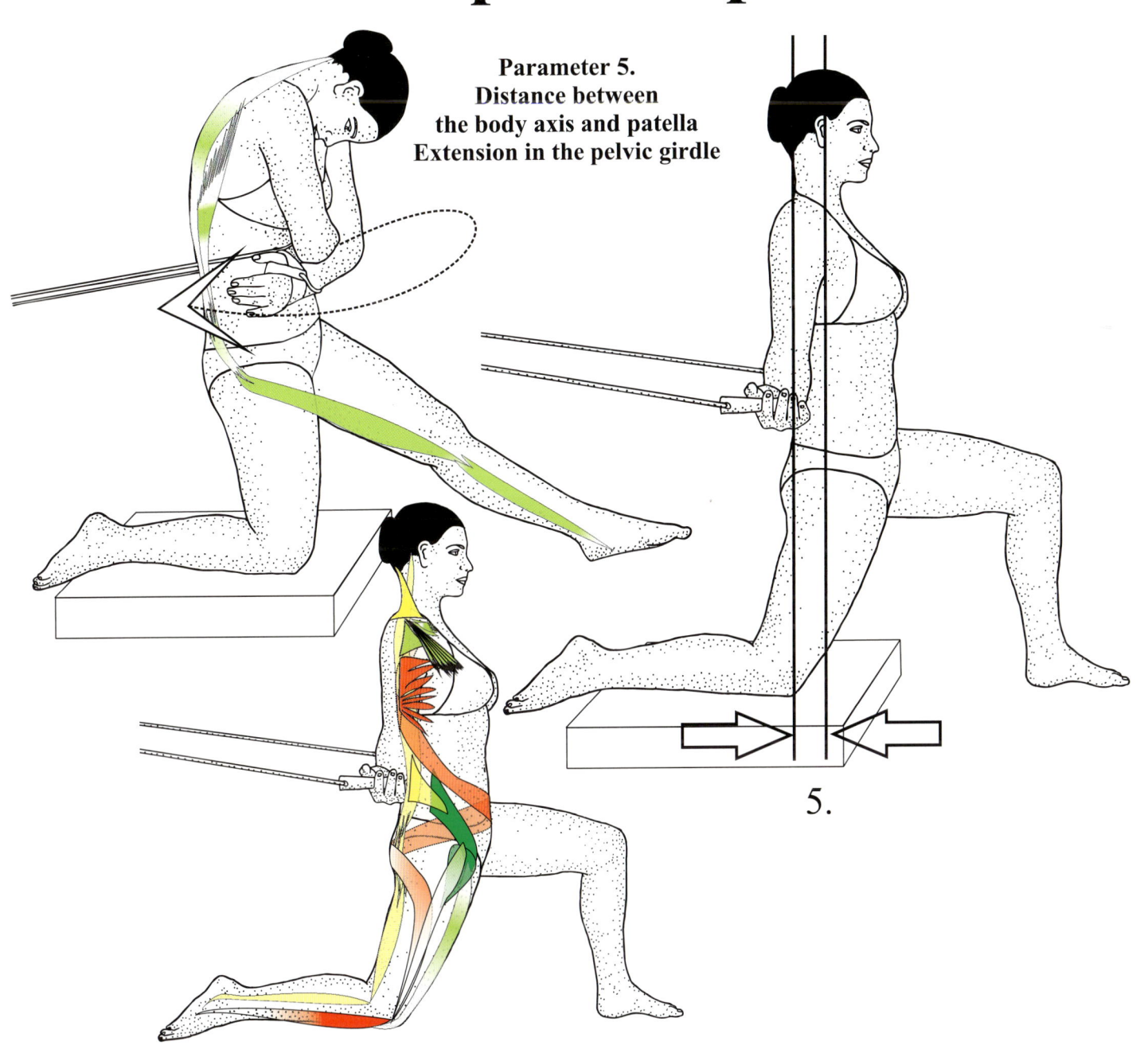

Parameter 5.
Distance between the body axis and patella
Extension in the pelvic girdle

5.

Parameter 5: Distance between the body axis and patella.
  Movement: Extension in the pelvic girdle in a spirally stabilized body.
  Norm: + 20 cm
Distance between the body axis and patella (kneecap).
The body axis runs in the upper part through the outer ear perpendicularly to the ground (plumb line) through the centre of the pelvis.
A pole is placed against the back. This does not allow lordosis greater than 2.5 cm (the width of a thumb).
This parameter assesses the ability to extend the step through extension in the hip and SI joint.

Stretched muscles
Pelvic girdle:
- m. iliopsoas
- m. gluteus medius (anterior part)
- m. tensor fasciae latae
- m. rectus femoris

Shoulder girdle:
- m. subclavius
- m. pectoralis minor
- m. pectoralis major
- m. serratus anterior

The muscles in the upper side of the shoulder girdle relax:
- m. trapezius pars descendens
- m. levator scapulae
- mm. scaleni
- m. semispinalis capitis, cervicis etc.

Activated muscles
The interscapular muscles are strengthened:
- m. trapezius
- m. latissimus dorsi
- mm. rhomboidei

Linking the muscle chains
The exercise is stabilized by the spiral muscle chains:
TR-B, C - trapezius,
LD-A, B - latissimus dorsi.
The vertical muscle chain ES - erector spinae
relaxes in reciprocal inhibition.
Part of the TR and LD muscles chains are the oblique abdominal muscles and, above all, the m. gluteus maximus, which reciprocally inhibits the hip flexors.

Parameter 1.
Stretching the distance between the outer ear and the anterior edge of the acromion
Extension in the shoulder girdle

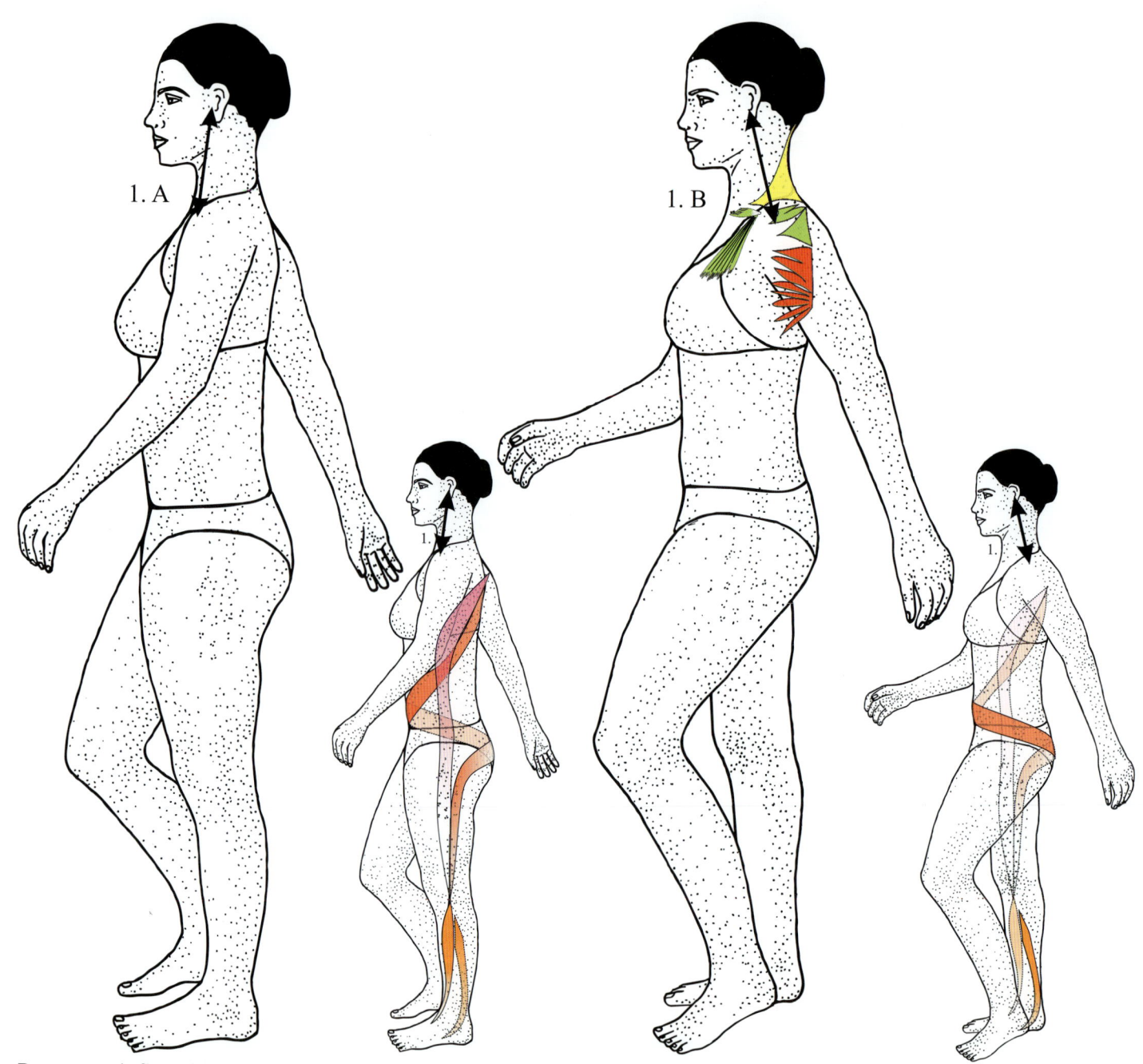

1. A

1. B

Parameter 1: Stretching the distance between the outer ear and the anterior edge of the acromion.
  Movement: Extension in the shoulder girdle with lower fixation of the shoulder blade, marking time.
  Norm: + 5 cm

The distance between the outer ear and anterior part of the acromion.
The change in the distance in the anterior position and posterior position is assessed.
This parameter assesses the ability for lower fixation of the shoulder blade and activation of the TR - trapezius and LD - latissimus dorsi spirals. At the same time, the cervical spine is stretched.

Stretched muscles
The muscles in the anterior side
of the shoulder girdle are stretched:
- m. subclavius
- m. pectoralis minor
- m. pectoralis major
- m. serratus anterior

The muscles in the upper side of the shoulder girdle relax:
- m. trapezius, pars descendens
- m. levator scapulae
- mm. scaleni
- m. semispinalis capitis, cervicis and other muscles.

Activated muscles
The interscapular muscles are strengthened:
- m. trapezius
- m. latissimus dorsi
- mm. rhomboidei

Linking the muscle chains
The exercise is stabilized by the muscle chains:
TR-B, C - trapezius,
LD-A, B - latissimus dorsi.

The vertical muscle chain ES - erector spinae relaxes in reciprocal inhibition.

Parameter 1.
Stretching the distance between the outer ear and the anterior edge of the acromion
Extension in the shoulder girdle

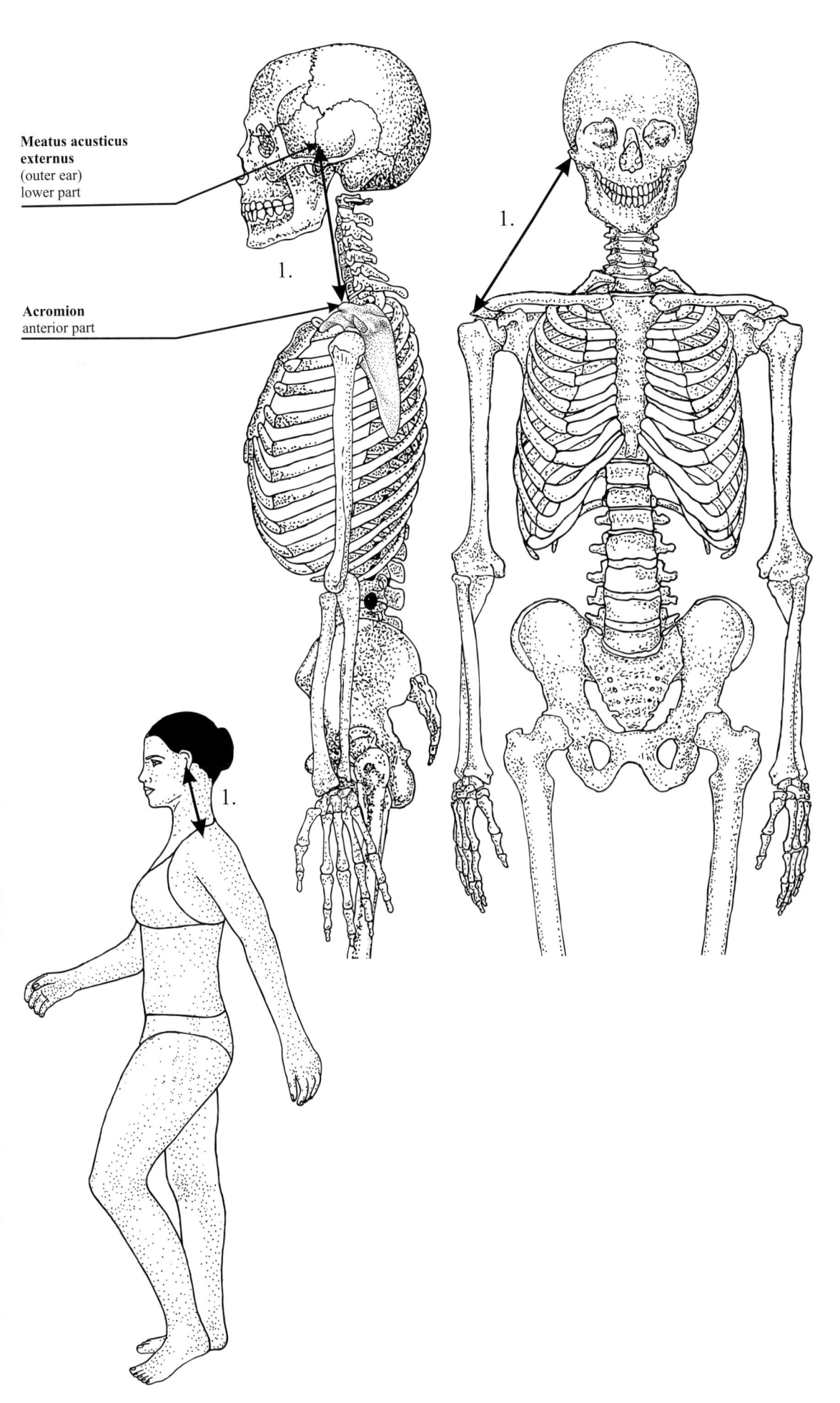

Meatus acusticus externus
(outer ear)
lower part

Acromion
anterior part

- 221 -

Parameter 2.
Distance between the hand and the level of the back
Extension in the shoulder girdle with outward rotation

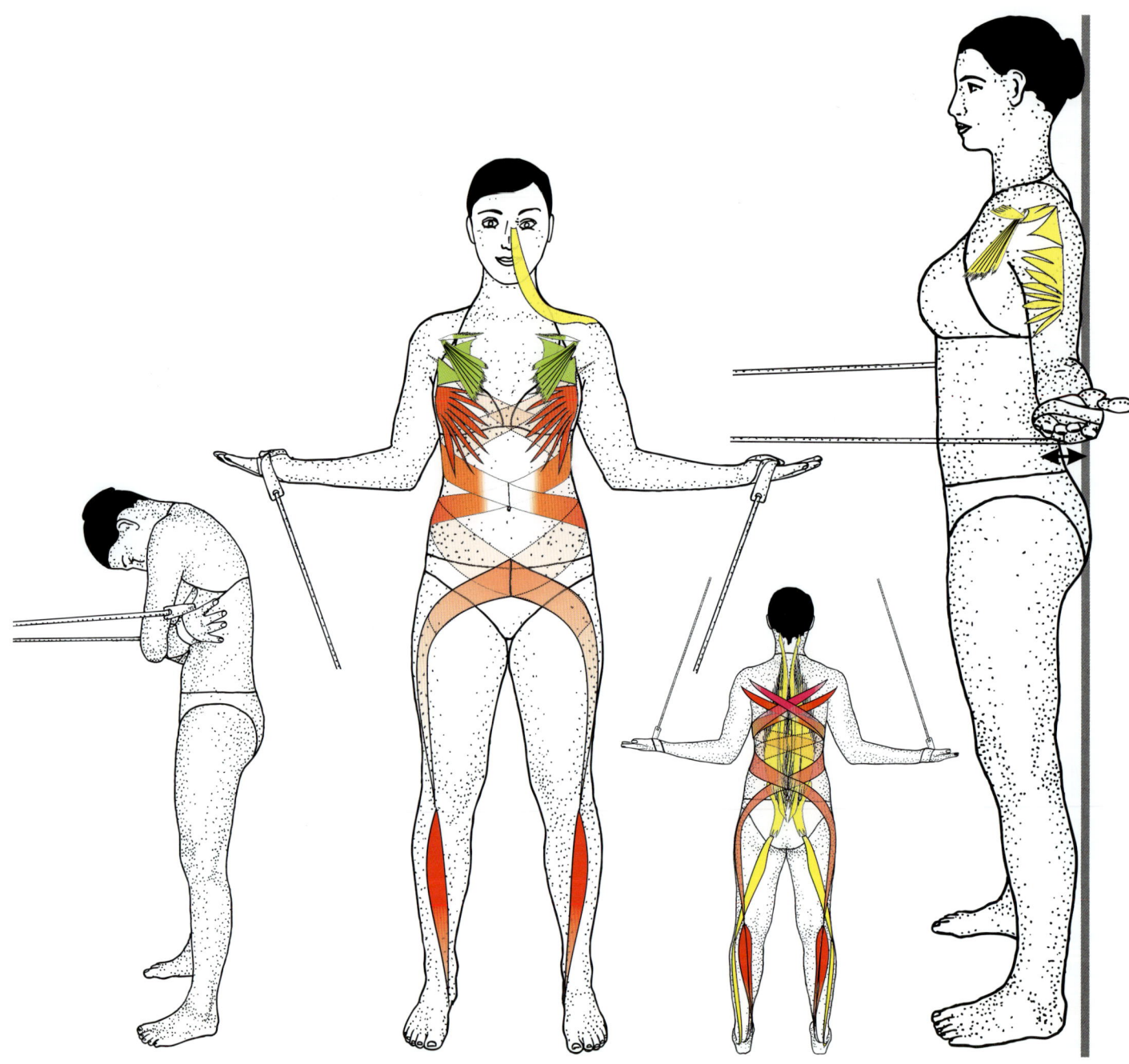

Parameter 2: Distance between the hand and the level of the back.
  Movement: Extension in the shoulder girdle with outward rotation.
  Norm: 0 cm
Distance between the arm and level of the back.
The distance in the anterior position of the arm is assessed.
This parameter assesses the ability to stretch the anterior muscle group of the shoulder girdle.

Stretched muscles
The muscles in the anterior side of the shoulder girdle are stretched:
- m. subclavius
- m. pectoralis minor
- m. pectoralis major
- m. serratus anterior
- m. subscapularis

The muscles in the upper side of the shoulder girdle relax:
- m. trapezius pars descendens
- m. levator scapulae
- mm. scaleni
- m. semispinalis capitis, cervicis and other muscles.

Activated muscles
The interscapular muscles are strengthened:
- m. trapezius
- m. latissimus dorsi
- mm. rhomboidei

Linking the muscle chains
The exercise is stabilized by the spiral muscle chains:
TR-B, C - trapezius,
LD-A, B - latissimus dorsi.
The vertical muscle chain ES - erector spinae relaxes in reciprocal inhibition.

Parameter 3.
Reducing the girth
Extension in the shoulder girdle, activation of the oblique abdominal muscles, breathing out

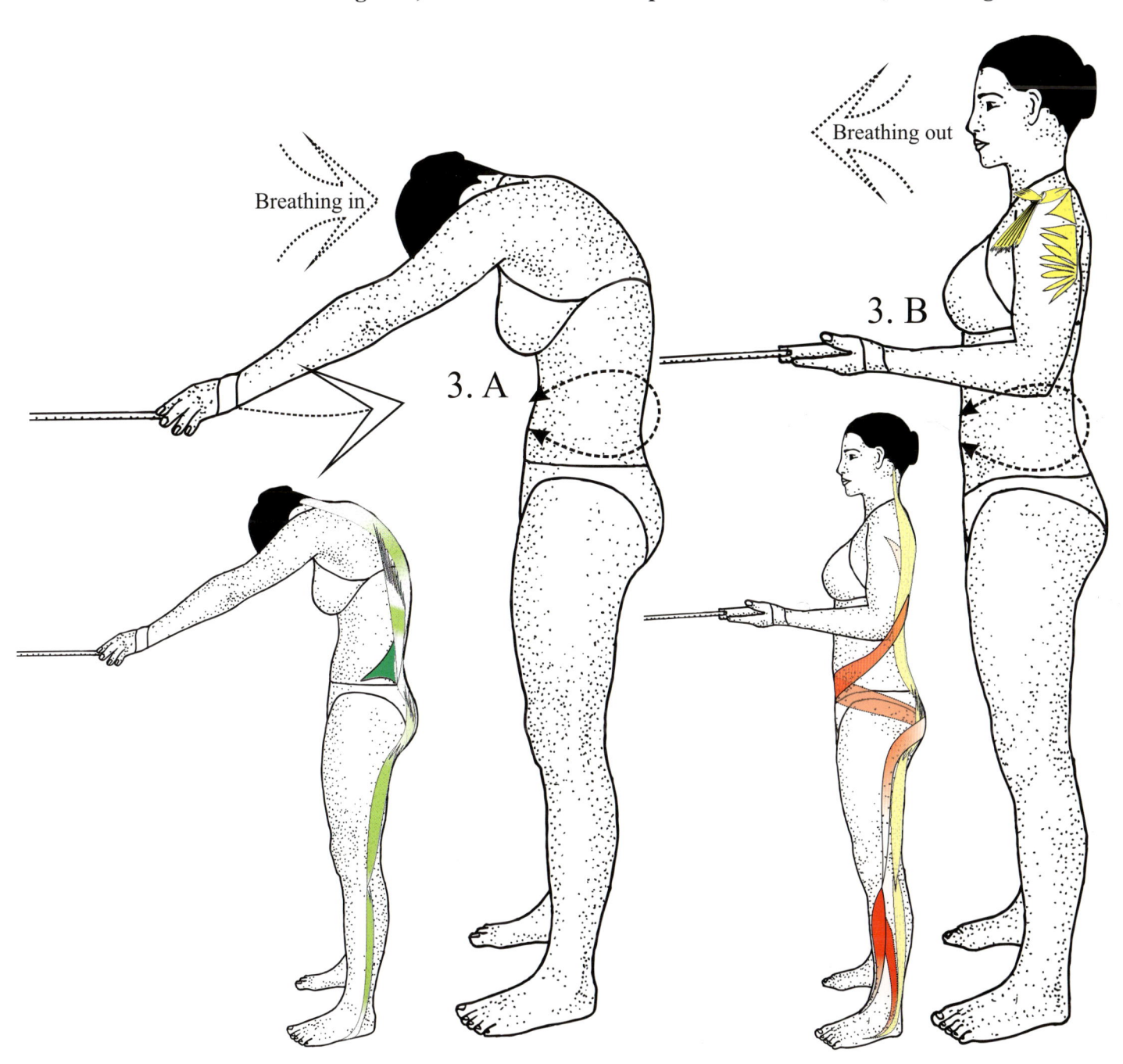

Parameter 3: Reducing the girth.
  Movement: **Extension in the shoulder girdle with lower fixation of the shoulder blade.**
  Norm: 5 cm
Change in the girth in the region of the navel.
This parameter assesses the ability to contract the girth by activating the oblique abdominal muscles and the transverse muscle within the TR - trapezius, LD - latissimus dorsi spiral.

Stretched muscles
The muscles in the anterior side of the shoulder girdle are stretched:
- m. subclavius
- m. pectoralis minor
- m. pectoralis major
- m. serratus anterior

The muscles in the upper side of the shoulder girdle relax:
- m. trapezius pars descendens
- m. levator scapulae
- mm. scaleni
- m. semispinalis capitis, cervicis and other muscles.

Activated muscles
The interscapular muscles are strengthened:
- m. trapezius
- m. latissimus dorsi
- mm. rhomboidei

Linking the muscle chains
The exercise is stabilized by the spiral muscle chains:
TR-B, C - trapezius,
LD-A, B - latissimus dorsi.
The vertical muscle chain ES - erector spinae relaxes in reciprocal inhibition.
Part of the TR and LD are the oblique abdominal muscles, which contract the girth.

Parameter 4.
Traction between the pelvis and the chest
Extension in the shoulder girdle, activation of the oblique abdominal muscles and the m. gluteus maximus

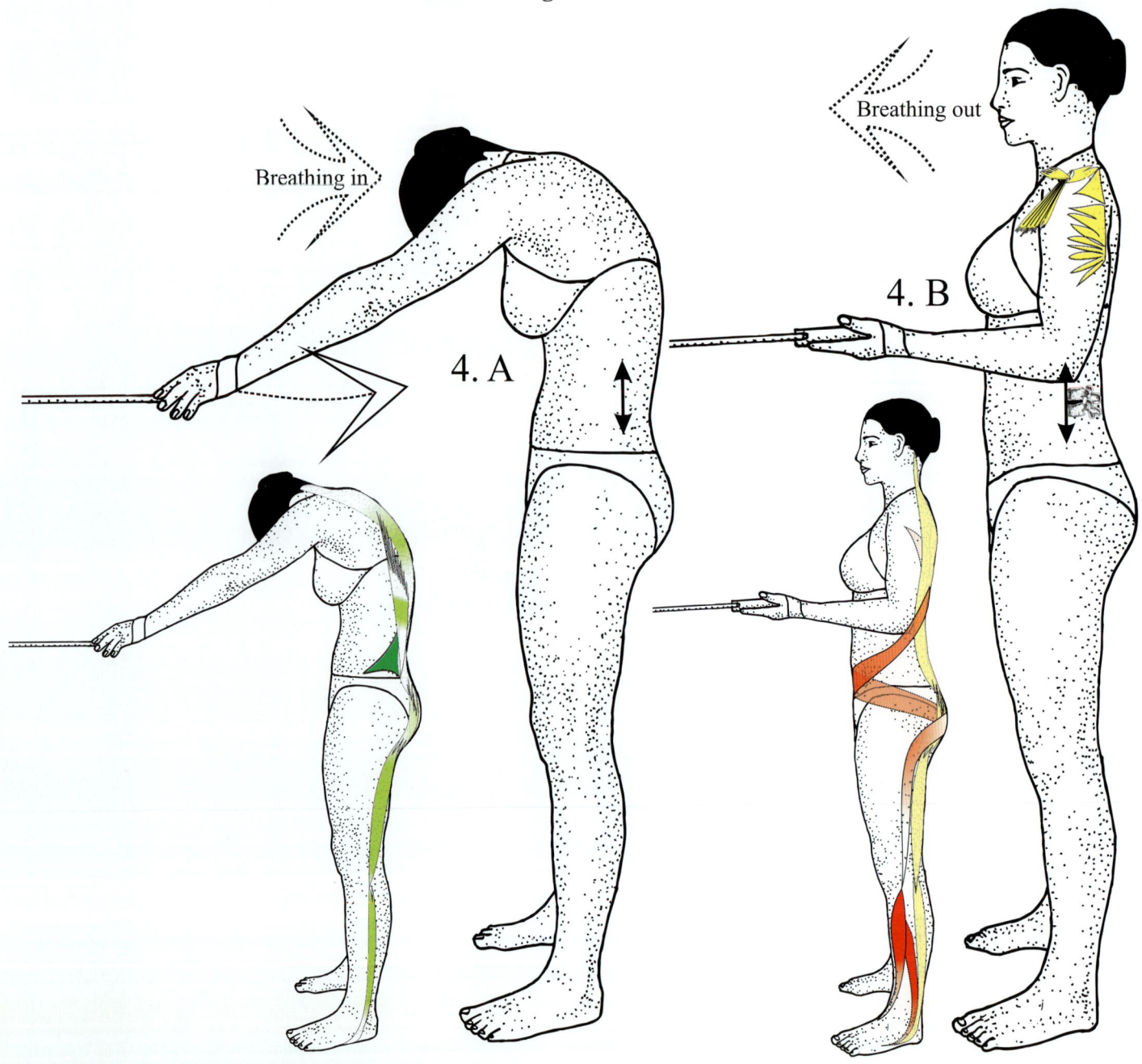

Breathing in

4. A

Breathing out

4. B

Parameter 4: Traction of the lumbar spine.
  Movement: Extension in the shoulder girdle with lower fixation of the shoulder blade.
  Norm: 1-2 cm
Elevation between the pelvis and the 10th rib.
A measurement is taken 8 cm from the posterior relief of the body, ie. on the anterior side of the vertebral units.
The parameter assesses the ability to straighten lordosis and stretch the intervertebral discs and joints.

Stretched muscles
The muscles in the anterior side
of the shoulder girdle are stretched:
- m. subclavius
- m. pectoralis minor
- m. pectoralis major
- m. serratus anterior

The muscles in the upper side
of the shoulder girdle are relaxed:
- m. trapezius, pars descendens
- m. levator scapulae
- mm. scaleni
- m. semispinalis capitis, cervicis and other muscles.

Activated muscles
The interscapular muscles are strengthened:
- m. trapezius
- m. latissimus dorsi
- mm. rhomboidei

Linking the muscle chains
The exercise is stabilized by the spiral muscle chains:
TR-B, C - trapezius,
LD-A, B - latissimus dorsi.
The vertical muscle chain ES - erector spinae relaxes in reciprocal inhibition.
Part of the TR and LD muscle chains are the oblique abdominal muscles and the m. gluteus maximus, which lift the chest.

Parameter 4.
Traction between the pelvis and the chest
Extension in the shoulder girdle, activation of the oblique abdominal muscles and the m. gluteus maximus

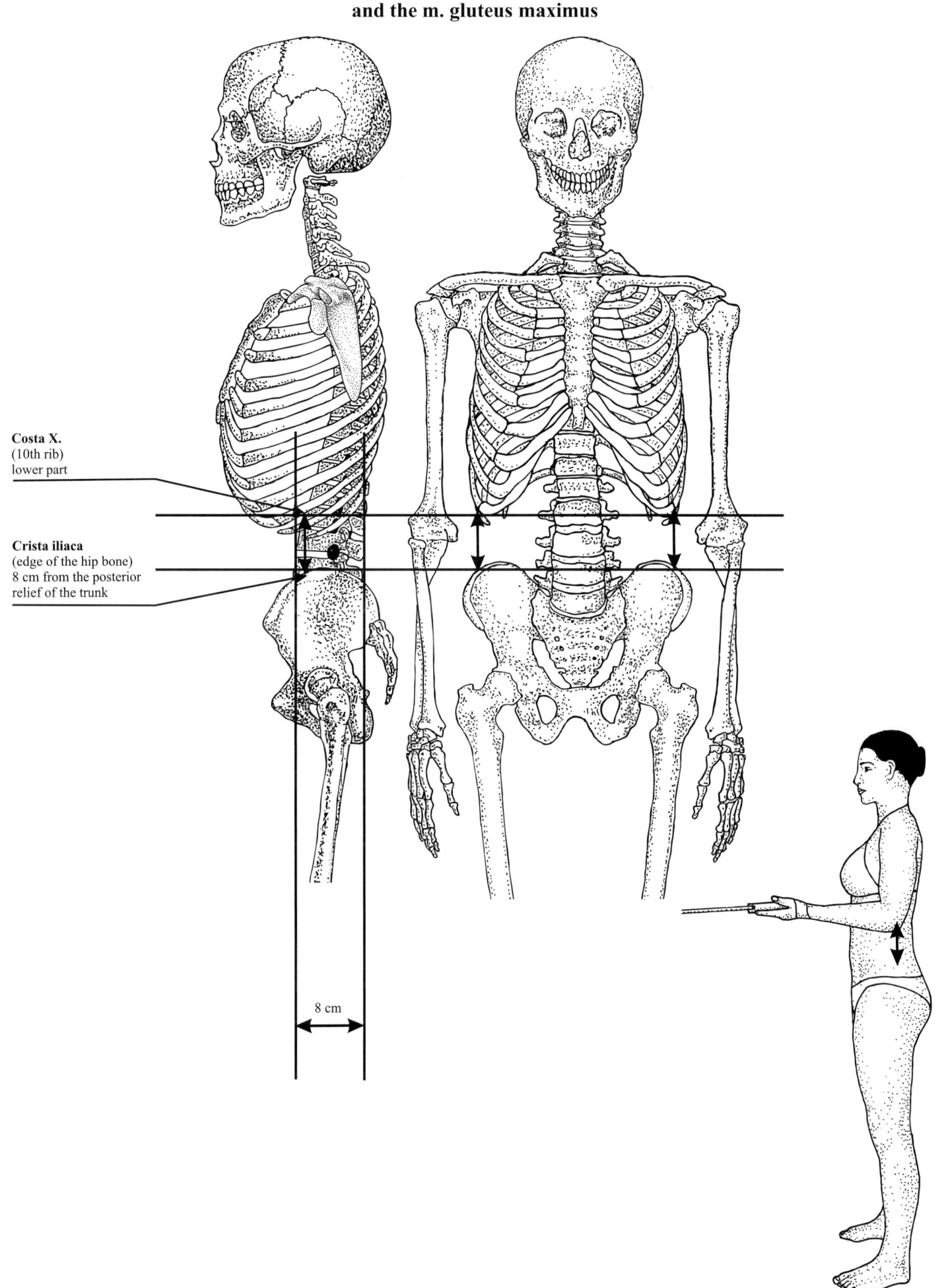

Costa X.
(10th rib)
lower part

Crista iliaca
(edge of the hip bone)
8 cm from the posterior relief of the trunk

8 cm

Parameter 5.
Distance between the body axis and patella
Extension in the pelvic girdle

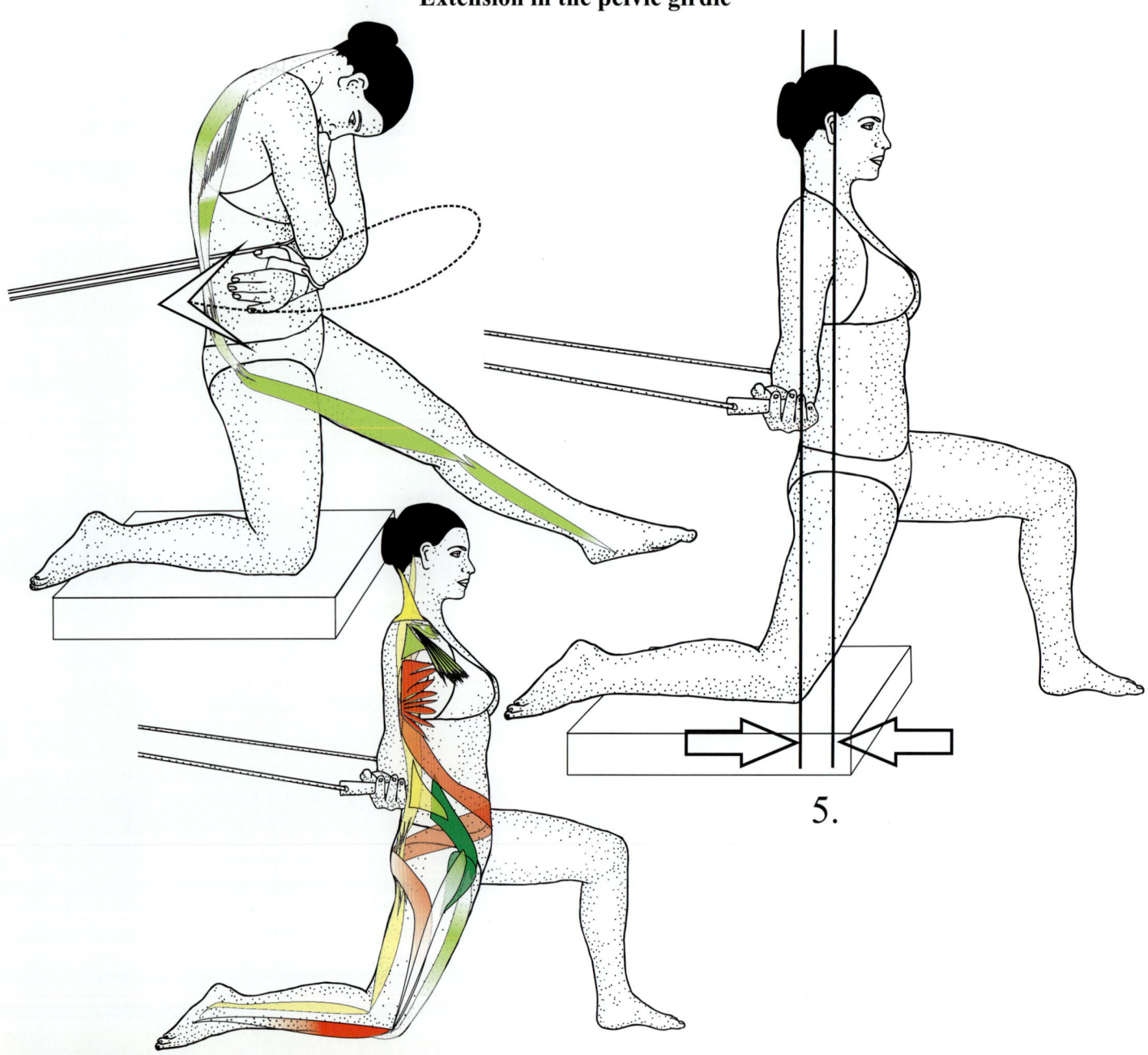

Parameter 5: Distance between the body axis and patella.
  Movement: Extension in the pelvic girdle in a spirally stabilized body.
  Norm: + 20 cm

Distance between the body axis and patella (kneecap).
The body axis runs in the upper part through the outer ear perpendicularly to the ground (plumb line) through the centre of the pelvis.
A pole is placed against the back. This does not allow lordosis greater than 2.5 cm (the width of a thumb).
This parameter assesses the ability to extend the step through extension in the hip and SI joint.

Stretched muscles
Pelvic girdle:
- m. iliopsoas
- m. gluteus medius (anterior part)
- m. tensor fasciae latae
- m. rectus femoris

Shoulder girdle:
- m. subclavius
- m. pectoralis minor
- m. pectoralis major
- m. serratus anterior

The muscles in the upper side of the shoulder girdle relax:
- m. trapezius pars descendens
- m. levator scapulae
- mm. scaleni
- m. semispinalis capitis, cervicis etc.

Activated muscles
The interscapular muscles are strengthened:
- m. trapezius
- m. latissimus dorsi
- mm. rhomboidei

Linking the muscle chains
The exercise is stabilized by the spiral muscle chains:
TR-B, C - trapezius,
LD-A, B - latissimus dorsi.
The vertical muscle chain ES - erector spinae relaxes in reciprocal inhibition.
Part of the TR and LD muscles chains are the oblique abdominal muscles and, above all, the m. gluteus maximus, which reciprocally inhibits the hip flexors.

Parameter 6.
Distance between the root of the nose and the patella
Flexion of the trunk with one leg extended

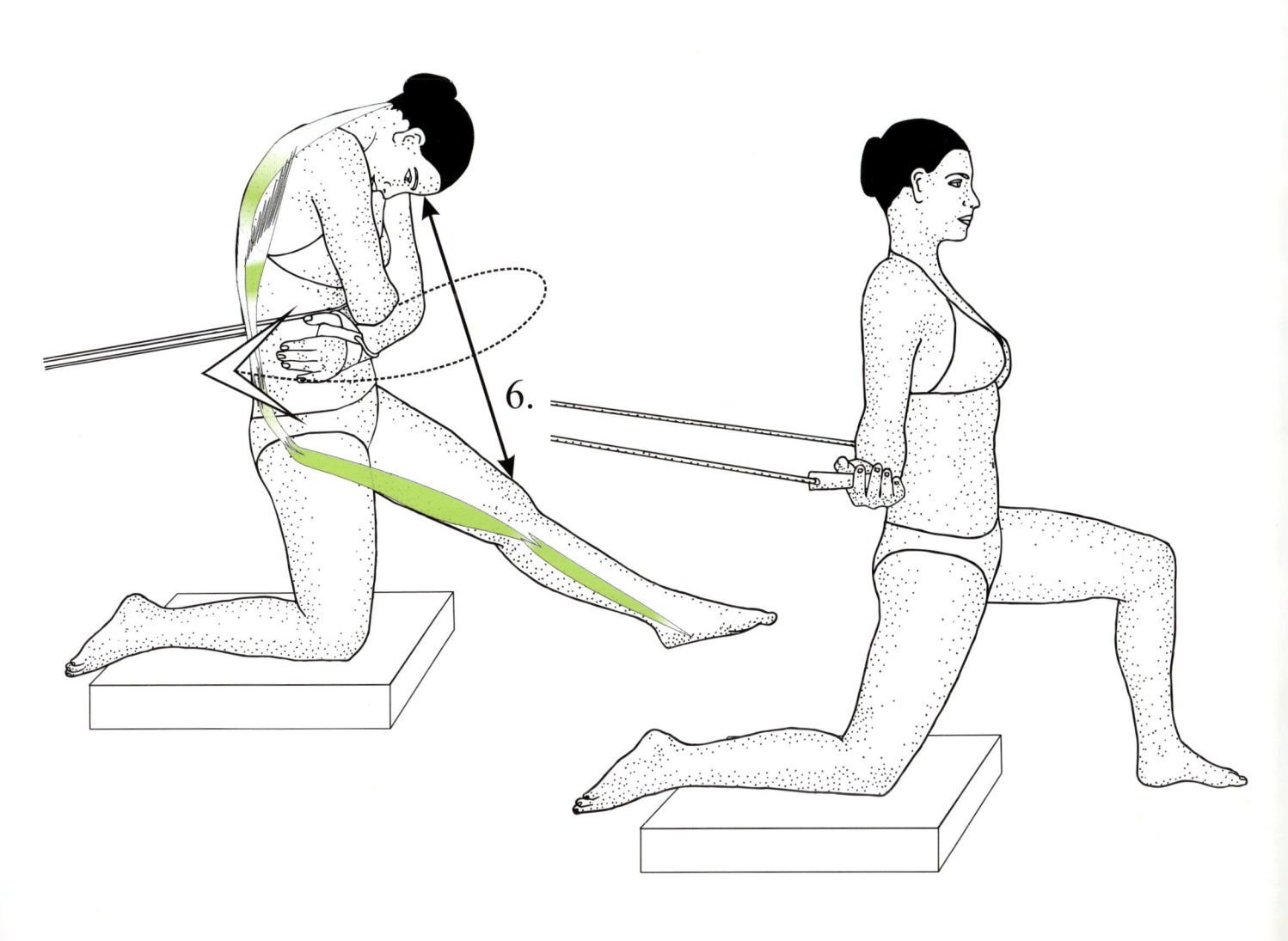

Parameter 6: Distance between the root of the nose and the patella.
  Movement: Flexion of the trunk in a kneeling position with one leg extended.
  Norm: + 30 cm
Distance between the root of the nose and the patella (kneecap).
This parameter assesses the ability to stretch the back muscles and ischiocrural muscles.

Stretched muscles
Back muscles:
- m. erector spinae
- m. quadratus lumborum
- m. multifidus

Ischiocrural muscles:
- m. biceps femoris
- m. semitendinosus
- m. semimembranosus
- m. adductor magnus

Parameter 7.
Stretching the distance between spinous processes C7 and S1
Stretching the back

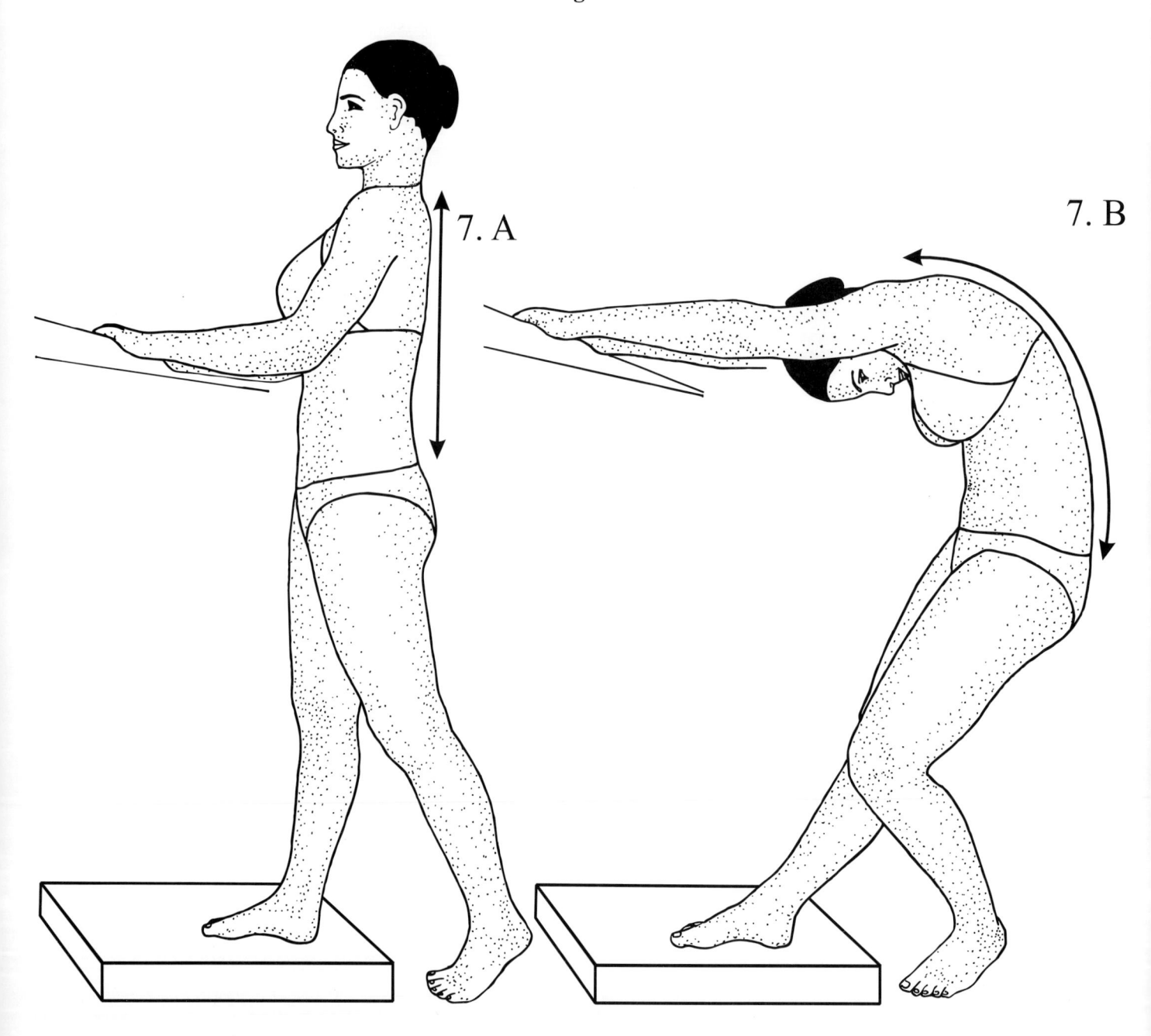

7. A

7. B

Parameter 7: Stretching the distance between spinous processes C7 and S1.
  Movement: Flexion of the trunk in a standing position with one leg extended.
  Norm: + 10 cm
Distance between spinous processes C7 and S1 - upper part of the sacral bone.
This parameter assesses the ability to stretch the back muscles and, partly, the ischiocrural muscles.

Stretched muscles
Back muscles:
- m. erector spinae
- m. quadratus lumborum
- m. multifidus

Ischiocrural muscles:
- m. biceps femoris
- m. semitendinosus
- m. semimembranosus
- m. adductor magnus

Parameter 7.
Stretching the distance between spinous processes C7 and S1
Stretching the back

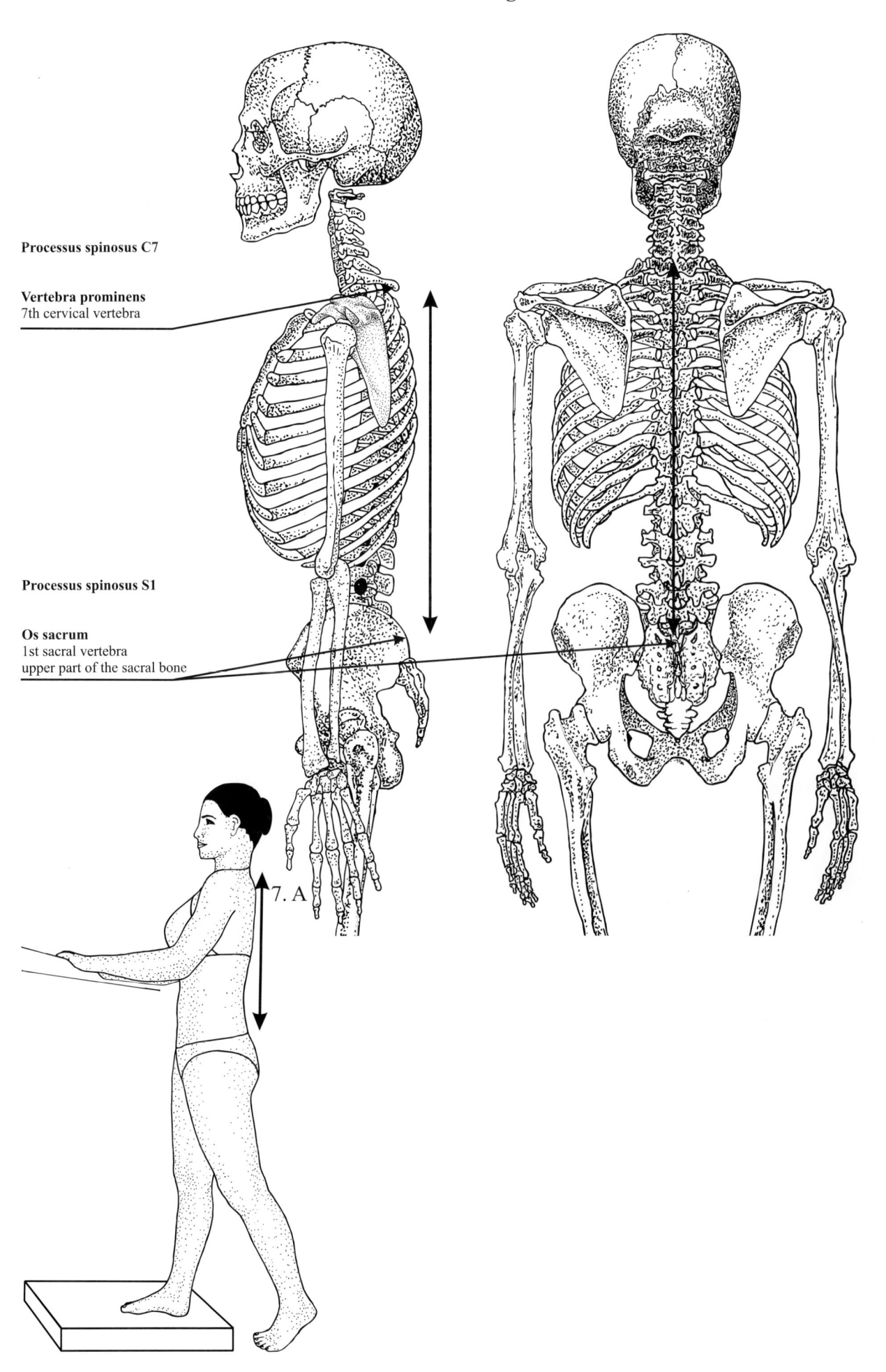

Processus spinosus C7

Vertebra prominens
7th cervical vertebra

Processus spinosus S1

Os sacrum
1st sacral vertebra
upper part of the sacral bone

7. A

Parameter 8.
Lateral mobility of spinous process Th5
Mobility of the chest when marking time

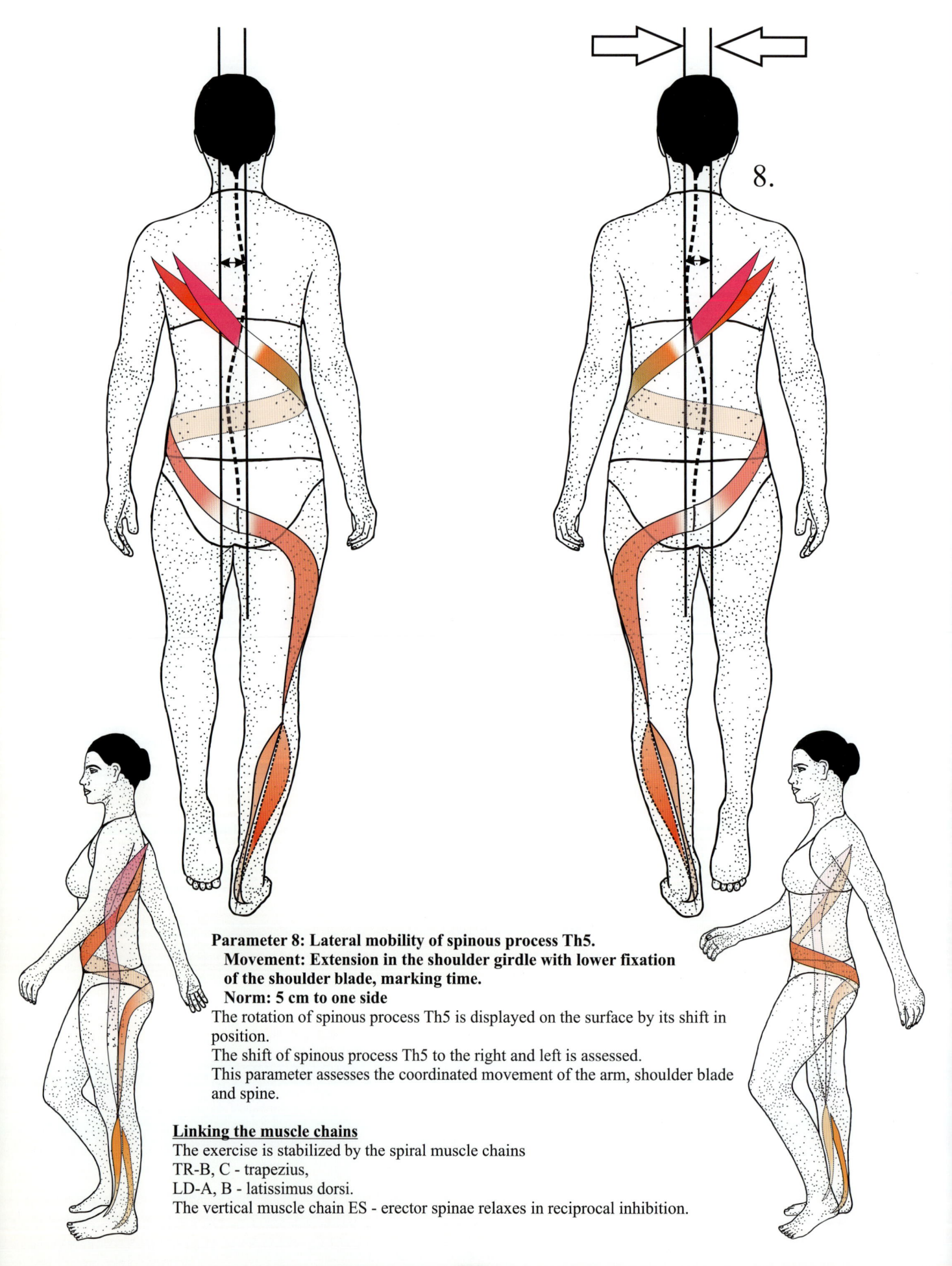

Parameter 8: Lateral mobility of spinous process Th5.
  Movement: Extension in the shoulder girdle with lower fixation of the shoulder blade, marking time.
  Norm: 5 cm to one side

The rotation of spinous process Th5 is displayed on the surface by its shift in position.
The shift of spinous process Th5 to the right and left is assessed.
This parameter assesses the coordinated movement of the arm, shoulder blade and spine.

<u>Linking the muscle chains</u>
The exercise is stabilized by the spiral muscle chains
TR-B, C - trapezius,
LD-A, B - latissimus dorsi.
The vertical muscle chain ES - erector spinae relaxes in reciprocal inhibition.

Parameter 9.
Rotation of the chest against the pelvis
Mobility of the chest and pelvis
in extension exercises for the arms and legs

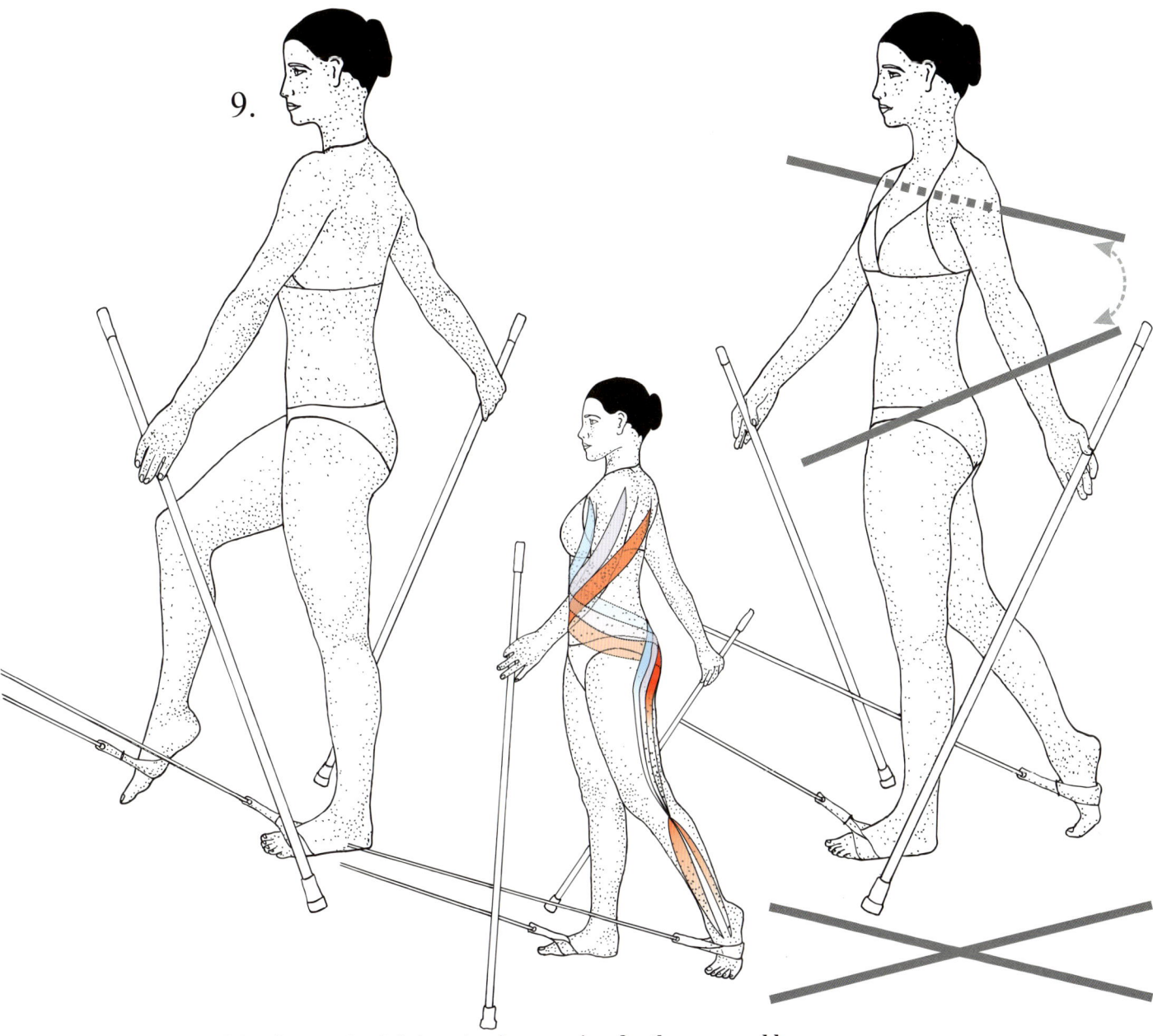

Parameter 9: Mobility of the chest and pelvis in extension exercises for the arms and legs.
  Movement: Rotation of the chest against the pelvis.
  Norm: 90°

The angle between the shoulder girdle and the pelvic girdle. The angle between the placed poles is measured while viewing the shoulder girdle and pelvic girdle from above. This parameter assesses the ability to extend the step by rotating the pelvis. A precondition for the correct performance of rotation is the activation of all four spirals (TR, LD, SA, PM) and inhibition of the vertical chains.

Stretched muscles
Pelvic girdle:
- m. iliopsoas
- m. gluteus medius (anterior part)
- m. tensor fasciae latae
- m. rectus femoris

Shoulder girdle:
- m. subclavius
- m. pectoralis minor
- m. pectoralis major
- m. serratus anterior

The muscles in the upper side of the shoulder girdle relax:
- m. trapezius pars descendens
- m. levator scapulae
- mm. scaleni
- m. semispinalis capitis, cervicis etc.

Activated muscles
The interscapular muscles are strengthened:
- m. trapezius
- m. latissimus dorsi
- mm. rhomboidei

Linking the muscle chains
The exercise is stabilized by the spiral muscle chains:
TR-B, C - trapezius,
LD-A, B - latissimus dorsi,
SA - B - serrtus anterior,
PM - B - pactoralis major.
The vertical spiral chain ES - erector spinae relaxes in reciprocal inhibition.
Part of the TR and LD muscle chains are the oblique abdominal muscles and, above all, the m. gluteus maximus, which reciprocally inhibits the hip flexors.

Cardiovascular training
A comprehensive whole-body global movement plan
Vertebrovisceral relations, psychosomatic factors

1. **Reducing increased muscle tone.**
   Reducing resistance to improve the blood supply to the muscles. Improving muscle nutrition.
   Improving the metabolism in the mitochondria of the muscles.
   Reducing the proprioceptive information from tense muscles
   (Increased proprioception unnecessarily employs the analyzer in the CNS - stress).

2. **Increased mobility of the chest and abdominal region.**
   Increased mobility of the diaphragm.
   Increased vital capacity of the lungs. Improved oxygen saturation of the blood.
   Occurrence of negative suction pressure in the chest. Promotion of venous return. Promotion of lymph drainage.

3. **Straightening the head in the axis position.**
   Reduction of increased tone in the neck muscles.
   Increased blood flow to the CNS.

4. **Mobilization of the zone of the cardiac sympathetic nerve, Th1-5 and neck region.**
   (ganglion cervicale superior, medius inferior).
   Relaxation of the muscles which cross this area.
   Adopting an axis position of the body and head.
   Mobilization of the neck in rotation.

5. **Alternating activation and relaxation of the large muscle groups.**
   Improving the blood supply and metabolism of the muscles. The muscle pump.

6. **Alternating engagement of the muscles of the legs, arms, neck and trunk.**
   Promotion of the activity of the muscle pump.
   Promotion of venous return. Promotion of lymph drainage.

7. **Exercising in a balanced position.**
   Opening the vascular flow in the groin and armpits.

8. **Proportionate, controlled, long-term, comprehensive exertion.**
   Control of the force and extent of movement, cardiovascular stress (pulse rate).

9. **Regeneration of the spine and large joints.**
   Spine: traction, centration, stabilization, mobilization
   Joints: - strengthening and stretching the muscles connected with the function of the joints
      - stabilization of the joints through rapid contraction of the stabilizing muscles
      - mobilization of the joints in unstressed movement

10. **Eliminating pain and the use of pain killers.**
    Pain in the regions of the muscles, discs and joints.
    Mental pain, lack of movement.

11. **Positive impact on the mind. Prevention of brain degeneration.**
    Eliminating the risk of the occurrence of psychosomatic illnesses.
    Endorphin rush.
    Good vascular supply to the brain. Supply of nutrients and oxygen. Promotion of the metabolism.
    Regeneration of the CNS and PNS.
    Elimination of stress, depression and the burnout syndrome.
    It is important to provide information about a clear concept of a solution to the problem.

Main goal:
To improve the metabolism in the mitochondria of the muscles

Eliminating the risk of ischemic heart disease
   Hypertension
   Hyperglycemia
   Dyslipoproteinemia
   Obesity

Positive impact on the locomotor apparatus

Pathway to the goal:
   Engaging the whole-body dynamic spiral muscle chains. Relaxing the vertical rest position muscle chains in reciprocal relations and stretching them. A life-long regular movement programme.

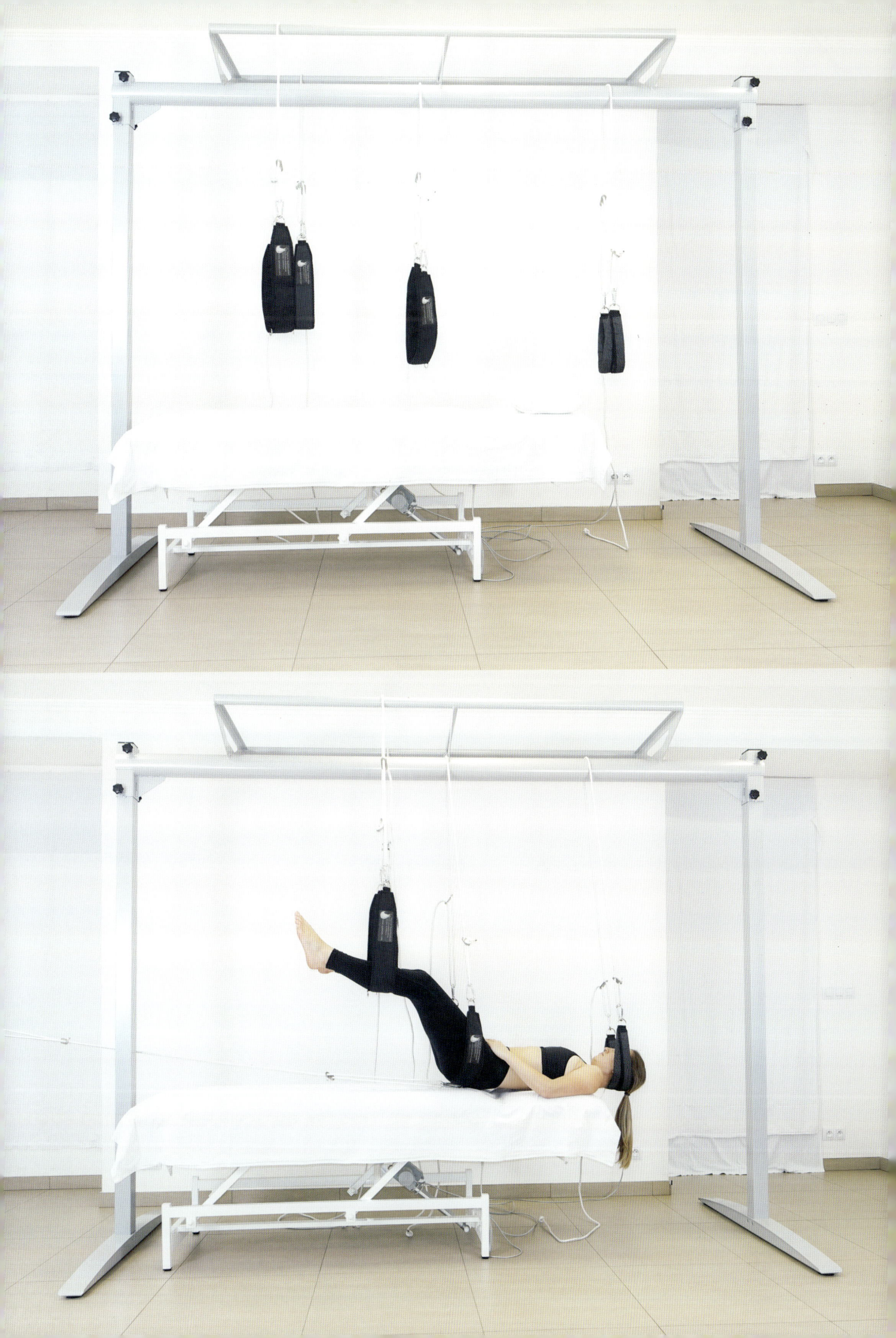

EXPANDER ERGO
A DESK AT WHICH YOUR BACK WON'T HURT.

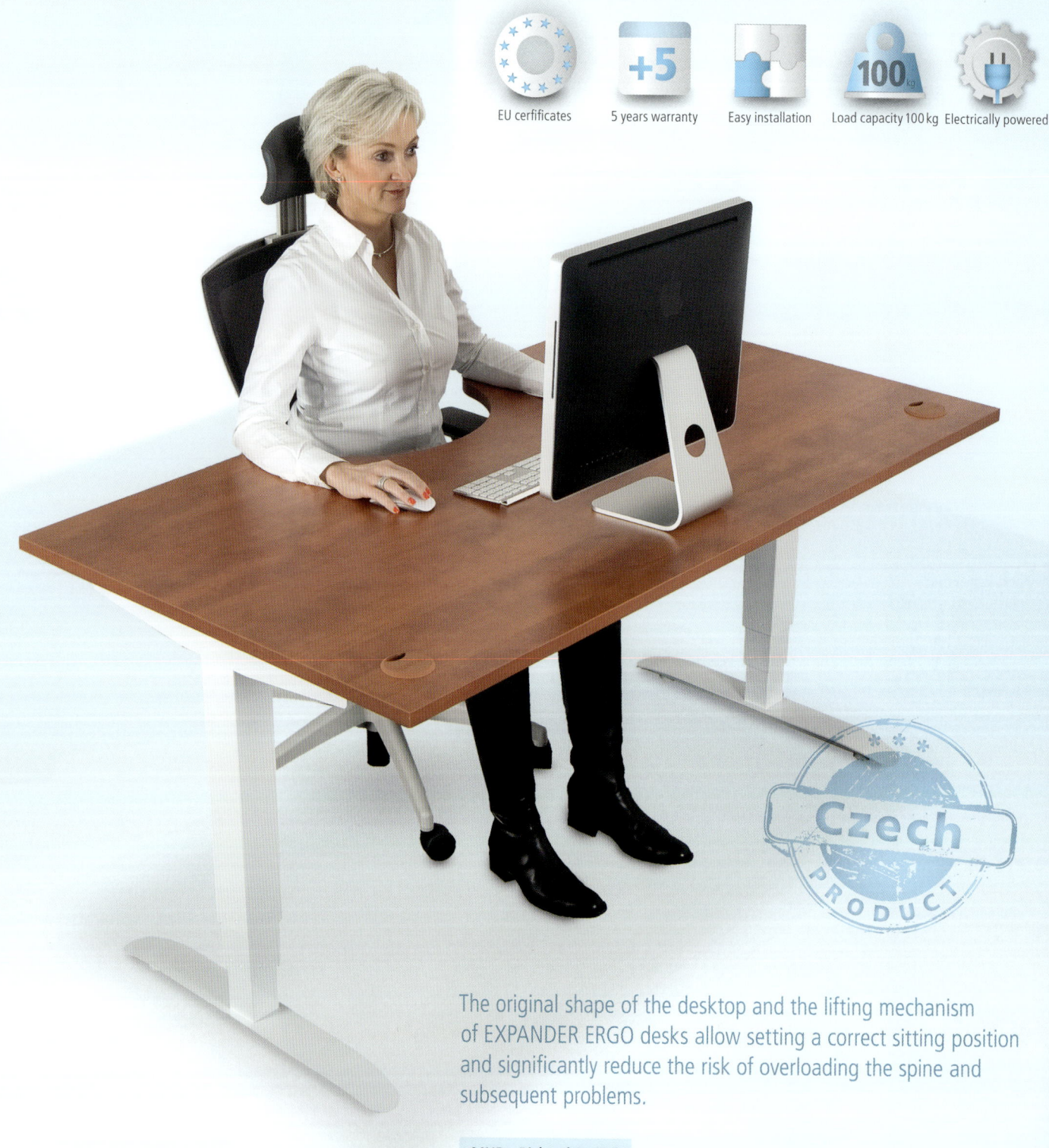

- EU cerfificates
- 5 years warranty
- Easy installation
- Load capacity 100 kg
- Electrically powered

Czech PRODUCT

The original shape of the desktop and the lifting mechanism of EXPANDER ERGO desks allow setting a correct sitting position and significantly reduce the risk of overloading the spine and subsequent problems.

MUDr. Richard Smíšek

- author of the original SM method of spiral spine stabilization
- founder of the Smíšek Rehabilitation and Educational Centre
- a top expert on the treatment and prevention of backache formation
- creator of the desktop shape of EXPANDER ERGO desks

HON move®

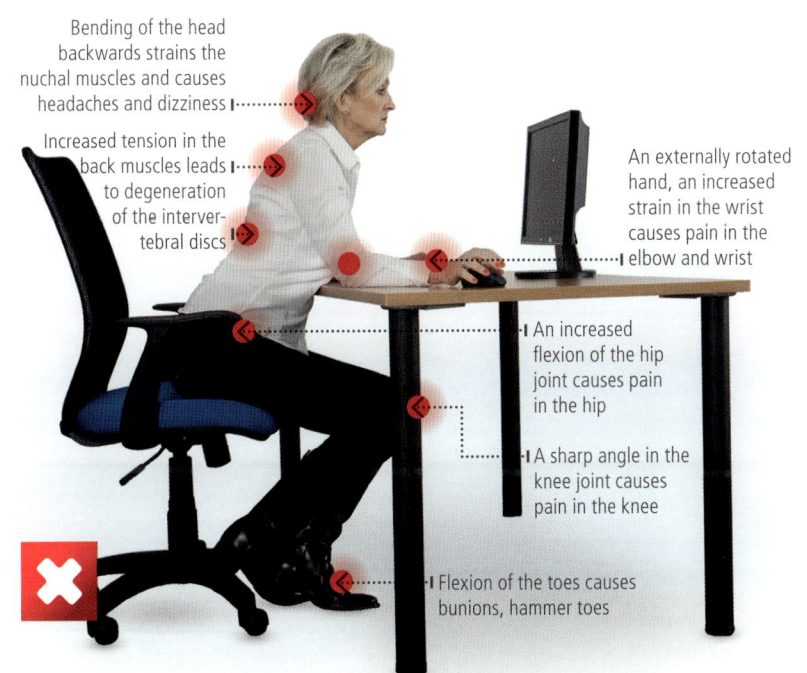

Bending of the head backwards strains the nuchal muscles and causes headaches and dizziness

Increased tension in the back muscles leads to degeneration of the intervertebral discs

An externally rotated hand, an increased strain in the wrist causes pain in the elbow and wrist

An increased flexion of the hip joint causes pain in the hip

A sharp angle in the knee joint causes pain in the knee

Flexion of the toes causes bunions, hammer toes

Incorrect and long-term sitting is today's disease of civilization, found already in children of school age. They carry bad habits acquired during incorrect sitting at school and at home at a PC forward into their adulthood. The body, and especially the spine, becomes affected by a one-sided load.

An incorrect sitting position causes intervertebral disc herniation in the lumbar and cervical spine, scoliosis, headaches, dizziness and chronic back pain.

HON move®

Tension of the nuchal muscles decreases

Trapezius muscles relax

Arm weight is transferred to the table top, allowing the back of the neck to relax

Tension in the wrist and forearm is significantly reduced

Body weight is transferred to the chair backrest, tension of the muscles along the spine decreases, pressure on the spine is reduced

The lifting mechanism of the EXPANDER ERGO desk enables you to set the correct height of the desktop in relation to your height, which is an essential condition for correct sitting. Thanks to the cut-out in the desktop, your arms are supported, thereby relieving the trapezius muscles and allowing nuchal relaxation.

Sitting is an unnatural position for humans. EXPANDER ERGO desks enable you to make a welcome change and continue working while standing. The arms remain supported and in contrast with sitting, the legs can be stretched. In general, blood circulation improves and you will certainly feel better.

www.hon-move.com

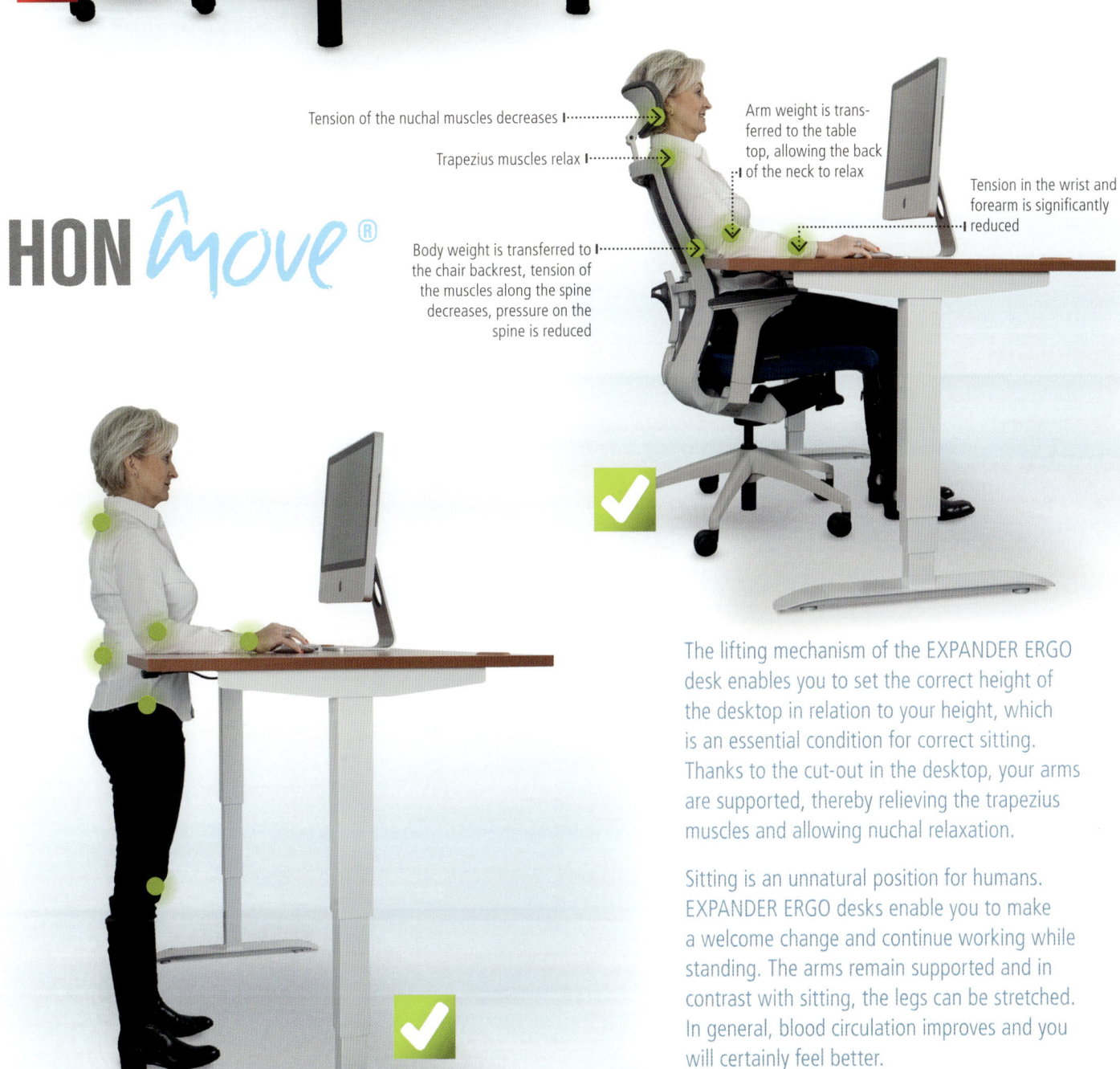

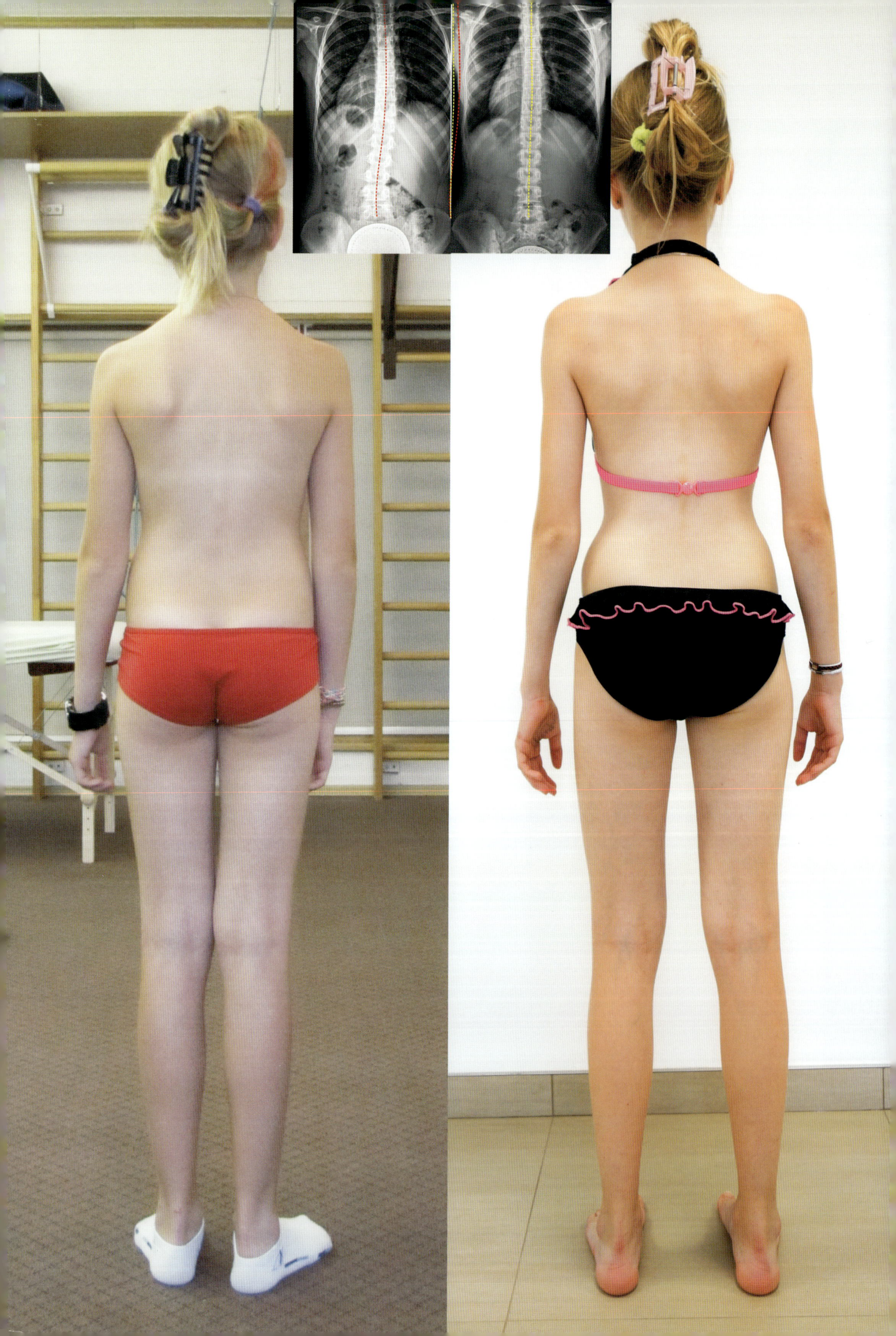

제3차 SSM 척추측만증 국제워크샵

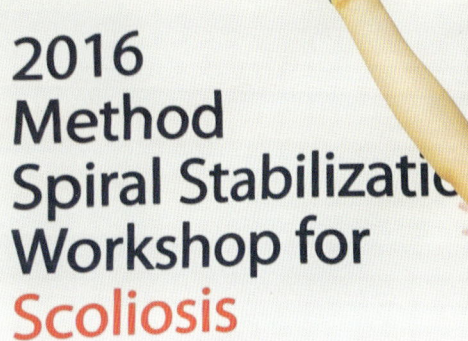

2016 Method Spiral Stabilization Workshop for Scoliosis

2016/01/29 - 02/03

Education partner in Korea
Davinch Academy
General Manager: Sangyong Ham
No.205, 2 complex, DMC XI, 223-28,
Jeungsan-dong, Eunpyeong-gu, Seoul,
Korea
Hamsand@empas.com
www.davinchxt.com
Phone: 0082-10-2581-7456

다빈치아카데미
부장 함상용
서울시 은평구 증산동
223-28 DMC자이 2단지 상가 205호

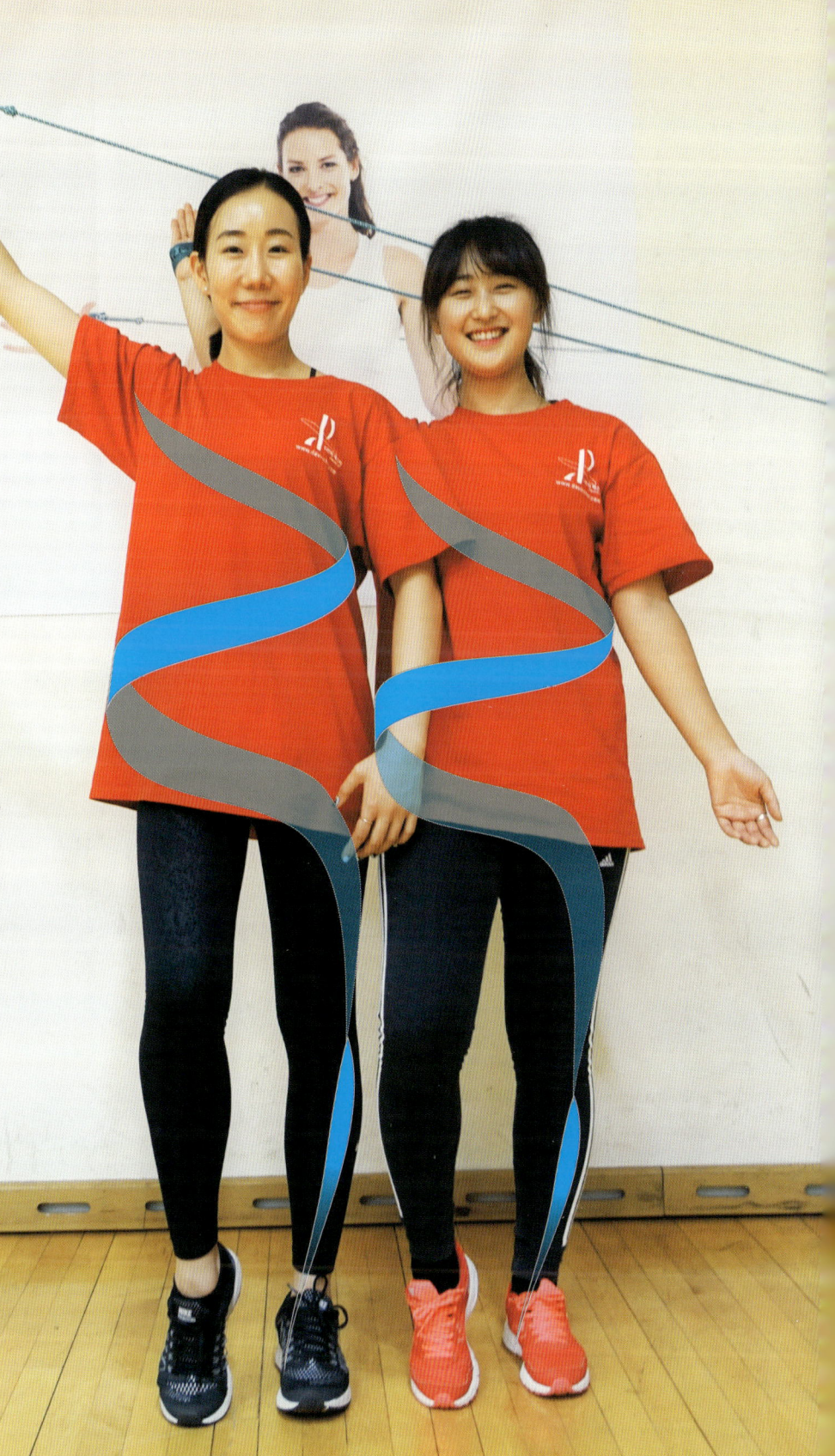

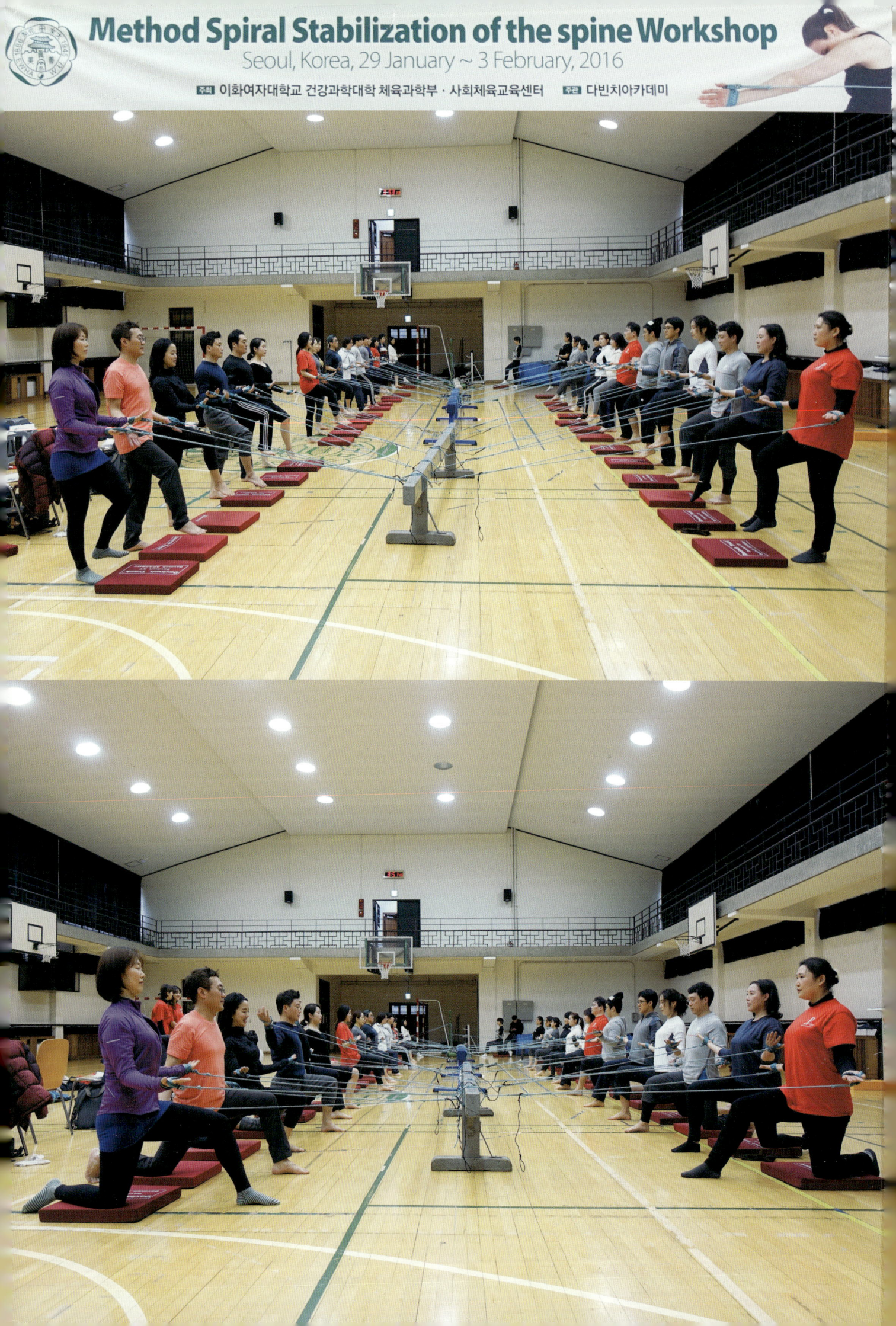

Method Spiral Stabilization of the spine Workshop
Seoul, Korea, 29 January ~ 3 February, 2016

주최 이화여자대학교 건강과학대학 체육과학부 · 사회체육교육센터   주관 다빈치아카데미